Family Nurse Practitioner Certification Intensive Review

Maria T. Codina Leik, MSN, ARNP, FNP-C, AGPCNP-BC, is the president and principal lecturer at National ARNP Services, Inc. (npreview.com). Well known for her ability to simplify complex concepts for her students, she is a popular speaker and educator. Ms. Leik taught previously in the nurse practitioner (NP) program at Florida International University Graduate School of Nursing. She is board certified by the American Nurses Credentialing Center (ANCC) and the American Academy of Nurse Practitioners Certification Board (AANPCB) in two specialties: family NP and adult-gerontology primary care NP. She is an experienced NP with more than two decades of clinical practice. In addition to her two NP certification review books published by Springer Publishing Company, Ms. Leik is the author of chapters in two NP textbooks and is a member of Sigma Theta Tau International Honor Society of Nursing.

Family Nurse Practitioner Certification Intensive Review

Fast Facts and Practice Questions

Third Edition, Revised Reprint

Maria T. Codina Leik, MSN, ARNP, FNP-C, AGPCNP-BC

SPRINGER PUBLISHING COMPANY

Springer Publishing Company, LLC
11 West 42nd Street
New York, NY 10036
www.springerpub.com

Acquisitions Editor: Margaret Zuccarini
Compositor: diacriTech

ISBN: 978-0-8261-3429-5
ebook ISBN: 978-0-8261-3428-8

19 20 21 / 5 4 3

Library of Congress Cataloging-in-Publication Data
Names: Codina Leik, Maria T., author.
Title: Family nurse practitioner certification intensive review : fast facts and practice questions / Maria T. Codina Leik.
Description: Third edition. | New York, NY : Springer Publishing Company, LLC, [2018] | Includes bibliographical references and index.
Identifiers: LCCN 2017044822 | ISBN 9780826134295 | ISBN 9780826134288 (e-book)
Subjects: | MESH: Nurse Practitioners | Family Practice | Certification | Examination Questions
Classification: LCC RT82.8 | NLM WY 18.2 | DDC 610.73076—dc23 LC record available at https://lccn.loc.gov/2017044822

Printed in the United States of America by Bradford & Bigelow.

To Edward, whose love and infinite support helped me on this grand adventure.

To TCL, FLC, and RCJ.

And to my awesome daughters, Maryfaye and Christina.

Contents

SECTION V: GERONTOLOGY REVIEW

SECTION VI: PROFESSIONAL ISSUES REVIEW

SECTION VII: PRACTICE QUESTIONS AND ANSWERS

Contributors and Reviewers

CONTRIBUTORS

Julie Adkins, DNP, APN, FNP-BC, FAANP
Certified Family Nurse Practitioner
Adkins Family Practice, LLC
West Frankfort, Illinois

Jill C. Cash, MSN, APN, FNP-BC
Nurse Practitioner
Vanderbilt Medical Group Westhaven Family Practice
Franklin, Tennessee, and
Vanderbilt University Medical Center
Nashville, Tennessee

Susanne W. Gibbons, PhD, C-AGNP
Assistant Professor
Daniel K. Inouye Graduate School of Nursing
Uniformed Services University of the Health Sciences
Bethesda, Maryland

Cheryl A. Glass, MSN, WHNP, BC
Clinical Research Specialist
KEPRO Peer Review
Medical Solutions Unit
Nashville, Tennessee

Susanne J. Pavlovich-Danis, MSN, ARNP-C, CDE, CRRN
Director of Clinical Continuing Education
TeamHealth
Advanced Practice Registered Nurse
Plantation Medical Clinic
Nursing Professor, University of Phoenix,
South Florida Campus
Miramar, Florida

Elizabeth Johnston Taylor, PhD, RN
Professor
School of Nursing
Loma Linda University
Loma Linda, California

REVIEWERS

Donna Bowles, EdD, MSN, RN, CNE
Associate Professor
Indiana University Southeast
New Albany, Indiana

Linda Carman Copel, PhD, RN, PMHCNS, BC, CNE, NCC, FAPA
Professor
Villanova University College of Nursing
Philadelphia, Pennsylvania

Jill C. Cash, MSN, APN, FNP-BC
Nurse Practitioner
Vanderbilt Medical Group Westhaven Family Practice
Franklin, Tennessee, and
Vanderbilt University Medical Center
Nashville, Tennessee

Lucille R. Ferrara, EdD, MBA, RN, FNP-BC
Assistant Professor and Director
Family Nurse Practitioner Program
Lienhard School of Nursing
New York, New York

Frank L. Giles, PhD, CRC, CCM, NCC, LMFT
President
Giles & Associates, Inc.
Madison, Mississippi

Cheryl A. Glass, RN, MSN, WHNP, BC
Clinical Research Specialist
KEPRO Peer Review
Medical Solutions Unit
Nashville, Tennessee

Pamela L. King, PhD, FNP, PNP
MSN Program Director
Spalding University
Louisville, Kentucky

Liza Marmo, RN-BC, MSN, CCRN, ANP-C
Director, Clinical Services
Lehigh Valley Health Network
Allentown, Pennsylvania

JoAnne M. Pearce, MS, RNC, APRN-BC
Nursing Education Consultant
Idaho State University
Pocatello, Idaho

Sue Polito, RN, MSN, ANPC, GNPC
Specialist Professor
Monmouth University
West Long Branch, New Jersey

Dana R. Sherman, DNP, ARNP, ANP-BC, FNP-BC
Clinical Adjunct Faculty
Florida International University
Advanced Practice Registered Nurse
Emergency Department
Mount Sinai Medical Center
Miami Beach, Florida

Cirese Webster, RN, CPN, FNP-BC
Nurse Practitioner
Metro Medical and Midwest Physicians
Certified Pediatric Nurse
St. Louis Children's Hospital
St. Louis, Missouri

Preface

Welcome to the third edition of *Family Nurse Practitioner Certification Intensive Review*. This review book is designed to help you study effectively and efficiently for the family nurse practitioner certification exams of both the American Nurses Credentialing Center (ANCC) and the American Academy of Nurse Practitioners Certification Board (AANPCB).

The goal for all of my nurse practitioner (NP) certification review books is to provide you, the student and/or NP test-taker, with a tool to effectively and rapidly review for both the ANCC and the AANPCB certification exams. This book is also a good resource for current NP students. Many students credit these books with helping them pass not only their certification exam, but also quizzes and tests when they were students. Students report that the review book has helped them successfully pass their school's dreaded "exit" exam.

New disease topics, tables, procedures, and updated clinical content in this edition relate to the latest exam questions. There are new photographs of dermatological diseases and other conditions. The text now includes three new chapters: (a) Professional Roles and Reimbursement, (b) Culture and Spiritually Related Health Beliefs, and (c) Evidence-Based Medicine and Epidemiology. These new chapters will help those who are taking the ANCC and the AANPCB exam. In addition, there is an increase in the total number of practice questions and answers, which include rationales. New-format questions are included, and the question dissection section has been expanded.

The book's format remains the same as in the popular and best-selling first two editions, which were also published by Springer Publishing Company. The book is styled as a "mega-review" study guide because it combines six different resources in one: (a) certification exam information that is highly specific for both the ANCC and AANPCB exams, (b) test-taking techniques, (c) a question dissection and analysis section that breaks down questions for further study, (d) a review of primary care diseases and conditions, (e) a review of pertinent normal physical exam findings, and finally (f) questions with rationales to practice your new skills.

This book and my *Adult-Gerontology Nurse Practitioner Certification Intensive Review* have become the most sought-after and relied-upon review books for use in studying for both the ANCC and the AANPCB certification exams. The contents and procedures in this book are designed for review purposes only. They are not intended for use in clinical practice.

If you have any comments or suggestions for this book, or want me to teach a review course at your school, please contact me at npreviews@gmail.com. If you want to attend one of my webinars or live-review courses, please visit my website at www.npreview.com. I will post updates and new treatment guidelines on my website at www.npreview.com.

Maria T. Codina Leik

Acknowledgments

The role of the nurse practitioner can be difficult, but it is also a rewarding one. As NPs, we can touch so many lives. When we care for our patients, we are combining nursing with medicine. I think as NPs, we have the best of both worlds. But before we can practice, we must first pass the NP certification exam. So, as usual, this book is dedicated to all my review course students, past and present, who worked so hard to pass the certification exam.

To my editor, Margaret Zuccarini, thank you for your infinite patience. I want to extend my gratitude to Springer Publishing Company, New York, and their staff who helped make this book a reality. Extra kudos to Donna Frassetto, Martha Cushman, and Lindsay Claire.

Thank you, Angelica Rundell, for your support of our review course students. Last, but not least, I want to extend my deep gratitude to my dear parents, Ricardo G. Codina and Thelma Y. Codina.

Family Nurse Practitioner Certification Intensive Review

I

Exam and Health Screening Overview

1

Certification Exam Information

AMERICAN NURSES CREDENTIALING CENTER

www.nursecredentialing.org
Credentials: FNP-BC, AGPCNP-BC
Toll-Free Phone: (800) 284-2378
Mobile App: "MYANCC" (Apple Store/Google Play)
Electronic Transcripts: aprnvalidation@ana.org

The American Nurses Credentialing Center (ANCC) is the independent credentialing body of the American Nurses Association (ANA). It is the largest nurse credentialing organization in the United States. The current edition of the ANCC Family Nurse Practitioner (FNP) exam was released on February 9, 2016, and the Adult-Gerontology Primary Care Nurse Practitioner (AGPCNP) exam was released on December 23, 2015.

The ANCC currently offers certification exams for the following nurse practitioner (NP) specialties: family NP (FNP-BC), adult-gerontology primary care NP (AGPCNP-BC), adult-gerontology acute care NP (AGACNP-BC), pediatric primary care NP (PPCNP-BC), and psychiatric–mental health NP (PMHNP-BC). It retired the adult NP and gerontologic NP exams in 2015. You must first establish an online account at the ANCC website before you can apply for the any of the exams. You can use the mobile app "MYANCC" to apply or renew your certification and keep track of your continuing-education (CE) hours in the mobile app.

Prometric Computer Testing Centers

ANCC Exams
Prometric Test Centers
www.prometric.com/ANCC
Toll-Free Phone: (800) 350-7076
Special Conditions Department (Special Accommodations): (800) 967-1139

The ANCC uses Prometric Testing Centers to administer its exams. Before you can schedule an appointment, you must have your candidate eligibility number; this is provided in the Authorization to Test Notice letter sent to qualified candidates who meet eligibility requirements and have completed their application documentation.

You can schedule, reschedule, cancel, and/or confirm an appointment at the website portal or by telephone. Prometric has 8,000 test centers in 160 countries, including the United States, Puerto Rico, the U.S. Virgin Islands, Canada, Venezuela, and the United Kingdom. There are also test centers in Africa, Asia, and Europe.

International Testing for Military Personnel

Military nurses who want to take the exam outside of the United States are allowed to take their exams at one of Prometric's "global" testing centers.

Qualifications

One must be a graduate of an approved master's, postgraduate, or doctoral degree program with a specialization in family NP (plus the required minimum of 500 faculty-supervised clinical practice hours) from an institution of higher learning. The program must be accredited by the Commission on Collegiate Nursing Education (CCNE) or the Accreditation Commission for Education in Nursing (formerly known as the National League for Nursing Accrediting Commission). In addition, the candidate must possess an active RN license in any state or territory of the United States. The ANCC will, on an individual basis, accept the professional legally recognized equivalent (of NP status) from another country if the applicant meets its certification criteria. If he or she is educated and/or licensed outside the United States, there are additional requirements.

AMERICAN ACADEMY OF NURSE PRACTITIONERS CERTIFICATION BOARD

www.aanpcert.org
Credentials: FNP-C, AGNP-C
Toll-Free Phone: (855) 822-6727
Fax: (512) 637-0540
Certification Administration: (512) 637-0500
Email: certification@aanpcert.org
Electronic Transcripts: transcripts@aanpcert.org (via secure electronic transmission from registrar's office)

The American Academy of Nurse Practitioners Certification Board (AANPCB) is an independent organization that is affiliated with the American Association of Nurse Practitioners (AANP) and the American Academy of Emergency Nurse Practitioners (AAENP).

The AANPCB is currently offering three specialty exams: Family NP (FNP-C), Adult-Gerontology Primary Care NP (AGNP-C), and the Emergency NP (ENP-C) specialty exam. The current FNP and AGNP exams were both released in October 2016. Their Adult NP exam was retired in December 2015 and the Gerontologic NP exam was retired in December 2012.

You must first establish an online account at their website before you can apply for the exam. Applicants enrolled in an MSN or post-master's certificate program may begin the application process 6 months before completion of the program. If you are enrolled in a DNP program, you can begin the application process as early as 1 year prior to completion of the program. But you must complete all the NP program didactic courses and supervised clinical practice hour requirements before you can sit for the exam. In addition, an official transcript showing the DNP degree awarded and conferral date is required to release your exam score. The certification start date will be the date the score is released (not the date the examination was taken).

PSI Computer Testing Centers

AANPCB Exams
PSI Services LLC (PSI)
www.psiexams.com
Toll-Free Phone: (800) 733-9267
Fax: (702) 932-2666

The AANPCB's exams are administered by PSI Services LLC, which has more than 300 locations across the United States and Canada. Locations are listed on the PSI scheduling portal. Approved qualified candidates who have completed their applications (final transcripts included) are sent an authorization to test by email from the AANPCB. About 1 day after you receive the AANPCB email, PSI Services will send you your PSI Eligibility ID number from support@psionline.com providing a link to their online scheduling system (to schedule/reschedule/cancel/confirm). You can also register by phone (800-733-9276).

Important information about applying for the AANC and AANPCB exams is given in Table 1.1.

Table 1.1 Application Timeline for Certification Exams

Timeline	Recommended Activities Before Graduation
About 3 to 4 months before graduation	Open an account on the ANCC and/or the AANPCB website and start the application process. Find out about the certification requirements. Download and read the General Testing Booklet, Test Content Outline, and the Reference List. Visit your SBON website and read the licensure requirements for NPs in your state. Download the licensure application.
About 4 to 6 weeks before graduation	Order three to four copies of your official final transcript.
About 2 to 3 weeks before graduation	The NP director of your program needs to sign the ANCC Education Validation Form.

AANPCB, American Academy of Nurse Practitioners Certification Board; ANCC, American Nurses Credentialing Center; NP, nurse practitioner; SBON, state board of nursing.

EXAM BACKGROUND INFORMATION

The ANCC releases a new edition of their exams about every 2 years. The AANPCB is now releasing a new edition of their exam annually. There is more than one version of each exam—each ANCC exam edition has several versions, but the AANPCB exam only has two. If you have failed the exam and retake it, you will get a different version of the exam. The version of the exam that you are taking is assigned by the testing center computer system. What this means is that you may be taking a different version of the exam than your classmate even though both of you are taking the same edition of the exam on the same date and time at the same testing center.

Exam Format

New question formats for the ANCC and AANPCB exams were introduced beginning with the 2016 exams. There are more new-format questions on the ANCC exam than on the AANPCB exam. The new formats on the ANCC exam include "drag and drop," multiple-choice question with five or six answer options (you are asked to pick two or three correct answers), "hot spot" (a picture is presented that is divided into four quadrants and you click on the correct quadrant as the answer), colored photographs of skin and eye conditions, EKG strips, and chest x-ray films. These new formats are discussed in Chapter 2. Most questions on the ANCC exam are still multiple choice with four answer options.

Similarly, most AANPCB exam questions are the classic multiple-choice format with four answer options. There may be one EKG strip, a chest x-ray film, as well as some multiple-choice questions with five to six answer options (you are asked to pick two to three answers). The exams are computer-based tests (CBTs) unlike the NCLEX-RN® exam, which is a computer-adaptive test. The NP exams do not shut down automatically after you have earned enough points, as occurs with the NCLEX-RN exam.

Test Content Outline and Reference List

Both the ANCC and the AANPCB provide Test Content Outlines (TCOs) and a Reference List on their website. It is important that you read these documents. Read each carefully and concentrate your studies on the designated topic areas.

Total Number of Questions and Time

ANCC: FNP Exam (released February 2016)
ANCC: AGPCNP Exam (released December 2015)

There are 200 total questions (only 175 questions are graded). There are 25 questions that are not graded (for statistical data).

Total Time: Total counted testing time is 4 hours.

AANPCB: FNP Exam (released February 2018)
AANPCB: AGNP Exam (released February 2018)

There are 150 total questions (only 135 questions are graded). There are 15 questions that are not graded.

Total Time: Total counted testing time is 3 hours.

Computer Tutorial

For both exams, each testing session starts with a computer tutorial session of 10 to 15 minutes. This time is not counted as part of the testing time (it is "free" time). When the tutorial time expires, the computer will automatically start the exam and the first question will appear on the screen. The countdown clock (upper corner of the screen) will start counting down the time. The countdown clock will not stop for "breaks," but if you need a break, inform a testing center staff member who is monitoring the testing area. Watch the time clock closely because when the allotted testing time expires, the computer will automatically shut down the exam.

Time Allotted per Question

For both the ANCC and AANPCB certification exams, each question is allotted about 60 seconds. If you find yourself spending too much time on one question, pick an answer (best guess), then "mark" it so that you can return to it later. Never leave any question unanswered. If you guess correctly, it will get counted; if you leave it blank, it is marked as an error (0 points).

Sample Exam Questions

I highly recommend that you try the free sample exams at the ANCC's website even if you are planning to only take the AANPCB exam. The ANCC's sample exam is web-based and contains 25 questions. It can be taken as many times as desired at no charge (and it is scored every time). The AANPCB also has free questions, which are listed on the last two pages of their candidate handbook (no answer key is provided). If you want to familiarize yourself with the format of the AANPCB exam, you can purchase their 75-item Practice Examination (timed 90 minutes), which is taken online and graded. It can only be taken once. The ANCC also sells sample exam questions, but their free web-based sample exams provide a good opportunity to practice using their exam formats. If you are an FNP, you can take the free sample exams for the FNP, AGPCNP, and PNP. You will have a total of 75 questions from these three exams.

COMPARING THE ANCC VERSUS THE AANPCB EXAM

1. **What are the passing rates for the two exams?**
   For the exams released in 2016, the passing rates for the ANCC and AANPCB exams are as follows:
   FNP exam: 82% for the ANCC versus 80% for the AANPCB, or a difference of just 2%.
   AGPCNP/AGNP exam: 82% for the ANCC versus 76% for the AANPCB—a 6% difference, which is significant.
2. **What is the major difference between the two exams?**
   There are two major differences between the two exams. First, the ANCC exam contains more nonclinical questions than the AANPCB exam. Second, new question formats, such as drag and drop, photographs, EKG strip, chest x-ray film, and multiple-choice questions with five to six answer options, were added beginning with the 2016 ANCC exams.

   The vast majority of questions on the AANPCB exam are on clinical topics. Most of the questions are the classic multiple-choice format with four answer options, but there may be some multiple-choice questions that have five to six answer options (you are asked to pick two or three answers), an EKG strip, and a chest x-ray film.
3. **Are there apps from the Apple Store and the Google Play Store?**
   AANC: The ANCC has an app that can be used to apply for the exam.
   AANPCB: The AANPCB does not have an app currently, but it may have one in the near future.
4. **What are the new commands in the ANCC Prometric exams?**
   You can now "highlight" words (keywords) to help you concentrate on the best clues (that you picked). You can also use the "strikeout" command, which allows you to cross out (eliminate) the answer option(s) that you think is(are) wrong (distractors). These two new commands are not yet available for the PSI AANPCB exam.
5. **If I join their respective membership organizations, will I receive a discount on my fees?**
   ANCC: To be eligible, you need to be a member of the ANA. If you belong to a state nursing association, you may already be a member of the ANA. Check with your state's nursing association. To apply for membership, apply online at the ANA's website (www.nursingworld.org). A word of warning: If you are not a member, you only have 5 business days after you apply for the exam to claim the membership discount. Exam discount claims received after this time are not allowed, and "refunds will not be issued."
   AANPCB: To be eligible for the exam discount, you must be a member of the AANP (www.aanp.org). If you already applied for the exam as a nonmember, you have up to 30 days to apply for membership. To receive the membership discount (as a refund), you need to send an email to inform them that you are a member (certification@aanpcert.org).
6. **How do I apply for the ANCC or the AANPCB certification exam?**
   For both agencies, you must initially open an online account at their website. To avoid loss of information, it is best to complete your online application within 30 days once it is started. The application forms are in typeable PDF so you can fill them in directly on your computer and then print a hardcopy for your records.
   ANCC: The ANCC accepts applications online, by mail, expedited method (fax/email), and by their new mobile app "MYANCC" (Apple Store/Google Play).
   AANPCB: The AANPCB accepts applications online and by mail. Applying online does not expedite processing. The organization automatically charges a nonrefundable paper

application processing fee for all paper applications (email, mail, and fax). There is no charge for processing of supporting documents for certification and recertification (e.g., unofficial transcripts, RN license).

If you apply by mail, do not forget to photocopy the entire contents of your application package. If you plan on using the U.S. Postal Service to mail your package, I would recommend that you pay the extra fee for registered mail.

7. **How early can I apply for the certification exam?**
   Both the ANCC and AANPCB allow students to apply as early as 6 months before graduation.
   ANCC: The ANCC will not process an application until payment has cleared. A completed application must contain copy of your RN license, an official copy of your final transcripts, and the original copy of the Validation of Education form, signed by your NP program director.
   AANPCB: The AANPCB allows DNP students to apply up to 12 months before graduation, but it will not release the exam scores until the MSN or DNP degrees are issued. If you apply before you graduate, you are required to submit an official copy of your current transcript (the interim transcript). The interim transcript is your most recent transcript, which contains all the course work that you have completed up to that date. When the official final transcript is released, either you or the registrar's office of your school can mail or email it directly to the AANPCB.

   In addition, the AANPCB requires a hard copy of your RN license. Do not forget to download the State Board of Nursing Notification Form from the board's website so that it can release your exam scores to your state board of nursing (SBON).
8. **How long does it take to process a completed application?**
   ANCC: It takes about 4 to 6 weeks to process an application. Be warned that the ANCC will not process an application until it is complete and all required documents have been received (copy of RN license, original of the signed education validation form, final transcript). If there are problems with your application, an email will be sent to you. Answer all the questions on the forms, and do not leave any blanks.
   AANPCB: It generally takes between 4 to 6 weeks after you have paid the fees and submitted all the required documentation to process an application. Fill out all the questions, and do not leave any blanks or forget signatures. An error can delay your application significantly.
9. **What is the ANCC's "expedited application" process?**
   This option shortens the processing time to 5 business days ($200 nonrefundable fee). Download and print the Certification Expedite Review Request Form from the ANCC website and fax it to (301) 628-5233. If your school has not released your final transcript, it will delay the expedited application. The Validation of Advanced Practice Nursing Education form can be signed by electronic signature (give your NP director's email address) and an electronic copy of your final transcript can be emailed directly by secure transmission from your school's registrar (aprnvalidation@ana.org). Follow up by calling to verify that the ANCC has received your faxed application.

   Note: Mailing the ANCC "expedite" form will delay processing; it should be faxed. If you both fax and mail it, you will be charged the processing fee twice.

   The AANPCB does not expedite applications.
10. **What are the final transcript and the "official" transcript?**
    The final transcript is the one that is issued after you graduate from your NP program. It should indicate the type of degree you earned along with the NP specialty you graduated with (e.g., family or adult-gerontology NP).

A transcript is considered "official" only if it remains inside the sealed envelope in which it was mailed from your college registrar's office or if it is mailed directly from their office to the certifying agency. An electronic copy of your transcript can be transmitted directly by secure transmission from the registrars' office (aprnvalidation@ana.org). Order at least three to four copies of your final transcripts and keep the extras unopened to keep them official. Open one copy (yours) and check it for accuracy.

11. **What is the ANCC Validation of Education form?**
This one-page form is a requirement for ANCC applicants only. Most NP programs have this document signed in bulk by the current director of the NP program. Ideally, it should be distributed to the students before the final day of school. You must send the original signed form (not a copy) to the ANCC with your application.
Note: It is probably a good idea for all NP students to get this document signed, even if they plan to take only the AANPCB exam. Because the ANCC requires this form, it will save you precious time in the future if you decide to apply for their exam. You always have the option of applying quickly for the "other" certification exam if you fail the first. Do not forget that you will need another official final transcript (another good reason why you should have at least four copies of your transcript).

12. **Is it possible to take the exam at any time of the year?**
You can take both certification exams at any time of the year, whenever the Prometric and the PSI testing centers are open.

13. **When should I schedule my exam?**
Do not wait until the last minute to schedule your exam because the testing centers in your area may no longer have the date (or the time) that you desire. Morning time slots tend to get filled very quickly. Both Prometric and PSI testing centers allow test-takers to schedule, reschedule, or cancel an appointment on their website or by phone, but you should give them notice.
Prometric (ANCC): Processing fee is charged if less than 30-day notice is given and up to noon on the fifth business day of the appointment (Eastern Standard Time).
PSI (AANPCB): Requires a minimum of at least 2 days in advance to reschedule or cancel an exam (before 5:00 p.m. Pacific Standard Time).
Note: Avoid scheduling yourself at the time of the day when you tend to get tired or sleepy. For most, this is usually after lunchtime. Simply picking the wrong time of day can cause you to fail the exam, sometimes by as little as 2 points.

14. **What should I do if the time slot or date that I want is no longer available?**
Look for another testing center as soon as possible. For some, it may mean a long drive to another city, but it may well be worth the extra time and effort if your authorization-to-test letter is about to expire.

15. **What happens if I am late or miss my scheduled appointment?**
Table 1.2 presents important information about the AANPCB exams. If you are late or miss your appointment, you are considered a "no show" by the testing center staff. Your testing time period or "window" will automatically expire on that same day. Call the certifying agency as soon as possible for further instructions. Both the ANCC and the AANPCB will allow you to reschedule your exam (one time only), and you will be charged a rescheduling fee.

16. **If I have a disability, how can I obtain special testing accommodations?**
You can download the Special Accommodations Form from each organization's website (ANCC and AANPCB). It requires a description of the disability and limitations related to testing. It should be dated and signed by the provider. For example, if a student has severe test-taking anxiety, a special accommodation (if approved) is an extension of the testing time. Check the agency's website for further instructions.

Table 1.2 American Academy of Nurse Practitioners Certification Board: Important Information Regarding Testing

Candidate Actions	Consequences
■ Arrived late for exam appointment	■ Will not be allowed to take the examination as scheduled
■ Did not give at least 48 hours of notice (before canceling exam appointment)	■ Is responsible for paying any applicable testing center fee
■ Missed exam appointment	■ Will forfeit fee and require a new identification number
■ Did not have required mandatory primary ID	■ Will not be allowed to take the exam

Source: American Academy of Nurse Practitioners Certification Board (2016).

COMMON QUESTIONS ABOUT THE NURSE PRACTITIONER CERTIFICATION EXAMS

1. **What are the passing scores?**
   ANCC: The passing score is 350 points or higher. ANCC scores range from 100 to 500 points. *AANPCB*: The passing score is 500 points or higher. AANPCB scores range from 200 to 800 points.
2. **Will I find out immediately if I pass (or fail) the exam?**
   Yes, you will. After you exit the testing area, ask the proctor to print a copy of your results (pass or fail format). This is the "unofficial" score. If you pass the exam, you will not get a number score. According to the AANPCB, a preliminary "pass" score at the testing center is not considered official notification. It does not indicate active certification status, and it may not be used for employment or licensure as an NP. A letter with your official score will be mailed to you at a later date, indicating the type of certification and the starting date.

   If you fail the exam, you will receive a scaled number score with diagnostic feedback information for each domain such as:

   Low: Your score from this content area is below the acceptable level.

   Medium: Your score from this content area is marginally acceptable.

   High: Your score from this content area is above average.

   Concentrate your studies on the domain/category(s) in which you score "low" or "medium."
3. **How many times a year can I retake the FNP and AGNP certification exam?**
   ANCC: You can take this exam up to three times in a 12-month calendar period. You must wait at least 60 days between each exam. If you fail, you can reapply online (retest application), but wait about 5 days (after taking your exam) before you reapply online.

   AANPCB: You can take the exam up to two times per calendar year. Although there is no wait-time requirement prior to retesting, the AANPCB requires test-takers to take 15 contact hours in their area(s) with the weakest score (your "areas of weakness"). Reapply for the exam online by using the Retake Application form.

   Note: The continuing-education hours that you took before sitting for the certification exam are not eligible. The contact hours must be taken after you failed the exam. If you took a review course, it can be retaken again with the new dates. When you have completed the required 15 contact hours, email or fax the certificate of completion as proof. Call the AANPCB certification office first before faxing any documents.
4. **What happens if I fail the ANCC or AANPCB exam the second time?**
   You must resubmit a full application along with all the required documentation (like the first time) and pay the full test fee.

5. **What happens if my Authorization-to-Test letter expires and I have not taken the exam?**
Call the certifying agency for further instructions immediately. Both the ANCC and the AANPCB will allow you to reschedule your exam (one time only). You must pay a rescheduling fee. If you fail to test on your extended testing window, you must reapply like a new applicant and pay the full registration fee again.
6. **Is it possible to extend the testing window?**
ANCC: You can request (one time only) a new 90-day testing window. It must occur less than 6 months from the last day of the initial testing window. Your request for extension to the ANCC should be received before the initial 90-day testing period expires.
AANPCB: You can request an extension (one time only) by sending an email to certification@aanpcert.org. If an extension is granted, it will be for 60 days only. If you do not retake the exam during that time, you must reapply to take the examination (like the first time) and pay the full fee.
7. **Is there a penalty for guessing on the exam?**
No, there is no penalty for guessing. Therefore, if you are running out of time, answer the remaining questions at random. Do not leave any questions "blank" or without an answer, because this will be marked as an error (0 points). You may earn a few extra points if you guess correctly, which can make the difference between passing and failing the exam.
8. **Is it possible to return to a question later and change its answer?**
Yes, it is, but only if you "mark" the question. You will learn about this simple command during the computer tutorial time at the beginning of the exam. "Marking" a question allows the test-taker to return to the question at a later time (if you want to change or review your answer). On the other hand, if you indicate to the computer that your answer is "final," then you will not be allowed to change the answer. Do not worry about forgetting to "unmark" the questions if you run out of time. As long as a question has an answer, it will be graded by the computer.
9. **Does the certifying agency inform the SBON of my certification status?**
The AANPCB and the ANCC will not automatically send your scores to your SBON. For both certifying agencies, you must sign their Release of Scores consent form, which is one of the documents required when you apply for the exam.
10. **How can I obtain an "official" verification of my national certification for my employer?**
Both agencies have verification request forms on their websites. If you just took the exam, the AANPCB recommends you wait at least 10 days after your testing date. A nominal fee is charged.
11. **I am getting married (or divorced). Is there a problem with changing my legal name after I applied for the exams using my maiden or married name?**
Yes, there may be a problem. The name that you use in your application must be the same name as the one listed on your primary identification such as your unexpired driver's license, passport, or military ID. Check the agency's website or call for more details. If you get married after you applied for the exam, it is better to wait before changing the name on your driver's license until you have taken and passed the exam.

CERTIFICATION RENEWAL

1. **How long is my certification valid?**
Certification from the ANCC as well as the AANPCB is valid for 5 years. A few months before your certification expires, both the ANCC and the AANPCB will send you a reminder letter. "Failure of the certificant to receive (his or her) renewal notice does not relieve the certificant of his or her professional responsibility for renewing their certification."

2. **Can I still use my professional designations after my certification expires because I forgot to renew it?**
   No, the ANCC states that credentials cannot be used, once they have expired.
3. **What should I do if I change my legal name, have a new email address, new telephone contact number, or move to a new address?**
   You need to update your online account at the ANCC or at the AANPCB website within 30 days if there are any changes in your contact information, such as your legal name, residence address, email, or phone number.
4. **Is there a time period that must be followed to renew certification?**
   Yes, there is. All of the contact hours and practice hours must be completed within the current 5-year certification period.
5. **When should I submit my renewal application?**
   The process can be started as early as 12 months before your certification expires. It is best to start early because if you do not have enough continuing-education/clinical/pharmacology contact hours, you still have enough time to obtain them. Recertification applications should be submitted no later than 12 weeks prior to the expiration date of the current certification to allow time for reviewing, processing, and issuing the new certificate before the expiration of the current certification.
   Note: Save a digital or hard copy (or other proof) of all your continuing-education hours and clinical practice hours. If you are audited, you will be asked to submit proof of your continuing-education hours (e.g., certificates) and clinical practice hours.
6. **How many clinical hours of practice are required to renew my certification every 5 years?**
   The ANCC no longer requires clinical practice hours for recertification, although the AANPCB does require 1,000 hours of clinical practice in your area of specialty (completed in the previous 5 years before recertification), plus 100 hours CE, of which 25 hours must be pharmacology CE. If you plan to use your clinical volunteer hours as an NP, keep a notebook to record each clinical site's address, the number of hours that you practiced, and the name/signature of the supervising NP/physician. If you do not have enough clinical hours, another method you can use to recertify is to retake the examination combined with the required continuing-education hours. For ANPs and GNPs, you do not have the option to recertify by retaking the examination because the exams for your specialty have been retired.
7. **How many continuing-education contact hours are required for recertification?**
   ANCC: 75 contact hours of continuing education are required. You also need one or more of the eight ANCC renewal categories (e.g., academic credits, presentations, preceptor hours, quality improvement project, professional service, practice hours, retake exam, publication or research).
   AANPCB: 100 contact hours of continuing education are required.
8. **How many pharmacotherapeutic contact hours are required per renewal cycle?**
   ANCC: Of the 75 contact hours, 25 of those hours must be in pharmacotherapeutics. If you double the 75 (150 contact hours), only 25 contact hours are required.
   AANPCB: Of 100 contact hours, 25 contact hours of advanced pharmacology are required.
9. **What happens if my certification lapsed (I forgot to renew it)?**
   There is no "grace period" or backdating. On the day when your certification expires, you are prohibited from using your designation after your name. In addition, you will have a gap in your certification dates. The ANCC recommends that you check with your state licensing board to determine whether you can continue to practice as an NP. They also recommend that you check with your employer and with the agencies that are reimbursing your services.

10. **If my specialty certification exam was retired (ANP, GNP), can I continue with my specialty designation?**
    Yes, you may. You can renew your certification through continuing education and clinical hours. If you let your certification lapse, you no longer have the examination option. Unless there are other options in the future (check the websites for updates), only students who have graduated from an AGNP program are permitted to take that exam. ANPs and GNPs are not allowed to take the AGNP exam.
11. **Is there any reciprocity between the ANCC and the AANPCB?**
    No, there is not. Both the ANCC and the AANPCB discontinued their reciprocity program many years ago.

EXAM QUESTION CLASSIFICATION

American Nurses Credentialing Center

AGPCNP and FNP Certification Exams

Both the FNP and the AGPCNP exams have a total of 200 questions, but only 175 of the questions will be graded. The AGPCNP exam contains more nonclinical topics than the FNP exam. On the AGPCNP exam, the Professional Roles domain comprises 29% of questions, but on the FNP exam, the same domain comprises only 17% (see Table 1.3). For both exams, the true percentage of clinical questions is actually higher because many nonclinical topics are mixed into the two clinical domains (Foundations of Advanced Practice Nursing and Independent Practice. The nonclinical topics inserted under these two predominantly clinical domains include advocacy, theory, community needs assessment, research methodology, critiquing research findings, and ethical issues, among others. On the FNP exam, approximately 33% of the questions are likely to cover nonclinical topics (about 58 questions; see Table 1.4 for more information.) On the AGPCNP exam, about 20% of the questions (about 35 questions) are likely to cover nonclinical topics. The ANCC, unlike the AANPCB, does not release age-group statistics.

Table 1.3 ANCC AGPCNP Exam Domains

AGPCNP Exam (released December 2015)	%	Number of Questions
Foundations of Advanced Practice Nursing	29	51
Professional Roles	29	51
Independent Practice	42	73
TOTAL	100	175 graded questions

AGPCNP, Adult-Gerontology Primary Care Nurse Practitioner; ANCC, American Nurses Credentialing Center.

Adapted from the ANCC Adult-Gerontology Primary Care NP Certification Exam Test Content Outline (2016).

Table 1.4 ANCC FNP Exam Domains

FNP Exam (released February 2016)	%	Number of Questions
Foundations of Advanced Practice Nursing	37	64
Professional Practice	17	30
Independent Practice	46	81
TOTAL	100	175 graded questions

ANCC, American Nurses Credentialing Center; FNP, family nurse practitioner.

Summary

1. There are only three domains in the ANCC FNP and AGPCNP certification exams.
2. Almost all the questions on the AANPCB exam have to do with clinical topics.

3. For the FNP exam, about one out of four questions cover nonclinical topics
4. For the AGPCNP exam, about one out of three questions cover nonclinical topics.
5. Test-takers who score low in two of the three domains will fail the exam.

American Academy of Nurse Practitioners Certification Board

AGNP and FNP Certification Exams

The AANPCB FNP and AGNP exams were both released in October 2016. The exams have a total of 150 questions, but only 135 of these are graded. The AANPCB releases the domain as well as the age breakdown of their exams. There are four domains in the AANPCB exams. The largest domain is Assessment (36%), followed by Diagnosis (24%), Plan (23%), and Evaluation (17%). Percentage breakdown by age group of the AANPCB's FNP exam questions is detailed in Table 1.5. The percentage for the AGNP exam is detailed in Table 1.6. There is a big difference between the FNP and AGNP exams regarding the percentage of questions on adolescents: On the FNP exam, 18% (24 questions) focus on adolescents, but in the AGNP exam, it is only 7% (nine questions).

Table 1.5 Age Groups by Percentage (FNP Exam)

Age Group	%	Number of Questions
Adults (21–64 years)	37	50
Geriatrics	21	29
Frail Elderly	7	9
Early/Late Adolescence (12–20 years)	18	24
Pediatrics (birth–11 years)	14	19
Prenatal (pregnancy)	3	4
TOTAL	100	135 graded questions

FNP, family nurse practitioner.

Source: *AANPCB Family Nurse Practitioner and Adult-Gerontology Primary Care Nurse Practitioner Candidate Handbook* (2017).

Table 1.6 Age Groups by Percentage (AGNP Exam)

Age Group	%	Number of Questions
Adults (21–64 years)	43	58
Geriatrics	38	51
Frail Elderly	17	23
Early/Late Adolescence (12–20 years)	2	3
TOTAL	100	135 graded questions

AGNP, adult-gerontology nurse practitioner.

Summary

1. On the AANPCB FNP exam, the age group with the largest number of questions is adults (50 questions). The next largest group is geriatrics (29 questions).
2. When these two age groups are combined (age 21 years and older), they make up about 66% of questions (88 questions) in the FNP exam. Therefore, at least one out of two questions will relate to a patient who is 21 years of age or older.
3. There will be very few questions on the prenatal period and obstetrics (four questions). Keep this in mind when you are reviewing, and do not spend too much time on this content.
4. On the AANPCB AGNP exam, the age group with the least number of questions is adolescents (nine questions).

5. On the AANPCB AGNP exam, the questions are centered mostly on adult and geriatric age groups (126 questions).
6. As is usual for the AANPCB exams, almost all the questions are clinically based.

FAST FACTS: ANCC AND AABPCB EXAMS

1. The current ANCC AGPCNP exam (2016) probably has about 33% nonclinical questions—about one out of three questions.
2. The ANCC FNP exam probably has about 20% nonclinical questions or about one out of four questions.
3. The current AANPCB FNP and AGNP exams contain very few nonclinical questions.
4. The ANCC and AANPCB NP certification tests are designed for entry-level (not expert-level) practice. Most test-takers who sit for the NP certification exams are new graduates.
5. There are 25 pilot-test questions on the ANCC exam and 15 pilot-test questions on the AANPCB exam. These questions are not graded. There is no way to identify the pilot test questions from the graded questions.
6. New clinical information (treatment guidelines or new drugs) released within the previous 10 months prior to the current exam will most likely not be included.
7. Keep in mind that the questions will be on primary care disorders (e.g., primary care clinics, public health clinics). If you are guessing, avoid picking an exotic diagnosis as an answer.
8. The AANPCB exams will list the normal lab results when they are pertinent to a question, but they will be listed only once. Write them down on some scratch paper (or a whiteboard). When a related question comes up later, these pertinent lab values will not be listed again.
9. Follow the norms given by the AANPCB. For example, they may list their mean corpuscular volume (MCV) normal value between 82 and 102 fL (femtoliters). The usual norm taught in NP schools is an MCV between 80 and 100 fL (use this norm for the ANCC exam).
10. Unlike the AANPCB, the ANCC does not list the normal lab results. If you are taking the ANCC exam, it is important to memorize some normal lab results and to write them down on scratch paper during the computer tutorial time period.
11. Learn the significance of abnormal lab results and the type of follow-up needed to further evaluate the patient.
    - *Example*: An elderly male patient complains of a new-onset, left-sided temporal headache accompanied by scalp tenderness and indurated temporal artery. The NP suspects temporal arteritis. The screening test is the sedimentation rate, which is expected to be much higher than normal (elevated value).
    - *Example*: A patient with an elevated white blood cell (WBC >11,000/mm^3) count accompanied by neutrophilia (>70%) and the presence of bands ("shift to the left") most likely has a serious bacterial infection.
12. Expect to find many culture-related questions on the ANCC exam.
    - *Example*: If a traditional Muslim woman refuses to undress and use a hospital gown, an alternative is to examine her with her clothes on (modified physical exam).
13. The other cultures that may be addressed on the ANCC exam are Mexicans, Cubans, Chinese, Cambodians/Filipinos, and Native Americans (e.g., Navajo). Cultural topics are covered in this book in the nonclinical chapters.
    - *Example*: A Navajo woman has an appointment for a follow-up visit, but she does not show up for the appointment. The most common cause for Navajo patients to skip health visits and follow-up visits is the lack of transportation.
14. Sometimes there will be one unexpected question relating to a dental injury.
    - *Example*: A completely avulsed permanent tooth should be reimplanted as soon as possible. It can be transported to the dentist in cold milk (not frozen milk).

15. There may be a question on epidemiologic terms.
    - *Example*: *Sensitivity* is defined as the ability of a test to detect a person who has the disease. *Specificity* is defined as the ability of a test to detect a person who is healthy (or to detect the person without the disease).
16. Learn the definition of some of the research study designs.
    - *Example*: A cohort study follows a group of people who share some common characteristics to observe the development of disease over time (e.g., the Framingham Nurses' Health Study).
17. Several emergent conditions that may present in the primary care area will be on the exam.
    - *Example*: Navicular fracture, acute myocardial infarction (MI), cauda equina syndrome, anaphylaxis, angioedema, meningococcal meningitis, etc.
18. Become familiar with the names of some anatomic areas.
    - *Example*: Trauma to Kiesselbach's plexus will result in an anterior nosebleed.
19. Some questions may ask about the "gold-standard test" or the diagnostic test for a condition.
    - *Example*: The diagnostic or gold-standard test for sickle cell anemia, glucose-6-phosphate dehydrogenase (G6PD) anemia, and alpha or beta thalassemia is the hemoglobin electrophoresis.
20. Distinguish between first-line and second-line antibiotics. (For adult-gerontology NPs, the age in the example that follows can be changed to an adolescent or an adult.)
    - *Example*: A 7-year-old child with acute otitis media (AOM) who is treated with amoxicillin returns in 48 hours without improvement (complains of ear pain, bulging tympanic membrane). The next step is to discontinue the amoxicillin and start the child on a second-line antibiotic such as amoxicillin-clavulanate (Augmentin) BID (twice a day) × 10 days.
21. Become knowledgeable about alternative antibiotics for penicillin-allergic patients. If the patient has a gram-positive infection, the possible alternatives are macrolides, clindamycin, or quinolones with gram-positive activity such as levofloxacin or moxifloxacin.
22. If a patient has an infection that responds well to macrolides, but she thinks she is "allergic" to erythromycin (symptoms of nausea or gastrointestinal [GI] upset), inform her that she had an adverse reaction, not a true allergic reaction (hives, angioedema).
    - *Example*: Switch the patient from erythromycin to azithromycin (usually a Z-Pack).
23. If a patient fails to respond to the initial medication, add another medication (follow the steps of the treatment guideline).
    - *Example*: A patient with chronic obstructive pulmonary disease (COPD) is prescribed ipratropium bromide (Atrovent) for dyspnea. On follow-up, the patient complains that his symptoms are not relieved. The next step would be to prescribe an albuterol inhaler (Ventolin) or to prescribe a combination inhaler.
24. Disease states are usually presented in their full-blown "classic" textbook presentations.
    - *Example*: In a case of acute mononucleosis, the patient will most likely be a teen presenting with the classic triad of sore throat, prolonged fatigue, and enlarged cervical nodes. If the patient is older, but has the same signs and symptoms, it is still mononucleosis (reactivated type).
25. Ethnic background may give a clue for some diseases.
    - *Example*: Alpha thalassemia is more common among Southeast Asians (such as Filipinos). Beta thalassemia is more common in Mediterranean people.
26. No asymptomatic or "borderline" cases of disease states are presented in the test.
    - *Example*: In real life, most patients with iron-deficiency anemia are asymptomatic and do not have either pica or spoon-shaped nails. In the exam, they will probably have these clinical findings plus the other findings of anemia.

27. Become familiar with lupus or systemic lupus erythematosus (SLE).
    - *Example*: A malar rash (butterfly rash) is present in most patients with lupus. These patients should be advised to avoid or to minimize sunlight exposure (photosensitivity).
28. Become familiar with polymyalgia rheumatica (PMR).
    - *Example*: First-line treatment for PMR includes long-term steroids. Long-term, low-dosed steroids are commonly used to control symptoms (pain, severe stiffness in shoulders and hip girdle). PMR patients are also at higher risk for temporal arteritis.
29. The gold-standard exam for temporal arteritis is a biopsy of the temporal artery. Refer the patient to an ophthalmologist for management.
30. Learn the disorders for which maneuvers are used and what a positive report signifies.
    - *Example*: Finkelstein's test—positive in De Quervain's tenosynovitis. Anterior drawer maneuver and Lachman maneuver—positive if anterior cruciate ligament (ACL) of the knee is damaged. The knee may also be unstable. McMurray's sign—positive in meniscus injuries of the knee.
31. Some conditions need to be evaluated with a radiologic test.
    - *Example*: Damaged joints: Order an x-ray first (but MRI is the gold standard).
32. The abnormal eye findings in diabetes (diabetic retinopathy) and hypertension (hypertensive retinopathy) should be memorized. Learn to distinguish each one.
    - *Example*: Diabetic retinopathy (neovascularization, cotton wool spots, and microaneurysms). Hypertensive retinopathy (atrioventricular [AV] nicking, silver and/or copper wire arterioles).
33. Become knowledgeable about physical exam "normal" and "abnormal" findings.
    - *Example*: When checking deep tendon reflexes (DTRs) in a patient with severe sciatica or diabetic peripheral neuropathy, the ankle jerk reflex (Achilles reflex) may be absent or hypoactive. Scoring: absent (0), hypoactive (1), normal (2), hyperactive (3), and clonus (4).
34. There are only a few questions on benign or physiologic variants.
    - *Example*: A benign S4 heart sound may be auscultated in some elderly patients. Torus palatinus and fishtail uvula may be seen during the oral exam in a few patients.
35. Some commonly used drugs have rare (but potentially life-threatening) adverse effects.
    - *Example*: A rare but serious adverse effect of angiotensin-converting enzyme inhibitors (ACEIs) is angioedema. A common side effect of ACEIs is a dry cough (up to 10%).
36. Learn about the preferred and/or first-line drug used to treat some diseases.
    - *Example*: ACEI or angiotensin receptor blockers (ARBs) are the preferred drugs to treat hypertension in diabetics and patients with mild to moderate renal disease because of their renal-protective properties.
37. When medications are used in the answer options, they will be listed either by name (generic and brand name) or by drug class alone.
    - *Example*: Instead of using the generic/brand name of ipratropium (Atrovent), it may be listed as a drug class (an anticholinergic).
38. Most of the drugs mentioned in the exam are the well-recognized drugs.
    - *Example*:

      Penicillin: Amoxicillin (broad-spectrum penicillin), penicillin VK

      Macrolide: Erythromycin, azithromycin (Z-Pack), or clarithromycin (Biaxin)

      Cephalosporins: First-generation (Keflex), second-generation (Cefaclor, Ceftin, Cefzil), third-generation (Rocephin, Suprax, Omnicef)

      Quinolones: Ciprofloxacin (Cipro), ofloxacin (Floxin)

      Quinolones with gram-positive coverage: Levofloxacin (Levaquin), moxifloxacin (Avelox), gatifloxacin (Tequin)

Sulfa: Trimethoprim-sulfamethoxazole (Bactrim, Septra), nitrofurantoin (Macrobid)
Tetracyclines: Tetracycline, doxycycline, minocycline (Minocin)
Nonsteroidal anti-inflammatory drug (NSAID): Ibuprofen, naproxen (Aleve, Anaprox)
COX-2 inhibitor: Celecoxib (Celebrex)

- Other examples are listed in both Chapters 2 and 3.

39. Category B drugs are allowed for pregnant or lactating women.
    - *Example*: For pain relief, pick acetaminophen (Tylenol) instead of NSAIDs such as ibuprofen (Advil) or naproxen (Aleve, Anaprox). Avoid nitrofurantoin and sulfa drugs during the third trimester (these increase risk of hyperbilirubinemia).
40. The preferred treatment for cutaneous anthrax is ciprofloxacin 500 mg orally BID for 60 days or for 8 weeks. If the patient is allergic to ciprofloxacin, use doxycycline 100 mg BID. Cutaneous anthrax is not contagious; it comes from touching fur or animal skins that are contaminated with anthrax spores.
41. There are some questions on theories and conceptual models.
    - *Example*: Stages of change or "decision" theory (Prochaska) includes concepts such as precontemplation, contemplation, preparation, action, and maintenance (see Chapter 26).
42. Other health theorists who have been included on the exams in the past are (not inclusive): Alfred Bandura (self-efficacy), Erik Erikson, Sigmund Freud, Elisabeth Kübler-Ross (grieving), and others.
    - *Example*: If a small child expresses a desire to marry a parent of the opposite sex, the child is in the oedipal stage (Freud). Child's age is about 5 to 6 years (preschool to kindergarten).
43. Starting at the age of about 11 years, most children can understand abstract concepts (early abstract thinking) and are better at logical thinking.
    - *Example*: When performing the Mini-Mental State Exam, when the NP is asking about "proverbs," the nurse is assessing the patient's ability to understand abstract concepts.
44. Keep these good communication rules in mind: Ask open-ended questions, do not reassure patients, avoid angering the patient, and respect the patient's culture. There may be two to three questions relating to "abuse" (child abuse, domestic abuse, elderly abuse).
45. Follow national treatment guidelines for certain disorders. Following is a list of treatment guidelines used as references by the ANCC and the AANPCB.*
    - ***Asthma***: National Asthma Education and Prevention Program. (2007). *Expert Panel Report 3: Guidelines for the Diagnosis and Management of Asthma–Full Report 2007.* Bethesda, MD: National Institutes of Health.
    - ***COPD***: Global Initiative for Chronic Obstructive Lung Disease. (2016). *Global Strategy for the Diagnosis, Management, and Prevention of Chronic Obstructive Pulmonary Disease, Updated 2014.*
    - ***Diabetes***: American Diabetes Association Clinical Practice Recommendations. (2016). FNP exam. *Diabetes Care, 37*(Suppl. 1).
    - ***Ethics***: *Guide to the Code of Ethics for Nurses with Interpretive Statements: Development, Interpretation, and Application.* (2015). (2nd ed.). Silver Spring, MD: Nursesbooks.org.
    - ***Healthy People***: Office of Disease Promotion and Health Prevention. (2010). *Healthy People 2020* (3rd ed.). McLean, VA: International Medical Publishing.
    - ***Health Promotion***: *The Guide to Clinical Preventive Services 2014: Recommendations of the U.S. Preventive Services Task Force.* (2014). Rockville, MD: Agency for Healthcare Research & Quality.

---

*Not an all-inclusive list.

- ***Hyperlipidemia***: 2014 ACC/AHA Release Updated Guideline on the Treatment of Blood Cholesterol to Reduce ASCVD Risk: A Report of the American College of Cardiology/American Heart Association Task Force on Practice Guidelines. (2014). *Journal of the American College of Cardiology*, *63*(25-PA), 2889–2934.
- ***Hypertension***: 2014 Evidence-Based Guideline for the Management of High Blood Pressure in Adults: Report from the Panel Members Appointed to the Eighth Joint National Committee (JNC 8). (2014). *Journal of the American Medical Association*, *311*(5), 507–520.
- ***Mental Health***: American Psychiatric Association. (2013). *Diagnostic and Statistical Manual of Mental Disorders* (5th ed.). Arlington, VA: American Psychiatric Publishing.
- ***Pediatrics***: American Academy of Pediatrics. (2008). *Bright Futures: Guidelines for Health Supervision of Infants, Children, and Adolescents* (3rd ed.). Elk Grove Village, IL: Author.
- ***Sexually Transmitted Diseases (or Sexually Transmitted Infections)***: Centers for Disease Control and Prevention. (2015). Sexually Transmitted Diseases Treatment Guidelines. U.S. Department of Health and Human Services.

46. The ANCC exam has several questions about evidence-based medicine that are designed in the drag-and-drop format. For important facts, review Chapter 2 to become familiar with this format, as well as the new chapter in this book on Evidence-Based Medicine and Epidemiology for important facts.
47. If the question is asking for the initial or screening lab test, it will probably be a "cheap" and readily available test such as the CBC (complete blood count (CBC) to screen for anemia.

MAXIMIZING YOUR SCORE

1. The first answer that "pops" in your head is usually the correct answer.
2. If you are guessing, pick an answer at random. Try not to change it unless you are sure.
3. Use the "mark" command so that you can return to the question later when you complete the exam.
4. Avoid changing too many answers. If you are not sure, then leave the answer alone. I advise my students not to change more than three answers.
5. Avoid choosing exotic diseases as answers if you are guessing. Remember, these are tests for primary care conditions.
6. One method of guessing is to look for a pattern. Pick the answer that does not fit the pattern. Another is to pick the answer that you are most "attracted" to. Go with your gut feeling, and do not change the answer unless you are very sure.
7. Remind yourself to read slowly and carefully throughout the test. Avoid reading questions too rapidly. Make sure that you understand the stem of the question (usually the last sentence of a question).
8. If you are having problems choosing or understanding the answer options, try to read them from the bottom up (from option D to A, or from 4 to 1).
9. Eliminate the wrong answers after you read all the answer options. If an answer option contains all-inclusive words ("all," "none," "every," "never," "none"), then it is probably wrong.
10. Be careful with certain words such as "always," "exactly," "often," "sometimes," and "mostly."

11. Assume that each question has enough information to answer it correctly. Questions and answers are carefully designed. Take the facts at face value.
12. The first few questions are usually harder to solve. This is a common test design. Do not let it shake your confidence. (Guess the answer and "mark" it so that you can return to it later.)
13. Save yourself time (and mental strain) by reading the last sentence (or stem) of long questions and case scenarios *first*. Then read the question again from the beginning. The advantage of this "backward reading" technique is that you know ahead of time what the question is asking for. When you read it again "normally," it becomes easier to recognize important clues that will help you answer the question.
14. Just because a statement or an answer is true does not mean that it is the correct answer. If it does not answer the stem of the question, then it is the wrong answer.
15. Design and memorize your "scratch paper" a few weeks before you take the exam. Choose what you want on it wisely. Remember to keep it brief.
16. Use the time left from the "free" computer tutorial time to write down the facts that you memorized for your scratch paper. If you run out of time, skip this step.
17. Some suggestions of facts to write down on the scratch paper are lab results (hemoglobin, hematocrit, MCV, platelets, WBC count, neutrophil percentage, potassium, urinalysis, etc.). Other popular choices are the murmurs, mnemonics, and cranial nerves.
18. Do not leave any of the questions unanswered because there is no penalty for guessing. Questions that are left blank are marked as errors (0 points). If you have only 30 minutes left and you are not done, quickly answer the remaining questions at random.
19. If you spend more than 60 seconds on a question, you are wasting time. Answer it at random and then "mark" it so that you can return to it later (after you finish the entire test).
20. Consider a quick break (if you have enough time) if you get too mentally fatigued. Solving 200 questions is pretty intense. If you feel "fuzzy" or tired, go to the bathroom and get a drink of water, and splash cold water on your face. This can take less than 5 minutes. You can bring bottled water, but you have to leave it outside the testing area.
21. The countdown clock in the computer does not stop for breaks. Do not use more than 5 minutes for your quick bathroom break.
22. If you have failed the test before, try not to memorize what you did on the previous exam you took. The answers you remember may be wrong. Pretend that you have never seen the test before so that you can start out fresh mentally.
23. Do not panic or let your anxiety take over. Learn to use a calming technique, such as deep breathing, to calm yourself quickly before you take the exam.
24. Consider using a test-anxiety hypnosis CD and use it every night for at least 2 to 3 weeks for maximum effect.
25. One of the most important advice that I can give you is to make sure that you get enough sleep the night before the exam. Aim for at least 7 to 8 hours of sleep. Better yet, make sure that you get enough sleep a few nights before, not just the night before.
26. Before the test, practice answering questions and check the rationales afterward. The ANCC has free questions per specialty that you can take online and score. Buy practice questions from the ANCC or the AANPCB (depends on which test you are taking).
27. Check out the website allnurses.com and search for examination tips from other who have taken/failed the FNP certification exam. You can also do this directly by using a Google, Bing, or other search engine.

PREPARING FOR THE EXAM

Review Timeline

1. Start seriously reviewing for the exam at least 3 months in advance. Study time can range from 2 to 3 hours per session or you can break it up into 1-hour segments. Be consistent. The best time to study is the time of day you are most alert.
2. Prepare a study schedule by organ system. Photocopy the table of contents of your primary care textbook. Place check marks next to the diseases that you want to concentrate on and then schedule the date and time period for each organ system.
3. Concentrate your studies on your weaker areas. For example, if orthopedics is one of your weak areas, devote more time to it. Spend 3 days on orthopedics versus 1 day for the "easy" organ systems (easy since you understand them better).
4. I highly recommend that you attend at least one quality review course and buy CDs of another review course. I teach review courses live and by webinar. You can view my class schedule at my website at www.npreview.com.
5. Buy a new notebook. If you find that you are having a problem understanding a concept, write it down in your notebook, then research it and find the answer to your question.
6. Meet with someone in your local area or by phone who is also taking the exam. Practice quizzing each other.
7. Note the disease and topics that I have highlighted in this review book. Some organ systems have more "weight" on the exam than others. Become more familiar with these areas.
8. If you are taking the ANCC exam, I highly recommend that you devote at least 30% of your study time learning about the nonclinical topics.
9. If you learn better in a group, organize one. Decide ahead of time what organ systems or diseases to cover together so that you do not waste time.

Testing Center Details

1. Call the testing center or confirm your appointment online 4 weeks before to verify your appointment date and time.
2. Locate and drive to the testing center 1 to 2 weeks before taking the exam. Save the address of the testing center on your GPS or map app.
3. Arrive at least 45 to 60 minutes before your scheduled time so that you have enough time to park your car, locate the testing center, and check in for your appointment.
4. Acceptable forms of primary identification (photo with signature). If you do not have the proper forms of identification, you will not be allowed to take the exam.
   - Driver's license issued by the Department of Motor Vehicles (DMV)
   - State ID card issued by the DMV
   - Passport
   - U.S. military ID
   - Your secondary ID (nonphoto): Card with your name and signature (e.g., credit card, ATM card, Social Security card, Voter Registration card, employee ID)
   - Expired IDs are not acceptable
   - The name that is printed on your primary ID must match the name that you used when you applied for the exam
   - Check that both your primary and secondary IDs and the letter with your Prometric identification number match; make sure that all your IDs are inside your wallet/handbag
5. Biometrics are used for enhanced security. Your fingerprint is scanned before testing and every time you reenter the test area (it is erased in 24 hours to ensure privacy). The test-taking room is also monitored closely by videotape and microphones.

6. A whiteboard (8.5 × 11 inches) with the pen, or scratch paper and pencil, is given to you by the testing center staff (and collected after you are done). If you are given paper and tend to write a lot, ask for extra paper.
7. You can request noise-reducing headsets or ear plugs; consider this option if you are sensitive to noise.
8. Cell phones, watches, cameras, pagers, jewelry (except for engagement and/or wedding ring) and food or drink are not allowed inside the testing area.
9. Testing computers are predetermined. Each test-taker is assigned one small cubicle with one computer. If you are having problems seeing the computer screen, bring it to the proctor's attention as soon as possible.
10. Verify that you are given the correct examination as soon as you sit down. Check that the title and the examination code on the screen match the information sent by the testing agency for your NP specialty.
11. No food or drink is allowed inside the testing room. But you can bring in a drink and food (e.g., snack bar) and place it outside the locker (top of the locker) so that you do not have to open your locker. You are not permitted to unlock your locker during the testing period.
12. If you need to go to the restroom, you must first sign out with the proctor/testing staff. Remember, the time clock will continue to count down the time. It does not stop for breaks.
13. Do not forget your glasses if you need them to read text on the computer.

The Night Before the Exam

1. Avoid eating a heavy meal or consuming alcoholic drinks the night before the exam. Avoid eating 3 to 4 hours before bedtime (prevents heartburn).
2. Get enough sleep. Aim for at least 7 to 8 hours. Getting adequate sleep is probably one of the most important things you can do to help you pass the exam.
3. If you are scheduled to take your exam in the morning, set two alarms to wake you up on time. Give yourself extra time if it is a weekday (traffic congestion).

The Day of the Exam

1. Avoid eating a heavy breakfast or eating only simple carbs. The best meals are a combination of a protein with a complex carbohydrate (eggs, whole-wheat bread, nuts, cheese, etc.). If you eat only simple carbs, you can become hypoglycemic within 1 hour.
2. If you get drowsy and "fuzzy" during the exam, there are several ways to "wake up" rapidly. Excuse yourself and go the bathroom to drink cold water and to splash cold water on your face. You can perform 10 to 20 "jumping jacks." Drinking a caffeinated beverage or coffee can be very helpful. (However, don't drink too much.)
3. Avoid drinking too much fluid and do not forget to empty your bladder before the exam.
4. Wear comfortable clothing and dress in layers in case of temperature changes.
5. Jewelry is not allowed inside the testing area except for wedding and/or engagement rings. .

OTHER TEST-TAKING ISSUES

Test Anxiety

It is normal to feel anxious before taking an exam. A little anxiety helps us to become alert and vigilant, but too much anxiety can wear you down both emotionally and physically.

Your internal perception about how well you will do on the exam is very important. If you tend to become very anxious (or you are now more anxious because you previously failed the exam), there are calming methods that may prove helpful in controlling your anxiety. Following are some suggestions to help reduce test-taking anxiety a few weeks before the exam.

1. Make sure that you have devoted enough time for your review studies. If you feel in your gut that you have not studied "enough" or that you are not ready, it will worsen anxiety.
2. Consider signing up for both the ANCC and AANPCB exams. It can help to reduce your anxiety level because you feel like you have a "backup" exam.
3. If you have a firm job offer, I also recommend that you sign up for both exams to decrease test-taking anxiety.
4. Consider taking one to two review courses. My review courses and webinars are listed at my website www.npreview.com.
5. Avoid negative "self-talk." When you catch yourself doing it, silently tell yourself to "Stop it! Right now!"
6. Improve the nutritional content of your diet, especially about 2 weeks before the exam. Vitamins and supplements that may be helpful to the brain are omega-3 capsules (fish oil); B-complex vitamins; vitamins C, D, and E; choline; and others.
7. Hypnotherapy audio files are sold online for use in portable-player devices. For maximum effectiveness, it is best to listen to them daily for 2 to 4 weeks.
8. "Tapping" is another method used to counteract test anxiety (or increase self-confidence). The technique is demonstrated in videos posted to YouTube.

Your Panic Button

If you find yourself feeling panicky during the exam, try the following calming technique. Practice this exercise at home until you feel comfortable doing it.

Breathing Exercise

1. Close your eyes. During inhalation, tell yourself gently, "I am breathing in calmness." Then hold your breath and count from 1 to 3.
2. During exhalation, tell yourself gently "I am breathing out fear" while counting from 1 to 5.
3. Inhale deeply through your nose and exhale slowly through your mouth.
4. Complete one cycle of three inhalations and three exhalations. Repeat as needed.

2

Question Dissection and Analysis*

EVIDENCE-BASED MEDICINE (EBM)

I. Discussion

Questions about EBM are typically designed in "drag-and-drop" format on the American Nurses Credentialing Center exam. They are presented as two boxes with three sections each. The example that follows illustrates this format. On the left side, three types of article summaries (or research studies) are marked A, B, or C (in the exam, they will appear as yellow boxes). On the right side, you will see the rankings from 1 to 3 (in the exam, they will be blue boxes). You "drag" one of the articles from the left-hand box into the correct ranking or hierarchy in the right-hand box. Your job is to rank the three research article summaries as 1, 2, or 3 (best evidence, moderate evidence, weakest evidence).

II. Example

Article Summaries	Strength of Evidence (strongest to weakest)
A) A meta-analysis on Medline and Cochrane databases that found 53 RCTs about gingko biloba use in patients with early dementia	1.
B) A specialty society opinion paper regarding the effectiveness of gingko biloba supplementation in dementia	2.
C) An experimental study on 500 patients with early dementia who were given gingko biloba daily for 6 months versus the control group, which given placebo pills	3.

RCTs, randomized controlled trials.

III. Correct Answer:

Article A is ranked 1, Article C is ranked 2, and Article B is ranked 3.

IV. Question Dissection

Best Clues

I teach a three-step system to students in my review courses.

- First, identify the research study that has the highest/best level of evidence (#1 ranking). An easy way to do this is by searching for keywords in the question such as "meta-analysis," "systematic review" or "randomized controlled trials" combined with "Cochrane

*For additional information, see http://ancc.nursecredentialing.org/certification/ExamResources/SampleQuestions/FamilyNP/demo/item3.htm database," "Medline database," and/or Cumulative Index to Nursing and Allied Health Literature ("CINAHL").

- Next, look for the research study that has the weakest evidence (#3 ranking). It usually contains keywords such as "expert opinion" or "specialty society."
- Therefore, view the study that is leftover as having the middle ranking (#2 ranking). In addition, keep in mind that if the choices do not include a meta-analysis or systemic review, then the study with the highest ranking would be an RCT or an experimental study. The ANCC exams usually have several of this type of question. Further discussion about EBM appears in the chapter on Evidence-Based Medicine and Epidemiology later in this book.

  The levels of evidence rankings are:
  - Meta-analysis and/or systematic reviews (Cochrane/Medline/CINAHL/PubMed)
  - RCTs (used for testing medical treatment effectiveness, subjects assigned at random to either a control or treatment group)
  - Experimental studies (control group, intervention group, randomization)
  - Cohort/case control studies
  - Retrospective chart reviews
  - Expert/specialty society opinions

PHOTOGRAPHS

I. Discussion

On the ANCC exam, expect to see several colored photographs of skin conditions and a few on the eye/fundi. In the future, there may be pictures from other organ systems. The stem of the question usually will ask for the possible diagnosis, differential diagnosis, or type of treatment. If you plan to take the ANCC exam, you need to memorize how a skin condition or eye finding appears in colored photos/pictures. It is a good idea to use a search engine (e.g., Google, Bing, Yahoo) to look for the images. For example, you want to become familiar with skin cancers, such as basal cell and melanoma, and with funduscopic findings in diabetes and hypertension.

II. Example

The nurse practitioner (NP) is performing a routine physical exam on a 54-year-old White male farmer who is an immigrant from Australia. The NP notices a shiny round, ulcerated skin lesion on the patient's head. It has a firm texture with indurated edges and telangiectasia.

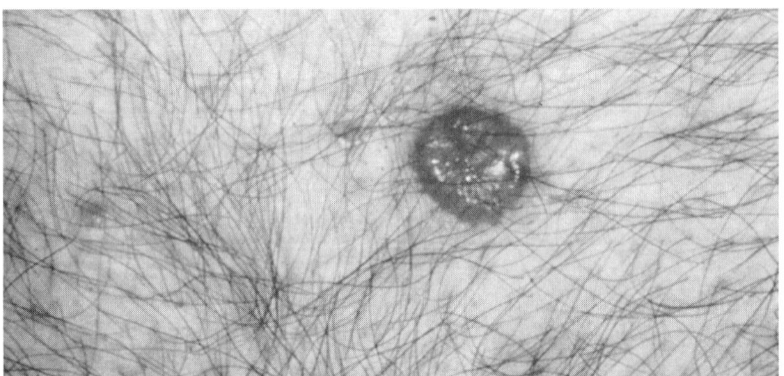

Figure 2.1 Sample exam photograph. This image can be found in color in the app.

Source: Courtesy of National Cancer Institute.

See Figure 2.1. The patient reports that the lesion does not itch, but it has slowly enlarged over the past few years. Which of the following conditions is most likely in this patient?

A) Nodular melanoma
B) Squamous cell carcinoma
C) Basal cell carcinoma
D) Actinic keratosis

III. Correct Answer: Option C

C) Basal cell carcinoma

IV. Question Dissection

Best Clues

- Notice that the skin lesion has a pearly or wax-like (shiny) appearance with telangiectasia, which is "classic" for basal cell carcinoma; some lesions may show central ulceration
- Patient has risk factors for skin cancer, such as light-colored skin, and he is from Australia, which has high rates of skin cancer
- The skin lesion is located on a sun-exposed area
- It is probably not nodular melanoma, which usually has pigment such as brown or black color with irregular borders
- Actinic keratosis is a precancer of squamous cell carcinoma and is usually located on the scalp (males), face, and the back of the hands (dorsum); they appear as a crusty/scaly growth that slowly enlarges over time
- The gold-standard test for skin cancer is the skin biopsy

MULTIPLE-CHOICE QUESTIONS WITH MORE THAN ONE CORRECT RESPONSE

I. Discussion

Expect to see some multiple-choice questions with five to six answer options in both the ANCC and American Academy of Nurse Practitioners Certification Board (AANPCB) exams. The question will ask for two to three correct answers. For example, you may be asked to pick two or three differential diagnoses for a case of skin rash. The clues are given in the presentation of the signs and symptoms.

II. Example

A 75-year-old woman with mild dementia, hyperlipidemia, and emphysema is brought in by her middle-aged daughter as a walk-in patient in a community clinic with a complaint of the sudden onset of red rashes on her left lower arm and hand. During the skin exam, the NP notes that there are a few blisters. When the NP touches one of the blisters, it ruptures and drains clear serous fluid. Which of the following three conditions should the NP consider in the differential diagnosis?

A) Contact dermatitis
B) Erysipelas
C) Psoriasis
D) Impetigo
E) Thermal burn

III. Correct Answer: Options A, D, and E

A) Contact dermatitis
D) Impetigo
E) Thermal burn

IV. Question Dissection

Best Clues

- Easily ruptured blisters (fragile) is a classic finding for bullous impetigo, an acute bacterial skin infection caused by *Staphylococcus* or *Streptococcus.*
- Contact dermatitis can present with just red skin or red skin with blisters. The rash can be located anywhere on the body and it may have a pattern (like a belt) or no pattern.
- The timing of the rash is very important. Is it acute or chronic? Rule out option C (psoriasis), which is a chronic skin disease.
- Erysipelas is a type of cellulitis caused by strep. It resembles a bright-red, warm, raised rash (plaque-like) with discrete borders usually located on the face or the shins. Blistering is not present.
- A thermal burn is a burn caused by heat (fire, heat). Consider a second-degree burn in the differential diagnosis because of its acute onset. Also, the patient has mild dementia, which puts her at a higher risk for accidents.

DIAGNOSTIC IMAGING

I. Discussion

Questions about diagnostic imaging tests may appear on the exam. You may get a multiple-choice question alone or a question that is accompanied by a chest x-ray film. I recommend that you use a search engine (Google, Bing, Yahoo) to search for images of chest films with lobar consolidation due to community-acquired pneumonia (CAP), right middle lobe pneumonia, pulmonary tuberculosis (TB) infection, and emphysema/chronic obstructive pulmonary disease [COPD]).

II. Example

A 34-year-old male smoker presents in an urgent care clinic complaining of a productive cough, chest congestion, fever, chills, and poor appetite for 1 week. Cough is productive of greenish sputum, which is sometimes tinged with a small amount of blood. Vital signs are temperature of 101.2°F, pulse of 100 beats/min, respirations of 24 breaths/min, and BP 122/88 mmHg. A radiograph of the chest is obtained (see Figure 2.2). What is the most likely diagnosis in this patient?

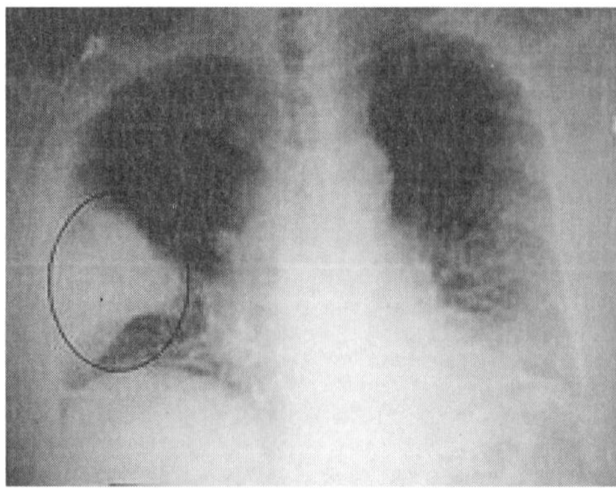

Figure 2.2 Sample exam photo.

A) Acute bronchitis
B) Right middle lobe pneumonia
C) Right lower lobe pneumonia
D) Legionella pneumonia

III. Correct Answer: Option B

B) Right middle lobe pneumonia

IV. Question Dissection

Best Clues

- Presence of signs and symptoms of CAP such as fever, cough productive of green sputum with small amount of blood (or rust-colored sputum). Rust-colored sputum is associated with *Streptococcus pneumoniae* infection.
- Most of the middle lobe of the right lung is in the anterior chest by the right nipple area. Notice that lobar consolidation is located in the same area.
- Patients with acute bronchitis may have chest congestion but not fever, chills, or productive cough with purulent sputum.
- Legionella pneumonia (Legionnaire's disease) is uncommon in primary care. Look for a history of exposure to "nebulized" water sources such as air conditioners, fountains, etc. Presents with pneumonia signs/symptoms that are accompanied by GI symptoms (diarrhea, nausea/vomiting).

CULTURE

I. Discussion

There will be several questions on the ANCC exam that address culture. The questions will address knowledge of cultural practices that influence health-seeking behavior. Some of the cultures that may be included in the ANCC exam are Hispanic/Latino, Muslim, Chinese, Native American (Navajo), and Southeast Asian (Vietnamese, Hmong, Filipinos, and others).

II. Example

An elderly woman immigrant from Vietnam who recently has been diagnosed with hypertension is returning for a 4-week follow-up visit. The patient is on a prescription of hydrochlorothiazide 12.5 mg daily. Her blood pressure during the visit is 150/94 mmHg. The NP queries the patient whether she is taking her medication. The patient looks down at the floor and does not directly answer the question. Which of the following statements regarding the health behaviors of Southeast Asians is incorrect?

A) The patient may have difficulty verbalizing questions about his or her treatment
B) The patient may ask to consult with an older family member about major health decisions
C) If the patient is not compliant with taking medications, he or she will not directly communicate it with the health provider
D) The patient will directly verbalize his or her disagreement in a loud voice

III. Correct Answer: Option D

D) The patient will directly verbalize his or her disagreement in a loud voice.

IV. Question Dissection

Best Clues

- The patient's behavior (aggressive, loud) is considered rude in most Asian cultures

Notes

1. The Hmong ethnic group that immigrated to the United States came from several countries (e.g., Laos, Vietnam, Thailand). A traditional household has a male (i.e., father) who is the head of the household. The family identifies with a clan group, which is headed by an older male.
2. For major health decisions, the head of the family is always involved in the health decision. If the father is dead, then another older male relative (e.g., uncle) may be consulted.
3. Most Asians have high regard for physicians (and college education). Because of this cultural value, they may not directly disagree or question the health care provider.
4. Asian Americans and Pacific Islanders are eight to 13 times more likely to develop liver cancer than other groups due to higher rates of chronic hepatitis B infection.

LAB RESULTS AND DIAGNOSTIC TESTS

I. Discussion

Laboratory tests, such as hemoglobin and hematocrit, mean corpuscular volume (MCV), total white blood cell (WBC) count, percentage of neutrophils in the WBC differential, thyroid-stimulating hormone (TSH), prostate-specific antigen (PSA), and urinalysis (UA), are commonly encountered in the exams. Learn the significance of the abnormal results and the follow-up tests that are needed to evaluate them further.

The AANPCB exam does list the norms for some of the common laboratory tests. They will appear only when needed to answer a question (such as an anemia question). It is important that you copy the lab norm that is given (on your scratch paper) because it will be listed only once.

In contrast, the ANCC does not list any of the normal results in its certification exams. Therefore, if you plan to take the ANCC exam, it is important that you memorize the normal results of these laboratory tests.

Be warned that lab results are also used as distractors; the labs listed may not be necessary to solve the exam question correctly. The normal results for these labs are also included in the pertinent review chapters of this book (e.g., TSH will be found in Chapter 9.

II. Example

An elderly man of Mediterranean descent has a routine CBC done for an annual physical. The following are his lab test results: hemoglobin is 12.0 g/dL, hematocrit is 39%, and MCV is 72 fL. His PSA result is 3.2 ng/mL. UA shows no leukocytes and few epithelial cells. Which of the following laboratory tests are indicated for this patient?

A) Serum iron, serum ferritin, total iron-binding capacity (TIBC), and the red cell distribution width (RDW)
B) Serum vitamin B_{12} and folate level with a peripheral smear
C) CBC with white cell differential and UA
D) Urine culture and sensitivity with microscopic exam of the urine (Tables 2.1 and 2.2)

III. Correct Answer: Option A

A) Serum iron, serum ferritin, total iron-binding capacity (TIBC), and the red cell distribution width (RDW)

Table 2.1 List of Laboratory Norms

CBC	Reference Ranges
Hemoglobin	
Males	13.0–17.5 g/dL
Females	12.0–16 g/dL
Hematocrit	
Males	40%–50%
Females	36%–45%
MCV	80–100 fL
RDW	>14.5%
Platelet count	<150,000/mm³ (increased risk of bleeding, disseminated intravascular coagulation)
Reticulocytes	0.5%–1.5% of red cells (↑ acute bleeding, starting treatment for vitamin deficiencies (iron, B_{12}, folate), acute hemolytic episodes
Total WBC count	4,500–11,000/mm³ (↑ bacterial infections)
Neutrophils (or segs)	>50% (↑ bacterial infections)
Band forms (immature WBCs)	>6% (↑ severe bacterial infections) Also called "shift to the left"
Eosinophils	>3% (↑ allergies, parasitic diseases, cancer)

CBC, complete blood count; MCV, mean corpuscular volume; RDW, red cell distribution width; WBC, white blood cell.

Table 2.2 List of Blood Chemistries

Laboratory Test	Reference Ranges
TSH	>5.0 mU/L (hypothyroidism) <0.4 mU/L (hyperthyroidism)
PSA	<4.0 ng/mL (benign prostatic hyperplasia [BPH, prostate cancer)
Ferritin	<15 mcg/L (iron-deficiency anemia)
ESR; sed rate	Men 0–22 mm/hr Women 0–29 mm/hr Elevated (giant cell arteritis, rheumatoid arthritis [RA], lupus, inflammation)
CRP	Elevated (inflammation, autoimmune diseases, a risk factor for heart disease)
cTnT	Elevated in myocardial infarction, heart damage, heart failure Sensitive test for myocardial cell damage
B-type natriuretic peptide	Elevated (elevated in heart failure)
Potassium	<3.0 or >5.5 mEq/L (risk of arrhythmia)

CRP, c-reactive protein; cTnT, cardiac troponins; ESR, erythrocyte sedimentation rate; PSA, prostate-specific antigen; TSH, thyroid-stimulating hormone.

IV. Question Dissection

Best Clues

- Low hemoglobin and hematocrit for gender (male) and age (abnormal CBC result)
- An MCV of 72 fL, which is indicative of microcytic anemia (assessment)
- The ethnic background of the patient (demographics)
- Ignore the UA and PSA tests because they are not necessary to solve the problem

Notes

1. You must go through three steps to answer this question correctly:
   First step: A hemoglobin of less than 13.5 g/dL in males (but not in females) is indicative of anemia. An MCV of 72 fL is indicative of microcytic anemia (norm 80–100 fL).
   Second step: The MCV will direct you in the differential diagnosis (microcytic, normocytic, or macrocytic).
   Third step: The differential diagnosis for microcytic anemia is iron deficiency and alpha/beta thalassemia trait or minor for the exams.
2. In iron-deficiency anemia, the following results are found:
   - Decreased (serum ferritin and serum iron levels)
   - Elevated (TIBC and RDW)
3. In alpha or beta thalassemia trait or minor, the following results are found:
   - Normal to high (serum ferritin and serum iron levels)
   - Normal (TIBC)
4. The gold-standard test to diagnose any anemia involving abnormal hemoglobin (thalassemia, sickle cell, etc.) is the hemoglobin electrophoresis.
5. The RDW is a measure of the variability in size of RBCs (or anisocytosis). An elevated RDW is one of the earliest indicators of iron-deficiency anemia.
6. In clinical practice, rule out iron-deficiency anemia first (most common anemia in the world for all ages/races/gender) before ordering a hemoglobin electrophoresis.

HEALTH INSURANCE PORTABILITY AND ACCOUNTABILITY ACT (HIPAA)

I. Discussion

One common topic that is frequently included in the certification exam is the HIPAA of 1996. The questions are designed to determine whether you know how to apply HIPAA regulations in primary care practice. Your job is to determine whether the activity is compliant (or not) with HIPAA regulations.

II. Example

According to the HIPAA of 1996, which of the following examples demonstrates noncompliance?

A) The sign-in sheet on the front desk is covered so that other patients' names are not visible to new patients

B) The medical assistant calls the patient who is in the waiting room using his or her first name

C) A patient's chart that is hanging on the door of the exam room is turned backward

D) The NP calls the daughter of an elderly diabetic patient and leaves a detailed message on the answering machine regarding her mother's lab results

III. Correct Answer: Option D

D) The NP calls the daughter of an elderly diabetic patient and leaves a detailed message on the answering machine regarding her mother's lab results

IV. Question Dissection

Best Clues

- In option D, the phrase "detailed message on the answering machine" is a good clue of HIPAA noncompliance
- The question does not specify whether the patient authorized that her information could be released to her daughter. Therefore, assume that no authorization was given by the patient
- Option B shows HIPAA compliance because only the patient's first name is used

Notes

1. Option D demonstrates two examples of HIPAA noncompliance. First, there is no mention that the patient gave consent for her daughter to have access to her medical information. Second, the NP did not follow the "minimum necessary requirement" rule when leaving a detailed message on the daughter's answering machine.
2. The best action in this case is for the NP to call the elderly patient's home and to leave only his or her name, the name of the clinic, and a phone number that the patient can call.
3. When speaking to a patient in the waiting room area (or any public area), use only the patient's first name. If both the patient's first and last names are used, then option C would be an example of HIPAA noncompliance.

WOMEN'S HEALTH

I. Discussion

Expect to see several questions addressing gynecological conditions. The topics that are covered include recognizing and treating sexually transmitted infections or diseases (STIs or STDs), oral contraceptive issues, abnormal Pap smears, menopausal conditions, threatened abortion or early pregnancy, and many more. For example, there will be questions about vaginal disorders such as bacterial vaginosis (BV), candida vaginitis, trichomoniasis, and atrophic vaginitis, and when a pregnancy would have to be established to make a choice of medications.

Be aware that a clinical finding can be described in detail instead of using its common name. For example, the term *clue cell* is not used in the question that follows. Instead, it is described in detail ("mature squamous epithelial cells with numerous bacteria noted on the cell surface and borders").

II. Example

An 18-year-old female student presents in the college health clinic complaining of a strong odor in her vagina. She reports that she had an abortion about 3 weeks ago and recently completed her prescription of antibiotics. The NP performs a vaginal speculum exam and notes a large amount of gray to off-white discharge coating the patient's vaginal walls. It has a milk-like consistency. During microscopy, the slide reveals mature squamous epithelial cells with numerous bacteria on the cell borders. The vaginal pH is 6.0. Which of the following conditions is most likely?

A) Trichomoniasis
B) Bacterial vaginosis
C) Candida vulvovaginitis
D) Hormonal changes

III. Correct Answer: Option B

B) Bacterial vaginosis

IV. Question Dissection

Best Clues

- The vaginal pH is alkaline (pH of 6.0).
- Rule out *Candida* because it is classified as a yeast organism (not a bacteria).
- Rule out *Trichomonas* because it is a protozoan or unicellular flagellated organism.
- The odor and discharge are not due to hormonal changes in an 18-year-old.

Notes

1. BV has an alkaline pH (vagina normally has acidic pH of 3.5–4.5). BV is the only vaginal condition with an alkaline pH for the exam.
2. BV is not considered an STD (it is caused by an imbalance of vaginal bacteria). The sex partner does not need to be treated. It is a vaginosis (not a vaginitis).
3. BV does not cause inflammation (the vulvovagina will not be red or irritated). The microscopy slide will have very few WBCs and a large number of clue cells.
4. The vaginal discharge in *Candida* infection is a white color with a thick and curd-like consistency. It frequently causes redness and itching in the vulvovagina due to inflammation.
5. The microscopy in candidiasis will show a large number of WBCs, pseudohyphae, and spores ("spaghetti and meatballs").
6. Candida yeast is normal flora of the GI tract and in some women's vaginas.
7. *Trichomonas* infection (or trichomoniasis) vaginal discharge is copious, bubbly, and green in color. It causes a lot of inflammation, resulting in itching and redness of the vulvovagina. It is considered to be an STI. The sex partner also needs treatment.
8. Microscopy (wet smear) is the gold standard of diagnosis for BV, candida vaginitis, and trichomoniasis for the exam.

MEDICATIONS

I. Discussion

When studying pharmacology for the exam, it is generally not important to memorize the specific drug doses. What is more important is to study a drug's "safety" issues such as contraindications, major drug/food interactions, and the well-known side effects.

You will need to be familiar with the drug's indications and the duration of treatment. Become familiar with a "first-line drug" and the alternative drug (if applicable). For example, the first-line (or preferred) drug for treating "strep" throat is still penicillin VK (V potassium) PO for 10 days. If the patient has a penicillin allergy, macrolides can be used instead.

The majority of the medicines seen on the exam are the well-known drugs that have been in use for a few years to many decades (i.e., doxycycline, penicillin, amoxicillin). Memorize the drug class and some representative drugs from that class. For example, in the quinolone drug class are the drugs such as ofloxacin (Floxin), moxifloxacin (Avelox), and levofloxacin (Levaquin). You can memorize a drug either by its generic name or by both its generic and brand name. In addition, you need to become familiar with some of the Food and Drug Administration (FDA) category X drugs (listed in Chapter 3).

II. Examples

Example A

Using the drug class as the answer option:

A previously healthy 30-year-old complains of an acute onset of fever and chills accompanied by a productive cough with purulent sputum and a loss of appetite. The patient denies receiving an antibiotic in the previous 3 months. The NP diagnoses community-acquired pneumonia (CAP). The Infectious Diseases Society of America (IDSA) and the American Thoracic Society (ATS) treatment guidelines recommend which of the following as the preferred first-line treatment for this patient?

A) Macrolides
B) Antitussives
C) Cephalosporins
D) Fluoroquinolones with gram-positive bacteria activity

Example B

Which of the following antibiotics is preferred treatment for healthy adults diagnosed with uncomplicated community-acquired pneumonia (CAP)?

A) Azithromycin (Zithromax Z-Pak 250 mg) 500 mg on day 1, then 250 mg daily for 4 days
B) Dextromethorphan with guaifenesin (Robitussin DM) 1 to 2 teaspoons PO QID as needed
C) Cephalexin (Keflex) 500 mg PO QID × 10 days
D) Levofloxacin (Levaquin) 500 mg PO daily × 7 days

Example C

The following is an example of a question about a common side effect:

Possible side effects that may be seen in a patient who is being treated with hydrochlorothiazide for hypertension are:

A) Dry cough and angioedema
B) Swollen ankles and headache
C) Hyperuricemia and hyperglycemia
D) Fatigue and depression

III. Correct Answers

Example A: Option A

A) Macrolides

Example B: Option A

A) Azithromycin (Zithromax Z-Pak 250 mg) 500 mg on day 1, then 250 mg daily for 4 days

Example C: Option C

C) Hyperuricemia and hyperglycemia

IV. Question Dissection

Best Clues

- Lack of comorbidity ("healthy adults") is an important clue in Examples A and B
- Your knowledge of the latest IDSA and the ATS treatment guidelines helps to correctly answer Examples A and B (covered in Chapter 8)
- For Example C, you must memorize the adverse side effects of the thiazide diuretics

Notes

1. According to the IDSA and the ATS treatment guidelines, outpatient treatment of CAP in healthy patients (no comorbidities) involves the macrolides (azithromycin, clarithromycin, or erythromycin).
2. Example A is caused by angiotensin-converting enzyme (ACE) inhibitors. Look for a sudden or new onset of a dry cough in a patient with hypertension (without signs of the common cold). Angioedema is a rare adverse effect and can be life-threatening.
3. Example B is caused by calcium channel blockers (CCBs). Look for a hypertensive patient with swollen ankles (not associated with heart failure) and headache.
4. Example C is caused by the thiazide diuretics (hyperuricemia and hyperglycemia).
5. Example D is caused by beta-blockers. Look for a patient with history of myocardial infarction (MI), heart failure and/or hypertension who complains of increased fatigue and depression (avoid if possible in depressed patients, pulse <50 beats/min, second- or third-degree heart block).

U.S. CENTERS FOR DISEASE CONTROL AND PREVENTION STATISTICS

I. Discussion

It is important that you memorize these U.S. Centers for Disease Control and Prevention (CDC) statistics. The questions will be short and to the point. Determine whether a question is asking about the most common cause of death (mortality) or whether it is asking about the most common cause of a certain disease in a population (prevalence). For example, the most common cause of cancer death overall is lung cancer (mortality), but the most common cancer overall (prevalence) is skin cancer. The most common type of skin cancer is basal cell skin cancer.

Sometimes, a question will ask about a gender-specific cause. For example, the most common cancer in females is breast cancer and the most common cancer in males is prostate cancer (prevalence). But the cancer causing the most deaths overall for both males and females is still lung cancer (mortality).

Mortality Statistics

- Disease causing the most deaths overall: heart disease
- Cancer with the highest mortality: Lung cancer
- Cancer with the highest mortality in males (lung cancer) and in females (lung cancer)
- Most common cause of death in adolescents: Motor vehicle crashes

Prevalence

- Most common cancer in females: Breast cancer
- Most common cancer in males: Prostate cancer
- Most common type of cancer overall (males/females): Skin cancer
- Most common type of skin cancer (males/females): Basal cell cancer
- Skin cancer with the highest mortality: Melanoma
- Gynecological cancer (vulva, vagina, cervix, uterus, ovary)
    - Uterine/endometrial cancer (most common gynecological cancer)
    - Ovarian cancer (second most common gynecological cancer)

II. Example

What is the most common type of gynecological cancer?

A) Uterine cancer
B) Cervical cancer
C) Breast cancer
D) Ovarian cancer

III. Correct Answer: Option A

A) Uterine cancer

IV. Question Dissection

Best Clues

- This question is based on your recall of facts that you memorized (rote memory)
- Rule out breast cancer because it is not considered a gynecological cancer

Notes

1. There may be a question about the gynecological cancers (see example). These types of cancers are located in the pelvis (labia, vagina, uterus, fallopian tubes, ovaries).
2. Breast cancer is not classified as a gynecological cancer.

BENIGN PHYSIOLOGICAL VARIANTS

I. Discussion

A benign variant is a physiological abnormality that does not interfere with bodily process or function. There are very few questions on benign variants. Some examples of the benign variants that have been seen on the exams include the geographic tongue, torus palatinus, and a split or fishtail uvula (listed in Chapter 5). Benign variants are listed under the appropriate organ system.

II. Example

A 45-year-old female patient complains of a sore throat. Upon examination, the NP notices a bony growth midline at the hard palate of the mouth. The patient denies any changes or pain. It is not red, tender, or swollen. She reports a history of the same growth for many years without any change. Which of the following conditions is most likely?
A) Torus palatinus
B) Geographic tongue
C) Acute glossitis
D) Leukoplakia

III. Correct Answer: Option A

A) Torus palatinus

IV. Question Dissection

Best Clues

- The description of a chronic bony growth located midline in the hard palate
- Rule out glossitis, geographic tongue, and hairy leukoplakia because they are all located on the tongue and not on the hard palate (roof of the mouth)

Notes

1. A torus palatinus is a benign growth of bone (an exostosis) located midline on the hard palate and covered with normal oral skin. It is painless and does not interfere with function.
2. A "geographic tongue" has multiple fissures and irregular smoother areas on its surface that makes it look like a topographic map. The patient may complain of soreness on the tongue after eating or drinking acidic or hot foods.
3. Leukoplakia is not a benign variant. It appears as a slow-growing white plaque that has a firm to hard surface that is slightly raised on the tongue or inside the mouth. It is considered a precancerous lesion. It is due to chronic irritation of the skin or to precancerous changes on the tongue and inside the cheeks. Its causes include poorly fitting dentures, chewing tobacco (snuff), and using other types of tobacco. Refer the patient for a biopsy because it can sometimes become malignant.
4. Oral hairy leukoplakia (OHL) of the tongue is a painless white patch (or patches) that appears corrugated. It is usually located on the lateral aspects of the tongue (or other areas inside the mouth) and is associated with HIV and AIDS infection. It is caused by Epstein–Barr virus (EBV) infection of the tongue. It is not considered a premalignant lesion.

U.S. PREVENTIVE SERVICES TASK FORCE SCREENING GUIDELINES

I. Discussion

USPSTF screening guidelines are graded as A, B, C, D, or I (insufficient evidence or evidence is lacking or of poor quality). The highest rating is a Grade A (routine screening is advised—high certainty that the net benefit is substantial). A rating of Grade D means that the harm outweighs the benefits (or there is no benefit) to the service and the use of the service is discouraged.

Both the ANCC and the AANPCB exams use the USPSTF screening recommendations. Regarding breast cancer screening, the USPSTF (2016) currently recommends that a screening baseline mammogram (with or without clinical breast exam) start at age 50 years, then every 2 years until the age of 74 years. For women aged 40 to 49 years, mammograms should be based on individual factors (such as risk factors, preferences, risk vs. benefits of mammograms).

II. Example

What is the USPSTF screening recommendation for ovarian cancer?

A) Annual bimanual pelvic exam with pelvic ultrasound
B) Pelvic and intravaginal ultrasound
C) Intravaginal ultrasound with CA-125 tumor marker
D) The USPSTF does not recommend routine screening of women for ovarian cancer

III. Correct Answer: Option D

D) The USPSTF does not recommend routine screening of women for ovarian cancer

IV. Question Dissection

Best Clues

- Do not "overread" the question. Assume that the question is asking about routine screening of the general population.
- Transvaginal ultrasound and CA-125 are not used for routine screening.
- Although the bimanual pelvic exam is "low tech," it is being used as a distractor.

Notes

1. The USPSTF (2018) is against routine screening for ovarian cancer in asymptomatic women who are not known to have a high risk of hereditary cancer syndrome.
2. If there is a case scenario of an older woman who complains of vague abdominal/pelvic symptoms (stomach bloating, low-back ache, constipation) and is found to have a palpable ovary during the bimanual exam, rule out ovarian cancer.
3. Always rule out ovarian cancer in a postmenopausal woman who has a palpable ovary.
4. The next step is to order a pelvic and intravaginal ultrasound with CA-125. Refer to oncologist.
5. The strongest risk factor for ovarian cancer (or breast cancer) is genetic predisposition, such as *BRCA1* or *BRCA2* mutations and positive family history (Table 2.3). Absolute risk of developing ovarian cancer is 35% to 45% in women with *BRCA1* mutation. Other risk factors are age, obesity, clomiphene (Clomid) use, or endometriosis.

Table 2.3 USPSTF Screening Guidelines

Disease	Screening Test
Breast cancer (2016)	Baseline mammogram at age 50 years Screen every 2 years until age 74 years (biennial) After age 75 years (insufficient evidence)
Cervical cancer (2012)	Baseline Pap smear/cytology at age 21 years Screen every 3 years until age 65 years Do not screen women younger than 21 years even if sexually active
Lung cancer (2013)	Aged 55–80 years with 30 pack-year history of smoking or quit smoking up to 15 years previously Annual screening with LDCT
Hysterectomy (no cervix)	Do not screen (if no history of precancer or cervical cancer)
Prostate cancer (2012)	Routine screening is not recommended
Testicular cancer (2011)	Routine screening is not recommended
Colon cancer (2016)	Baseline screening at age 50 years Use *high-sensitivity* fecal occult blood test (yearly) or sigmoidoscopy (every 5 years) or colonoscopy (every 10 years) from age 50–75 years
Skin cancer (2012)	Aged 10–24 years Educate fair-skinned persons to avoid sunlight (10 a.m.–3 p.m.) and use sunblock ≥SPF 15
Tobacco smoking (2015)	Ask all adolescents and adults about tobacco use, advise them to stop smoking, and provide behavioral interventions/smoking cessation
Fall prevention in community-dwelling older adults (2012)	Aged 65 years or older: Exercise and vitamin D dose is from 600 to 800 IU Ask about falls, balance or gait problems
Ovarian cancer (2016)	Routine screening is not recommended High-risk (*BRCA* mutation, family history breast/ovarian cancer) are screened by specialist; refer for genetic counseling
Abdominal aortic aneurysm (2014)	One-time screening (men aged 65–75 years) for cigarette smokers or those who have quit but smoked previously Screening test is ultrasound of abdomen

LDCT, low-dose, computed tomography; SPF, sun protection factor; USPSTF, U.S. Preventive Services Task Force.

FOLLOWING UP ON A PRESCRIPTION MEDICINE

I. Discussion

In these cases, a patient who is taking prescription medicine is running out of his or her supply or does not have refills left. The test-taker must decide what type of initial follow-up is needed. Depending on the case scenario, for a patient who is fully symptomatic due to the abrupt cessation of medicine (either due to running out of refills or discontinuation of health insurance), a reasonable initial action is to continue the prescription medicine.

II. Example

A 65-year-old female smoker presents with a history of Barrett's esophagus and gastroesophageal reflux disease (GERD). The patient reports that her gastroenterologist's prescription for esomeprazole (Nexium) 40 mg daily ran out a few days ago. She is complaining of severe heartburn and a sore throat. During the physical exam, the NP notes an erythematous posterior pharynx without tonsillar discharge and mild dental enamel loss on the rear molars. What is the best initial action for the NP to follow?

A) Refer the patient to an oncologist for a biopsy to rule out esophageal cancer
B) Give the patient a refill of her proton-pump inhibitor (PPI) prescription and advise her to schedule an appointment with her gastroenterologist
C) Recommend that the patient take over-the-counter (OTC) ranitidine (Zantac) twice a day until she can be seen by her gastroenterologist
D) Switch the patient's prescription to another brand of PPI because her symptoms are not improving

III. Correct Answer: Option B

B) Give the patient a refill of her proton-pump inhibitor (PPI) prescription and advise her to schedule an appointment with her gastroenterologist

IV. Question Dissection

Best Clues

- Rule out option A because the patient is already under the care of a gastroenterologist.
- OTC ranitidine (Zantac) is not potent enough to control the symptoms of erosive esophagitis. A PPI is the preferred treatment for erosive esophagitis.
- Do not switch the patient to another brand of PPI. Her worsening symptoms are caused by rebound caused by abrupt cessation of PPI.
- The best initial action in this case is to refill the PPI prescription because the patient is fully symptomatic (erosive esophagitis) until she can see her gastroenterologist.

Notes

1. The patient's severe symptoms are caused by the sudden discontinuation of the high-dose PPI (rebound-type of reaction).
2. Barrett's esophagus is the "precancerous" lesion of esophageal cancer. It is best managed by a gastroenterologist (not an oncologist).
3. Patients diagnosed with Barrett's esophagus typically have endoscopic examinations with biopsy by a gastroenterologist annually (or every 6 months for high-grade lesions).
4. Patients with Barrett's esophagus are treated with high-dose PPIs for a "lifetime."
5. The first-line treatment of mild, uncomplicated GERD is lifestyle changes (avoid eating 3 to 4 hours before bedtime, dietary changes, weight loss if overweight, etc.).
6. If a patient is at high risk for esophageal cancer (aged 50 years or older, smoker, chronic GERD for decades), consider referral to a gastroenterologist for an upper endoscopy.

TANNER STAGES

I. Discussion

Expect to see at least one to two questions regarding Tanner stages in girls and boys. Because Tanner stage I is prepuberty and Tanner stage V is the adult pattern for both boys and girls, the only stages to memorize for the exams are Tanner stage II to Tanner stage IV.

For girls, memorize the pattern of breast development and for boys, the genital development (testes and penis). It is not as important to memorize pubic hair development for both.

Tanner Stages

Girls:

Stage I: Prepubertal pattern
Stage II: Breast bud and areola starts to develop
Stage III: Breast continues to grow with nipples/areola (one mound/no separation)
Stage IV: Nipples and areola become elevated from the breast (a secondary mound)
Stage V: Adult pattern

Boys:

Stage I: Prepubertal pattern
Stage II: Testes and scrotum start to enlarge (scrotal skin starts to get darker/more rugae)
Stage III: Penis grows longer (length) and testes/scrotum continues to become larger
Stage IV: Penis become wider and continues growing in length (testes are larger with darker scrotal skin and more rugae)
Stage V: Adult pattern

II. Example

A 14-year-old boy is brought in by his mother for a physical exam. Both are concerned about his breast enlargement. The teen denies breast tenderness. On physical exam, the NP palpates soft breast tissue that is not tender. No dominant mass is noted. The skin is smooth and there is no nipple discharge with massage. The teen has a body mass index (BMI) of 29. Which of the following statements is correct?

A) Advise the mother that the patient has physiological gynecomastia and should return for a follow-up exam
B) Order an ultrasound of both breasts to further assess the patient's breast tissue development
C) Reassure the mother that the patient's breast development is within normal limits
D) Educate the mother that her son has pseudogynecomastia

III. Correct Answer: Option D

D) Educate the mother that her son has pseudogynecomastia

IV. Question Dissection

Best Clues

- The boy is very overweight (BMI 29) and is almost obese.

- The clinical breast exam does not show palpable breast tissue. Instead, the breast palpation reveals soft fatty tissue.
- It is wrong to "reassure" a patient or a family member in the exam (poor therapeutic communication technique).

Notes

1. Physiological gynecomastia physical exam findings will show disk-like breast tissue that is mobile under each nipple/areola, the breast may be tender, and the breast can be asymmetrical (one breast larger than the other).
2. A BMI of 25 to 29.9 is considered overweight. Obesity is a BMI of 30 or higher.
3. Overweight to obese males are at highest risk for pseudogynecomastia.

QUESTIONS ABOUT FOOD

I. Discussion

There are basically three kinds of food-related questions on the exam. You may be asked to pick the foods that have high levels of certain minerals, such as potassium, calcium, or magnesium. Other questions will address food interactions (tetracycline and dairy), drug interactions (monoamine oxidase inhibitor [MAOI] and high tyramine-containing foods such as fermented foods), or foods that should be avoided for a particular disease (e.g., wheat products in the case of celiac disease).

Certain foods are recommended for certain diseases (e.g., salmon/omega-3 for heart disease) because of their favorable effect. In contrast, certain foods are contraindicated for some conditions because of adverse or dangerous effects.

II. Example

Which of the following foods are known to have high potassium content?

A) Low-fat yogurt, soft cheeses, and collard greens
B) Aged cheese, red wine, and chocolate
C) Potatoes, apricots, and brussels sprouts
D) Black beans, red meat, and citrus juice

III. Correct Answer: Option C

C) Potatoes, apricots, and brussels sprouts

IV. Question Dissection

Best Clues

- First, look at the answer option pairs for inconsistencies in the list of foods.
- Rule out option A because it is inconsistent and these foods do not contain high levels of potassium: low-fat yogurt and soft cheeses (calcium) with collard greens (vitamin K).
- Rule out option B because these foods have high a tyramine, not potassium, content.
- Rule out option D because it is inconsistent. Although citrus juices are high in potassium, both black beans and red meat are not (iron).
- If options A, B, and D are incorrect, then the only one left is option C (potatoes, apricots, and brussels sprouts. A large number of fruits and vegetables are rich in potassium and vitamins.

Notes

1. Foods with high tyramine content can cause dangerous food–drug interactions with MAOI inhibitors (e.g., isocarboxide [Marplan], phenelzine [Nardil], and tranylcypromine [Parnate]).
2. Foods and supplements containing stimulants, such as caffeine and ephedra, are best avoided by patients with hypertension, arrhythmias, high risk for MI, hyperthyroid disease, albuterol use, amphetamine use, etc.
3. If one of the food choices in an answer option is incorrect, rule out this option because all of the foods on the list have to be correlated.

Examples of Food Groups

1. Gluten (avoid with celiac disease/celiac sprue): Wheat (including spelt and kamut), rye, barley (breads, cereals, pasta, cookies, cakes)
   - Gluten-free (safe carbohydrates): Corn, rice, potatoes, quinoa, tapioca, soybeans
2. Plant sterols and stanols (reduce cholesterol, LDL, triglycerides): sterol-fortified spreads (Benecol spread), sterol-fortified foods, wheat germ, sesame oil
3. Monounsaturated fats/fatty acids (decrease risk of heart disease):
   - Olive oil, canola oil, some nuts (almonds, walnuts), sunflower oil/seeds
   - Mediterranean diet, which is high in monounsaturated fats
4. Saturated fats or trans fats (increase risk of heart disease): Lard, beef fat (fatty steak), deep-fried fast foods
5. Omega-3 or fish oils (decrease risk of heart disease): Fatty cold-water marine fish (salmon), fish oils, flaxseed oil, and krill oil
6. Magnesium (decreases BP, dilates blood vessels): Some nuts (almonds, peanuts, cashews), some beans, whole wheat; also found in laxatives, antacids, milk of magnesia
7. Potassium (helps decrease BP): Most fruits (especially apricot, banana, orange, prune juice), some vegetables
8. Folate (decreases homocysteine levels and fetal neural tube defects): Breakfast cereals fortified with folate, green leafy vegetables (i.e., spinach), liver
9. Iron (treats iron-deficiency anemia): Beef, liver, black beans, black-eyed peas
10. Vitamin K (should control intake if on anticoagulants): Green leafy vegetables (kale, collard greens, spinach), broccoli, cabbage
11. High sodium content (increases water retention, can increase BP): Cold cuts, pickles, preserved foods, canned foods, hot dogs, chips
12. Calcium (helps with osteopenia and osteoporosis, helps decrease BP): Low-fat dairy, low-fat milk, low-fat yogurt, cheeses

Common Disorders Associated With Certain Foods

1. Celiac disease
   - Lifetime avoidance of gluten-containing cereals such as wheat, rye, and barley
   - Gluten-free: Rice, corn, potatoes, peanuts, soy, beans, meat, dairy, all fruits/vegetables; most people with celiac disease can eat oats
2. Hypertension
   - Maintain an adequate intake of calcium, magnesium, and potassium
   - Calcium: Low-fat dairy, low-fat yogurt, cheeses
   - Magnesium: Wheat bread, nuts (almonds, peanuts, cashews), some beans
   - Potassium: Most fruits (apricot, banana, oranges, cantaloupes, raisins), green vegetables
   - Avoid high-sodium foods: Cold cuts, pickles, preserved foods, canned foods, preservatives

3. Migraine headaches and MAOIs (Marplan, Nardil, and Parnate)
   - High-tyramine foods: Aged cheeses/meats, red wine, fava beans, draft beer, fermented foods
4. Anticoagulation therapy (i.e., warfarin sodium or Coumadin)
   - Keep daily intake of vitamin K-containing foods such as green leafy vegetables (kale/collard greens, spinach, cabbage), broccoli stable; vitamin K decreases the effectiveness of warfarin sodium; avoid excessive intake of vitamin K-rich foods

CASE MANAGEMENT

I. Discussion Only

Medical case managers are experienced RNs who work for hospitals, health care plans, and health insurance companies. Their job is essentially to coordinate the outpatient health care of patients with high-cost chronic conditions. The goal of case management is to decrease disease exacerbations and decrease the risk of hospitalization.

Asthma

A good outcome for children with asthma is their ability to attend school full time and to play normally every day. A poor case management outcome is if the child misses school and/or is unable to play due to poor control of asthma symptoms.

Notes

1. With asthma, a good case outcome is for the child (or adult) to return to normal function. For children, it means the child is attending school and can play daily. If the child is not able to attend school full time (frequent absences), this is a poor case management outcome.
2. The risk factors for asthma fatality include a history of ED visits, frequent use of short-acting beta-agonist use (i.e., albuterol), nocturnal awakenings, increased dyspnea and wheezing, respiratory viral infection, etc.
3. Diseases that are selected for case management are usually chronic conditions such as asthma, congestive heart failure (CHF), HIV infection, chronic psychiatric conditions, and so on. A good outcome will show good symptom control, no exacerbations or hospitalizations.

ALL QUESTIONS HAVE ENOUGH INFORMATION

I. Discussion Only

Assume that all the questions on the exams contain enough information to answer them correctly. Do not read too much into a question or assume that it is missing some vital information. As far as the ANCC and AANPCB exams are concerned, all questions contain enough information to allow you to solve them correctly. Unless indicated otherwise, consider a patient is in good health unless a disease or other health condition is mentioned in the test question.

EMERGENT CASES

I. Discussion

The ability to recognize and initially manage emergent conditions that may present in the primary care arena is a skill that is expected of all NPs. It is important to memorize not only the presenting signs and symptoms of a given condition, but also its initial management in primary care.

Learn how these conditions present so that you can recognize them in the exam. The following is a list of emergent conditions that will be on the exam. (They are discussed in detail in the "Danger Signals" sections of Chapters 5 through 17.)

Danger Signals

Cardiovascular System

- Acute myocardial infarction (MI)
- Congestive heart failure (CHF)
- Bacterial endocarditis
- Abdominal aortic aneurysm (AAA)

Skin and Integumentary System

- Angioedema/anaphylaxis
- Stevens–Johnson syndrome
- Meningococcemia
- Rocky Mountain spotted fever (RMSF)
- Lyme disease
- Herpes zoster opthalmicus
- Melanoma
- Basal cell carcinoma

Gastrointestinal System

- Acute abdomen (surgical abdomen)
- Acute appendicitis
- Acute pancreatitis
- Acute diverticulitis
- Acute cholecystitis
- *Clostridium difficile infection*
- Colon cancer

Men's Health

- Testicular torsion
- Priapism
- Prostate cancer

Psychosocial Mental Health

- Depression with suicidal plan
- Acute serotonin syndrome
- Malignant neuroleptic syndrome

Nervous System

- Cerebrovascular accident (CVA)
- Temporal arteritis headache
- Subarachnoid bleeding
- Acute bacterial meningitis
- Subdural hematoma

Head, Eyes, Ears, Nose, and Throat

- Retinal detachment
- Orbital cellulitis
- Optic neuritis
- Peritonsillar abscess

- Battle sign
- Herpes keratitis
- Temporal arteritis
- Acute angle-closure glaucoma

Pulmonary System

- Anaphylaxis
- Severe asthmatic exacerbation (impending respiratory failure)
- Pulmonary emboli
- Community-acquired pneumonia
- Lung cancer

Renal System

- Acute pyelonephritis
- Acute renal failure
- Bladder cancer

Women's Health

- Dominant breast mass attached to surrounding tissue
- Ruptured tubal ectopic pregnancy
- Paget's disease of the breast
- Ovarian cancer

II. Example

An asthmatic male patient complains of a sudden onset of itching and coughing after taking two aspirin tablets for a headache in the waiting room. The patient's lips and eyelids are becoming swollen. The patient complains of feeling hot. Bright-red wheals are noted on his chest and arms and legs. Which of the following is the best initial intervention to follow?

A) Call 911
B) Check the patient's blood pressure, pulse, and temperature
C) Give an injection of aqueous epinephrine 1:1000 (1 mg/mL) 0.5 mg IM into the vastus lateralis muscle immediately
D) Initiate a prescription of a potent topical steroid and a Medrol Dose Pack

III. Correct Answer: Option C

C) Give an injection of aqueous epinephrine 1:1000 dilution (1 mg/mL) 0.5 mg IM into the vastus lateralis muscle immediately.

IV. Question Dissection

Best Clues

- The quick onset of symptoms, such as angioedema, after taking aspirin
- The classic signs and symptoms of anaphylaxis described in this case
- Severe anaphylactic episodes occur almost immediately or within 1 hour after exposure

Notes

1. Treatment of anaphylaxis (in primary care):
    - If only one clinician is present: Give an injection of epinephrine 1:1000 dilution 0.3 to 0.5 mg IM *stat*, and then call 911. May repeat dose within 5 minutes in case of poor response.

(continued)

2. ED treatment medications: Administer epinephrine IM, 100% oxygen by face mask, an antihistamine (H1 blocker) such as diphenhydramine (Benadryl), an H2 antagonist such as ranitidine, a bronchodilator such as albuterol (short-acting beta-2 agonist), and systemic glucocorticosteroids such as prednisone.
3. Patients with an atopic history (asthma, eczema, allergic rhinitis) with nasal polyps are at higher risk for aspirin and nonsteroidal anti-inflammatory drug (NSAID) allergies.
4. Anaphylaxis is classified as a type I IgE-dependent reaction.
5. Biphasic anaphylaxis occurs in up to 23% of cases (symptoms recur within 8–10 hours after initial episode). This is the reason why these patients are prescribed a Medrol Dose Pack and a long-acting antihistamine after being discharged from the ED.
6. The most common triggers for anaphylaxis in children are foods. Medications and insect stings are the most common triggers in adults.

PRIORITIZING OTHER EMERGENT CASES

I. Discussion

During life-threatening situations, managing the airway, breathing, and circulation (the ABCs) is always the top priority. If the question does not describe conditions requiring the ABCs, then the next level of priority is the acute or sudden change in the mental status and the level of consciousness (LOC). One of the most important clues in such problems is the acute timing of onset of symptoms or the sudden change of the LOC from the patient's "baseline."

II. Example

A 16-year-old boy presents to a community clinic accompanied by his grandmother, who reports that he fell off his bike this morning. The patient now complains of a headache with mild nausea. The patient's grandmother reports that he was not wearing a helmet. The health history is uneventful. Which of the following statements is indicative of an emergent condition?

A) The patient complains of multiple painful abrasions that are bleeding on his arms and legs
B) The patient complains of a headache that is relieved by acetaminophen (Tylenol)
C) The patient makes eye contact occasionally and answers with brief statements
D) The patient is having difficulty with following normal conversation and answering questions

III. Correct Answer: Option D

D) The patient is having difficulty with following normal conversation and answering questions

IV. Question Dissection

Best Clues

- History of recent trauma that is followed by a headache with nausea.
- The patient did not wear a bicycle helmet.

Notes

1. Any recent changes in LOC, even one as subtle as difficulty with normal conversation, should ring a bell in your head.

(*continued*)

2. Notice the words "normal conversation." Do not overread the question and ask yourself what they mean by "normal conversation." Take it at face value.
3. Changes in LOC on the test are usually subtle changes. Signs to watch for include difficulty answering questions, slurred speech, apparent confusion, inability to understand instructions/conversation, being sleepy/lethargic, and so forth.
4. Even though the patient is bleeding, note that he has "abrasions," which are superficial.
5. The behavior described in option C is considered "normal" for an adolescent male (or female).

GERIATRICS

I. Discussion

The ANCC does not give any information about the number of questions by age group, but the AANPCB does. Elderly patients are divided into two age categories on the AANPCB exam. Those between the ages of 65 and 84 years are the "young gerontologicals." Those from the age of 85 years and older are the "frail elderly."

The AANPCB's FNP exam has a total of 38 questions (29%) on gerontological topics. The AANPCB Adult-Gerontology NP exam has a total of 67 questions (50%) on gerontological topics.

II. Example

Which of the following drug classes is considered as first-line treatment for unipolar depression in the elderly?

A) Selective serotonin reuptake inhibitors (SSRIs)
B) Selective norepinephrine reuptake inhibitors (SNRIs)
C) Tricyclic antidepressants (TCAs)
D) Monamine oxidase inhibitors (MAOIs)

III. Correct Answer: Option A

A) Selective serotonin reuptake inhibitors (SSRIs)

IV. Question Dissection

Best Clues

- There are no obvious clues in this question. Answering it correctly is based on your recognizing that unipolar depression is the same disease entity as major/minor depression. Depression in bipolar patients is called *bipolar depression.*
- SSRIs are the first-line treatment for unipolar/major depression. They carry an FDA warning that they increase suicidality in children and young adults up to age 23 years.
- TCAs have many anticholinergic effects (dry mouth, sedation, arrhythmias, confusion, urinary retention, etc.).
- MAOIs have major food and drug interactions and are not first-line drugs.

CHOOSING THE BEST INITIAL INTERVENTION

I. Discussion

Numerous questions on the exam will ask test-takers about the best initial intervention to perform in a given case scenario. The question may ask you to pick out the best initial evaluation, treatment, or statement to say to a patient.

One reason why some test takers answer these questions incorrectly is because they skip a step in the "SOAPE" process (subjective, objective, assessment, planning, and evaluation). The first step of the patient evaluation is to find "subjective" information such as asking about the patient's symptoms and other historical/demographic information. The next step is to find "objective" information. This means performing a physical examination or other tests. It is best to start out "low tech," such as performing a neurological exam for PVD or another low-tech maneuver.

For example, in a case of peripheral vascular disease (PVD), it makes sense to check the pulse and BP first on the lower and upper extremities before ordering an expensive test such as an ultrasound Doppler flow study. The following are examples of actions that can be done using the "SOAPE" mnemonic as a guide.

S: Look for Subjective Evidence

1. Interview the patient and/or family member about the history of the present illness.
2. Ask about the presentation of the illness (timing, signs and symptoms, etc.).
3. Ask whether the patient is on any medication, inquire about the past medical history, diet, etc.
4. Be alert for the historical findings because they provide important clues that help point to the correct diagnosis (or differential diagnosis).

O: Look for Objective Evidence

1. Perform a physical exam (general or targeted to the present complaints; examine associated systems in the differential, e.g., diabetic foot exams).
2. If applicable, perform a physical maneuver (Tinel's, Kernig's, drawer, etc.).
3. Order laboratory/other tests to "rule in" (or "rule out") the differential diagnosis.
4. If the laboratory test result is abnormal, you may be asked about the next step (such as a follow-up lab test that is more sensitive or specific).

A: Diagnosis or Assessment

1. What is the most likely diagnosis based on the history, disease presentation, and physical exam findings?
2. If applicable, figure out whether the lab or other testing results point to a more specific diagnosis (or rule out a diagnosis).
3. Decide whether the condition is emergent or not (if applicable).

P: Treatment Plan

1. Initiate or prescribe medications and symptomatic treatment (if applicable).
2. Educate the patient.
3. Recommend a follow-up visit to assess response to treatment, etc.

E: Evaluate Response to the Treatment/Intervention or Evaluate the Situation

1. Decide where there is poor or no response to treatment (or worsens).
2. Decide whether a situation is emergent.

II. Example

A 13-year-old girl with a history of mild persistent asthma and allergic rhinitis complains of a cough that has been waking her up very early in the morning. She reports that she is wheezing more than usual. She is accompanied by her mother. Her last office visit was 8 months ago. Which of the following is the best initial course of action?

A) Initiate a prescription of a short-acting beta-2 agonist QID PRN
B) Refer the patient to an allergist for a scratch test
C) Discuss her symptoms and other factors associated with the asthmatic exacerbation
D) Perform a thorough physical exam and obtain blood work

III. Correct Answer: Option C

C) Discuss her symptoms and other factors associated with the asthmatic exacerbation

IV. Question Dissection

Best Clues

- The patient's asthma appears to be getting worse (wheezing more than usual, early-morning cough).
- There is a need to find out about precipitating factors, medication compliance, comorbid conditions, what is precipitating the asthma, and so on.
- Always obtain a history (subjective) before performing a physical exam and labs.
- The adolescent age group starts at age 13 years (ANCC).

Notes

The correct order of actions to follow in this case scenario is the following:

1. Interview the patient/parent to find out more about the symptoms, etc. (subjective).
2. Perform a thorough physical exam (objective).
3. Administer a nebulizer treatment. Check peak expiratory flow (PEF) before and after treatment to assess for effectiveness.
4. Initiate a prescription of a short-acting beta-2 agonist QID PRN and a low-dosed steroid inhaler BID.
5. Refer the patient to an allergist for a scratch test if you suspect the patient has allergic asthma (evaluation).
6. Patients with asthmatic exacerbations whose PEF is less than 50% of predicted value after being given nebulized albuterol/saline treatments should not be discharged. Consider calling 911.
7. The differential diagnosis for an early-morning cough includes postnasal drip, allergic rhinitis, sinusitis, GERD, and so forth.

SIGNS AND SYMPTOMS

I. Discussion Only

It is very common for a question to ask for the sign(s) and/or symptom(s) of a disease process. After a description of a disease's signs and symptoms, you may be asked about the diagnosis or about the laboratory or follow-up tests for the disease.

PICK OUT THE MOST SPECIFIC SIGN/SYMPTOM

I. Discussion

Always pick out the most specific answer to a question when it is asking about the signs and/or symptoms of a disease. Learn the unique or the most specific signs/symptoms associated with the disease. The following question is a good example of this concept.

II. Example

Which of the following is *most likely* to be found in patients with a long-standing case of iron-deficiency anemia?

A) Pica
B) Fatigue
C) Pallor
D) Irritability

III. Correct Answer: Option A

A) Pica

IV. Question Dissection

Best Clues

- The diagnosis (iron-deficiency anemia)
- Knowledge that pica is also associated with iron-deficiency anemia

Notes

1. If you are guessing, use common sense. Fatigue and irritability are found in many conditions.
2. Pallor is also seen in many disorders such as shock, illness, and anemia.
3. By the process of elimination, you are left with option A, the correct choice.
4. Another specific clinical finding in iron-deficiency anemia is spoon-shaped nails (or koilonychia). Do not confuse this finding with pitted nails (psoriasis).

DERMATOLOGY QUESTIONS

I. Discussion

Many of the questions from this area are also accompanied by a colored photograph (ANCC). The AANPCB does not use photographs yet but may do so in the future. One of the problems that students have with these questions is their unfamiliarity with the dermatologic terms used to describe the skin condition. A list and description of the primary and secondary skin lesions are available in Chapter 6.

- Maculopapular: A skin rash that has both color (macular) and texture (small papules or raised skin lesions—the color ranges from red [erythematous] to bright pink)
- Maculopapular rash in a lace-like pattern (fifth disease)
- Maculopapular rashes with papules, vesicles, and crusts (varicella zoster, herpes simplex)
- Maculopapular rashes that are oval shaped with a herald patch (pityriasis rosea)
- Vesicular rashes on an erythematous base (herpes simplex, genital herpes)

II. Example

A male nursing assistant who works in a nursing home is complaining of multiple pruritic rashes that have been disturbing his sleep at night for the past few weeks. He reports that several of the residents are starting to complain of pruritic rashes. On physical exam, the NP notices multiple small papules, some vesicles, and maculopapular excoriated rashes on the sides and the webs of the fingers, on the waist, and on the penis. Which of the following is the most likely diagnosis?

A) Scarlatina
B) Impetigo
C) Erythema migrans
D) Scabies

III. Correct Answer: Option D

D) Scabies

IV. Question Dissection

Best Clues

- History (pruritic rashes disturb sleep at night, and individual works in a higher risk area [nursing home])
- Classic location of the rashes (finger webs, waist, penis)

Notes

1. Assume that a patient has scabies if excoriated pruritic rashes are located in the finger webs and the penis until proven otherwise. Higher risk groups are health care providers or people who work with large populations such as those in schools, nursing homes, group homes, or prisons.
2. The usual recommendation is that all family members and close contacts be treated at the same time as the patient (spread by skin-to-skin contact). Used clothes/sheets should be washed in hot water and then dried or ironed with high heat.
3. The rash of scarlatina has a sandpaper-like texture and is accompanied by a sore throat, strawberry tongue, and skin desquamation (peeling) of the palms and soles. It is not pruritic.
4. The rash of impetigo initially appears as papules that develop into bullae. These rupture easily, becoming superficial, bright-red "weeping" rashes with honey-colored exudate that becomes crusted as it dries. The rashes are very pruritic and are located on areas that are easily traumatized, such as the face, arms, or legs. Insect bites, acne lesions, and varicella lesions can also become secondarily infected, resulting in impetigo.
5. Cutaneous larva migrans (creeping eruption) rashes are shaped like red raised wavy lines (serpiginous or snake-like) that are alone or a few may be grouped. They are red and very pruritic, and they become excoriated from scratching (appears maculopapular).
6. The areas of the body that are commonly exposed directly to contaminated soil and sand, such as the soles of the feet, extremities, or the buttocks, are the most common locations for larva migrans.
7. Systemic treatment with either ivermectin once a day (for 1–2 days) or albendazole (for 3 days) is the preferred therapy for larva migrans.

CHOOSING THE CORRECT DRUG

I. Discussion

Test-takers are expected to know not only a drug's generic and/or brand name, but also its drug class. If you are familiar only with the drug's brand name or generic form, you will still be able to recognize the drug on the test because both names will be listed.

In addition, the drug's action, indication(s), common side effects, drug interactions, and contraindications are important to learn. Drugs may only be listed as a drug class.

II. Example

A 10-year-old female student complains of pain and decreased hearing in her left ear that is getting steadily worse. She has a history of allergic rhinitis and is allergic to dust mites. On physical exam, the left tympanic membrane is bulging and red with displaced landmarks. The tympanogram exam reveals a flat line. The student denies frequent ear infections, and the last antibiotic she took was 8 months ago for a urinary tract infection. She is allergic to sulfa and tells the NP that she will not take any erythromycin because it makes her very nauseated. Which of the following is the best choice of treatment for this patient?

A) Amoxicillin 500 mg PO three times a day for 7 days
B) Pseudoephedrine (Sudafed) 20 mg PO as needed every 4 to 6 hours
C) Fluticasone (Flonase) nasal inhaler 1 to 2 sprays each nostril every 12 hours
D) Clarithromycin (Biaxin) 500 mg PO two times a day for 10 days

III. Correct Answer: Option A

A) Amoxicillin 500 mg PO three times a day for 7 days

IV. Question Dissection

Best Clues

- Red bulging tympanic membrane with cloudy fluid inside and displaced landmarks
- Last antibiotic taken was 8 months ago and ear infections were infrequent (lack of risk factors for beta-lactamase–resistant bacteria)

Notes

1. This question is more complicated compared with the first example. Although the question is asking about the correct drug treatment, it also lists the signs/symptoms of the disease. In order to answer this question correctly, you must first arrive at the correct diagnosis, which is acute otitis media (AOM).
2. Amoxicillin is the preferred first-line antibiotic for both AOM and acute sinusitis in children (for patients with no risk factors for resistant organisms).
3. The ideal patient is someone who has not been on any antibiotics in the past 3 months and/or does not live in an area with high rates of beta-lactam–resistant bacteria.
4. If the patient is a treatment failure, or was on an antibiotic in the previous 3 months, then a second-line antibiotic, such as amoxicillin-clavulanate (Augmentin) BID or cefdinir (Omnicef) BID, should be given.
5. If penicillin-allergic, an alternative is azithromycin (Z-Pack) and clarithromycin (Biaxin) BID.
6. Pseudoephedrine (Sudafed) is for symptoms only. Do not use for infants, young children, or patients with hypertension.
7. A nasal steroid spray BID is a good adjunct treatment for this patient because of allergic rhinitis, which causes the eustachian tube to swell and get blocked.

DIAGRAMS

I. Discussion

The only diagram seen on the test at the moment is one of a chest with the four cardiac auscultatory areas (aortic, pulmonic, tricuspid, and mitral) marked. The diagram is used for questions on either cardiac murmurs or the heart sounds.

II. Example

Which of the following is the best location to auscultate for the S3 heart sound?

A) Aortic area
B) Pulmonic area
C) Tricuspid area
D) Mitral area

III. Correct Answer: Option D

D) Mitral area

IV. Question Dissection

Best Clues

- Memorization of the S3 heart sound facts

Notes

1. The mitral area, sometimes called the cardiac apex, is the optimal location to hear the S3.
2. This area is located at the left fifth intervertebral space, along the mid-clavicular line.
3. The left lateral recumbent position brings the apex closer to the chest wall and improves the practitioner's ability to hear the left ventricular S3.

"GOLD STANDARD" TESTS

I. Discussion

Learn to distinguish between a screening test and a diagnostic test (the "gold standard"). Depending on the disease process, the preferred diagnostic test might be a biopsy (e.g., melanoma), blood culture (e.g., septicemia), or an MRI scan (e.g., meniscus cartilage damage).

In contrast, screening tests are generally more available and cost-effective. Some examples of screening tests are the CBC (anemia), BP (hypertension), Mantoux test (TB), or a UA (UTI). The ideal screening test is one that can detect a disease at an early-enough stage so that it can help to decrease the morbidity and mortality. A good example of a disease with no approved screening test is ovarian cancer. The CA-125 is not sensitive enough to detect ovarian cancer during the early stages of the disease when it is potentially curable.

II. Example

A middle-aged male nurse is having his Mantoux test result checked. A reddened area of 10.5 mm is present. It is smooth and soft and does not appear to be indurated. During the interview, the patient denies fever, cough, and weight loss. Which of the following is a true statement?

A) The Mantoux test result is negative
B) The Mantoux test result is borderline
C) The Mantoux test should be repeated in 2 weeks
D) A chest x-ray and sputum culture are indicated

III. Correct Answer: Option A

A) The Mantoux test result is negative

IV. Question Dissection

Best Clues

- Knowledge that skin induration, not the red color, is the best indicator of a positive reaction
- Lack of signs or symptoms of TB

Notes

1. When some test-takers see the 10.5-mm size and the red color, they assume automatically that it is a positive result.
2. The Mantoux test (TB skin test) result is negative because of the description of the soft and smooth skin (it is not indurated). Erythema alone is not an important criterion. The area must be indurated (firm texture) and of the correct size to be positive for TB.
3. For pulmonary TB, a sputum culture is the gold standard. Treatment is started with at least three antitubercular drugs because of high rates of resistance. When the sputum culture and sensitivity result are available, the antitubercular antibiotic treatment can be narrowed down or changed. Another drug can be added.
4. TB is a reportable disease. Noncompliant patients who refuse treatment can be quarantined to protect the public.
5. A baseline LFT level and follow-up testing are recommended for patients on isoniazid (INH).

ARE TWO NAMES BETTER THAN ONE?

I. Discussion

Some diseases and conditions are known by two different names that are used interchangeably in both the clinical area and the literature. Sometimes the alternate name is the one being used in the exam questions. This can fool the test-taker who is familiar with the disease but only recognizes it under its other name.

II. Examples

1. Degenerative joint disease (DJD), or osteoarthritis
2. Atopic dermatitis, or eczema
3. Senile arcus, or arcus senilis
4. Lupus, or systemic lupus erythematosus (SLE)
5. Otitis media with effusion (OME), or middle ear effusion (MEE)
6. Group A beta *Streptococcus*, or *Streptococcus pyogenes*
7. Tinea corporis, or ringworm
8. Enterobiasis, or pinworms
9. Vitamin B_{12}, or cobalamin, or cyanocobalamin
10. Vitamin B_1, or thiamine
11. Scarlet fever, or scarlatina
12. Otitis externa, or swimmer's ear
13. Condyloma acuminata, or genital warts
14. Tic douloureux, or trigeminal neuralgia
15. Tinea cruris, or jock itch
16. Thalassemia minor, or thalassemia trait (either alpha or beta)
17. Giant cell arteritis, or temporal arteritis
18. Psoas sign, or iliopsoas muscle sign
19. Tinea capitis, or ringworm of the scalp
20. Light reflex, or the Hirschberg (corneal reflex) test
21. Sentinel nodes, or Virchow's nodes
22. Mantoux test or TB skin test (TST)

23. Erythema migrans, or early Lyme disease
24. Sinusitis, or rhinosinusitis
25. Major depression, or unipolar depression

SUICIDE RISK AND DEPRESSION

I. Discussion

All depressed patients should be screened for suicidal and/or homicidal ideation. This is true in the clinical arena as well as on the exam. Avoid picking statements that do not directly address the patient's suicidal and homicidal plans. Risk factors for suicide and depression are discussed in Chapter 15.

Incorrect answers are statements that are judgmental, reassuring to the patient, vague, disrespectful, or do not address the issue of suicide (or homicide) in a direct manner.

II. Example

An NP working in a school health clinic is evaluating a new student who has been referred by a teacher. The student is a 16-year-old boy with a history of attention deficit disorder (ADD). He complains that his parents are always fighting and he thinks that they are getting divorced. He reports that he is failing two classes. During the interview, he stares at the floor and avoids eye contact. He reports that he is having problems falling asleep at night and has stopped seeing friends, including his girlfriend. Which of the following statements is the best choice to ask this teen?

A) "Do you want me to call your parents after we talk?"
B) "Do you have any plans for killing or hurting yourself or other people?"
C) "Do you have any close male or female friends?"
D) "Do you want to wait to tell me about your plans until you feel better?"

III. Correct Answer: Option B

B) "Do you have any plans for killing or hurting yourself or other people?"

IV. Question Dissection

Best Clues

- Classic behavioral cues (avoidance of eye contact, insomnia, social isolation)
- Parents fighting and getting divorced

Notes

1. Option B is the most specific approach in the evaluation for suicide in this case.
2. Although option C ("Do you have any close male or female friends?") is a common question asked of depressed patients, it is incorrect because it does not give specific information about specific plans of suicide or of homicide.
3. Always avoid picking answer choices in which an intervention is delayed. The statement "Do you want to wait to tell me about your plans until you feel better?" is a good example. This advice is applicable to all areas of the test.
4. Teenagers are separating from their parents emotionally and value their privacy highly. When interviewing a teen, do it privately (without parents) and also with the parent(s) present.

OTHER PSYCHIATRIC DISORDERS

I. Discussion

Other psychiatric disorders, such as obsessive compulsive disorder (OCD), bipolar disorder, minor depression, anxiety, panic disorder, alcohol addiction, attention deficit hyperactivity disorder (ADHD), ADD, and posttraumatic stress disorder (PTSD) may be included in the exams. Not all of these disorders are usually seen together in one exam. The most common psychiatric conditions on the exam are major depression, alcohol abuse, and suicide risk. The question may be as straightforward as querying about the correct drug treatment for the condition, as illustrated in this example.

II. Example

Which of the following drug classes is indicated as first-line treatment of both major depression and OCD?

A) Selective serotonin reuptake inhibitors (SSRIs)
B) Tricyclic antidepressants (TCAs)
C) Mood stabilizers
D) Benzodiazepines

III. Correct Answer: Option A

A) Selective serotonin reuptake inhibitors (SSRIs)

IV. Question Dissection

Best Clues

- Rule out benzodiazepines, which are used to treat anxiety or insomnia (process of elimination)
- Mood stabilizers, such as lithium salts, are used to treat bipolar disorder (process of elimination)
- The stem is asking for the "first-line treatment" for depression, which is the SSRIs

Notes

1. TCAs are not first-line treatment for depression (SSRIs are first-line treatment).
2. TCAs are also used as prophylactic treatment for migraine headaches, chronic pain, and neuropathic pain (i.e., tingling, burning) such as postherpetic neuralgia. Examples of TCAs are amitriptyline (Elavil) and nortriptyline (Pamelor).
3. Do not give suicidal patients a prescription for TCAs because of the high risk of hoarding the drug and overdosing. Overdose of TCAs can be fatal (cardiac and CNS toxicity).
4. SSRIs are also first-line treatment for OCD, generalized anxiety disorder (GAD), panic disorder, social anxiety disorder (extreme shyness), posttraumatic stress disorder (PTSD, and premenstrual mood disorder (fluoxetine or Prozac). Examples of SSRIs are citalopram (Celexa), escitalopram (Lexapro), fluoxetine (Prozac), sertraline (Zoloft), and paroxetine (Paxil).
5. Anticonvulsants, such as carbamazepine (Tegretol), are also used for chronic pain and trigeminal neuralgia.

ABUSIVE SITUATIONS

I. Discussion

Health care workers are required by law to report suspected and actual child abuse to the proper authorities. Abuse-related topics may include domestic violence, physical abuse, child abuse, child neglect, elderly abuse, elderly neglect, and sexual abuse.

II. Example

A 16-year-old teenager with a history of attention deficit hyperactivity disorder (ADHD) is brought in to the ED by his mother. She does not want her son to be alone in the room. The NP doing the intake notes several burns on the teen's trunk. Some of the burns appear infected. The NP documents the burns as mostly round in shape and about 0.5 cm (centimeter) in size. Which of the following questions is most appropriate to ask the child's mother?

A) "Your son's back looks terrible. What happened to him?"
B) "Does your son have more friends outside of school?"
C) "Did you burn his back with a cigarette?"
D) "Can you please tell me what happened to your son?"

III. Correct Answer: Option D

D) "Can you please tell me what happened to your son?"

IV. Question Dissection

Best Clues

- Option D is the only open-ended question in the group
- In addition, it is not a judgmental statement

Notes

1. In general, open-ended questions are usually the correct answer in cases in which an NP is trying to elicit the history in an interview.
2. "Your son's back looks terrible. What happened to him?" and "Did you burn his back with a cigarette?"
   - Both are considered judgmental questions and are always the wrong choice.
3. These types of questions are more likely to make people defensive and/or hostile and cause them to end the conversation.
4. "Does your son have more friends outside of school?"
   - This question does not address the immediate issue of the burn marks on the boy's back.
5. Communication tips:

   Questions on Abuse:
   - If a history is being taken, pick the open-ended question first. Interview both the patient and possible "abuser" together, and then interview the patient separately.

   Questions on Depression:
   - Pick the statement that is the most specific to find out whether the patient is suicidal or homicidal.
   - Any answer considered judgmental or confrontational is wrong.

(*continued*)

- Do not pick answers that "reassure" patients about their issues, because this discourages them from verbalizing more about it.
- In addition, do not ignore cultural beliefs. Integrate them into the treatment plan if they are not harmful to the health of the patient.

THE "CAGE" MNEMONIC

I. Discussion

The CAGE is a screening tool used to screen patients for possible alcohol abuse. A positive response to two out of four questions is highly suggestive of alcohol abuse. In the exam, you are expected to use higher level cognitive skills and apply the concepts of CAGE. Examples of this concept are the questions that ask you to pick the patient who is most likely (or least likely) to abuse alcohol.

CAGE Screening Tool (Two or More Positive Answers Is Suggestive of Alcoholism)

C: Do you feel the need to **c**ut down?
A: Are you **a**nnoyed when your friends/spouse comment about your drinking?
G: Do you feel **g**uilty about your drinking?
E: Do you need to drink **e**arly in the morning? (eye-opener)

II. Example

Which of the following individuals is least likely to have an alcohol abuse problem?

A) A woman who gets annoyed if her best friend talks to her about her drinking habit
B) A carpenter who drinks two cans of beer when playing cards with friends
C) A nurse who feels shaky when she wakes up and drinks one glass of wine to feel better.
D) A college student who tells his friend that he drinks only on weekends but feels that he should be drinking less

III. Correct Answer: Option B

B) A carpenter who drinks two cans of beer nightly when playing cards with friends

IV. Question Dissection

Best Clues

- Lack of risk factor (two cans of beer at night is considered normal consumption for males); for females, the limit is one drink per day (one 12 oz. beer, 5 oz. wine)
- There is no description of any negative effects on the carpenter's daily functioning, social environment, or mental state

Notes

Any person who feels compelled to drink (or use drugs) no matter what the consequences are to his or her health, finances, career, friends, and family is addicted to the substance.

1. "A woman who gets annoyed if her best friend talks to her about her drinking habit." This is the "A" in CAGE ("annoyed"), a good example of an alcohol abuser getting annoyed when someone close remarks about her drinking problem.

(continued)

2. "A nurse who feels shaky when she wakes up and drinks one glass of wine to feel better." This is the "E" in CAGE ("eye-opener"). The patient is having withdrawal symptoms and must drink in order to feel better.
3. "A college student who tells his friend that he drinks only on weekends but feels that he should be drinking less." This fits the "C" in CAGE ("cut down"). This student is aware that he is drinking too much.

PHYSICAL ASSESSMENT FINDINGS

I. Discussion

Questions about physical exam findings are plentiful. Learn the classic presentation of disease and emergent conditions. The knowledge of normal findings, as well as some variants, is important for the exam. In addition, if the question style used is negatively worded, careful reading is essential.

II. Example

An older woman complains of a new onset of severe pain in her right ear after taking swimming classes for 2 weeks. On physical exam, the right ear canal is red and swollen. Purulent green exudate is seen inside. Which of the following is an incorrect statement?

A) Pulling on the tragus is painful
B) The tympanic membrane is translucent with intact landmarks
C) The external ear canal is swollen and painful
D) Tenderness of the mastoid area during palpation

III. Correct Answer: Option B

B) The tympanic membrane is translucent with intact landmarks

IV. Question Dissection

Best Clues

- Positive risk factor (history of swimming)
- Classic signs (reddened and swollen ear canal with green exudate)

Notes

1. Acute otitis externa is a superficial infection of the skin in the ear canal. It is more common during warm and humid conditions such as swimming and summertime.
2. The most common bacterial pathogen is *Pseudomonas* (bright-green pus).
3. Otitis externa does not involve the middle ear or the tympanic membrane (translucent tympanic membrane with intact landmarks, no redness, no bulging).
4. Acute mastoiditis is a possible complication of AOM.

TWO-PART QUESTIONS

I. Discussion

There may be case scenarios that are followed by two questions. These questions are problematic because the two questions are dependent on each other.

To solve both correctly, the test-taker must answer the first portion by figuring out the diagnosis in order to solve the second question correctly.

II. Example

Part One

An adolescent male reports the new onset of symptoms 2 weeks after returning from a hiking trip in North Carolina. He presents with complaints of high fever, severe headache, muscle aches, lack of appetite and nausea. The symptoms are accompanied by a generalized red rash that is not pruritic. The rash initially appeared on both ankles and wrists and then spread toward the patient's trunk. The rash involves both the palms and the soles. Which of the following conditions is most likely?

A) Meningococcemia
B) Rocky Mountain spotted fever (RMSF)
C) Idiopathic thrombocytopenic purpura (ITP)
D) Lyme disease

Part Two

Which of the following is the best treatment plan to follow?

A) Refer the patient to the hospital ED
B) Refer the patient to an infectious disease specialist
C) Initiate a prescription of oral glucocorticoids
D) Collect a blood specimen for culture and sensitivity

III. Correct Answers

Part One: Option B

B) Rocky Mountain spotted fever (RMSF)

Part Two: Option A

A) Refer the patient to the hospital ED

IV. Question Dissection

Best Clues

Part One

- Location and activity (south-central United States, outdoor activity)
- Classic rash (red rash on both wrists and ankles that spreads centrally with involvement of the palms and the soles)
- Systemic symptoms (high fever, headache, myalgia, nausea)

Part Two

- Knowledge of the emergent nature of RMSF (can cause death if not treated within the first 8 days of symptoms)

Notes

1. Early treatment is important, and empiric treatment should be started early if RMSF is suspected. Refer the patient to the closest ED as soon as possible.
2. It may be difficult to distinguish RMSF from meningococcemia before the blood culture results and the CSF culture results are available.
3. Doxycycline is the preferred agent for both children and adults.
4. RMSF:
   - Dog/wood tick bite; spirochete called *Rickettsia rickettsii*
   - Treat with doxycycline 100 mg PO/IV for a minimum of 7 days or longer

(continued)

5. Early Lyme disease (erythema migrans rash stage):
   - Ixodes (deer) tick bite; spirochete called *Borrelia burgdorferi*
   - Treat with doxycycline × 21 days
   - Majority of the cases are in the mid-Atlantic and New England states (i.e., CT, MA, NY, NJ, PA).
6. ITP severity ranges from mild to severe (platelet count <30,000/µL). Platelets are broken down by the spleen, causing thrombocytopenia. Look for easy bruising, petechiae, purpura, epistaxis, and gingival bleeding (combined with low platelet count).
7. Initial treatment for ITP is glucocorticoids (i.e., prednisone) based on platelet response.

NORMAL PHYSICAL EXAM FINDINGS

I. Discussion

A good review of normal physical exam findings and some benign variants is necessary. Pertinent physical exam findings are discussed at the beginning of each organ system review.

A good resource to use in your review is the advanced physical assessment textbook that was used in your program. Keep in mind that sometimes questions about normal physical findings are written as if they were a pathological process. This is important to remember when you encounter these types of questions.

II. Example

A 13-year-old girl complains of an irregular menstrual cycle. She started menarche 6 months ago. Her last menstrual period was 2 months ago. She denies being sexually active. Her urine pregnancy test is negative. Which of the following would you tell the child's mother?

A) Consult with a pediatric endocrinologist to rule out problems with the hypothalamic–pituitary–adrenal (HPA) axis

B) Advise the mother that irregular menstrual cycles are common during the first year after menarche

C) Advise the mother that her child is starting menarche early and has precocious puberty

D) Ask the medical assistant to get labs drawn for thyroid-stimulating hormone (TSH), follicle-stimulating hormone (FSH), and estradiol levels

III. Correct Answer: Option B

B) Advise the mother that irregular menstrual cycles are common during the first year after menarche

IV. Question Dissection

Best Clues

- Patient recently started menarche 6 months ago (knowledge of pubertal changes); the ovaries may not ovulate monthly (resulting in irregular periods) when starting menarche
- The teen is not sexually active (rule out pertinent negative, such as the negative pregnancy test)

Notes

1. This question describes normal growth and development in adolescents.
2. When girls start menarche, their periods may be very irregular for several months up to 2 years.

ADOLESCENCE

I. Discussion

During this period of life, numerous changes are occurring, both physically and emotionally. Adolescents are thinking in more abstract ways and are psychologically separating from their parents. The opinions of peers are more important than those of the parents. Privacy is a big issue in this age group and should be respected.

II. Example

Which of the following is the second highest cause of mortality among adolescents and young adults in this country?

A) Suicide
B) Smoking
C) Homicide
D) Illicit drug use

III. Correct Answer: Option A

A) Suicide

IV. Question Dissection

Best Clues

- Rote memory (suicide is the second highest cause of mortality among adolescents)

Notes

1. According to the CDC, the number one cause of mortality in this age group is motor vehicle crashes.
2. The second most common cause of mortality in adolescents in the United States is suicide and the third is homicide.
3. Screening for depression in all adolescents is recommended. Signs of a depressed teen include falling grades, acting out, avoiding socializing, moodiness, and so forth.
4. Smoking is ruled out because its health effects take decades (i.e., COPD).
5. Mortality from illicit drug use is more common among adults.

DIFFERENTIAL DIAGNOSIS

I. Discussion

Differential diagnoses are the conditions whose presentations share many similarities. For example, the differential diagnoses to consider for chronic cough (a cough lasting more than 8 weeks) are asthma, GERD, ACE inhibitors, chronic bronchitis, lung cancer, and lung infections such as TB (and many more). As a clinician, your ability to apply differential diagnosis is important for patient safety. In this type of question, the differential diagnoses are the distractors.

II. Example

A 67-year-old man walks into an urgent care center. The patient complains of episodes of chest pain in his upper sternum when he is climbing up stairs in his apartment building. When he stops the activity, the pain goes away. He reports that once when he was eating a steak dinner, he also experienced the chest pain. A fasting total lipid profile is ordered. The result reveals total cholesterol of 250 mg/dL, LDL of 180 mg/dL, and high-density lipoprotein (HDL) of 25 mg/dL. Which of the following is most likely?

A) Acute esophagitis
B) Myocardial infarction (MI)
C) Gastroesophageal reflux disease (GERD)
D) Angina

III. Correct Answer: Option D

D) Angina

IV. Question Dissection

Best Clues

- Classic presentation (chest pain that is precipitated by exertion and is relieved by rest)
- History (several episodes of the same chest pain)
- Positive risk factors (low HDL, elevated lipid levels, age, and gender)

Notes

All four answer options are some common conditions that can mimic angina (differential diagnoses). Rule out the pertinent negatives.

- Pain is relieved by rest (angina). If pain not relieved by rest, then rule out angina.
- Risk factors for heart disease and chest pain (angina, MI) are present.
- Physical activity aggravates the condition (angina, MI).
- There is a lack of history of aggravating factors such as intake of certain meds such as NSAIDs, aspirin, bisphosphonates, or alcohol (rule out esophagitis).
- Chest pain is not related to meals (rule out GERD).

CLASSIC PRESENTATION

I. Discussion

Because certification exams are administered all over the country, the questions are written to conform to the classic "textbook presentation." This allows the test to be valid and statistically sound. All of the questions on the exam are referenced by at least two to three reliable sources. For both exams, a large number of clinical questions are referenced by popular medical and nursing textbooks.

The disease process is described at its height, although in real-life practice, the signs and/or symptoms are dependent upon the stage of the illness. For example, for the majority of disease processes, usually the prodromal period, or the early phase, is asymptomatic or mildly symptomatic, while during the height of the illness, the full signs and symptoms are usually present.

II. Example

While performing a routine physical exam on an older White male patient with a history of cigarette smoking, hyperlipidemia, and hypertension, the NP palpates a pulsatile mass in the patient's midabdominal area. A bruit is auscultated over the soft mass. Which of the following is the recommended imaging method?

A) CT scan
B) Abdominal ultrasound

C) Radiography of the chest
D) Plain film of the abdomen

III. Correct Answer: Option B

B) Abdominal ultrasound

IV. Question Dissection

Best Clues

- Pulsatile mass located in the middle of the abdomen that is associated with a bruit
- Patient demographics

Notes

1. This question describes the classic case of an abdominal aortic aneurysm (AAA).
2. Some of the risk factors for AAA are male gender (age older than 60 years), smoker, uncontrolled hypertension, White race, genetic diseases such as Marfan syndrome, and family history.
3. Signs and symptoms of AAA rupture are abrupt onset of severe abdominal pain with low-back pain and abdominal distension with signs and symptoms of shock.
4. The initial imaging diagnostic test to order is the abdominal ultrasound.

ETHNIC BACKGROUND

I. Discussion

Ethnic background is an important clue for certain genetic disorders. For example, Tay-Sachs, a rare and fatal genetic disorder, is most common among Eastern European (Ashkenazi) Jews.

A warning about ethnic background: It can also be used as a distractor. In most medical conditions, the patient's ethnic background does not affect the treatment plan or the patient's response to treatment. The next question is an example of this concept.

II. Example

Which of the following laboratory tests is a sensitive indicator of renal function in people of African descent?

A) Serum blood urea nitrogen (BUN)
B) Serum creatinine concentration
C) Estimated glomerular filtration rate (eGFR)
D) Serum BUN-to-creatinine ratio

The question in this example can also be phrased as: Which of the following laboratory tests is a sensitive indicator of renal function in people of Hispanic descent? Or Asian descent?

III. Correct Answer: Option C

C) Estimated glomerular filtration rate (eGFR)

IV. Question Dissection

Best Clues

- Knowledge that the eGFR is a better test of renal function compared with the serum creatinine concentration

Notes

1. A GFR value of 60 mL/min/1.73 m^2 or less is a sign of kidney damage (refer to a nephrologist).
2. The eGFR is an "estimated" value (it is not measured directly) and is computed by using specific formulas (Modification of Diet in Renal Disease [MDRD] study equation, Cockcroft–Gault, others).
3. The serum creatinine is affected by age (less sensitive in elderly), gender (higher in males), ethnicity (higher with African background), and other factors.
4. The BUN is a waste product of the protein from foods that you have eaten. If you eat more protein before the test, it will increase (or decrease with low protein intake).
5. Dehydration will elevate the BUN value.

SENTINEL EVENTS

I. Discussion

The Joint Commission adopted a Sentinel Event Policy in 1996 to assist ambulatory care centers and hospitals improve patient safety. A sentinel event is defined as "a patient safety event (not primarily related to the natural course of patient's illness or underlying condition) that reaches a patient and results in any of the following: death, permanent harm, or severe temporary harm" (The Joint Commission, 2016). Sentinel events require immediate investigation.

II. Example

All of the following are considered sentinel events except:

A) Unanticipated death of a full-term infant
B) Abduction of any patient who is receiving treatment or services
C) Suicide of a patient who is receiving around-the-clock care
D) Nausea and vomiting caused by a prescription of oral erythromycin

III. Correct Answer: Option D

D) Nausea and vomiting caused by a prescription of oral erythromycin

IV. Question Dissection

Best Clues

- If you are not sure of the answer, one way to guess is to look for a pattern or for contextual clues
- Notice that options A, B, and C all have something in common; they are all serious patient safety events
- Option D is not considered a serious patient event. GI side effects, such as nausea/vomiting, anorexia, and abdominal pain, are not life-threatening
- An example of a sentinel event involving medications is when a patient who is allergic to a drug (e.g., macrolides) is prescribed erythromycin, resulting in death of the patient due to anaphylaxis

3

Pharmacology Review

During your review, memorize both the drug class and the representative drug(s) for that particular class. The reason is that sometimes drugs are listed by class only. Memorizing drug doses is generally not emphasized to the same extent as on the NCLEX-RN® examination. Higher level thinking skills, such as knowledge of drug indications and drug safety issues, are considered more important in the nurse practitioner (NP) examinations.

Learn about clinically important drug "safety" issues, such as drug–drug interactions, disease–drug interactions, and the adverse reactions that are seen in the primary care area. For example, one of the most common drug interactions in the primary care area is between warfarin sodium (Coumadin) and trimethoprim–sulfamethoxazole (Bactrim). Sulfa drugs will interact with warfarin (increases the blood level), which results in an elevation of the INR and the risk of bleeding.

The most common question about drugs (prescription and over-the-counter [OTC]) is related to disease management. These questions involve the correct drug(s) used to treat a condition.

The drugs that are included in the examinations are usually the "older" drugs that have been in use for several years to several decades (e.g., doxycycline, amoxicillin). Drugs that have been recently released (past 6 months or less) will not be included on the examinations. Lately, there have been a few questions about pharmacokinetics (e.g., first-pass metabolism, excretion).

This section is not meant to be a comprehensive review of pharmacology. The goal is to help you understand pharmacologic concepts, drug names, drug class, drug interactions, disease–drug interactions, types of laboratory tests needed for certain medications in order to help you pass your American Nurses Credentialing Center (ANCC) or American Academy of Nurse Practitioners Certification Board (AANPCB) certification exam. Do not use the contents of this review book for clinical practice.

ORAL DRUGS: FIRST-PASS HEPATIC METABOLISM (OR FIRST-PASS EFFECT)

All oral drugs must go through "first-pass metabolism" before they can be used by the body. When a drug is swallowed, it is absorbed through the small intestine where it enters the portal circulation. Inside the liver, the cytochrome P450 (CYP450) system is responsible for the biotransformation of not only many drugs, but other substances such as alcohol, herbs, and some foods and toxins.

Drugs that have extensive first-pass metabolism cannot be given by the oral route simply because there is not enough of the active drug left. A good example is insulin, which, if given by the oral route, is completely broken down in the GI tract (by enzymes). To bypass first-pass metabolism, insulin must be given by injection.

DRUG METABOLISM (BIOTRANSFORMATION)

The most active organ is the liver (CYPP450 enzyme system). The CYP450 system can either be induced (increase drug metabolism) or it can be inhibited (slow down drug metabolism). Genetic variants of the CYP450 system and receptors determine how an individual's body breaks down and reacts to a drug. The other organ systems that are involved in biotransformation of drugs are the kidneys, the GI tract (breakdown by gut bacteria), and the lungs (CO_2).

DRUG EXCRETION

Almost all drugs/chemicals are broken down by the liver and excreted from the body in the bile, urine, feces, respiratory gas (CO_2), and as sweat (sweat glands). It is unusual to have a drug that is totally (100%) broken down by only one organ (e.g., kidneys only). Most drugs are excreted by both the hepatobiliary system and the kidneys.

PHARMACOLOGY TERMS

- *Half-life (t½):* The amount of time in which drug concentration decreases by 50%
- *Area under the curve (AUC):* The average amount of a drug in the blood after a dose is given it is a measure of the availability (bioavailability) of a drug after it is administered
- *Minimum inhibitory concentration (MIC):* The lowest concentration of an antibiotic that will inhibit the growth of organisms (after overnight incubation)
- *Maximum concentration*: The highest concentration of a drug after a dose
- *Trough (minimum concentration)*: The lowest concentration of a drug after a dose

POTENT INHIBITORS: CYP450 SYSTEM

The following are some "problematic" drugs. These drugs are responsible for a large number of drug–drug interactions. Drugs that act as inhibitors slow down drug clearance (increase drug concentration). When this happens, the patient is at high risk for a drug overdose and adverse effects. When a test question is asking about a drug interaction, think of these drugs and drug classes.

- Macrolides (erythromycin, clarithromycin)
- Antifungals (ketoconazole, fluconazole)
- Cimetidine (Tagamet)
- Citalopram (Celexa)

Although not a drug, grapefruit juice affects the CYP450 system. Drugs that are adversely affected by grapefruit juice include statins, erythromycin, calcium channel blockers (nifedipine, nisoldipine), antivirals (indinavir, saquinavir), amiodarone, benzodiazepines (diazepam, triazolam), cisapride, carbamazepine, buspirone, others.

NARROW THERAPEUTIC INDEX DRUGS (see Table 3.1)

- Warfarin sodium (Coumadin): Monitor INR
- Digoxin (Lanoxin): Monitor digoxin level, EKG, electrolytes (potassium, magnesium, calcium)
- Theophylline: Monitor blood levels

- Carbamazepine (Tegretol) and phenytoin (Dilantin): Monitor blood levels
- Levothyroxine: Monitor TSH
- Lithium: Monitor blood levels, TSH (risk of hypothyroidism)

Table 3.1 Safety Issues With Some Prescription Drugs*

Drug Class and Generic and Trade Names	Safety Issues
Proton-pump inhibitors (PPIs)	Increased risk of fractures (postmenopausal women), pneumonia, *Clostridium difficile* infection, hypomagnesemia, B_{12} and iron malabsorption, atrophic gastritis, and kidney disease
Omeprazole (Prilosec)	Interacts with warfarin (Coumadin), diazepam (Valium), carbamazepine (Tegretol), phenytoin (Dilantin), ketoconazole (Nizoral)
Vitamin K antagonist Warfarin (Coumadin)	Interacts with "G" herbs such as garlic, ginger, gingko, and ginseng; other herbs/supplements: Feverfew, green tea, and fish oil; numerous drug interactions Discontinue 7 days before surgery
TZDs	*Black Box Warning*: Cause or exacerbate congestive heart failure in some patients; do not use if New York Health Association Class III or IV heart failure
Pioglitazone (Actos)	Stop if causes dyspnea, weight gain, cough (heart failure)
Atypical antipsychotics Risperidone (Risperdal) Olanzapine (Zyprexa)	High risk of weight gain, metabolic syndrome, and type 2 diabetes; monitor weight every 3 months *Black Box Warning*: Higher mortality in elderly patients
Quetiapine (Seroquel)	Monitor TSH, lipids, weight/body mass index
Bisphosphonates	Erosive esophagitis, abdominal pain, stop immediately if symptoms of esophagitis (chest pain, difficulty swallowing, burning midback) or jaw pain (osteonecrosis); take alone upon awakening with 8-oz glass water (*not* juice) before breakfast; do not lie down for 30 minutes afterward; do not mix with other drugs; take first thing in the morning before breakfast
Alendronate (Fosamax) Risedronate (Actonel)	Contraindications: Active GI disease (GERD, PUD), CKD, esophageal stricture/varices
Statins	Do not mix with grapefruit juice; drug-induced hepatitis or rhabdomyolysis higher if mixed with azole antifungals
Atorvastatin (Lipitor)	
Lovastatin (Mevacor)	
Rosuvastatin (Crestor)	
Simvastatin (Zocor)	High-dose Zocor (80 mg) has highest risk of rhabdomyolysis (muscle pain/tenderness) Chinese descent: Higher risk myopathy or rhabdomyolysis when taking simvastatin 40 mg/d (or higher) with niacin Creatine kinase level goes up
Lincosamides Clindamycin (Cleocin)	Higher risk of CDAD

*List is not all inclusive.

BID, twice a day; CDAD, *Clostridium difficile*–associated diarrhea; CKD, chronic kidney disease; GERD, gastroesophageal reflux disease; PUD, peptic ulcer disease; TID, three times a day; TSH, thyroid-stimulating hormone TZDs, thiazolidinediones.

DRUGS USED TO TREAT HEART DISEASE

Cardiac Glycosides: Digoxin (Lanoxin)

- Treats certain supraventricular tachyarrhythmias and heart failure (HF) due to left ventricular [LV] systolic dysfunction
  - Digoxin has a narrow therapeutic range (0.5–2.0 ng/mL). Not a first-line drug for heart rate control in most patients with atrial fibrillation
- Signs and symptoms of digoxin overdose:
  - Initial symptoms are gastrointestinal (anorexia, nausea/vomiting, abdominal pain). Others are arrhythmias, confusion, and visual changes (yellowish green tinged-color vision, scotomas)
- What laboratory tests should be ordered if digoxin toxicity is suspected?
  - Order a digoxin level, electrolytes (potassium, magnesium, calcium), creatinine, and serial EKGs
- Treatment: Digoxin-specific antibodies are immunoglobulin G (IgG) antidigoxin antibodies that bind free digoxin in blood (Digibind, DigiFab).
- Potassium values (adult to elderly):
  - Critical: Values that are less than 2.5 or greater than 6.5 mEq/L
  - Normal: Values that are 3.5 to 5.0 mEq/L

Anticoagulants: Warfarin Sodium (Coumadin)

- FDA Pregnancy Category X
- Vitamin K antagonist (VKA)
- Indications: Prophylaxis and treatment thromboembolic events associated with atrial fibrillation or heart valve replacement (pulmonary embolism [PE], deep venous thrombosis [DVT], stroke, thromboemboli)
- Duration of action: 2 to 5 days (single dose)
- For atrial fibrillation, target INR is 2.0 to 3.0 (ideal INR 2.5)
- Initial dose (outpatients): Starting dose 2 to 5 mg orally once a day (maintenance dose 2 to 10 mg per day based on INR value); may start lower doses if elderly patient, liver disease, etc; do not forget to check baseline PT, APTT, creatinine, LFTS, and INR
  - On day 3 (outpatient): Periodically check INR (dose changes are based on INR value); consult with clinic's or hospital's warfarin-dosing protocols.
- Contraindications: See Table 3.3.

Table 3.2 Drugs That Increase Bleeding Risk

Drug Class	Name
Coumarins	Warfarin sodium (Coumadin); reversal/antidote is vitamin K (phytonadione)
Direct thrombin inhibitors	Dabigatran (Pradaxa) oral; reversal/antidote is idarucizumab (Praxbind)
Factor Xa inhibitor	Rivaroxaban (Xarelto), apixaban (Eliquis)
Heparins	Heparin, low-molecular-weight heparin (Lovenox); reversal/antidote is protamine sulfate
Antiplatelet	Clopidogrel (Plavix); no reversal agent yet, but fresh frozen plasma or cryoprecipitate seem effective
Salicylate Other meds that contain salicylate	Aspirin, magnesium salicylate (Doan's Pills), salsalate (Disalcid), bismuth subsalicylate (Pepto-Bismol)
NSAIDs	Ketorolac (Toradol); do not exceed 5 days of use Naproxen (Aleve, Naprosyn), ibuprofen (Advil, Motrin), indomethacin (Indocin) Mefenamic acid (Ponstel) is indicated for dysmenorrhea

NSAIDs, nonsteroidal anti-inflammatory drugs.

Table 3.3 Drug Contraindications*

Drug Class and Generic and Trade Names	Contraindications and Notes
Vitamin K antagonist Warfarin (Coumadin)	Pregnancy (category X), large esophageal varices, thrombocytopenia, recent eye/brain/trauma surgery, within 72 hours of major surgery, blood dyscrasias Careful if history of GI bleeding
ACE inhibitors	Avoid mixing with potassium supplements
Enalapril (Vasotec)	Careful with potassium-sparing diuretics
Captopril (Capoten)	ACE inhibitor cough—new onset of dry cough (not accompanied by upper respiratory infection symptoms), switch to ARB
ARBs	Avoid mixing with potassium supplements
Valsartan (Diovan)	Do not combine ACEI with ARBS
Losartan (Cozaar)	
Potassium-sparing diuretics	Higher risk of hyperkalemia if combined with ACEI, potassium, or ARBs and with severe renal disease
Triamterene (Dyrenium)	
	Diuretics may worsen urinary incontinence
Triamterene + hydrochlorothiazide (Dyazide)	
Amiloride (Midamor)	
Spironolactone (Aldactone)	Avoid combining with ACEI, ARBS, high potassium diet/ supplements, salt substitutes, chronic NSAIDs (risk of hyperkalemia); gynecomastia may occur Aldosterone antagonist activity
Beta-Blockers	Contraindicated if patient has chronic lung diseases (asthma, COPD, emphysema, chronic bronchitis)
Propranolol (Inderal), atenolol (Tenormin), metoprolol (Lopressor), pindolol (Visken)	Do not discontinue beta-blockers abruptly due to severe rebound (hypertensive crisis)
Phosphodiesterase 5 (PDE5) inhibitors Sildenafil (Viagra)	Do not mix with nitrates (nitroglycerine, isosorbide dinitrate) and some alpha-blockers; erection greater than 4 hours—refer to ED
Tadalafil (Cialis) Vardenafil (Levitra)	Do not give within 3 to 6 months of a myocardial infarction, stroke
SSRIs Citalopram (Celexa)	Avoid doses greater than 40 mg/d; can prolong QT interval For patients older than 60 years of age, the maximum dose is 20 mg per day

*List is not all inclusive.

ACEI, angiotensin-converting enzyme inhibitor; ARB, angiotensin receptor blocker; COPD, chronic obstructive pulmonary disease; ED, emergency department; GI, gastrointestinal; HCTZ, hydrochlorothiazide; NSAIDs, nonsteroidal anti-inflammatory drugs; SSRIs, selective serotonin reuptake inhibitors.

Consistently Stable INR

- Check every 2 to 4 weeks up to every 12 weeks per the ACCP

Single Out-of-Range INR

- If patient has stable INR and has a single out-of-range INR equal to or less than 0.5 below or above therapeutic INR (2 to 3), experts suggest continuing current warfarin dose; retest INR within 1 to 2 weeks

INR of Less Than 5 With No Significant Bleeding Risk

- Omit one dose and/or reduce maintenance dose slightly; recheck INR

Signs and Symptoms: Elevated INR

Educate patient to call if prolonged bleeding from cuts, frequent nosebleeds, bloody/tarry stool, hematuria, petechiae, excessive bruising, excessive menstrual bleeding, persistent oozing/bleeding gums after brushing, sudden decrease in hemoglobin, new onset of severe headache especially after a fall (CNS bleed).

One Missed Dose

- Take the dose as soon as possible on the same day. Do *not* double dose the next day

Vitamin K

- The ACCP advises against routine vitamin K1 (phytonadione) supplementation
- Dietary issues: Do not forget to review patient's daily dietary intake of vitamin K foods (kale, spinach, collards/mustard/beet greens, broccoli raab); high intake of vitamin K will reduce anticoagulant effect of warfarin (will decrease INR)
- Contraindications: See Table 3.3

Alcohol

- Avoid drinking or limit to no more than one to two servings occasionally; increases risk of bleeding even if INR is in target range

Adverse Reaction

- "Purple toes syndrome" (rare); skin necrosis located in subcutaneous fat, breasts, extremities, trunk (within first few days of receiving large doses of warfarin)

CLINICAL PEARLS

- **After warfarin is discontinued, anticoagulant effects persist for 2 to 5 days.**
- **Be aware of increased bleeding risk with certain drugs (Table 3.2).**
- **Asian patients may require lower starting and maintenance doses of warfarin.**
- **Some genotypes require lower doses of warfarin.**
- **Persons older than 60 years are more likely to have larger increases in INR (after dose is increased) compared with younger patients.**
- **INR values lower than 2.0 increase stroke risk sixfold.**
- **Mayonnaise, canola oil, and soybean oil also have high levels of vitamin K.**
- **Warfarin algorithms and dosing calculators/programs are available online.**

DIURETICS

Thiazide Diuretics

- Hypertension, HF, edema, diabetes insipidus
- Hypertension accompanied by osteopenia or osteoporosis
- Hydrochlorothiazide (HCTZ)
- Chlorthalidone
- Indapamide (Lozol)
- Do not combine with lithium (increased risk of lithium toxicity)
- **Contraindication**: Sulfa allergy

Adverse Effects

- Elevates plasma glucose/hyperglycemia (careful with diabetics)
- Elevates cholesterol and LDL (careful if preexisting hyperlipidemia)
- Elevates uric acid (can precipitate a gout attack)
- Hypokalemia (severe muscle weakness, arrhythmias)

Pharma Notes

- Chlorthalidone is longer acting and more "effective" than HCTZ. Preferred by Eighth Joint National Committee (JNC 8).
- Patients with both hypertension and osteoporosis have an extra benefit from thiazides.
- Thiazide diuretics reduce calcium excretion by the kidneys and stimulate the osteoblasts. This helps build bone.
- Patients with serious sulfa allergies should avoid thiazide and loop diuretics. Potassium-sparing diuretics, such as triamterene and amiloride (Midamor), are the alternative options for these patients.

Potassium-Sparing Diuretics

- Hypertension, alternative diuretic for patients with severe sulfa allergy
- Triamterene (Dyrenium)
- Amiloride (Midamor)
- Combination: Triamterene and HCTZ (Dyazide), amiloride and HCTZ (Moduretic)
- *Black Box Warning*: Hyperkalemia, which can be fatal; higher risk with renal impairment, diabetes, elderly, severely ill
- Monitor serum potassium (baseline, during, dose changes, illness)
- Contraindications: See Table 3.3.

Mineralcorticoid Receptor Antagonists

- Spironolactone (Aldactone): Hypertension, HF, hirsutism (also considered as a potassium-sparing diuretic)
- Eplerenone (Inspra)

Pharma Notes

- Do not give potassium supplement. Avoid using salt substitutes that contain potassium.
- Be careful with combinations of angiotensin-converting enzyme inhibitors (ACEIs)/ angiotensin-receptor blockers (ARBs) or NSAIDs; increases risk of hyperkalemia.
- Avoid with severe renal disease (increases risk of hyperkalemia).
- Spironolactone adverse effects: Gynecomastia (13%) and hyperkalemia.
  - *Black Box Warning*: There is increased risk of both benign and malignant tumors.

Loop Diuretics

- Edema from heart failure, cirrhosis, renal disease, and hypertension
- Loop diuretics are excreted via the loop of Henle of the kidneys and are more potent than HCTZ
- Furosemide (Lasix)

- Bumetanide (Bumex)
- More potent than thiazides but with shorter duration of action
- *Black Box Warning*: Excessive amounts of furosemide may lead to profound diuresis; medical supervision required, individualized dose schedule
- **Contraindication**: Sulfa allergy

Adverse Effects

- Electrolytes (hypokalemia, hyponatremia, hypomagnesemia, and low levels of chlorine)
- Hypovolemia and hypotension (dizziness, lightheadedness)
- Pancreatitis, jaundice, and rash
- Ototoxicity (worsens aminoglycoside ototoxicity effect if combined)

DRUGS USED TO TREAT HYPERTENSION

Beta-Blockers (Beta-Antagonists)

- Hypertension, postmyocardial infarction (MI), angina, arrhythmias, and migraine prophylaxis
- Beta-blockers are preferred for treating angina pectoris and postacute MI (unless contraindicated such as shock, hypotension, severe bradycardia, heart block greater than first-degree block, chronic pulmonary disease)
- Adjunctive treatment: Hyperthyroidism/thyrotoxicosis (decreases heart rate, and anxiety)
- Propranolol and carvedilol (Coreg) are noncardioselective beta blockers (blocks beta-1 and beta-2)
    - Propranolol immediate release (Inderal) or extended release (Inderal LA)
- Cardioselective beta-blockers are more potent because they block beta-1 receptors, which are found mainly in the heart
    - Atenolol (Tenormin) daily
    - Metoprolol immediate release (Lopressor) or extended release (Toprol XL)
- Timolol oral (Blocadren) or timolol ophthalmic drops (glaucoma)
- **Contraindications**: See also Table 3.3
    - Asthma (causes bronchoconstriction)
    - Chronic obstructive pulmonary disease (COPD; causes bronchoconstriction)
    - Chronic bronchitis (causes bronchoconstriction)
    - Emphysema (causes bronchoconstriction)
    - Bradycardia and atrioventricular (AV) block (second- to third-degree block)

Adverse Effects

- Bronchospasm (blocks beta-2 receptors in the lungs)
- Bradycardia (blocks beta-1 receptors in the heart)
- Depression, fatigue (careful with elderly)
- Erectile dysfunction
- Blunts hypoglycemic response (warn diabetic patients)
- HF

ACE Inhibitors and Angiotensin Receptor Blockers (Colucci, 2018)

- Hypertension, diabetes (renal), chronic kidney disease (CKD), post-MI, heart failure
- Improve left ventricular ejection fraction (LVEF) and survival post-MI
- Preferred agents for patients with heart failure with reduced ejection fraction (HFrEF) are the ACEIs or ARBs, and mineral corticoid receptor antagonist (spironolactone, eplerone)

- Category C (first trimester) and category D (second to third trimesters)
- ACE inhibition blocks conversion of angiotensin I to angiotensin II (potent vasoconstrictor); ACEI suffix of "pril"
- ARBs block angiotensin II (less aldosterone); ARB suffix of "sartan"
- *Black Box Warning*: ACEIs can cause death/injury to the developing fetus during the second and third trimesters; discontinue ACEIs and ARBs immediately if pregnant
- **Contraindications**: See Table 3.3; ACEI-/ARB-associated angioedema, hereditary angioedema

ACEIs

- Ramipril (Altace)
- Lisinopril (Zestril, Prinivil)
- Benazepril (Lotensin)
- Captopril (Capoten)
- Enalapril (Vasotec)
- Combination: Lisinopril and HCTZ (Zestoretic), enalapril and HCTZ (Vaseretic), captopril and HCTZ (Capozide), benazepril and amlodipine (Lotrel)

ARBs

- Losartan (Cozaar)
- Irbesartan (Avapro)
- Valsartan (Diovan)
- Candesartan (Atacand)
- Combination: Losartan and HCTZ (Hyzaar), valsartan and HCTZ (Diovan HCT), valsartan and amlodipine (Exforge)

Adverse Effects

- Angioedema and anaphylactoid reactions
- ACEI cough
- Hyperkalemia

Direct Renin Inhibitor

- Aliskiren (Tekturna) blocks the catalytic action of renin, JNC 8 does not recommend aliskiren as initial treatment for hypertension.
- **Contraindications**: Concomitant use of ACEI or ARBs, angioedema, pregnancy/breastfeeding, age younger than 2 years

Pharma Notes

- ACEI cough occurs within the first few months of treatment. It is a dry and hacking cough (without other symptoms of upper respiratory infection). Stop ACEI and switch to an ARB.
- ACEIs and ARBs are preferred drugs for hypertension in diabetics (diabetic nephropathy), and for patients with CKD.
- Avoid using salt substitutes that contain potassium.
- Captopril is associated with agranulocytosis, neutropenia, leukopenia (rare). Monitor CBC.
- Both ACEIs and ARBs are excreted in breast milk (breastfeeding mothers should avoid them).

CLINICAL PEARLS

- **JNC 8 encourages use of chlorthalidone (longer acting, more effective). If your patient is already on HCTZ and doing well, do not change. But if you have a new hypertensive patient or one with a BP that is hard to control, consider chlorthalidone 12.5 to 25 mg alone or combined with ACEI or ARBs (or another antihypertensive drug class). Baseline electrolytes, such as sodium, potassium, and calcium, are needed.**
- **Be careful prescribing ACEIs/ARBs to sexually active, reproductive-aged females who are not consistently using birth control (categories C and D during the second and third trimester). Warn patients taking salt substitutes that some contain potassium.**

Calcium Channel Blockers (Calcium Antagonists)

- Hypertension, angina, arrhythmias, Raynaud's phenomenon (first line)
- Amlodipine (Norvasc)
- Diltiazem (Cardizem)
- Nifedipine (Procardia)
- Verapamil (Calan): Do not mix with erythromycin and clarithromycin (drug interaction)
- **Contraindications**
  - AV block (second- to third-degree block)
  - Bradycardia
  - Congestive heart failure (CHF)

Pharma Notes

- Careful/limit use of short-acting acting calcium blockers such as nifedipine (increases mortality). Long-acting CCBs show no increased risk.
- Up to 25% patients on verapamil develop constipation.

Adverse Effects

- Headache (vasodilation)
- Peripheral edema (not due to fluid overload)
- Bradycardia
- HF and heart block
- Hypotension, QT prolongation
- Constipation is the most commonly reported side effect

Alpha-Blockers

- Hypertension with coexisting benign prostatic hyperplasia (BPH); alpha blockers are initial therapy for symptomatic BPH
- Terazosin (Hytrin) 1 mg PO at bedtime
- Doxazosin (Cardura)

Adverse Effects

- Orthostatic hypotension
- Dizziness, syncope
- Priapism (Flomax)
- Do not give during cataract/glaucoma surgery (floppy iris syndrome)

Pharma Notes

- This is not a first-line choice except for males with both hypertension and BPH.
- Potent vasodilator. Common side effects are dizziness and hypotension. Give at bedtime at very low dose and slowly titrate up. Careful with frail elderly (risk of syncope and falls).
- Some experts recommend taking some antihypertensive medications (except diuretics) in the evening. The physiologic increase in BP occurs in early morning (3 to 5 a.m.) and peaks in early afternoon.

CLINICAL PEARLS

- **In the United States, most heart attacks occur during the morning hours (6 a.m. to 12 p.m.).**
- **The day of the week when most MIs occur is Monday, and the season when most MIs occur is in winter.**

ANTIBIOTICS

Antibiotics are either bacteriostatic or bactericidal. Bactericidal antibiotics kill bacteria. Bacteriostatic antibiotics limit bacterial growth and replication. The result is a lower bacterial count, which helps the immune system clear the infection.

Tetracyclines (Category D)

Tetracyclines are bacteriostatic. They may cause permanent discoloration of teeth (brown to yellow) and skeletal defects if taken during the last half of pregnancy, in infancy, or by children younger than 9 years of age.

Generally, tetracyclines are not used in children who are younger than 9 years of age. Treat acne starting at age 13 to 14 years. By this age, all permanent teeth have erupted (except wisdom teeth).

- Doxycycline
- Minocycline
- Tetracycline

Adverse Reactions

- Photosensitivity reaction (severe sunburns) occurs with minimal sunlight exposure; avoid or minimize sunlight exposure; use sunblock, wide-brim hats, and sunglasses
- Esophageal ulcerations are rare; swallow tablet completely using a full glass of water
- **Contraindications**: Avoid in pregnancy, infancy, and in children aged 8 years or younger

Pharma Notes

- Do not use oral tetracycline for mild acne (comedones). Start with OTC topicals such as salicylic acid (Noxzema, Stridex) and benzoyl peroxide.
- For mild acne not responding to OTC drugs, try prescription topicals (benzoyl peroxide and erythromycin/Benzamycin), tretinoin (Retin-A), azelaic acid cream.

(continued)

(continued)

- Consider adding tetracycline if a patient with moderate inflammatory acne is not responding to topical prescriptions (Benzamycin, Retin-A, azelaic acid) after 2 to 3 months.
- Another option to tetracycline is minocycline (Minocin).
- Tetracycline binds to some minerals (calcium, dairy products, iron, magnesium, zinc). It is best to take it on an empty stomach. Take 1 hour before or 2 hours after a meal.
- Tetracyclines may decrease effectiveness of oral contraceptive pills.
- Minocycline (Minocin) can cause vertigo (more common in females) that is dose related. It usually resolves in 1 to 2 days after discontinuation of the drug.
- Advise patients to throw away expired tetracycline pills (they degenerate and may cause nephropathy or Fanconi syndrome; Table 3.4).

Table 3.4 Macrolides and Tetracyclines

Generic Name (Trade Name)	Drug Interactions
Macrolides	
Erythromycin BID to QID	Many major drug interactions **Contraindication**: Myasthenia gravis (respiratory failure)
Azithromycin (Z-Pack)	Anticoagulants: Warfarin (Coumadin) Avoid mixing with antacids (decreased effectiveness)
Clarithromycin BID	QT prolongation/bradyarrhythmias: Verapamil (Calan), amlodipine (Norvasc), diltiazem (Cardizem), amiodarone, others Benzodiazepines: Triazolam (Halcion), midazolam (Versed) Asthma: Salmeterol (Serevent), theophylline Others: Anticonvulsants (carbamazepine [Tegretol], phenytoin), ergotamine, statins (rhabdomyolysis), and others
Ketolide	
Telithromycin (Ketek) once a day	*Black Box Warning*: Myasthenia gravis patients—do not use Do not use in children; causes liver failure; avoid if history of jaundice/hepatitis from macrolides Same drug interactions as macrolides
Tetracyclines	
Tetracycline QID	Photosensitivity reactions (use hat, sunblock)
Doxycycline BID	If taken without water and pill gets stuck in the esophagus, it can cause esophagitis/esophageal ulceration Binds with iron, calcium, magnesium, zinc
Minocycline (Minocin) BID	Antacids, sucralfate, and bile acid sequestrants markedly decrease absorption; oral contraceptives (may decrease effectiveness); can cause pseudotumor cerebri

BID, twice a day; QID, four times a day.

Macrolides (Category B)

Macrolides are bacteriostatic. They cover gram-positive cocci (except enterococci), *Staphylococcus aureus*, *Streptococcus pyogenes*, and atypical bacteria (i.e., mycoplasma, chlamydia). Compared with other antibiotic drug classes, macrolides (and quinolones) are associated with more drug interactions. Both erythromycin and clarithromycin (Biaxin) are potent CYP 34A inhibitors, but not azithromycin (which has fewer drug interactions). All macrolides are category B except clarithromycin and telithromycin (both are category C; avoid using in pregnancy).

- Erythromycin (Ery-Tab, E.E.S.) BID to QID
- Azithromycin (Z-Pack)
- Clarithromycin (Biaxin) BID

Adverse Effects

- GI distress (diarrhea, nausea, vomiting)
- Ototoxicity, cholestatic jaundice
- QT with prolongation (risk of torsades de pointes)

Pharma Notes

- Erythromycin's GI side effects are common (nausea, vomiting, abdominal pain, diarrhea).
- If a condition must be treated with a macrolide (i.e., atypical bacteria) and the patient cannot tolerate erythromycin, switch the patient to azithromycin (Z-Pack) or clarithromycin (Biaxin).
- Multiple drug interactions (anticoagulants, digoxin, theophylline, astemizole, carbamazepine, cisapride, triazolam, terfenadine).

CLINICAL PEARLS

- **Advise patients to use only one pharmacy so that all the drugs they take are on one database. This makes it easier for the pharmacy to check for drug interactions.**
- **May prolong INR and increase risk of bleeding if warfarin is mixed with erythromycin or clarithromycin.**

Cephalosporins (Category B)

- Cephalosporins and penicillins belong to the beta-lactam family of antibiotics.
- Beta-lactams are bactericidal and work by interfering with the cell wall synthesis of actively growing bacteria.
- There are five generations of cephalosporins. However, as the NP certification exams are about primary care conditions, only the first to the third generations are covered.

First-Generation Cephalosporins

- Activity against gram-positive cocci bacteria (group A streptococcus, *S. aureus*)
- Not effective against beta-lactamase producing strains and methicillin-resistant *Staphylococcus aureus* (MRSA)
- Poor anaerobic coverage; increased risk of cross-reactivity if allergic to penicillin

Second-Generation Cephalosporins

- Considered to be "broad-spectrum" antibiotics; used to treat infections caused by both gram-positive cocci (*Streptococcus. pneumoniae*) and gram-negative bacteria (i.e., *Haemophilus influenzae, Moraxella catarrhalis*) such as rhinosinusitis and otitis media

Third-Generation Cephalosporins

- Less effective against gram-positive infections compared to the first-generation cephalosporins
- Better protection against enterobacteria and gram-negative bacteria (i.e., *H. influenzae, Escherichia coli, Proteus mirabilis*) compared to first or second generation cephalosporins

Pharma Notes

- Rocephin (ceftriaxone) 250 mg IM is first-line treatment for gonorrheal infections.
- MRSA skin infections (boils, abscesses)—do not use cephalosporins. First-line therapy is either trimethoprim–sulfa (Bactrim DS), doxycycline or minocycline, and clindamycin. Treat for at least 5 to 10 days.
- Patients who have a true allergy to penicillin (history of anaphylaxis, angioedema) are more likely to have an allergic reaction to cephalosporins (especially first generation).
- Anaphylaxis and angioedema are type 1 IgE-mediated reactions (Table 3.5).

Table 3.5 Cephalosporins and Penicillins*

Generic Name (Trade Name)	Indications
Cephalosporins	
First generation	
Cephalexin (Keflex) PO QID	Pregnancy: Urinary tract infection (if sensitive) pregnancy Skin: Cellulitis (not caused by MRSA), impetigo
Second generation	
Cefuroxime axetil (Ceftin) PO BID	ENT: Rhinosinusitis, otitis media
Cefprozil (Cefzil) PO BID	Lungs: CAP, exacerbation chronic bronchitis
Cefaclor (Ceclor) PO BID	Avoid using cefaclor because it does not cover common pathogens
Third generation	
Ceftriaxone (Rocephin) IM	STDS: Gonorrhea infections, pelvic inflammatory disease Renal: pyelonephritis
Cefixime (Suprax) daily to BID	ENT: Acute otitis media in children, acute rhinosinusitis, otitis media
Cefdinir (Omnicef) daily to BID	Genitourinary: Pyelonephritis Lungs: CAP
Penicillins	
Penicillin VK PO QID	Strep throat (first line)
Amoxicillin BID to TID	Otitis media (first line), rhinosinusitis (first line)
Amoxicillin plus clavulanic acid (Augmentin PO BID)	Otitis media/rhinosinusitis (first to second line) Cystitis
Benzathine penicillin G IM	Syphilis (first line)
Dicloxacillin PO QID	Penicillinase-resistant penicillin; cellulitis (not caused by MRSA), impetigo, erysipelas

*List is not all inclusive.

BID, twice a day; CAP, community-acquired pneumonia; ENT, ear–nose–throat; IM, intramuscular; MRSA, methicillin-resistant Staphylococcus aureus; PO, by mouth; QID, four times a day; VK, V potassium.

Penicillins (Category B)

Penicillins are bactericidal and directly kill bacteria. Amoxicillin and ampicillin are broad-spectrum penicillins. They are effective against gram-positive bacteria as well some gram-negative bacteria (*H. influenzae, E. coli, P. mirabilis*).

- Penicillin VK PO TID to QID
- Amoxicillin PO BID to TID
- Amoxicillin plus clavulanic acid (Augmentin) PO BID
- Benzathine penicillin G IM
- Dicloxacillin PO QID

Adverse Reactions

- Diarrhea
- *Clostridium difficile*-associated diarrhea (CDAD)
- Vaginitis (usually candida)
- Stevens–Johnson syndrome

Pharma Notes

- Avoid using amoxicillin for patients with mononucleosis (causes a generalized rash not related to allergy). Use penicillin VK instead (if not allergic). If penicillin allergy, use a macrolide antibiotic.
- Dicloxacillin is for penicillinase-producing staph skin infections (mastitis and impetigo).
- Patients who have a true allergy to penicillin (history of anaphylaxis, angioedema) are more likely to have an allergic reaction to cephalosporins (especially, first generation).
- Anaphylaxis and angioedema are type 1 IgE-mediated reactions.
- Some women will complain of candida vaginitis with amoxicillin. Recommend probiotic capsules or eating yogurt daily.

Fluoroquinolones (Quinolones; Table 3.6)

Quinolones are bactericidal. Effective against gram-negative bacteria and some atypical bacteria (*Chlamydia, Mycoplasma, Legionella*). Newer generation quinolones (levofloxacin, moxifloxacin, gatifloxacin) are also active against gram-positive bacteria and have excellent activity against streptococcal pneumonia.

- Fluoroquinolones
  - Ciprofloxacin (Cipro, Ciloxan Opthalmic) PO BID
  - Ofloxacin (Floxin, Ocuflox Opthalmic) PO BID
- Broad-spectrum quinolones
  - Levofloxacin (Levaquin) PO daily
  - Moxifloxacin (Avelox) PO daily
  - Gemifloxacin (Factive) PO daily
- *Black Box Warnings*
  - Increased risk of Achilles tendon rupture. Avoid strenuous activity while on the drug. Stop drug if tendon pain/swelling develops.
  - The Food and Drug Administration (FDA) states "serious side effects associated with fluoroquinolones generally outweigh the benefits for patients with sinusitis, bronchitis, and uncomplicated urinary tract infections who have other treatment options … for

patients with these conditions, fluoroquinolones should be reserved for those who do not have alternative treatment options" (FDA, 2016).

- **Contraindications**:
  - Children (younger than 18 years of age)
  - Myasthenia gravis
  - Pregnancy, breastfeeding

Table 3.6 Quinolones*

Generic Name (Trade Name)	Indications
Ciprofloxacin (Cipro) BID	Anthrax infection and prophylaxis (Cipro)
	Traveler's diarrhea (Cipro)
Ofloxacin (Floxin) BID	Urinary tract infections, pyelonephritis, epididymitis, prostatitis
	Black Box Warning: Risk of tendinitis and Achilles tendinopathy/ rupture
Broad-spectrum quinolones:	Levofloxacin: Increased risk of hypoglycemia
Levofloxacin (Levaquin) daily	Community-acquired pneumonia, acute exacerbation of chronic bronchitis, pyelonephritis, epididymitis, prostatitis
Moxifloxacin (Avelox) daily	Osteomyelitis, sinusitis, acute otitis media
Gemifloxacin (Factive) daily	
Topical formulations	
Floxin Otic (gtts)	Otitis media with perforated tympanic membrane, otitis externa
Ocuflox ophthalmic (gtts)	Bacterial conjunctivitis

*List is not all inclusive.
BID, twice a day.

Drug Interactions

Avoid concomitant use of quinolones with other QT-prolonging drugs (amiodarone, macrolides, tricyclic antidepressants [TCAs], antipsychotics, others) or with electrolyte imbalance (hypomagnesemia, hypokalemia) because these will elevate the risk of sudden death from arrhythmias (torsades de pointes).

Coadministration of minerals and antacids (aluminum/magnesium/calcium) or sucralfate drastically reduces effectiveness of quinolones due to binding (inactivation).

Adverse Effects

- Hypoglycemia (monitor blood glucose in diabetics)
- CNS effects (confusion, dizziness, headache, insomnia, seizures)
- QT prolongation, torsades de pointes
- Peripheral neuropathy
- Phototoxicity (advise patients to avoid excessive sunlight or UV light)
- Double vision
- Tendon rupture, tendinitis

Pharma Notes

- Achilles tendon rupture is a serious complication of quinolone therapy and patients who are on steroids or older than 60 years are at higher risk.
- Do not use quinolones in children (younger than 18 years) or women who are pregnant or breastfeeding due to adverse effects on growing cartilage.

(continued)

(continued)

- If a patient on quinolone reports a new onset of difficulty in walking, order an ultrasound to rule out Achilles tendon rupture or peripheral neuropathy and discontinue the medicine.
- Bioterrorism-related inhalation of anthrax spores (postexposure prophylaxis) is treated with ciprofloxacin 500 mg every 12 hours × 60 days (treat within 48 hours.). In addition, a three-dose series of anthrax vaccine is recommended.
- Cutaneous anthrax is treated with ciprofloxacin 500 mg BID × 7–10 days.
- Traveler's diarrhea is treated with Cipro 500 mg BID × 3 days.
- Ciprofloxacin has the best activity against *Pseudomonas aeruginosa* (gram negative) and is the first-line drug for treating pseudomonal pneumonia for patients with cystic fibrosis.

CLINICAL PEARL

Moxifloxacin (Avelox) is more likely to cause a hypersensitivity reaction compared with levofloxacin or ciprofloxacin (Prescriber's Letter, 2013).

Sulfonamides (Category C)

- Sulfonamides are bacteriostatic
- Active against gram-negative bacteria (*E. coli, Klebsiella, H. influenzae*)
- Trimethoprim–sulfamethoxazole (TMP-SMX) Bactrim DS BID
- Erythromycin–sulfisoxazole (Pediazole)
- Other sulfa-type drugs:
  - Diuretics (furosemide, HCTZ)
  - Sulfonylureas (glyburide, glipizide, etc.)
  - COX-2 inhibitor (celecoxib or Celebrex)
  - Dapsone (for HIV)
  - Sulfasalazine (for rheumatoid arthritis, Crohn's disease, ulcerative colitis)
  - Nitrofurantoin
- **Contraindications**:
  - Glucose-6-phosphate dehydrogenase (G6PD) anemia (a genetic hemolytic anemia) causes hemolysis
  - Newborns and infants younger than 2 months of age
  - Pregnancy in late third trimester (increased risk of hyperbilirubinemia/kernicterus)
  - Hypersensitivity to sulfa drugs

Drug Interactions

- Warfarin (increases INR)
- Astemizole (Hismanal)
- Others

Adverse Effects

Fever and nonblistering morbilliform rash, Stevens–Johnson syndrome, and others

Pharma Notes

- Patients with a UTI who are on warfarin (Coumadin) should not be given TMP-SMX (increased risk of bleeding). Monitor INR closely.
- Pregnant women (or suspected pregnancy) with a UTI can be treated with amoxicillin or cephalosporins (FDA category B).

CLINICAL PEARLS

- **HIV patients are at high risk (25%–50%) for sulfa-related Stevens–Johnson syndrome.**
- **In the United States, the typical G6PD deficiency anemia patient is a person of African American (10%) descent. Usually asymptomatic, but may present with hemolysis/ jaundice secondary to being treated with a sulfa drug or after eating fava beans. Look for a low hemoglobin and hematocrit (H&H) and jaundice. G6PD anemia is also seen with Mediterranean ancestry.**
- **Sulfonamide antibiotics are the second most frequent cause of allergic drug reactions (penicillins and cephalosporins are the first; Table 3.7).**

Table 3.7 Sulfonamides

Generic Name	Indications
TMP-SMX, Bactrim DS BID	Prophylaxis/ treatment of PCP (HIV-patients) MRSA cellulitis Urinary tract infections, pyelonephritis
Topical and ophthalmic sulfas	Bacterial conjunctivitis
Sulfacetamide ophthalmic	
Silver sulfadiazine (Silvadene)	Burns

BID, twice a day; DS, double strength; MRSA, methicillin-resistant *Staphylococcus aureus*; PCP, *Pneumocystis carinii* pneumonia; TMP-SMX, trimethoprim-sulfamethoxazole.

ANTIBIOTIC CASE SCENARIOS

Case 1

Penicillin-Allergic Patient With Strep Throat

An 18-year-old female patient has a positive throat C&S for *Streptococcus pyogenes* (group A beta streptococci). The patient reports a history of an allergic reaction to penicillin with "swollen lips" accompanied by itchy hives. Which of the following is the most appropriate treatment?

A) Clarithromycin (Biaxin) 250 mg PO BID × 10 days
B) Gargle with salt water three times a day
C) Cephalexin (Keflex) 250 mg PO QID × 10 days
D) Doxycycline 100 mg PO BID × 10 days

Question Dissection

Correct answer is option A: **A)** Clarithromycin (Biaxin) 250 mg PO BID × 10 days

Best Clues

- Positive C&S for strep
- Report of a penicillin allergy
- Rule out the following options because:
  - Option B (gargling with salt water is for symptoms and will not eradicate strep)

- Option C (penicillin-allergic patients may also be allergic to cephalosporins)
- Option D (doxycycline not effective for gram-positive infections)

Pharma Notes

- Become familiar with alternative antibiotics for penicillin-allergic patients. A good alternative antibiotic for these patients with gram-positive bacterial infections are macrolides such as azithromycin × 5 days (Z-Pack) or clarithromycin (Biaxin) PO BID.
- Clindamycin (Cleocin) is also an alternative, but it is associated with slightly higher risk of *Clostridium difficile* colitis.
- If age 18 years or older, quinolones with gram-positive activity (levofloxacin, gatifloxacin) are an option for some infections.

Case 2

Patient With Both Mononucleosis and Strep Throat Infection

A 16-year-old high school athlete is returning for follow-up for a severe sore throat. During the physical exam, purulent exudate is noted on both tonsils. Tender lymph nodes that are 1 cm in diameter are palpable on the posterior cervical chains. The lungs are clear. The rapid strep antigen test is positive for group A beta hemolytic *Streptococcus*. The Monospot test (heterophile antibody test) is positive. What is the best *initial* clinical management of this patient?

A) Initiate a prescription of amoxicillin 500 mg PO BID × 10 days
B) Initiate a prescription of penicillin V 250 mg PO TID × 10 days
C) Order an Epstein–Barr virus titer to determine whether the patient has an acute or a reactivated mononucleosis infection
D) Write a prescription for an abdominal ultrasound to determine the size of the patient's liver and spleen

Question Dissection

Correct answer is option B: **B)** Initiate a prescription of penicillin V 250 mg PO TID × 10 days

Best Clues

- Positive test results (Monospot and strep)
- Rule out:
  - Option A (avoid using amoxicillin if a patient has mononucleosis because of the risk of an amoxicillin "drug rash" that is not due to an allergy)
  - Option C (not for initial management of uncomplicated mononucleosis)
  - Option D (not for initial management; only for cases in which the physical exam reveals an enlarged liver and/or spleen)

Pharma Notes

- In the case of rash in mononucleosis patients who are treated with amoxicillin, it is very hard to determine whether the rash is due to a true allergy or whether the patient has a benign nonallergic drug rash. About 70% to 90% of patients with mono taking amoxicillin may break out with a "nonallergic" generalized maculopapular rash (mechanism is not well understood).
- If a patient has both mono and strep throat, avoid using amoxicillin or ampicillin. Instead, use penicillin (if not allergic) or a macrolide to treat the patient.

CLINICAL PEARL

Of patients with true penicillin allergy, a small percentage (0.17%–8.4%) will also react to a cephalosporin.

Case 3

Young Adult With History of GI Symptoms After Taking Erythromycin

A 25-year-old healthy male who is a nonsmoker is diagnosed with atypical pneumonia. The patient reports a history of nausea, upset stomach, and vomiting with erythromycin. The vital signs are temperature of 99.8°F, pulse of 80/min, and respiratory rate of 16 breaths/min. What is the most appropriate treatment plan for this patient?

A) Initiate a prescription of azithromycin (Z-Pack) PO × 5 days
B) Initiate a prescription of trimethoprim–sulfamethoxazole (Bactrim) 1 tablet PO BID × 10 days
C) Order a CBC with differential
D) Order a sputum for culture and sensitivity

Question Dissection

Correct answer is option A: **A)** Initiate a prescription of azithromycin (Z-Pack) PO × 5 days

Best Clues

- The patient has atypical pneumonia but is a healthy young adult and a nonsmoker. He is not febrile or toxic (fever is temperature of 100.4°F).
- Rule out:
  - Option B (Bactrim is not effective against *Mycoplasma* or *Chlamydia* bacterial infections, but it is an excellent drug for some gram-negative infections such as urinary tract infections [UTIS])
  - Option C (ordering a CBC with differential is not necessary in this case)
  - Option D (for community-acquired pneumonia [CAP], ordering a sputum for C&S is not recommended by the American Thoracic Society/Infectious Diseases Society of America [ATS/IDSA] treatment guidelines for CAP)

Pharma Notes

- GI upset (nausea and vomiting, abdominal pain) is a common side effect of erythromycin—it is not an allergic reaction (such as angioedema, hives, anaphylaxis). If a patient who needs a macrolide is not allergic, azithromycin (Z-Pack) is a good choice. It usually does not cause GI side effects, has fewer drug interactions, and a broader spectrum of activity.
- If the patient is allergic to macrolides, an alternative is doxycycline PO BID or the new-generation quinolones (Levaquin, Avelox) if age 18 years or older.

CLINICAL PEARL

Consider macrolide-resistant *S. pneumoniae* if the patient was on a macrolide in the previous 3 months.

Case 4

Answer Options Listed by Drug Class

A 65-year-old male presents with a history of a chronic cough that is productive of large amounts of off-white-colored sputum. The patient reports a 30-pack-year history of cigarette smoking. The chest x-ray reveals hyperinflation with flattened diaphragms and two small bullae on the left lobe. Which of the following drug classes is the initial treatment of choice for this condition?

A) Short-acting beta-2 agonists
B) Anticholinergics
C) Pneumococcal polysaccharide vaccine (Pneumovax)
D) Oxygen by nasal cannula

Question Dissection

The correct answer is option A: **A)** Short-acting beta-2 agonists

Best Clues

- Arriving at the correct answer is based on your knowledge of the current COPD treatment guidelines (Global Initiative for COPD/GOLD, 2015).
- Notice that the stem of the question is asking for the "initial treatment" (rule out options B, C, and D).

Pharma Notes

- For COPD patients with mild dyspnea, the initial treatment choice is a short-acting beta-2 agonist (albuterol, levalbuterol) or a short-acting anticholinergic (ipratropium bromide), or both. If not effective, the next step is either a long-acting beta-2 agonist (salmeterol) or a long-acting anticholinergic (tiotropium), or both. If the question is asking you for the next step (if symptoms are not better with short-acting bronchodilators), then start on a long-acting beta-2 agonist alone or combined with a long-acting anticholinergic.
- Smoking cessation is important. The flu vaccine and Pneumovax is recommended for all with COPD—it is considered a primary prevention measure.
- "Pack year" is calculated by multiplying the number of packs smoked per day by the number of years a person has smoked. One pack contains 20 cigarettes.

OVER-THE-COUNTER (OTC) DRUGS AND HERBS

Topical Nasal Decongestants

Oxymetazoline Nasal Spray (Afrin) and Phenylephrine (Neo-Synephrine)

- Short-term use of topical nasal decongestants (BID PRN × 3 days) is considered safe treatment for nasal congestion (common cold, allergic rhinitis)
- Rhinitis medicamentosa is due to chronic use (>3 days) of nasal decongestants

Antihistamines (histamine antagonist or H1 blocker)

Diphenhydramine (Benadryl), Loratadine (Claritin), and Cetirizine (Zyrtec)

- Avoid using diphenhydramine (Benadryl) in the elderly, if possible
- For elderly patients, use loratadine (Claritin) because it has a lower incidence of sedation
- Zyrtec is more potent and long acting. It is very effective for acute and chronic urticaria

Topical Antihistamines

- Nasal sprays: Allergic rhinitis, seasonal allergic rhinitis, vasomotor rhinitis
- Azelastine (Astelin) nasal spray

Ophthalmic Drops

- Pruritus from allergic conjunctivitis
- Azelastine hydrochloride ophthalmic solution 0.5%

Cold, Cough, and/or Sinus Medicines

Decongestants

- Pseudoephedrine (Sudafed) and phenylephrine
- The Combat Methamphetamine Epidemic Act of 2005 restricts the amount of pseudoephedrine you can buy; you must log in and present your ID to the pharmacy

Antitussives

- Dextromethorphan (Robitussin, Delsym) and benzonatate (Tessalon)
- Dextromethorphan increases risk of serotonin syndrome (major drug interaction) with MAOIs, selegiline (Eldepryl), SSRIs, and SNRIs.

Mucolytics

- Guaifenesin and water (Hydration)

CLINICAL PEARLS

- **Decongestants are contraindicated with hypertension, CAD (angina, MI).**
- **Advise patients that mixing decongestants with other stimulants (caffeine, Ritalin, albuterol inhaler) will cause heart palpitations, tremors, and anxiety.**

NSAIDs

OTC NSAIDs

- Ibuprofen (Advil, Motrin), naproxen sodium (Aleve)

Prescription NSAIDs

- Naproxen (Naprosyn, Anaprox), diclofenac (Voltaren) oral and topical gel
- Indomethacin (Indocin), ketoprofen (Orudis), ketorolac (Toradol)
- Cyclo-oxygenase-2 (COX-2) inhibitors: Celecoxib (Celebrex)

Topical NSAIDs

- Skin topical: Joint pain from osteoarthritis/DJD
- Diclofenac gel 1% (Voltaren Gel), diclofenac solution 1.5% (Pennsaid), patch 1.3% (Flector)

Ophthalmic NSAIDs

- Seasonal allergic conjunctivitis (for itch), eye pain after cataract surgery ketorolac ophthalmic (Acular)

NSAID Warnings

- NSAIDs should be avoided in HF, severe heart disease, GI bleeding, severe renal disease and during the last 3 months of pregnancy
- Patients with nasal polyps and asthma can be sensitive to aspirin/NSAIDs
- Ketorolac (Toradol) IM, IV, or tablets are for short-term use only (up to 5 days)

- **Contraindications**: Ketorolac should not be used before surgery, with concurrent acetylsalicylic acid (ASA), pediatric patients, active or recent GI bleed, stroke, labor/delivery, and others.
- For long-term use, document informed consent such as the higher risk of serious MI, stroke, emboli, GI bleeds, acute renal failure.
- COX-2 inhibitors (celecoxib) have lower risk of GI bleeding compared with the other NSAIDs. They are not a first-line NSAID except for patients at high risk for GI bleeding.
- Increased risk of bleeding if NSAIDs are combined with warfarin, dabigatran (Pradaxa), steroids, aspirin, alcohol. For long-term use, consider prescribing concurrent proton-pump inhibitors (PPIs), H2-receptor antagonists, or misoprostol (Cytotec). Cytotec is a synthetic prostaglandin.
- Avoid long-term use of NSAIDs if patient is on aspirin prophylaxis (interferes with aspirin's cardioprotective effect).
- NSAIDs may worsen hypertension in patients who were previously well controlled.

Salicylates

- Aspirin (Bayer) 325 mg to 650 mg every 4 to 6 hours PRN
- Aspirin controlled/extended/delayed release (enteric-coated): 650 to 1,300 mg every 8 hours (do not exceed 3.9 g/d)
  - Acute coronary syndrome: 160 to 325 mg PO; chew nonenteric-coated tablet as soon as possible (within minutes of symptoms)
  - Secondary prevention (MI, stroke): 75 to 81 mg PO daily (up to 325 mg/d)
  - Aspirin 845 mg with caffeine (BC Powder): One powder sublingually every 6 hours PRN; drink or mix powder with full glass of water
- Topical: Methyl salicylate and menthol (BenGay gel/cream)
- Nonacetylated salicylates: Salsalate (Disalcid), namebutone (Relafen)
- Do not take aspirin under the age of 12 years (Reye's syndrome)

Capsaicin

- Capsaicin topical cream (Zostrix HP), capsaicin patch
  - For temporary relief of muscle and joint pain (arthritis, sprains/ strains, bruises)
  - For neuropathic pain (postherpetic neuralgia [PHN], trigeminal neuralgia)
- May take up to 4 weeks to work; may cause temporary burning sensation; do not use on broken skin; advise patient to wash hands with soap and water immediately after using capsaicin cream and to avoid touching the eyes, nose, and mouth

Acetaminophen (Tylenol)

- Adults and children 12 years of age or older; maximum dose ranges from 3,000 mg (3 g) to 3,250 mg/d or 3,900/day (almost 4 g/d)
- Considered first-line drug for pain from osteoarthritis/DJD
- Regular-strength Tylenol (325 mg): Take two tablets every 4 to 6 hours PRN; do not take more than ten tablets in 24 hours (maximum dose is 3,250 mg in 24 hr)
- Extra-strength Tylenol (500 mg each): Take two caplets every 6 hours PRN; do not take more than six caplets in 24 hours (maximum dose 3,000 mg [3 g] in 24 hr)
- Extended-release Tylenol (8 hr; 650 mg each): Take two caplets every 8 hr PRN; do not take more than six caplets in 24 hours (maximum dose is 3,900 mg [3.9 g] in 24 hr)
- Duration: Do not use for more than 10 days unless directed by health provider
- *Avoid if:* chronic hepatitis B/C/D, dehydration, liver disease, cirrhosis, heavy drinker

- Risk of severe liver damage if intake of three or more alcoholic drinks/day while using medication
- Antidote for overdose: Acetylcysteine (Mucomyst)

EXAM TIPS

- **Capsaicin cream can be used to treat pain in trigeminal neuralgia and PHN.**
- **Maximum number of days that ketorolac (Toradol) can be used is 5 days.**
- **The maximum dose for acetaminophen (Tylenol) ranges from 3 to 4 g/d.**
- **Aspirin irreversibly suppresses platelet function for up to 7 days (due to irreversible acetylation). Life span of platelets is about 7 to 10 days.**
- **Discontinue ASA if patient complains of tinnitus (possible aspirin toxicity).**

IMMUNE SYSTEM DRUGS

Glucocorticoids (Steroids)

- Rheumatoid arthritis, lupus, and other autoimmune disorders
- Polymyalgia rheumatica (dramatic relief of symptoms)
- Asthma or acute asthmatic exacerbations
- Temporal arteritis/giant cell arteritis (high doses × several weeks to months)
- Uveitis (complication of autoimmune diseases such as rheumatoid arthritis, lupus, polymyalgia rheumatica)
- Skin (eczema, psoriasis, contact dermatitis)

Oral Steroids

- Prednisone 40 to 60 mg/day (high-dosed) for 3 to 4 days; can be used for short-term treatment (i.e., asthma exacerbation); there is no need to taper if patient is not on chronic steroids (oral or inhalation)
- Methylprednisolone (Medrol Dose Pack) × 7 days; does not need to be weaned

Topical Steroids

- Classification: (Class 1 (superpotent) to Class 7 (least potent)
  - Superpotent (Class 1) —clobetasol (Temovate)
  - Potent—halcinonide (Halog)
  - Moderate—triamcinolone (Kenalog)
  - Least potent (Class 7)—hydrocortisone

Pharma Notes: Topical Steroids

- Be careful with using topical steroids on children and limit duration.
- Use low-potency steroid for the eyelids, face, intertriginous areas, and the genitals.
  - *Example*: Use hydrocortisone cream/ointment/lotions 0.5% to 1% (OTC) to prescription strength such as hydrocortisone 2.5% (Hytone Rx).
  - May need to use ophthalmic-grade ointments for rashes around the eyes/eyelids.
- Use moderate to high-potency steroids for thicker skin (scalp, soles of feet, palms of the hands) or for plaques (psoriasis). Taper potent-strength topical steroids (or will rebound).

(continued)

(*continued*)

- What is "occlusion"?
  - Thick resistant psoriatic plaques are sometimes treated by using occlusion (increases absorption). The topical steroid is applied to the plaque and is covered with plastic wrap. Ultrapotent steroids (Temovate, etc.) should not be occluded for more than 2 weeks (risk of hypothalamic–pituitary–axis [HPA] suppression).

Acutely inflamed joints (knees/hips/shoulders/elbows) can be treated with intraarticular triamcinolone (Kenalog) injections up to three times per year. Do not inject septic joint with steroids.

Side Effects of Glucocorticoids/Steroids (Chronic Use)

- HPA suppression
- Cushing's disease (dorsal hump, rounded face, etc.)
- Osteoporosis (advise weight-bearing exercises, vitamin D, calcium 1,200 mg/d, bisphosphonates)
- Immunosuppression (increased risk of infection)
- Skin changes from long-term topical therapy (skin atrophy, striae, telangiectasia, acne, pigmentation changes)

CLINICAL PEARLS

- **A severe case of poison ivy or poison oak rash may require 14 to 21 days of an oral steroid to clear.**
- **The most common cause of acute liver failure in the United States is acetaminophen overdose (Poison Control Center: (800) 222-1222)**

OTHER DRUGS AND SAFETY ISSUES

Drugs That Require Eye Examination

The following drugs require careful monitoring of vision due to adverse effects. Check that the patient has baseline examination with regular eye exams done by an ophthalmologist.

- Digoxin (yellow to green vision, blurred vision, halos if blood level too high)
- Ethambutol and linezolid (optic neuropathy)
- Corticosteroids (cataracts, glaucoma, optic neuritis)
- Fluoroquinolones (retinal detachment)
- Viagra, Cialis, Levitra (cataracts, blurred vision, ischemic optic neuropathy, others)
- Accutane (cataracts, decreased night vision, others)
- Topamax (acute angle-closure glaucoma, increased intracranial pressure, mydriasis)
- Plaquenil (neuropathy and permanent loss of vision)

Cisapride (Propulsid)

- Available only by limited-access protocol in the United States
- *Block box warning*: Serious cardiac arrhythmias (ventricular fibrillation/tachycardia, torsades de pointes, prolongation of QT interval); check: 12-lead EKG at baseline; check serum electrolytes and creatinine
- Numerous drug contraindications (macrolides, antifungals, TCAs, etc.)

Theophylline Drug Interactions

- Theophylline level (adults): 5 to 15 mcg/mL
- Drug interactions (cimetidine, alprazolam, macrolides, fluvoxamine, others)
- Avoid combining with other stimulants (theophylline, pseudoephedrine, caffeine, Ritalin)
- Disorders worsened by stimulants: Hypertension, arrhythmias, stroke, seizures
- BPH: Causes urinary retention, worsening of symptoms
- Suspect toxicity if persistent vomiting

Tapering (Weaning) Drugs

- Certain drugs that are used long term need to be tapered; abrupt discontinuation will cause the treated condition to flare up (exacerbation), rebound, and/or have adverse effects:
  - Beta-blockers (rebound hypertension or hypertensive crisis)
  - Benzodiazepines (severe anxiety, insomnia, seizures, tremors)
  - Oral steroids
  - Anticonvulsants (seizures)
  - Paroxetine or Paxil
  - Antiarrhythmics (refer to cardiologists)
  - Antipsychotics and many others
  - Digoxin

ILLEGAL DRUGS

Cannabis (Marijuana, Hash, Hashish, Marinol)

- Euphoria ("high"), more sociable, increased appetite, and slurred speech
- Ataxia, nystagmus, conjunctival injection (red eyes), and dilated pupils (mydriasis)
- Lowers sperm count; increases heart rate and blood pressure
- Psychomotor effects lasts 12 to 24 hours

Prescription Opiods (Fentanyl, Oxycodone, Meperidine, Hydromorphone, Amphetamines)

- Euphoria, drowsiness, slowed breathing, pupil constriction (miosis)
- Overdose or combining with alcohol may cause respiratory depression, coma, death
- Naltrexone can reverse effects

Dextromethorphan (Robo, Robo-Trip, Triple C)

- Obtained from OTC cough and cold medications
- Euphoria, speech slurred, tachycardia, possibly elevated BP and temperature, seizures, paranoia, confusion

Cocaine (Coke, Crack, Rock)

- Happy, mental alertness, paranoia, decreased appetite, insomnia, nosebleeds
- Pupil dilations (mydriasis), tachycardia, hypertension, angina/MI, strokes, seizures
- May cause midline nasal septum perforation and/or ulceration with chronic use

Methamphetamine (Meth, Crystal Meth, Ice, Methylphenidate)

- Chronic use results in severe dental carries with loss of front teeth on the upper jaw
- Anorexia results in drastic weight loss; pupils appear constricted

U.S. FDA DRUG ENFORCEMENT AGENCY (DEA)

Controlled Substances Act

- *Schedule I drugs* (heroin, Ecstasy/MDMA, PCP, etc.)
  - Illegal to prescribe; no currently accepted medical use; high abuse potential
- *Schedule II drugs* (Demerol, Dilaudid, OxyContin, cocaine, amphetamines, fentanyl, etc.)
  - Only the original prescription with the prescriber's signature (not stamped) is acceptable
  - The total number of pills must be indicated; no refills are allowed
- *Schedule III drugs* (Tylenol with codeine, Vicodin, anabolic steroids, testosterone, etc.)
- *Schedule IV drugs* (benzodiazepines, Ambien, Lunesta, Soma, etc.)
- *Schedule V drugs* (cough medicines with less than 200 mg of codeine, Lomotil, Lyrica)
- *Schedule IV, V*: Can be mailed to the patient; some states allow NPs to prescribe lower-level controlled substances
- For all controlled substances: Must have the prescriber's and the supervising prescriber's name/DEA number with the clinic address on the pad; cannot be predated or postdated; some states do not require a supervising prescriber's signature. Caution: Rules vary by state and the prescriber should keep abreast of the rules in the state where he or she practices.

List of FDA Category X Drugs

- Finasteride (Proscar, Propecia): Reproductive-aged or pregnant women should not handle crushed/broken finasteride tablets
- Isotretinoin (Accutane)
- Warfarin sodium (Coumadin)
- Misoprostol (Cytotec)
- Androgenic hormones: Birth control pills, hormone replacement therapy (HRT), testosterone
- Live virus vaccines (measles, mumps, rubella, varicella, rotavirus, FluMist)
- Thalidomide, diethylstilbestrol (DES), methimazole, and so on

FDA Category Classifications

The new FDA Pregnancy and Lactation Labeling Rule (PLLR) went into effect on June 30, 2015. It replaces the pregnancy letter categories A, B, C, D, and X. The new labeling categories are: Pregnancy, Lactation, and Females and Males of Reproductive Potential. Prescription drugs and biologics approved after June 30, 2015 will use the new format immediately. Drugs/biologics approved on or after June 30, 2001 will be phased in gradually. Drugs approved prior to June 29, 2001 are not subject to the PLLR rule; but the pregnancy letter category must be removed by June 29, 2018. Over-the-counter drugs are not subject to this rule.

- Pregnancy: Includes labor and delivery; it will include information about the potential risks to the developing fetus.
- Lactation: Includes nursing mothers and drugs that should not be used during breastfeeding, as well and the clinical effects on the infant. It may have information about the timing of breastfeeding to minimize infant exposure.
- Females and Males of Reproductive Potential: Includes information on the drug's effect on fertility, pregnancy testing/loss (if available), and birth control.

Pharma Notes

Almost all the drugs on the 2016 edition of the exams were released before the PLLR became effective. Therefore, FDA category X may still be in use in these exams. In general, FDA category X drugs are those that interfere with or block hormones (finasteride, misoprostol, Lupron), contain estrogen (birth control pills, HRT), are live virus vaccines, interfere with cell growth (methotrexate, chemotherapy, radiation), or are derivatives of vitamin A (e.g., Accutane, high-dosed vitamin A supplements).

PRESCRIPTION PADS

Tamper-resistant prescription pads/paper are required. If a prescription goes directly to the pharmacy (electronically, by fax, or by telephone), it does not have to be to tamper-resistant paper. It should contain the following information:

- Practitioner's name/designation/license number/NPI (National Practitioner Identification) number
- Supervising physician's name/designation (some states do not require a supervising physician)
- Clinic address (if multiple sites, the sites where the NP works should be listed on the pad) and phone number(s)

Writing a Prescription

- Date, name, and address of the patient
- Drug name, dosage strength, dosage form, frequency, and duration
- Directions for use: Quantity and number of refills (indicate how many times or none)
- For controlled drugs, a DEA number *must* be on the script if the prescription is for a controlled drug
- For FDA Schedule II drugs, the script must be handwritten or typed on a tamper-resistant prescription pad and manually signed
    - Schedule II drug prescriptions cannot be called in to the pharmacy
- Avoid using initials or shortcuts (e.g., use *daily* instead of QD).
- Write the quantity of the drug in both number and written word form.
- **Examples:**
    - *Lunesta tablets 3 mg by mouth at bedtime as needed*
        - Dispense: #20 (twenty)
        - Refills: 1 (one)
    - *Bactrim DS 1 (one) tablet by mouth twice a day for 10 (ten) days*
        - Dispense: #20 (twenty)
        - Refills: 0 (none)

The "Five Rights"

- There are "five rights" that help to prevent or decrease the chances of a medical error:
    1. Right patient
    2. Right drug
    3. Right dose
    4. Right time
    5. Right route
- What is "e-prescribing"? The process of sending and receiving prescriptions by electronic means. Preferred method for drug prescriptions for Medicare and Medicaid.

Clinicians write the prescription in their offices on a computer or tablet using e-prescribing software.

COMPLEMENTARY AND ALTERNATIVE MEDICINE

Conventional medicine (or allopathic medicine) is also known as *modern medicine* or *Western medicine.* Alternative medicine is the treatments and substances that are not part of standard medicine.

Examples: Herbal supplements, probiotics, chiropractic, homeopathy, meditation, yoga, massage therapy

Complementary and alternative medicine (CAM) is the term used when Western medicine is combined with alternative medicine or "medical products and practices that are not part of standard care" (National Institutes of Health, 2010). CAM is using both Western medicine with alternative medicines (herbs) or with another healing system such as homeopathy, ayurveda (from India), or traditional Chinese medicine (or TCM).

Herbal Supplements

- Feverfew: Migraine headache
- Cinnamon: Improves blood sugar (diabetes) and cholesterol
- Glucosamine (with/without chondroitin): Osteoarthritis
- Natural progesterone cream (from wild yam root extract): Premenstrual symptoms (hot flashes)
- Isoflavones (from soy beans): Estrogen-like effects
- Saw palmetto: Urinary symptoms of BPH
- Kava kava, valerian root: Anxiety and insomnia
- St. John's wort: Mild depression; do not use with selective serotonin reuptake inhibitor (SSRIS), sumatriptan, HIV protease inhibitors (indinavir), others
- Tumeric: Alzheimer's disease, arthritis, cancer

Homeopathy

The founder is the physician Samuel Hahnemann (1755–1843). This healing system is based on the "Law of Similars" or "Let likes be cured by likes."

- What is the Homeopathic *Pharmacopoeia of the United States?* The HPUS is a list of approved homeopathic substances used in this country.
- How are homeopathic substances made? Extremely small amounts of a substance are diluted (ultradilution). For example, the herb *Arnica montana,* which is used to prevent or treat bruises, can be diluted 30 times (e.g., *Arnica montana* 30× dilution).

Ayurveda

An ancient healing system from India. Food, spices, herbs, yoga, and lifestyle are believed to prevent and treat disease.

Systems Review

II

4

Health Screening and Health Promotion Review

U.S. HEALTH STATISTICS

Mortality Statistics*

Leading cause of death (all ages/genders):

1. Heart disease (or diseases of the heart)
2. Cancer (or malignant neoplasms)
3. Chronic lower respiratory diseases (i.e., chronic obstructive pulmonary disease [COPD])

Cancer Mortality

- Leading cause of cancer death:
  - Lung cancer
- Leading causes of cancer deaths in men:
  1. Lung cancer
  2. Prostate cancer
  3. Colorectal cancer
- Leading causes of cancer deaths in women:
  1. Lung cancer
  2. Breast cancer
  3. Colorectal cancer

Leading Causes of Death in Adolescents

Death rate for teen males is higher than for females:

1. Accidents/unintentional injuries (39.5%); the most common cause is motor vehicle crashes (risk is highest from 16 to 19 years of age)
2. Suicide (16.8%): Watch teens for signs of depression, excess stress, and suicidal behavior; open communication between the adolescent and the parents/caregivers (or persons they trust) is extremely important in preventing teenage suicide
3. Homicide (14.3%): Nonfatal and fatal violence are much higher among young people compared to any other age group.

Leading Cause of Mortality by Age Group

- Birth to 12 months:
  - Congenital malformations (20.3%)
- Ages 1 to 44 years:
  - Unintentional injuries

*National Vital Statistics Reports. Volume 25, Number 2, February 16, 2016.

- Ages 45 to 64 years:
  - Cancer (30.9%)
- Ages 65 and older:
  - Heart disease (25.6%)

Life Expectancy

Average life expectancy is 78.6 years (a decrease of 0.1 year from 2015; National Center for Health Statistics. Mortality in the United States, 2016. https://www.cdc.gov/nchs/products/databriefs/db293.htm).

CANCER STATISTICS

Prevalence

- Most common cancer:
  - Skin cancer (5.4 million)
- Most common type of skin cancer:
  - Basal cell carcinoma
  - Melanoma causes the majority of skin cancer deaths
- Most common cancer by gender (prevalence):
  - Men
    - Prostate cancer
    - In men, there are more cases of prostate cancer (prevalence), but the cancer that causes the most deaths (mortality) is lung cancer
  - Women
    - Breast cancer
    - In women, there are more cases of breast cancer (prevalence), but the cancer that causes the most deaths (mortality) is lung cancer
- Most common cancer among all children:
  - Acute lymphoblastic leukemia (ALL; 34% of all cancers in children)

SCREENING TESTS

Sensitivity

- A sensitive screening test is very good at identifying/detecting those people who have the disease (true positive).
- An easy way to remember is to think of "sensitivity—rule in" or "SSIN or SIN."

Specificity

- A specific screening test is very good at identifying/detecting those people without the disease (true negative).
- An easy way to remember is to think of "specificity—rule out" or "SPOUT."

HEALTH PROMOTION/DISEASE AND DEATH PREVENTION

Primary Prevention (Prevention of Disease/Injury)

- Individual actions (healthy individuals): Eat a nutritious diet, exercise, use seatbelts and helmets
- Gun safety: Use safety locks for guns; keep guns out of reach of children/teens
- National programs: Federal health-promotion/disease-prevention programs include immunizations, the Occupational Safety and Health Administration (OSHA)'s job safety laws, and Environmental Protection Agency (EPA) laws.

- Programs promote a healthy lifestyle for youth (healthy diet, exercise, etc.)
- Building a youth center in an urban high-crime area or a Habitat for Humanity (shelter).
- Aspirin prophylaxis for primary prevention of CVD and colon cancer in adults aged 50 to 59 years who have a 10% risk or higher.

Secondary Prevention (Early Detection of a Disease to Minimize Bodily Damage)

- Screening tests (Pap smears, mammograms, CBC for anemia, etc.)
- Screening for depression (interviewing a patient about feelings of sadness, hopelessness)
- Screening for sexually transmitted infections (STIs; asking about sexual history, partners, signs and symptoms)
- Screening for alcohol abuse (interviewing a patient using the CAGE questionnaire)
- Testing for hepatitis C virus infection in a person with risk factors
- Having a person with a history of MI, TIA, or stroke take an aspirin or statin daily (to prevent a future stroke or MI)

Tertiary Prevention (Prevention of Disease Progression, Rehabilitation, Support Groups, Education on Equipment)

- Support groups: Alcoholics Anonymous (AA), breast cancer support groups, HIV support groups
- Education for patients with preexisting disease (i.e., diabetes, hypertension): Avoidance of drug interactions, proper use of wheelchair or medical equipment, others
- Rehabilitation: Cardiac rehabilitation, physical therapy (PT), occupational therapy (OT)
- Treatment of a person with hepatitis C virus infection
- Treatment of a person who has already had a heart attack with daily aspirin (to prevent another heart attack)

U.S. PREVENTIVE SERVICES TASK FORCE

Aspirin Use to Prevent Cardiovascular Disease and Colorectal Cancer (April 2016)

- Age 50 to 59 years with equal or more than 10% risk (10-year cardiovascular disease risk)
- Initiate low-dose aspirin use for primary prevention of cardiovascular and colorectal cancer (in patients who are not at increased risk for bleeding) with life expectancy of at least 10 years and who are willing to take low-dose aspirin daily for at least 10 years)

Breast Cancer (January 2016)

- Baseline mammogram: Start at age 50 years and repeat every 2 years until the age of 74 years
- Age 75 years or older: Insufficient evidence for routine mammogram
- Does not apply to women with known genetic mutations (*BRCA1* or *BRCA2*), familial breast cancer, history chest radiation at a young age or previously diagnosed with high-risk breast lesion who may benefit from starting screening in their 40s

Note*

Age 40 to 49 years (individualize based on risk factors, if done). The American Cancer Society recommends starting routine screening at age 40 years.

*U.S. Preventive Services Task Force (USPSTF) Recommendation Statement (January 2016).

Cervical Cancer (Table 4.1)

Table 4.1 Cervical Cancer Screening

Age Group	Recommendations for Pap/Liquid Cytology
Age 20 years or younger	Do not screen (even if sexually active with multiple partners). Cervical cancer is rare before age 21 years.
Age 21 to 65 years	Baseline at age 21 years. Screen every 3 years.
Age 30 to 65 years	Another option starting at age 30 years is to screen with combination of cytology plus human papillomavirus (HPV) testing every 5 years.
Had hysterectomy with removal of cervix	If hysterectomy with cervical removal was not due to cervical intraepithelial neoplasia (CIN grade 2) or cervical cancer, then can stop screening.
Women older than 65 years who had adequate prior screening	Do not screen if history of adequate prior screening and is otherwise not at high risk for cervical cancer.

Source: USPSTF (2012).

Notes*

These recommendations do not apply to women who are immunocompromised (i.e., HIV infection), had in utero exposure to diethylstilbestrol (DES), or have a diagnosis of high-grade precancerous cervical lesion or cervical cancer.

*USPSTF Screening Recommendations for Cervical Cancer (July 2015).

Colorectal Cancer (June 2016)

- Baseline: Starting at age 50 years until the age of 75 (older age is the most common risk factor)
- Age 76 to 85 years: Against routine screening but "there may be considerations"; individualize screening as needed
- Older than age 85 years: Screening for colorectal cancer bot recommended

Notes

These three methods are all acceptable for colorectal cancer. The screening intervals of each method differ:

- High-sensitivity fecal occult blood test (gFOBT) for three consecutive stool samples annually (high-sensitivity version such as Hemoccult SENSA superior to older Hemoccult II test)
- Flexible sigmoidoscopy or CT colonography every 5 years
- Colonoscopy every 10 years

Lipid Disorders

- Total lipid profile after a 9-hour (minimum) fast
- The USPSTF recommends the use of low- to moderate-dose statin when all of the following criteria area met:
  - Aged 40 to 74 years
  - The patient has one or more CVD risk factors (i.e., dyslipidemia, DM, hypertension, smoking)
  - The patient has a calculated 10-year risk of a cardiovascular event of 10% or greater
  - Age 76 years and older without history of heart attack or stroke (insufficient evidence)

Lung Cancer (June 2013)

- Screening for persons who smoke (30 pack-years) or have quit in the past 15 years
- Age 55 to 80 years: Annual screening with low-dose CT (LDCT)
- Discontinue screening once person has not smoked for 15 years or develops a health problem that substantially limits life expectancy or the ability or willingness to have curative lung surgery

Prostate Cancer (May 2012)

- This topic is being updated in 2016. The USPSTF recommends against prostate-specific antigen (PSA) screening for prostate cancer. The recommendation "applies to men in the general U.S. population, regardless of age."
- Grade D: The benefits of PSA-based screening for prostate cancer do not outweigh the disadvantages.

Ovarian Cancer (September 2012)

- Grade D: Routine screening is not recommended.
- Very high-risk women with *BRCA1/BRCA2* mutations: Refer to specialists. If ovarian cancer screening is done, transvaginal ultrasound with serum cancer antigen (CA-125) is ordered. The screening starts at age 30 years (or 5–10 years before earliest age of first diagnosis of ovarian cancer in family).
  - Some experts recommend bilateral salpingo-oophorectomy (BSO) between age 35 to 40 years (after childbearing is complete). BSO has a significant effect in reducing ovarian cancer risk in at-risk women.
- High-risk women: Refer for genetic counseling. Look for family history of having two or more first- to second-degree relatives with a history of ovarian cancer or a combination of ovarian cancer; women of Ashkenazi Jewish ethnicity with first-degree relative (or second-degree relatives on the same side of the family) with breast or ovarian cancer.

Skin Cancer Counseling

- Recommended for children, adolescents, and young adults (ages 10–24 years) with fair skin
- Education includes avoidance of sunlight from 10 a.m. to 4 p.m., use of SPF 15 or higher sunblock, protective clothing, wide-brim hats

Other

Routine screening is not recommended by the USPSTF for the following conditions:

- Ovarian cancer
- Oral cancer
- Prostate cancer
- Testicular cancer (adolescents or adult males; Table 4.2)

Table 4.2 USPSTF Health Screening Recommendations

	Baseline	Notes
Abdominal aortic aneurysm (AAA; June 2014)	Men at age 65 to 75 years who have smoked	One-time screening with ultrasonography in men ages 65 to 75 years who have smoked; individualize for men who never smoked
Breast cancer (January 2016)	Start at age 50 years	Mammogram every 2 years (biennial) until age 74 years
	Age 75 years or older*	Stop routine screening. Individualize*
	Breast self-exam (BSE)	Against teaching BSE (Grade D recommendation)

(continued)

Table 4.2 USPSTF Health Screening Recommendations *(continued)*

	Baseline	**Notes**
Blood pressure in adults (hypertension; October 2015)	Start at age 18 years or older	Recommends obtaining measurements outside of clinical setting for diagnostic confirmation before starting treatment
Colon/colorectal cancer (June 2016)	Start at age 50 years continue until age 75 years	High-sensitivity fetal occult blood test (FOBT; every year), or sigmoidoscopy (every 5 years), or colonoscopy (every 10 years)
	Age 76 to 85 years	Individualize*
	Age older than 85 years	Stop routine screening
Depression	Adolescents (12–18 years)	Start screening for major depressive disorder starting at age 12 to 18 years
Depression (adults; January 2016)	General adult population	Include pregnant and postpartum women; use Beck Depression Inventory
Diabetes mellitus (DM) type 2 (October 2015)	Age 40 to 70 years if overweight or obese	Applies to adults in primary care settings who are not "high risk"; DM patients with risk factors (certain ethnicities, PCOS, GDM, etc.) can undergo screening at younger age
Latent tuberculosis (September 2016)	Asymptomatic adults	Screen asymptomatic adults who are at increased risk for infection
Lung cancer (December 2013)	Aged 55 to 80 years with history of smoking	Low-dose computed tomography (LDCT) if currently smokes with 30-pack-year history *or* quit in the previous 15 years
Obesity	Start at age 6 to 18 years	Offer or refer for intensive behavioral interventions
Sexually transmitted infections (STIs; September 2014)	Start at the onset of sexual activity	High-intensity behavioral counseling for sexually active adolescents and adults who are at high risk for STIs
Skin cancer(July 2016)	Insufficient evidence	Routine screening is not recommended; individualize recommendation
Osteoporosis (being updated)	Start at age 65 years or older	May start earlier if a younger woman has a fracture risk equal or greater than that of a 65-year-old White woman (i.e., chronic steroids)
Ovarian cancer (September 2012)	Against routine screening	Do not screen for ovarian cancer except high risk (as of September 2016)
Pancreatic cancer (February 2014)	Against routine screening	

*Decision to screen is based on risk factors, life expectancy (>10 years), risk versus benefits.
FOBT, fecal occult blood test; GDM, gestational diabetes mellitus; PCOS, polycystic ovary syndrome.

RISK FACTORS

Breast Cancer

- Older age: Age 50 years or older (most common risk factor)
- Previous history of breast cancer
- Two or more first-degree relatives with breast cancer
- Early menarche, late menopause, nulliparity (longer exposure to estrogen)
- Obesity (adipose tissue can synthesize small amounts of estrogen)

Cervical Cancer

- Multiple sex partners (defined as greater than four lifetime partners)
- Younger age onset of sex (immature cervix easier to infect)
- Immunosuppression and smoking

Colorectal Cancer

- History of familial polyposis (multiple polyps on colon)
- First-degree relative with colon cancer
- Crohn's disease (ulcerative colitis)

Prostate Cancer

- Age 50 years or older
- African ancestry
- First-degree relative with prostate cancer

Sexually Transmitted Infections (STIs) or Sexually Transmitted Diseases (STDs)

- Multiple sexual partners
- Earlier age onset of sex
- New partners (defined as <3 months)
- History of STD
- Homelessness

VACCINES AND IMMUNIZATIONS (TABLE 4.3)

Hepatitis B Vaccine

- Total of three doses (0, 1, 6 months). First vaccine given at birth (monovalent hepatitis B vaccine).
- Need a minimum interval of 4 weeks between doses one and two.
- If series is not completed, catch up until three-dose series is completed. The Centers for Disease Control and Prevention (CDC) does not recommend a restart of the hepatitis B series.

Vaccine Facts

1. *If a patient had only one dose of hepatitis B vaccine, what is recommended?*
   Do not restart the hepatitis B series again. If only one dose, give the second dose. Catch up until the three-dose series is completed.

Seasonal Influenza Vaccine

- Start giving the influenza injection at the end of October of each year (fall to winter season). It takes 2 weeks after the shot for a person to develop antibodies.
- As long as influenza viruses circulate, vaccination should continue to be offered, even into January or later. Most seasons, influenza activity peaks in January or later (CDC, 2017).
- Health care personnel who work with patients older than 50 years should be vaccinated.
- If a person with an egg allergy *only* experiences hives, an influenza vaccine can be administered.

- Pregnant women may receive any licensed, recommended, and age-appropriate flu vaccine.

Formulations

Inactivated and Recombinant Influenza Vaccines (Injectable)

- Trivalent influenza vaccine or quadrivalent vaccines given by intramuscular (IM) injection in the arm preferred. There are intradermal and nasal forms of these vaccines.
- High-dose trivalent influenza vaccine for people age 65 years or older (Fluzone High-Dose)
- Recombinant trivalent influenza vaccine that is egg-free approved for persons age 18 years and older (Flublok)
- Quadrivalent influenza vaccine: protects against four types flu virus (broader protection). Age 4 years or older.

Live Attenuated Inactivated Virus (LAIV)

- For the 2017 to 2018 influenza season, there is a CDC and Advisory Committee on Immunization Practices (ACIP) recommendation against use of LAIV vaccine for all age groups.
- Only for healthy persons aged 2 to 49 years
- Some antivirals (amantadine, rimantadine, zanamivir, or oseltamivir) should be avoided 48 hours before and 14 days after vaccination because they interfere with antibody production. Do not give aspirin to children within the 4 weeks following vaccination.

LAIV Contraindications

- Pregnancy, chronic disease (i.e., asthma, COPD, renal failure, diabetes, immunosuppression)
- Contraindicated in children on aspirin therapy (ages 2–17 years)

Contraindications (all types of influenza vaccine)

- Infants age 6 months or younger
- People with severe, life-threatening allergies to components of the influenza vaccine (gelatin, gentamicin, preservative), which is not related to an egg allergy, should not be given influenza vaccine (egg-allergy-related reactions are discussed in the text that follows).

Safety Issues

- If severe reaction (hypotension, wheezing, nausea/vomiting, reaction requiring epinephrine or emergency medical attention) occurs after eating eggs or food containing eggs, vaccine should be administered in an inpatient or outpatient medical setting (clinics, hospitals, health departments, physician offices) under the supervision of a health care provider who is able to recognize and manage severe allergic conditions.
- If patient experienced *only* hives previously, he or she can receive the influenza vaccine. People with egg allergies no longer need to be observed for an allergic reaction for 30 minutes after receiving the flu vaccine (CDC, 2016; Committee on Infectious Diseases, 2017).
- Age-appropriate recombinant (RIV) or cell cultured flu vaccines are an option for patients who refuse egg-based influenza vaccine.
- Use caution or avoid influenza vaccine if history of Guillain–Barré syndrome within 6 weeks of previous vaccination.

Vaccine Facts

1. *What is the youngest age at which influenza vaccine (injection) can be given?*
   At the age of 6 months
2. *Most flu vaccines (including nasal spray) are manufactured using egg-based technology. What are the implications for patients?*
   Egg allergy affects 1.3% of children but only 0.2% of adults

Tetanus Vaccines (Tdap and Td)

- Give every 10 years for lifetime
- Boosters: For "dirty"/contaminated wounds, give a booster if the last dose was more than 5 years prior
- Infancy and children younger than age 7 years: Use DTaP form
- Age 7 years and older: Use only tetanus and diphtheria (Td); and tetanus, diphtheria; or the tetanus, diphtheria, acellular pertussis (Tdap) forms of the vaccine; give one Tdap dose (lifetime) to replace one Td dose
- DTaP: Give by IM route to infants and children younger than age 7 years
- Td: Give by IM route. Start using this form at the age of 7 years
- Tdap: Give by IM route

Safety Issue

- History of Guillain–Barré syndrome within 6 weeks of previous dose. Be careful with pertussis component if progressive or unstable neurological disorder, uncontrolled seizures.

Vaccine Facts

1. *When can the Tdap be used as a booster in adolescents and adults?*
   The Tdap can be substituted for a single dose of Td (once in a lifetime) starting at age 11 to 12 years
2. *What is done if a patient has a tetanus-prone wound and vaccination status is unknown?*
   Administer immediate dose of Td/Tdap vaccine and the tetanus immunoglobulin (TIG) injection as soon as possible
3. *Which wounds are considered at highest risk for tetanus infection?*
   Puncture wounds, wounds with devitalized tissue, soil-contaminated wounds, crush injuries, and others are at high risk for tetanus infection

Pneumococcal Vaccine

- Pneumococcal polysaccharide vaccine (PPSV23 or Pneumovax): All adults age 65 years or older or if high risk for pneumococcal disease (ages 2–64 years)
  - PPSV23: 50% to 85% effective
- Pneumococcal conjugate vaccine (PCV13 or Prevnar): All children younger than 5 years of age or at high risk for pneumococcal disease; PCV13 is also recommended for all adults age 65 years or older
- Age 65 years or older: CDC recommends giving PCV13 first (if never had PPSV23); then 12 months after PCV13, administer PPSV23 (better immunogenic response)

- Highest risk (of fatal pneumococcal infection):
  - Chronic diseases (alcoholism, diabetes, cerebrospinal fluid [CSF] leaks, asthma, chronic hepatitis)
  - Anatomical or functional asplenia (including sickle cell disease)
  - If immunocompromised or on medications causing immunocompromised state
  - Generalized malignancy or cancers of the blood (leukemia, lymphoma, multiple myeloma)
  - Renal diseases (e.g., chronic renal failure, nephrotic syndrome)
  - History of organ or bone marrow transplant

Vaccine Facts

1. *What vaccine is recommended for persons who are 65 years of age?*
   Adults 65 years or older (who never received Pneumovax): Give Prevnar (PCV13) initially, followed at 12 months with Pneumovax (PPSV23); if person has already had PPSV23 previously, wait 12 months to give PCV13
2. *If a person is vaccinated before the age of 65 with Pneumovax, what is recommended?*
   Give a booster dose of Pneumovax 5 years after the initial dose

Shingles Vaccine

- Zoster vaccine (Zostavax) is a live attenuated virus vaccine.
- Age 60 years: Give one-time dose by subcutaneous (SC) route. A past history of shingles is *not* a contraindication for receiving the shingles vaccine.
- The shingles vaccine can be administered to persons even if they never had a chickenpox infection. However, even if a person has had shingles before, the CDC still recommends the vaccine.
- Certain antivirals (acyclovir, famciclovir, valacyclovir) can decrease immunological response if taken 24 hours before or 14 days after vaccination.
- May cause exacerbation of asthma and polymyalgia rheumatica (PMR).
- Risk factors (shingles):
  - Older age (60 years or older), immunocompromised (HIV, steroids, chemotherapy)
  - Leukemia, lymphoma
- Contraindications:
  - Pregnancy and breastfeeding
  - Leukemia, lymphomas, or other malignancies of the bone/bone marrow
  - Immunocompromise (high-dose steroids >2 weeks, antitumor necrosis factor medications such as etanercept)

Vaccine Facts

1. *What age group should receive the shingles vaccine?*
   Give a one-time dose at the age of 60 years or older (even if patient has already had shingles). A person with a history of shingles can be vaccinated with shingles vaccine (unless there is a contraindication). The youngest age that Zostavax can be given is 50 years of age.
2. *Can any person who has never had chickenpox develop shingles?*
   No, they cannot.

(continued)

(continued)

3. *How long are persons with shingles contagious?*
   Shingles is infectious until all the skin lesions are dry and crusted. Follow contact precautions. About half of cases of shingles occur in persons aged 60 years or older.
4. *Which vaccine, the shingles vaccine or the varicella vaccine, contains more varicella zoster virus (VZV)?*
   The shingles vaccine (Zostavax) contains about 14 times more VZV compared with the varicella vaccine (Varivax).

Varicella Vaccine

- Varicella live attenuated virus (Varivax): Given by SC route. Need two doses. First dose given in infancy: 12 to 15 months (do not give to infants younger than 12 months).
  - Advise women not to get pregnant for 1 month after getting vaccine.
- A new combination vaccine called the *MMRV* (ProQuad) contains both chickenpox and the MMR vaccines (only for ages 12 years or younger).
- Postexposure prophylaxis: Ideally, vaccine should be given within 72 hours postexposure but may be given up to 5 days (120 hours) after incident (healthy, previously unvaccinated).
- Reactions: Mild rash or several small chickenpox rashes can occur after vaccination (contagious, avoid immunocompromised people).
- Acceptable proof of varicella immunity:
  - Documentation of two doses of varicella vaccine
  - Written diagnosis of chickenpox or shingles based on health care provider diagnosis
  - Positive laboratory varicella titer (IgG ELISA)
- Do not administer the varicella vaccine to a person born in the United States before 1980.

Safety Issues

Avoid giving to pregnant patients, patients with immunosuppression or on drugs that affect the immune system (steroids, biologics such as Humira, Enbrel), patients having radiation treatment or with any type of cancer.

Health Care Personnel Vaccination Recommendations

These recommendations also apply to students who are in training to become health care providers.

Td or Tdap

Give one-time dose of Tdap for all health care personnel who have not received the Tdap when due for a tetanus booster. Continue giving Td boosters every 10 years for a lifetime.

MMR

Proof of immunity is necessary (born before 1957, laboratory confirmation such as positive titers). If not vaccinated for MMR, two doses are needed (at least 28 days apart).

Varicella

Proof of immunity is necessary (positive varicella titer, documentation of two doses of varicella vaccine or diagnosis of varicella by physician/health care provider).

Hepatitis B

If incomplete hepatitis B series (fewer than three doses), complete the series (do not restart). If job involves blood or body fluids, obtain anti-HBs serological testing 1 to 2 months after dose 3. If anti-HBs is less than 10 mIU/mL, three additional doses should be administered on the regular hepatitis B schedule followed by anti-HBs testing in 1 to 2 months.

Influenza

All health care personnel should have an annual influenza shot during the fall/winter.

Table 4.3 CDC Immunization Recommendations for Adults and Teens (2016)*

Vaccine	Schedule	Notes
Hepatitis B	Total of three doses	If incomplete series, do not restart; if had one dose, give the second dose during the visit; if had two doses, give the third dose
Tetanus/diphtheria (Td)	Every 10 years for lifetime	Substitute one-time dose of Tdap for Td booster (once in a lifetime)
Tetanus/diphtheria/ acellular pertussis (Tdap)		Dirty wounds, give tetanus booster if last dose more than 5 years
Flu (influenza)	Give once a year in the fall or winter	Give in fall/winter season
Trivalent flu vaccine		Give flu to everyone 6 months or older
Quadrivalent flu vaccine	Age 4 years or older	
Live attenuated influenza vaccine (LAIV) intranasal**	Do not use the LAIV flu vaccine during 2017–2018 season	Instead, use trivalent or quadrivalent flu vaccine
	Do not give FluMist to pregnant women; use injection form	For healthy persons (not pregnant) from age 2 years to 49 years
Varicella**	Give two doses at least 4 weeks apart	Age 12 months or older; need two doses
Shingles/zoster	Single dose at age 60 years	Give single dose at age 60 years or older (regardless if reports history of shingles)
Meningococcal conjugate vaccine quadrivalent (MCV4)	Preteens, teens, and young adults: start at age 11 to 12 years	First-year college students who will be living in residence halls are at higher risk
Pneumococcal conjugate vaccine (PCV13)	One dose lifetime for adults	Give at age 65 years, followed in 12 months by the PPSV23
Pneumococcal polysaccharide vaccine (PPSV23)	One dose at age 65 years	If vaccinated before age 65 years, give a booster in 5 years

*List is not all inclusive.

**Live virus vaccines contraindications apply.

Source: Centers for Disease Control and Prevention (2017).

Other Types of Vaccines

Bacillus Calmette-Guérin

Bacillus Calmette-Guérin (BCG) is a vaccine against tuberculosis (TB) infection. BCG is made from live attenuated (or weakened) *Mycobacterium tuberculosis*. Vaccination with BCG can produce a false positive with the TB skin test (Mantoux).

Vaccine Facts

1. *What is the follow-up if a person with a history of BCG immunization has a positive purified protein derivative (PPD)?*
   TB blood testing (QuantiFERON, T-SPOT) is preferred. Most people with a positive TB blood test have latent TB infection. TB blood tests (interferon-gamma release assays [IGRAs]), unlike the TB skin test, are not affected by prior BCG vaccination.
2. *What is the follow-up if a person has a positive TB skin test or TB blood test?*
   Evaluate the person for signs and symptoms of TB. Rule out latent or active TB infection. Order a chest x-ray and check for signs and symptoms of TB such as a "chronic" cough, weight loss, and night sweats. Preferred treatment for latent TB infection is isoniazid daily orally for 9 months. According to the CDC, there are four treatment regimens for latent TB infection (April 2016). Consult or refer to TB specialist if the source has drug-resistant TB.

The National Vaccine Injury Compensation Program (VICP)

The VICP is a federal program created to compensate people who have been injured by certain vaccines. Call 1-800-338-2382 or visit the VICP website at www.hrsa.gov/vaccinecompensation.

CLINICAL PEARLS

- **TB blood tests (IGRA) are preferred method of TB testing for people who have received the BCG vaccine.**
- **During recent influenza seasons, between 80% and 90% of influenza-related deaths occurred in people aged 65 years or older. Remind older patients to get the influenza vaccine starting in the fall season.**

5

Head, Ear, Eyes, Nose, and Throat Review

DANGER SIGNALS

EYES

Herpes Keratitis

Acute onset of severe eye pain, photophobia, tearing, and blurred vision in one eye. Diagnosed by using fluorescein dye. A black lamp in a darkened room is used to search for fern-like lines in the corneal surface. In contrast, corneal abrasions appear round or irregularly shaped. Infection permanently damages corneal epithelium, which may result in corneal blindness. There are two types of herpesvirus that can infect the eyes (herpes simplex and herpes varicella zoster or shingles). If infection is due to herpes simplex virus (due to self-inoculation "cold sore," herpes whitlow), it is called *herpes simplex keratitis*. If infection is due to shingles of the trigeminal nerve (cranial nerve [CN] V) ophthalmic branch, it is called *herpes zoster ophthalmicus*. Herpes zoster ophthalmicus has eye findings accompanied by the acute eruption of crusty rashes that follow the ophthalmic branch (CN V_1) of the trigeminal nerve (one side of forehead, eyelids, and tip of nose). Refer to ED.

Acute Angle-Closure Glaucoma

Elderly patient with acute onset of severe eye pain accompanied by headache, nausea/vomiting, halos around lights, and decreased vision. Examination reveals a mid-dilated pupil(s) that is oval shaped. The cornea appears cloudy. Funduscopic examination reveals cupping of the optic nerve. This is an ophthalmological emergency. If the rise in intraocular pressure (IOP) is slower, patient may be asymptomatic. Refer to ED.

Multiple Sclerosis (Optic Neuritis)

Young adult with new or intermittent loss of vision of one eye (optic neuritis) alone or accompanied by nystagmus or other abnormal eye movements. May be accompanied by other neurological symptoms (aphasia, paresthesia, abnormal gait, spasticity, etc.). Complains of daily fatigue on awakening that worsens as day goes on. Heat exacerbates and worsens symptoms (heat sensitivity). Has recurrent episodes. Refer to neurologist.

Orbital Cellulitis

Acute onset of erythematous swollen eyelid with proptosis (bulging of the eyeball) and eye pain on affected eye. Unable to perform full range of motion (ROM) of the eyes (abnormal extraocular movement [EOM] exam) with pain on eye movement. Look for history of recent rhinosinusitis or upper respiratory infection (URI).

Caused by acute bacterial infection of the orbital contents (fat and ocular muscles). More common in young children than adults. Serious complication. Refer to ED.

Retinal Detachment

Sudden onset of a shower of floaters associated with "looking through a curtain" sensation with sudden flashes of light (photopsia). Refer to ED.

EARS, NOSE, AND SINUSES

Cholesteatoma

"Cauliflower-like" growth accompanied by foul-smelling ear discharge. Hearing loss on affected ear. On examination, no tympanic membrane or ossicles are visible because of destruction by the tumor. History of chronic otitis media infection. The mass is not cancerous, but it can erode into the bones of the face and damage the facial nerve (CN VII). Treated with antibiotics and surgical debridement. Refer to otolaryngologist.

Battle Sign

"Raccoon eyes" (periorbital ecchymosis) and bruising behind the ear (mastoid area) that appears about 2 to 3 days after trauma. Physical exam (after trauma) does not show these two clinical signs immediately. Search for a clear golden serous discharge from the ear or nose (described next). Rule out basilar and/or temporal bone skull fracture. Basilar skull fractures can cause intracranial hemorrhage. Refer to ED.

Clear Golden Fluid Discharge From the Nose/Ear

Indicative of a basilar skull fracture. Cerebrospinal fluid (CSF) slowly leaks through the fracture. Testing the fluid with a urine dipstick will show that it is positive for glucose, whereas plain mucus or mucopurulent drainage will be negative. Refer to ED.

PHARYNX

Peritonsillar Abscess

Severe sore throat and difficulty swallowing, odynophagia (pain on swallowing), trismus (jaw muscle spasm making it difficult to open mouth), and a "hot potato" voice. Unilateral swelling of the peritonsillar area and soft palate. Affected area is markedly swollen and appears as a bulging red mass with the uvula displaced away from the mass. Accompanied by malaise, fever, and chills. Refer to ED.

Diphtheria

Sore throat, fever, and markedly swollen neck ("bull neck"). Low-grade fever, hoarseness, and dysphagia. The posterior pharynx, tonsils, uvula, and soft palate are coated with a gray- to yellow-colored pseudomembrane that is hard to displace. Very contagious. Contact prophylaxis required. Refer to ED.

☑ NORMAL FINDINGS

EYES

- *Fundi:* The veins are larger than arteries; veins are darker (in color) than arteries
- *Cones:* For color perception, 20/20 vision, sharp vision
- *Rods:* For detecting light and shadow, night vision

- *Macula (and fovea):* The macula is the area responsible for central vision; the fovea (which contains large numbers of cones) is set in the middle, the area of the eye that determines 20/20 vision (sharpest vision)
- *Presbyopia:* Age-related visual change due to a decreased ability of the eye to accommodate stiffening of the lenses; usually starts at the age of 40 years; near vision is affected with decreased ability to read small print at close range

EARS

- *Bones (ossicles) of the ear:* Malleus, incus, and stapes. The stapes is the smallest bone in the body.
- *Tympanic membrane (TM):* Appears as translucent off-white to gray color with the "cone of light" intact.
- *Tympanogram:* This is the most objective measure to test for presence of fluid inside middle ear (results in a straight line vs. a peaked shape). Acute otitis media and serious otitis media will show a straight line on testing.
- *Pinna:* Has a large amount of cartilage. Refer injuries to plastic surgeon.
- *Tragus:* A small cartilage flap of tissue that is on front of the ear.
- *Cartilage:* Is found on the nose and the ears. Does not regenerate. Refer injuries to plastic surgeon.
- *Cerumen:* Ear wax; the color can range from yellow to dark brown.

NOSE

- Only the inferior nasal turbinates are usually visible. The medial and superior turbinates are not visible without special instruments.
- Bluish, pale, and/or boggy nasal turbinates are seen in allergic rhinitis.
- Lower third of the nose is cartilage. Cartilage tissue does not regenerate; if damaged, refer to plastic surgeon.

SINUSES

Sinuses are air-filled cavities in the skull. There are four: ethmoid and maxillary sinuses (both present at birth), frontal (age 5 years), and sphenoid (age 12 years). By age 12 years, a child's sinuses are nearly at adult proportions.

MOUTH

Mucous membranes are pink to dark pink and moist. Look for ulcers, fissures, leukoplakia, and inflammation. If the gums are red and swollen, the patient may have gingivitis (gums may bleed when brushing teeth) or be taking phenytoin (Dilantin) for seizures (gingival hyperplasia). The tongue should not be red or swollen (glossitis). A normal adult has 32 teeth (except wisdom teeth).

- *Leukoplakia:* White to light-gray patch that appears on tongue, floor of mouth, or inside cheek. Rule out oral cancer. Chewing or smoking tobacco and alcohol abuse are risk factors for oral cancer.
- *Aphthous stomatitis (canker sores):* Painful shallow ulcers on soft tissue of the mouth that usually heal within 7 to 10 days. Cause is unknown. Treat symptoms with

"Magic mouthwash" (combination of liquid diphenhydramine, viscous lidocaine, and glucocorticosteroid). Swish, hold, and spit every 4 hours as needed. See Figure 5.1.

- *Avulsed tooth:* Store in cool milk (no ice) and see dentist as soon as possible for reimplantation.
- *Vermillion border:* Vermillion border is the edges of the lips. The corners of the lips are called the *oral commissure* (cheilosis, perleche).

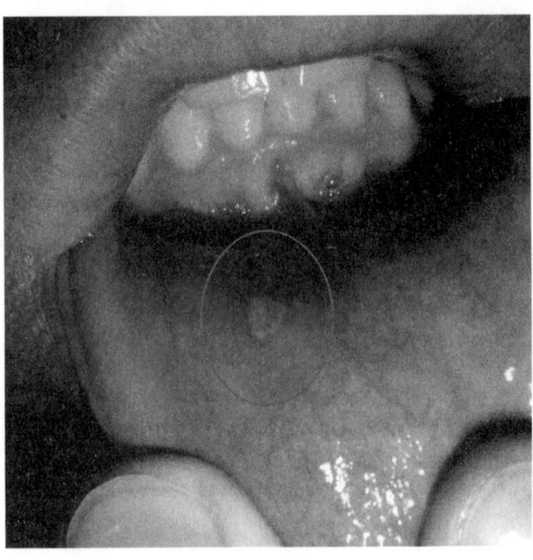

Figure 5.1 Aphthous stomatitis (canker sore). This image can be found in color in the app.

Source: Courtesy of Pfiffner Pascal.

SALIVARY GLANDS

There are three salivary glands (parotid, submandibular, and sublingual). The glands may become infected (sialadenitis, sialadenosis, mumps) or can become blocked with calculi or "stone" (sialolithiasis).

TONSILS

Also known as the *palatine tonsils*; tonsils are made up of lymphoid tissue. Butterfly-shaped glands with small pore-like openings that may secrete thick white exudate (mononucleosis) or purulent exudate that is a yellow to green color (strep throat).

POSTERIOR PHARYNX

- Look for postnasal drip (acute sinusitis, allergic rhinitis). Laying down supine worsens a postnasal drip cough. Sometimes, chronic sinusitis causes a chronic cough.
- Posterior pharyngeal lymph nodes that are mildly enlarged and distributed evenly on the back of the throat (allergies, allergic rhinitis).
- Hard palate: Look for any openings (cleft palate), ulcers, redness.
- Uvula: Should be in midline position; is displaced if infected and abscessed.

BENIGN VARIANTS

Geographic Tongue

- Tongue surface has a map-like appearance; patches may move from day to day
- Patient may complain of soreness with acidic foods, spicy foods

Torus Palatinus

- Painless bony protuberance midline on the hard palate (roof of the mouth); may be asymmetrical; skin should be normal
- Does not interfere with normal function

Fishtail or Split Uvula

- Uvula is split into two sections and resembles a fish tail
- May be a sign of an occult cleft palate (rare)

Physiological Gaze-Evoked Nystagmus

- On prolonged extreme lateral gaze, a few beats of nystagmus that resolve when the eye moves back toward midline in healthy patients, is normal
- Can also be caused by brain lesions

ABNORMAL FINDINGS

Papilledema

- Optic disc swollen with blurred edges due to increased intracranial pressure (ICP) secondary to bleeding, brain tumor, abscess, pseudotumor cerebri

Hypertensive Retinopathy (Figure 5.2)

- Copper and silver wire arterioles (caused by arteriosclerosis)
- Arteriovenous nicking (when arteriosclerotic arteriole crosses retinal vein, it indents the vein)
- Retinal hemorrhages

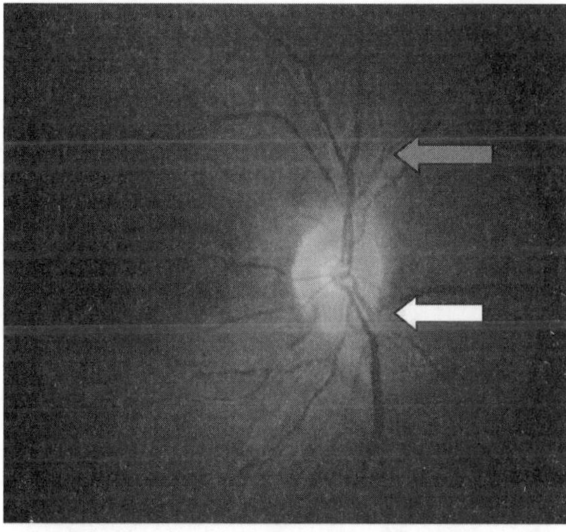

Figure 5.2 Hypertensive retinopathy. The gray arrow indicates a silver wire arteriole, and the white arrow indicates arteriovenous nicking. This image can be found in color in the app.

Source: Courtesy of Frank Wood.

Diabetic Retinopathy

- Microaneurysms (small bulges in retinal blood vessels that often leak fluid) caused by neovascularization (new fragile arteries in the retina that rupture and bleed)
- Cotton wool spots (fluffy yellow-white patches on the retina)

Cataracts

- Opacity of the lens of the eye, which can be central (nuclear cataract) or on the sides (cortical cataract)
- Up to 20% of older adults (aged 65–74 years) are affected; however, cataracts can appear at any age from birth (congenital cataracts) through adulthood to the elderly
- Symptoms include difficulty with glare (with headlights when driving at night or sunlight), halos around lights, and blurred vision

Allergic Rhinitis

- Blue-tinged or pale and swollen (boggy) nasal turbinates associated with increased in clear nasal discharge
- May be accompanied by itchy nose and nasal congestion

Koplik's Spots (Figure 5.3)

- Clusters of small-sized red papules with white centers inside the cheeks (buccal mucosa) by the lower molars
- Pathognomonic for measles

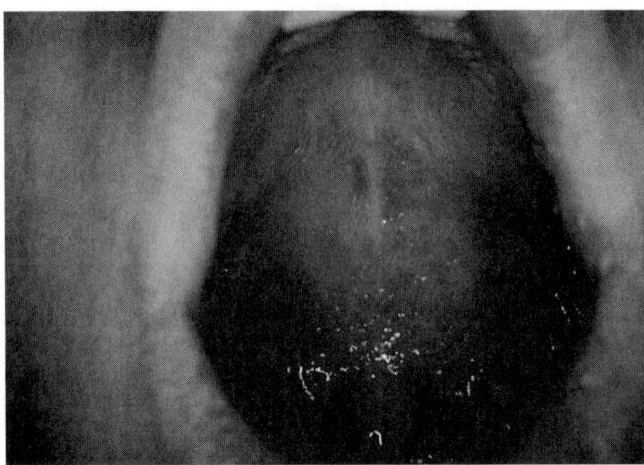

Figure 5.3 Koplik's spots. This image can be found in color in the app.

Source: Heinz F. Eichenwald, MD/Centers for Disease Control and Prevention. Retrieved from https://phil.cdc.gov/Details.aspx?pid=3187

Nasal Polyps

- Painless and soft round growths inside the nose. Look for fleshy mass inside nasal cavity. May have blockage on one side of the nose.
- There is increased risk of aspirin sensitivity or allergy.

Hairy Leukoplakia (Figure 5.4)

- Elongated papilla on the lateral aspects of the tongue that is pathognomonic for HIV infection
- Caused by Epstein–Barr virus (EBV) infection of tongue

Leukoplakia of the Oral Mucosa/Tongue

- Bright-white plaque caused by chronic irritation, such as from chewing tobacco or snuff (rule out oral cancer) or on the inner cheeks (buccal mucosa)

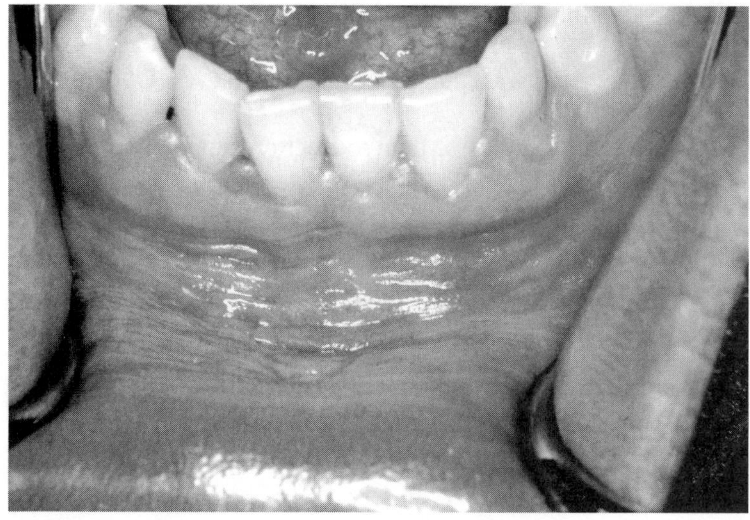

Figure 5.4 Oral hairy leukoplakia. This image can be found in color in the app.

Source: National Cancer Institute.

Cheilosis (Angular Cheilitis, Perleche)

- Painful skin fissures and maceration at the corners of the mouth due to excessive moisture. More common in elderly with dentures. Can be acute or chronic.
- Secondary infection with *Candida albicans* (yeast) or bacteria (*Staphylococcus aureus*). Multiple etiologies such as oversalivation, poorly fitting dentures, nutritional deficiencies, lupus, autoimmune disease, irritant dermatitis, squamous cell carcinoma, and pacifier use in children.

Treatment Plan

- Check B12 level to rule out pernicious anemia with cheliosis
- Remove underlying cause. Check if dentures fit correctly; if loose, refer to dentist.
- If yeast infection is suspected, microscopy with KOH. If positive (pseudohyphae and spores), treat with topical azole ointment (e.g., clotrimazole, miconazole) BID.
- If suspect staphylococcal infection, C&S. If positive, treat with topical mupirocin ointment BID.
- When infection has cleared, use barrier cream with zinc or petroleum jelly applied at night. High rate of recurrence.

EENT TERMINOLOGY

- *Palpebral conjunctiva:* Mucosal lining inside eyelids
- *Bulbar conjunctiva:* Mucosal lining covering the eyes
- *Buccal mucosa:* Mucosal lining inside the mouth
- *Soft palate:* Refers to the area where uvula, tonsils, anterior of throat are located
- *Hard palate:* "Roof" of the mouth
- *Hyperopia:* "Farsightedness"; distance vision is intact, but near vision is blurry
- *Myopia:* "Nearsightedness"; near vision intact, but distance vision is blurry
- *Cobblestoning:* Hyperplastic lymphoid tissue on the posterior pharynx

EVALUATION AND TESTING

VISION TESTING

Distance Vision

- The Snellen chart measures central distance vision.

  - If the person is illiterate, use the Tumbling E chart. Patient must stand 20 feet away from the chart.
  - If the patient wears glasses, test the vision with the glasses with both eyes (OU), the right eye (OD), and the left eye (OS).
- *Abnormal:* Two-line difference between each eye; less than four letters out of six correct.

Near Vision

- Ask patient to read small print.

Peripheral Vision

- Use the "visual fields of confrontation" exam.
- Look for blind spots (scotoma) and peripheral visual field defects.

Color Blindness

- Use the Ishihara chart.

Visual Test Results

- Definition of a Snellen test result 20/60:
  - *Top number (or numerator):* The distance in feet at which the patient stands from the Snellen or picture eye chart (always 20 feet and never changes).
  - *Bottom number (or denominator):* The number of feet that the patient can see compared to a person with normal vision (20/20 or less). Number changes, dependent on patient's vision. In this example, the patient can see at 20 feet what a person with normal vision can see at 60 feet.
- *Legal blindness:* Defined as a best corrected vision of 20/200 or less or a visual field less than 20 degrees (tunnel vision).

Children

By the age of 6 years, visual acuity (retina or CN II) is 20/20 in both eyes. Use the Snellen chart with the child standing 20 feet away from the chart. If the child's vision is not at least 20/30 in either eye by age 6 years, refer to ophthalmologist.

HEARING TESTS (TABLE 5.1)

Table 5.1 Types of Hearing Loss: Results of Weber and Rinne Tests

Results	Weber Test	Rinne Test
Normal	No lateralization (hears sound equally in both ears)	AC > BC
Sensorineural loss Presbycusis Ménière's disease	Lateralization to "good" ear (sound is heard louder in the ear that is normal)	AC > BC
Conductive loss Otitis media Serous otitis media Ceruminosis Perforation of tympanic membrane	Lateralization to "bad" ear (sound is heard louder in the "bad" or affected ear)	BC > AC

AC, air conduction; BC, bone conduction.

Weber Test (Figure 5.5)

- Place the tuning fork midline on the forehead.
- *Normal finding:* No lateralization. If lateralization (hears the sound in only one ear), abnormal finding.

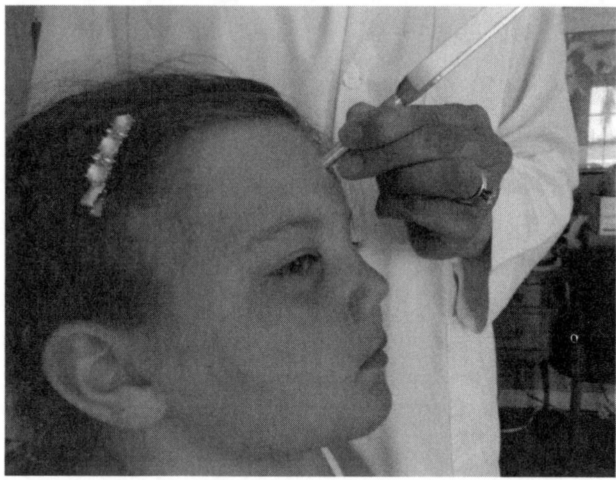

Figure 5.5 Weber test.

Rinne Test

- Place tuning fork first on mastoid process, then at front of the ear. Time each area.
- *Normal finding:* Air conduction (AC) lasts longer than bone conduction (BC; i.e., can hear longer in front of ear than on mastoid bone).

Types of Hearing Loss

Conductive Hearing Loss (Outer Ear and Middle Ear)

Any type of obstruction (or conduction) of the sound waves will cause conductive hearing loss. Other causes include blockage of the outer ear (ceruminosis, otitis externa) or fluid inside the middle ear (otitis media, serous otitis media).

Sensorineural Hearing Loss (Inner Ear)

Damage (or aging) of the cochlea/vestibule (presbycusis, Ménère's disease) and/or to the nerve pathways (CN VIII or acoustic nerve) causes sensorineural hearing loss. Other causes are ototoxic drugs (oral aminoglycosides, erythromycin, tetracyclines, high-dose aspirin, sildenafil, etc.) and stroke. Usually results in permanent hearing loss.

EXAM TIPS

- The Weber and Rinne test results are complete opposites of each other. For example, in sensorineural hearing loss, Rinne is AC greater than BC. In conductive hearing loss, it is Rinne BC greater than AC. During the exam, you could write this on your scratch paper (discussed in Chapter 1).

DISEASE REVIEW

EYES

Corneal Abrasion

Complains of acute onset of severe eye pain with tearing. Reports feeling of a foreign body sensation on the surface of the eye. Always ask any patient with eye complaints whether he or she wears contact lenses.

Herpes Keratitis

Complains of acute onset of severe eye pain, photophobia, and blurred vision in affected eye. Diagnosed by using fluorescein dye. A black lamp in a darkened room is used to search for fern-like lines in the corneal surface. (Corneal abrasions appear more linear or round.) Infection permanently damages corneal epithelium, which may result in corneal blindness.

Contact Lens-Related Keratitis

Complains of acute onset of red eye, blurred vision, watery eyes, photophobia, and sometimes a foreign-body sensation in affected eye. History of using contacts past prescribed time schedule, sleeping with contact lens, bathes/showers or swims with contacts, extended lens use, and use of tap/well water or poor disinfection practices.

Objective Findings

Use fluorescein dye strips with Wood's lamp (black lamp) in darkened room. Contact lens–associated abrasions are usually in the center and are round. Herpes keratitis appears as fern-like or branching curved lines (in contrast, corneal abrasions usually appear round or linear).

Treatment Plan

- Always check visual acuity and check pupils with penlight. Rule out penetrating trauma, retained foreign body, and contact lens-associated eye infections. If suspect bacterial infection, obtain C&S of eye discharge.
- Flush eye with sterile normal saline to remove foreign body. Evert eyelid to look for foreign body. If unable to remove, refer.
- Use topical ophthalmic antibiotic with pseudomonal coverage (especially if contact lens user) such as ciprofloxacin (Ciloxan), ofloxacin (Ocuflox), trimethoprim–polymyxin B (Polytrim) applied to affected eye × 3 to 5 days.
- Do not patch eye. Follow up in 24 hours. If not improved, refer to ED or ophthalmologist *stat* (Zovirax or Valtrex BID).
- Avoid steroid ophthalmic drops for herpes keratitis.
- Consider eye pain prescription (hydrocodone with acetaminophen; prescribe enough for 48 hours of use).
- Topical pain medication Acular 1 gtts QID (contraindication: allergy to nonsteroidal anti-inflammatory drugs [NSAIDs])

Hordeolum (Stye)

An external hordeolum is an abscess of a hair follicle and sebaceous gland in the upper or lower eyelid. An internal hordeolum involves inflammation of the meibomian gland. May have history of blepharitis.

Classic Case

Complains of acute onset of a swollen, red, and warm abscess on the upper or lower eyelid involving one hair follicle that gradually enlarges. May spontaneously rupture and drain purulent exudate. Infection may spread to adjoining tissue (preseptal cellulitis).

Treatment Plan

- Hot compresses × 5 to 10 minutes BID to TID until it drains
- If infection spreads (preseptal cellulitis), systemic antibiotics such as dicloxacillin or erythromycin PO QID. Refer to ophthalmologist for incision and drainage (I&D).

Chalazion

A chronic inflammation of the meibomian gland (specialized sweat gland) of the eyelids. It may resolve spontaneously in 2 to 8 weeks.

Classic Case

Complains of a gradual onset of a small superficial nodule on the upper eyelid that feels like a bead and is discrete and movable. Painless. Can slowly enlarge over time. If chalazion is large, it can press on the cornea and cause blurred vision.

Treatment Plan

Treatment is I&D, surgical removal, or intrachalazion corticosteroid injections by ophthalmologist.

Pinguecula

A raised yellow to white small round growth in the bulbar conjunctiva (skin covering eyeball) next to the cornea. Located on the nasal and temporal side of the eye. Caused by chronic sun exposure.

Pterygium (Figure 5.6)

A yellow triangular (wedge-shaped) thickening of the conjunctiva that extends across the cornea on the nasal side. Results from chronic sun exposure. Sometimes called *surfer's eye*. Can be red or inflamed at times. May complain of foreign body sensation on the eye.

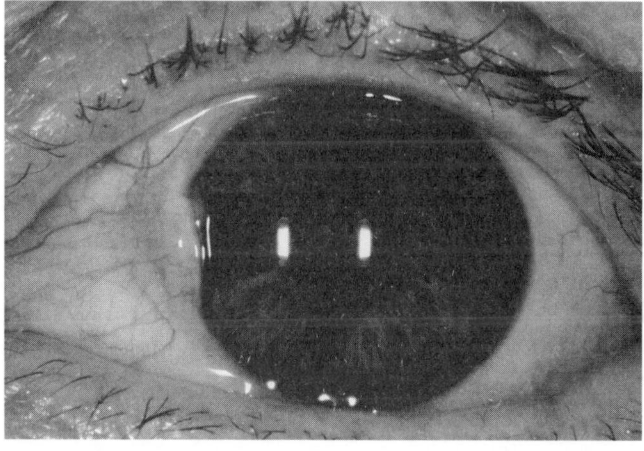

Figure 5.6 Severe pterygium. This image can be found in color in the app.

Source: Courtesy of Sciencia58.

Treatment Plan (Both Pinguecula and Pterygium)

- If inflamed, refer to ophthalmologist for prescription of weak steroid eye drops only during exacerbations. Use artificial tears PRN for irritation.
- Recommend use of good-quality sunglasses (100% against UVA and UVB).
- Remove surgically if encroaches on cornea and affects vision.

Subconjunctival Hemorrhage

Blood that is trapped underneath the conjunctiva and sclera secondary to broken arterioles. Can be caused by coughing, sneezing, heavy lifting, vomiting, local trauma, or can occur spontaneously. Resolves within 1 to 3 weeks (blood reabsorbed) like a bruise, with color changes from red, to green, to yellow. Increased risk if on aspirin, anticoagulants, and patient has hypertension.

Classic Case

Complains of sudden onset of bright-red blood in one eye after an incident of severe coughing, sneezing, or straining. May also be due to trauma such as a fall. Denies visual loss and pain.

Treatment Plan

Watchful waiting and reassurance of patient. Follow up until resolution.

Primary Open-Angle Glaucoma

Gradual onset of increased IOP greater than 22 mmHg due to blockage of the drainage of aqueous humor inside the eye. The retina (CN 2) undergoes ischemic changes and, if untreated, becomes permanently damaged. Most common type of glaucoma (60%–70%).

Classic Case

Most commonly seen in elderly patients, especially those of African or Caucasian ancestry or diabetics. Usually asymptomatic during early stages. Gradual changes in peripheral vision (lost first) and then central vision. May complain of missing portions of words when reading. If funduscopic exam shows cupping, IOP is too high. Refer to ophthalmologist.

Treatment Plan

- Check IOP (use tonometer). Normal range: 8 to 21 mmHg.
- IOP of 30 mmHg or more is considered very high. Urgent referral within 24 hours or less to ophthalmologist or refer to ED.

Medications

- *Betimol 0.5 % (timolol):* Beta-blocker eyedrops (decrease aqueous production)
- *Latanoprost (Xalatan):* Topical prostaglandin eyedrops (increase aqueous outflow)
- *Side effects and contraindications:* Same as oral form; include bronchospasm, fatigue, depression, heart failure, bradycardia
- *Contraindicated:* Asthma, emphysema, chronic obstructive pulmonary disease (COPD), second- to third-degree heart block, heart failure

Complication

- Blindness due to ischemic damage to retina (CN II)

Primary Angle-Closure Glaucoma

Sudden blockage of aqueous humor causes marked increase of the IOP, resulting in ischemia and permanent damage to the optic nerve (CN II).

Classic Case

Older patient complains of acute onset of decreased/blurred vision with severe eye pain and frontal headache that is accompanied by nausea and vomiting.

Objective Findings

- *Eyes:* Fixed and mid-dilated cloudy pupil (4–6 mm) that looks more oval than round. Pupil reacts slowly to light. Conjunctival injection with increased lacrimation.

Treatment Plan

Refer to ED.

Anterior Uveitis (Iritis)

Insidious onset of eye pain with conjunctival injection (redness; note that injection of the eye means the superficial blood vessels of the conjunctiva are prominent [red eyes]) located mainly on the limbus (junction between cornea and sclera) that is a complication of autoimmune disorders (rheumatoid arthritis [RA], lupus, ankylosing spondylitis), sarcoidosis, syphilis, others.

No purulent discharge (as in bacterial conjunctivitis). Refer to ophthalmologist for management as soon as possible within 24 hours. Anterior uveitis can result in blindness.

Age-Related Macular Degeneration (AMD)

Usually asymptomatic during the early stages. Caused by gradual damage to the pigment of the macula (area of central vision) that results in severe visual loss to blindness. Leading cause of blindness in the elderly. More common in smokers.

AMD can either be atrophic (dry form) or exudative (wet form). The dry form of AMD is more common (85%–90%) and is "less severe" compared to the wet form. The wet form of AMD is responsible for 80% of vision loss (choroidal neovascularization).

Classic Case

Elderly smoker complains of gradual or sudden and painless loss of central vision in one or both eyes. Reports that straight lines (doors, windows) appear distorted or curved. Peripheral vision is usually preserved.

Treatment Plan

- Refer to ophthalmologist. Patient is given a copy of the Amsler grid (focus eye on center dot and view grid 12 inches from eyes). Patient checks visual field loss daily to weekly (center of grid is distorted, blind spot or scotoma, or wavy lines).
- "Ocular" vitamins are lutein and zeaxanthin with zinc. Patients should consult their ophthalmologist before taking ocular vitamins.

Sjögren's Syndrome

Chronic autoimmune disorder characterized by decreased function of the lacrimal and salivary glands. It can occur alone or with another autoimmune disorder (i.e., with rheumatoid arthritis).

Classic Case

The classic symptoms are persistent daily symptoms of dry eyes and dry mouth (xerostomia) for longer than 3 months. Complains of chronic "dry eyes" and that both eyes have sandy or gritty sensation (keratoconjunctivitis sicca). Has used over-the-counter (OTC) artificial tears more than three times per day. Marked increase in dental caries; oral examination shows swollen and inflamed salivary glands.

Treatment Plan

- Use OTC tear-substitute eye drops three times/day. Refer to ophthalmologist (keratoconjunctivitis sicca). Refer to dentist (dental caries).
- Refer to rheumatologist for management.

Blepharitis

Chronic condition caused by inflammation of the eyelids (hair follicles, meibomian glands). Associated with seborrheic dermatitis and rosacea. Lid may be colonized by staphylococcal bacteria. Intermittent exacerbations. Complains of itching or irritation in the eyelids (upper/lower or both), gritty sensation, eye redness, and crusting.

Treatment Plan

- *Johnson's Baby Shampoo with warm water:* Gently scrub eyelid margins until resolves. Consider topical antibiotic solution (erythromycin eye drops) to eyelids two to three times/day (lid hygiene). Commercial eye lid scrub products are available.
- Warm compress to eyelids two to four times/day during exacerbations to soften debris and relieve itching.

NOSE

Allergic Rhinitis

Inflammatory changes of the nasal mucosa due to allergy. Increases risk of sinusitis. May have intermittent, seasonal, or daily symptoms. Atopic family history (asthma, eczema). May be allergic to dust mites (daily symptoms), mold and grasses (summer), ragweed pollen (fall), cockroach dander (older buildings in urban areas), others. May affect sleep and quality of life. Affects 10% to 30% of adults and children in the United States.

Classic Case

Complains of chronic or seasonal nasal congestion with clear mucus rhinorrhea or postnasal drip. Coughing due to postnasal drip worsens when supine. Accompanied by nasal itch and, at times, frequent sneezing. Some people produce a clicking sound to clear mucus inside their throat (palatal click).

Objective Findings

Nose has blue-tinged or pale boggy nasal turbinates. Mucus clear. Posterior pharynx reveals thick mucus, with colors ranging from clear, white, yellow, or green (rule out sinusitis). Undereye "circles" (venodilation). Children may have transverse nasal crease from frequent rubbing (allergic salute). Posterior pharynx may show cobblestoning (hyperplastic lymphoid tissue).

Treatment Plan

- First-line treatment: Topical nasal sprays
  - Use nasal steroid sprays daily (OTC): Fluticasone (Flonase) BID, triamcinolone (Nasacort Allergy 24HR), one to two sprays once a day.
  - If only partial relief, another option is topical antihistamine nasal spray azelastine (Astelin) daily or BID.
  - If no relief, consider combination product (azelastine and fluticasone nasal spray).
  - Use cromolyn sodium nasal spray TID (less effective than steroids).
- Use decongestants (i.e., pseudoephedrine, or Sudafed) PRN. Do not give to infants/young children.
- Consider oral antihistamines PRN. Second-generation antihistamines (OTC) are less sedating: cetirizine (Zyrtec), loratadine (Claritin) PO one daily or PRN. Be careful with diphenhydramine (Benadryl); it causes sedation.
- Ideally, eliminate environmental allergens.
- Dust mite allergies: Avoid using ceiling fans, no stuffed animals or pets in bed, use a HEPA filter for air conditioners, room filters, and the like. Refer to allergist.

Complications

- Acute sinusitis
- Acute otitis media

Rhinitis Medicamentosa

- Prolonged use of topical nasal decongestants (>3 days) causes rebound effects that result in severe and chronic nasal congestion.

- Patients present with daily severe nasal congestion and nasal discharge (clear, watery, mucus).

Epistaxis (Nosebleeds)

Anterior nasal bleeds are milder and more common than posterior nasal bleeds. Most episodes are self-limiting. Anterior nasal bleeds are the result of bleeding from Kiesselbach's plexus (vascular area). Posterior nasal bleeds can lead to severe hemorrhage. Aspirin use, NSAIDs, cocaine abuse, severe hypertension, and anticoagulants (i.e., warfarin sodium or Coumadin) place patients at higher risk. (Intranasal cocaine use can cause nosebleeds and nasal septum perforation.)

Classic Case

Complains of acute onset of nasal bleeding secondary to trauma (i.e., nose picking). Bright-red blood may drip externally through the nasal passages and/or the posterior pharynx. Profuse bleeding can result in vomiting of blood.

Treatment Plan

- Apply direct pressure on the front of the nose for several minutes. Use of nasal decongestants (i.e., Afrin) to shrink tissue helps to stop bleeding.
- Apply triple antibiotic ointment or petroleum jelly in front of the nose using cotton swab for a few days.

Complications

- Posterior nasal bleeds may hemorrhage. Refer to ED.

THROAT

Streptococcal Pharyngitis/Tonsillopharyngitis ("Strep" Throat)

An acute infection of the pharynx and/or palatine tonsils caused by group A streptococcal bacteria (*Streptococcus pyogenes*). Keep in mind that the most common pathogen is viral (rhinovirus, adenovirus, respiratory syncytial virus [RSV], etc.). Suspect viral etiology (or coinfection) if cough and symptoms such as stuffy nose, rhinitis with clear mucus, and watery eyes (coryza).

Classic Case

All ages are affected, but is most common in children. Abrupt onset of fever, sore throat, pain on swallowing, and mildly enlarged submandibular nodes. May have purulent exudate on tonsils. Anterior cervical nodes mildly enlarged and tender (anterior cervical adenitis). Adult may report having a child attending preschool.

> **Note**
>
> Centor criteria are a clinical decision tool used to help diagnose "strep" throat. Criteria for strep throat include tonsillar exudate, tender anterior cervical adenopathy, history of fever, and absence of cough.

Objective Findings

- Pharynx dark pink to bright red. Adults usually afebrile (or mild fever).
- May have tonsillar exudate that is yellow to green color. May have petechiae on the hard palate (roof of the mouth). Anterior cervical lymph nodes mildly enlarged.

Treatment Plan

- Rapid antigen detection testing (RADT) is a rapid "strep" test or throat C&S
- First line: Oral penicillin V 500 mg BID to TID × 10 days
- Alternative: Amoxicillin 500 mg BID × 10 days
  - Penicillin or beta-lactam allergy: Azithromycin (Z-Pak) × 5 days
- Throat pain and fever: Ibuprofen (Advil) or acetaminophen (Tylenol)
- Symptomatic treatment: Salt water gargles, throat lozenges; drink more fluids
- Repeat C&S after antibiotic treatment (test-of-cure): History of mitral valve prolapse or heart valve surgery

Complications

- *Scarlet fever (scarlatina):* Sandpaper-textured pink rash with sore throat and strawberry tongue (red sore tongue). Rash starts on the head and neck and spreads to the trunk, then the extremities. Next, the skin desquamates (peels off). Increased risk of acute rheumatic fever.
- *Acute rheumatic fever:* Inflammatory reaction to strep infection that may affect the heart and the valves, joints, and the brain.
- *Peritonsillar abscess:* Displaced uvula, red bulging mass on one side of anterior pharyngeal space, dysphagia, fever. Refer to ED *stat*.
- *Poststreptococcal glomerulonephritis*: Abrupt onset of proteinuria, hematuria, dark-colored urine, and RBC casts (urine) accompanied by hypertension and edema.

EARS AND SINUSES

Acute Otitis Media (AOM; Purulent or Suppurative Otitis Media)

Most cases occur in childhood. An acute infection of the middle ear cavity with bacterial pathogens due to mucus that becomes trapped in the middle ear secondary to temporary eustachian tube dysfunction. The infection is usually unilateral, but may at times involve both ears. Most have middle ear effusion (MEE).

Organisms

Adult infections usually due to *S. pneumoniae*. High rates of beta-lactamase resistance.

- *S. pneumoniae* (gram positive; up to 40% of cases
- *Haemophilus influenzae* (gram negative; up to 50% of cases)
- *Moraxella catarrhalis* (gram negative; up to 20% of cases)

Classic Case

Complains of ear pain (otalgia), popping noises, muffled hearing. Recent history of a cold or flare-up of allergic rhinitis. Adult infections usually develop much more slowly than in children. Afebrile or low-grade fever. May be accompanied by rupture of the TM (reports blood and pus seen on pillowcase on awakening with relief of ear pain).

Bullous Myringitis

Type of AOM infection that is more painful due to the presence of blisters (bullae) on a reddened and bulging tympanic membrane. Conductive hearing loss. Caused by different types of pathogens (mycoplasma, viral, bacteria). Treat the same as bacterial AOM.

Objective Findings

- Weber exam shows lateralization to the "bad"/affected ear (conductive hearing loss).
- Rinne test result is BC > AC (conductive hearing loss).

- TM: Bulging or retraction with displaced light reflex (displaced landmarks); may look opaque
- Erythematous TM
- Decreased mobility with flat-line tracing on tympanogram (most objective finding)
- If TM is ruptured, purulent discharge from affected ear (and relief of ear pain)

Treatment Plan

First Line

- Amoxicillin is first-line treatment for any age group (if no antibiotics in the prior month). Give amoxicillin 500 mg PO TID × 5 to 7 days.
  - Mild to moderate disease: Treat 5 to 7 days. Severe disease: Treat 10 days.
  - Most patients will respond in 48 to 72 hours. If no response to treatment, switch to second-line drug such as amoxicillin–clavulanate (Augmentin) TID, cefdinir (Omnicef) or cefprozil (Ceftin) BID, or levofloxacin (Levaquin) or moxifloxacin (Avelox) daily × 5 days.
- In addition to antibiotic, treat symptoms of ear pain (otalgia) and eustachian tube dysfunction (becomes swollen due to inflammation and cannot drain.). Patient will complain of a "plugged up" ear (MEE) and decreased hearing in affected ear (temporary). When fluid in the middle ear drains, hearing will become normal.

CLINICAL PEARLS

- **MEEs can persist for 8 weeks or longer after treatment of AOM.**
- **Allergy pillow covers, allergy mattresses, and HEPA allergy filters for air conditioners are recommended for patients with allergic rhinitis. Many are allergic to dust mites, an indoor allergen.**

ACUTE BACTERIAL RHINOSINUSITIS (ABRS)

- The maxillary and frontal sinuses are most commonly affected. Reports a history of a "bad cold" or flare-up of allergic rhinitis. Fluid is trapped inside the sinuses, causing secondary bacterial (*S. pneumoniae, H. influenzae*) or viral infection.

Classic Case

Complains of unilateral facial pain or upper molar pain (maxillary sinus) with nasal congestion for 10 days or longer with purulent nasal and/or postnasal drip. If frontal sinusitis, pain is located over the frontal sinus. May report hyposmia (reduced ability to smell). Postnasal drip cough worsens when supine and may interfere with sleep. Self-treatment with OTC cold and sinus remedies provides no relief of symptoms.

Objective Findings

- Posterior pharynx: Purulent dark yellow- to green-colored postnasal drip
- Sinuses: Are tender to palpation on the front cheek (maxillary) or on frontal sinus area above the inner canthus of the eye
- If seen with allergy flare-up, possible boggy swollen nasal turbinates
- Fever seen more often in children than adults
- Transillumination (frontal and maxillary sinuses: Positive ("glow" of light on infected sinus is duller compared with normal sinus); in transillumination, turn off the light (darken room). Place a bright light source directly on the surface of the cheek (on maxillary sinus). Instruct patient to open mouth and look at the roof of the mouth (hard

palate) for a round glow of light. Compare both sides. The "affected" sinus has no glow or duller glow compared with the normal sinus. For frontal sinusitis, place the light under the supraorbital ridge in the medial aspect and compare glow of light.

Treatment Plan

- There are two options when treating sinusitis:
  - Symptomatic treatment without antibiotics if mild, uncomplicated ABRS in healthy patient). Follow up in 10 days (if better, no antibiotics needed). If symptoms are worse (or have not resolved) on follow-up visit, initiate antibiotic treatment.
  - Treat with antibiotics if there are severe symptoms (toxic, high fever, pain, purulent nasal or postnasal drip for 2 to 3 days or longer), patient is immunocompromised, symptoms present for longer than 10 days (or have worsened).
- There is a high rate of spontaneous resolution in acute sinusitis (Gilbert, Chambers, Eliopoulos, Saag, & Pavia, 2016).

Antibiotic Treatment

First-Line (Adults)

- Amoxicillin–clavulanate (Augmentin) 1,000/62.5 mg or 2,000 mg/125 mg one tablet PO BID × 5 to 7 days. Treatment of children is covered in Section IV, Pediatrics and Adolescents Review.

Penicillin Allergy or Alternative Antibiotics

- Type 1 allergy (e.g., anaphylaxis, angioedema): Levofloxacin 750 mg PO daily or doxycycline BID × 5 to 7 days
- Type 2 allergy (e.g., skin rash): Cefdinir (Omnicef), cefpodoxime (Vantin), cefuroxime (Ceftin) PO BID × 5 to 7 days

Symptomatic or Adjunct Treatment (Rhinosinusitis or Otitis Media)

- Pain or fever
  - Naproxen sodium (Anaprox DS) PO BID or ibuprofen (Advil) PO QID PRN
  - Acetaminophen (Tylenol) every 4 to 6 hours PRN
- Drainage
  - Oral decongestants such as pseudoephedrine (Sudafed) or pseudoephedrine combined with guaifenesin (Mucinex D)
  - Topical decongestants (i.e., Afrin): Use only for 3 days maximum or will cause rebound
  - Saline nasal spray (Ocean spray) one to two sprays every 2 to 3 hours PRN
  - Steroid nasal spray (Flonase, Vancenase) if allergic rhinitis
  - Mucolytic (guaifenesin) and increase fluid to thin mucus
- Cough
  - Dextromethorphan (Robitussin) QID
  - Benzonatate (Tessalon Perles) prescription: Swallow pills with water; do not crush, suck, or chew; toxic for children younger than age 10 years (seizures, cardiac arrest, death)
  - Increase intake of fluids, avoid exposure to cigarette smoke and alcohol
  - The use of systemic steroids is not recommended

Treatment Failure

If symptoms persist despite treatment (purulent nasal discharge, sinus pain, nasal congestion, fever), switch to another antibiotic. If on amoxicillin, change antibiotic to amoxicillin–clavulanate (Augmentin) PO q12h × 10 to 14 days or levofloxacin (Levaquin) 750 mg daily. Recurrent sinusitis, refer to otolaryngologist.

Serious Complications of Otitis Media and Rhinosinusitis

- Refer to ED *stat*.
- *Mastoiditis:* Red and swollen mastoid that is tender to palpation.
- *Preorbital or orbital cellulitis (more common in children):* Swelling and redness at periorbital area, double vision or impaired vision and fever. Abnormal EOM (extraorbital muscles) movement of affected orbit (check cranial nerves, EOM). Altered level of consciousness (LOC) or mental status changes.
- *Meningitis:* Acute onset of high fever, stiff neck, severe headache, photophobia, toxic. Positive Brudzinski's or Kernig's sign.
- *Cavernous sinus thrombosis:* Complains of acute headache, abnormal neurological exam, confused, febrile. Life-threatening emergency with high mortality.

Otitis Media With Effusion (OME; Serous Otitis Media)

May follow AOM. Can also be caused by chronic allergic rhinitis. Complains of ear pressure, popping noises, and muffled hearing in affected ear. Sterile serous fluid is trapped inside middle ear.

Objective Findings

- TM may bulge or retract. Tympanogram abnormal (flat line or no peak).
- TM should not be red.
- A fluid level and/or bubbles may be visible inside the tympanic membrane.

Treatment Plan

- Oral decongestants (pseudoephedrine or phenylalanine)
- Steroid nasal spray BID to TID × few weeks or saline nasal spray (Ocean spray) PRN
- Allergic rhinitis, steroid nasal sprays with long-acting oral antihistamine (Zyrtec)

Otitis Externa (Swimmer's Ear)

Bacterial infection of the skin of the external ear canal (rarely fungal). More common during warm and humid weather (i.e., summer).

Organisms

- *Pseudomonas aeruginosa* (gram negative)
- *S. aureus* (gram positive)

Classic Case

Complains of external ear pain, swelling, discharge, pruritus, and hearing loss (if ear canal is blocked with pus). History of recent activities that involve swimming or getting ears wet.

Objective Findings

Ear pain with manipulation of the external ear or tragus. Purulent green discharge. Erythematous and swollen ear canal that is very tender to touch.

Treatment Plan

- Polymyxin B-neomycin-hydrocortisone (Cortisporin Otic) suspension 4 gtts QID × 7 days. Ofloxacin otic or ciprofloxacin otic ear drops BID × 7 days
- Keep water out of ear during treatment. If patient has recurrent episodes, prophylaxis is Otic Domeboro (boric) or alcohol and vinegar (VoSol).

Infectious Mononucleosis

Infection by the EBV (herpesvirus family). Peak ages of acute infection in the United States are between ages 15 and 24 years. After acute infection, EBV virus lies latent in oropharyngeal tissue. Can become reactivated and cause symptoms. Virus is shed mainly through saliva. *Classic triad:* Fever, pharyngitis, lymphadenopathy (> 50% cases).

Classic Case

Teenage patient presents with history of sore throat, enlarged posterior cervical nodes, and fatigue (several weeks). Fatigue may last weeks to months. May have abdominal pain due to hepatomegaly and/or splenomegaly. History of intimate kissing.

Objective Findings

- *CBC:* Atypical lymphocytes and lymphocytosis (greater than 50%); repeat CBC until resolves
- *LFTs:* Abnormal for 80% for several weeks
- *Heterophile antibody test (Monospot):* Positive (80%–90% of adults)
- *Nodes:* Large cervical nodes that may be tender to palpation
- *Pharynx:* Erythematous
- *Tonsils:* Inflamed, sometimes with cryptic exudate (off-white color)
- *Hepatomegaly (20%) and splenomegaly (50%):* Avoid vigorous palpation of the abdomen until resolves
- *Skin:* Occasionally a generalized red maculopapular rash is present

Treatment Plan

- Acute stages: Limit physical activity (sports, contact sports, weightlifting) for 4 weeks to reduce risk of splenic rupture. Order abdominal ultrasound if splenomegaly/hepatomegaly is present, especially if patient is an athlete, a physically active adult, or an athletic coach. Repeat abdominal ultrasound in 4 to 6 weeks if abnormal to document resolution.
- Treat symptoms.
- Avoid using amoxicillin if patient has "strep" throat (drug rash from 70% to 90%). Avoid close contact, kissing, sharing toothbrush, fork, spoon, knife, or using the same glass.

Complications

- Splenomegaly/splenic rupture is a rare but serious complication of mononucleosis.
- If airway obstruction, hospitalize and give high-dose steroids to decrease swelling.
- Neurological complications: Guillain–Barré, aseptic meningitis, optic neuritis, others.
- Blood dyscrasias (atypical lymphocytes) have repeat CBC until lymphocytes normalized.

EXAM TIPS

- **Seasonal allergic rhinitis: Topical steroid nasal spray (e.g., Flonase) is first-line treatment.**
- **New-onset urticaria: Benadryl or Zyrtec work well. Benadryl causes sedation and effect lasts several hours. Zyrtec is nonsedating and lasts 24 hours.**
- **Acute or reactivated mononucleosis can present with generalized maculopapular rash, enlarged tonsils with cryptic exudate (white or darker color), sore throat, enlarged cervical nodes that are tender to touch.**
- **Treatment for otitis externa is Cortisporin Otic drops (topical antibiotic combined with a steroid).**
- **Common bacterial pathogen in otitis externa is *P. aeruginosa*.**
- **Ruptured spleen is a catastrophic event. Avoid contact sports (i.e., 4 weeks) until ultrasound documents resolution.**
- **Betimol (timolol) ophthalmic drops have the same contraindications as oral beta blockers.**

- Cholesteatoma presents in affected ear with hearing loss, no TM, purulent exudate with odor, and yellowish to whitish cauliflower-like mass inside the middle ear.
- Penicillin-allergic patients, use macrolides, gram-positive coverage quinolones (avoid cephalosporins if had class I reaction or anaphylaxis from penicillins).
- Learn to recognize a description of eye findings such as pinguecula, pterygium, chalazion.
- Rinne test result of BC greater than AC with conductive hearing loss (i.e., ceruminosis, AOM).
- Weber test result is lateralization to the "bad" or affected ear with conductive hearing loss.
- Weber or Rinne are tests of the acoustic nerve or CN VIII.
- Lateralization (hearing sound louder on one side) on the Weber exam is an abnormal finding.
- Normal finding and sensorineural hearing loss results with the Rinne test is air conduction that lasts longer than bone conduction (AC > BC).
- Remember what 20/40 vision means: Patient can see at 20 feet what a person with normal vision can see at 40 feet.
- Carbamide peroxide (similar to hydrogen peroxide) is one of the most common OTC treatments for ceruminosis.
- Recognize herpes keratitis; cause is either herpes simplex or varicella zoster (shingles of trigeminal nerve ophthalmic branch). If herpes keratitis, refer to ED, ophthalmologist *stat.*
- Use fluorescein strips to check for corneal abrasions, keratitis.

6

Skin and Integumentary System Review

⚠ DANGER SIGNALS

Rocky Mountain Spotted Fever (RMSF)

Patient presents with abrupt onset of high fever, chills, severe headache, nausea/vomiting, photophobia, myalgia, and arthralgia followed by a rash that erupts 2 to 5 days after onset of fever. The rash consists of small red spots (petechiae) that start to erupt on both the wrist, forearms, and ankles (sometimes the palms and soles). It rapidly progresses toward the trunk until it becomes generalized (approximately 10% RMSF patients do not develop a rash). Most cases of RMSF occur from April to September (spring to summer). Highest frequency among males, Native Americans, and people aged 40 years or older. Higher mortality if not treated during the first 5 days of the infection. First-line treatment is doxycycline (both children and adults). More than 60% of cases occur in five states (NC, OK, AK, TN, MO). Use of DEET-containing repellent on skin and permethrin on clothing and gear can repel dog and deer ticks. See Figure 6.1 and Table 6.1.

Brown Recluse Spider Bites

Brown recluse spiders (*Loxosceles reclusa*) are found mostly in the midwestern and southeastern United States. Systemic symptoms include fever, chills, nausea, and vomiting. Deaths are rare but have occurred in young children (younger than age 7 years). Any child with systemic signs should be hospitalized (may cause hemolysis).

Most spider bites are located on the arms, upper legs, or the trunk (underneath clothing). Bite may feel like a pinprick (or be painless). The bitten area becomes swollen, red, and tender, and blisters appear within 24 to 48 hours. Central area of bite becomes necrotic (purple-black eschar). When the eschar sloughs off, it leaves an ulcer, which takes several weeks to heal.

Erythema Migrans (Early Lyme Disease)

The classic lesion is an expanding red rash with central clearing that resembles a target. The "bulls-eye" or target rash usually appears within 7 to 14 days after a deer tick bite (range, 3–30 days). The rash feels hot to the touch and has a rough texture. Common locations are the belt line, axillary area, behind the knees, and in the groin area. It is accompanied by flu-like symptoms. The lesion spontaneously resolves within a few weeks. It is most common in the northeastern regions of the United States. Use of DEET-containing repellent on skin and permethrin on clothing and gear can repel deer ticks. See Table 6.1.

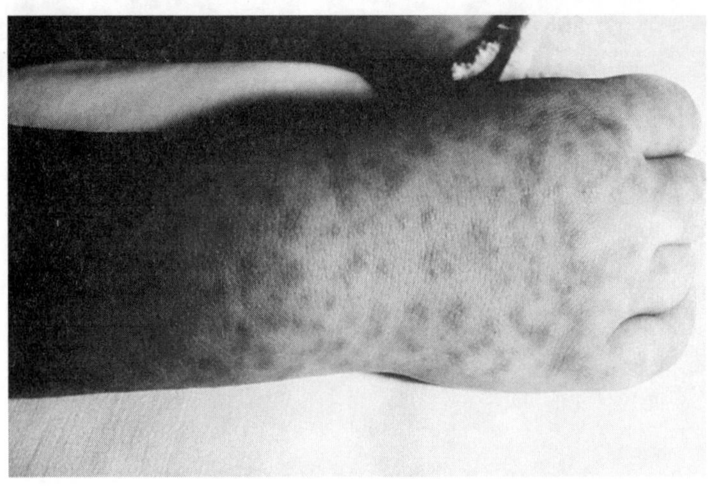

Figure 6.1 Rocky Mountain spotted fever (later stage rash). This image can be found in color in the app.

Source: Centers for Disease Control and Prevention. Retrieved from https://phil.cdc.gov/Details.aspx?pid=1962

Table 6.1 Skin Rashes

Disease	Description
Impetigo	"Honey-colored" crusts; fragile bullae; pruritic
Measles	Koplik's spots are small, white, round spots on a red base on the buccal mucosa by the rear molars
Scabies	Very pruritic, especially at night; serpiginous rash on interdigital webs, waist, axilla, penis
Scarlet fever	"Sandpaper" rash with sore throat (strep throat)
Tinea versicolor	Hypopigmented round to oval macular rashes; most lesions on upper shoulders/back; not pruritic
Pityriasis rosea	"Christmas tree" pattern rash (rash on cleavage lines); "herald patch" largest lesion, appears initially
Molluscum contagiosum	Smooth papules 1-mm size that are dome-shaped with central umbilication with a white "plug"
Erythema migrans	Red target-like lesions that grow in size; some central clearing; early stage of Lyme disease
Meningococcemia*	Purple-colored to dark-red painful skin lesions all over body; acute-onset high fever; headache; level of consciousness changes; rifampin prophylaxis for close contacts
Rocky Mountain spotted fever* (*Rickettsia rickettsii* from tick bite)	Red spot-like rashes that first break out on the hand/palm/wrist and on the feet/sole/ankles; acute-onset high fever; severe headache; myalgias

*These are life-threatening and are CDC reportable diseases.

Meningococcemia (Meningitis)

Symptoms include sudden onset of sore throat, cough, fever, headache, stiff neck, photophobia, and changes in level of consciousness (LOC; drowsiness, lethargy to coma). In some cases, there is abrupt onset of petechial to hemorrhagic rashes (pink to purple colored) in the axillae, flanks, wrist, and ankles (50%–80% of cases). Rapid progression in fulminant cases results in death within 48 hours. The risk is higher for first-year college students residing in dormitories and individuals with asplenia (no spleen), defective spleen (sickle cell anemia), HIV infection, or complement immune system deficiencies (Centers for Disease Control and

Prevention [CDC] recommends vaccination for these higher risk groups). Aerosol droplet precautions. Rifampin (BID for 2 days) prophylaxis is recommended for close contacts. See Table 6.1.

Shingles Infection of the Trigeminal Nerve (Herpes Zoster Ophthalmicus)

A sight-threatening condition caused by reactivation of the herpes zoster virus that is located on the ophthalmic branch of the trigeminal nerve (CN V). Patient reports sudden eruption of multiple vesicular lesions (ruptures into shallow ulcers with crusts) that are located on one side on the scalp, forehead, and the sides and the tip of the nose. If herpetic rash is seen on the tip of the nose, assume it is shingles until proven otherwise. The eyelid on the same side is swollen and red. The patient complains of photophobia, eye pain, and blurred vision. This is more common in elderly patients. Refer to an ophthalmologist or the ED as soon as possible.

Melanoma

Dark-colored moles with uneven texture, variegated colors, and irregular borders with a diameter of 6 mm or larger are observed. They may be pruritic. If melanoma is in the nail beds (subungual melanoma), it may be very aggressive. Lesions can be located anywhere on the body, including the retina. Risk factors include family history of melanoma (10% of cases), extensive/intense sunlight exposure, blistering sunburn in childhood, tanning beds, high nevus count/atypical nevus, and light skin/eyes. See Figure 6.2.

Acral Lentiginous Melanoma

This is the most common type of melanoma in African Americans and Asians, and it is a subtype of melanoma (<5%). These dark-brown to black lesions are located on the nail beds (subungual), palmar, and plantar surfaces, and rarely the mucous membranes. Subungual melanomas look like longitudinal brown to black bands on the nail bed.

Basal Cell Carcinoma (BCC)

Superficial form (30%) of BCC looks like a pearly or waxy skin lesion with an atrophic or ulcerated center that does not heal. The color could be white, light pink, brown, or flesh colored. It may bleed easily with mild trauma. This is more common in fair-skinned individuals with long-term daily sun exposure. An important risk factor is severe sunburns as a child. See Figure 6.3.

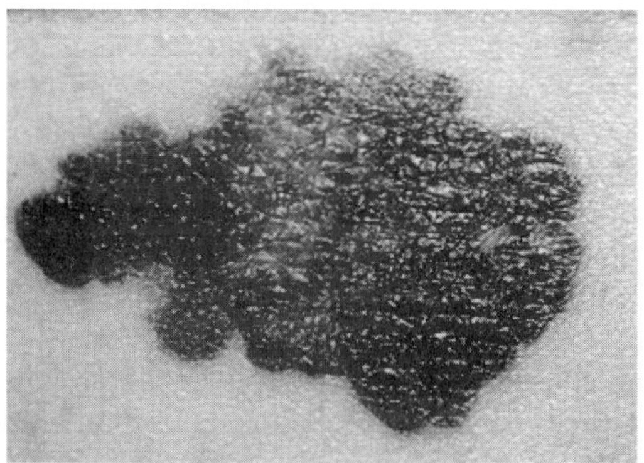

Figure 6.2 Melanoma. This image can be found in color in the app.

Source: National Cancer Institute (1985). Retrieved from https://visualsonline.cancer.gov/details.cfm?imageid=9186

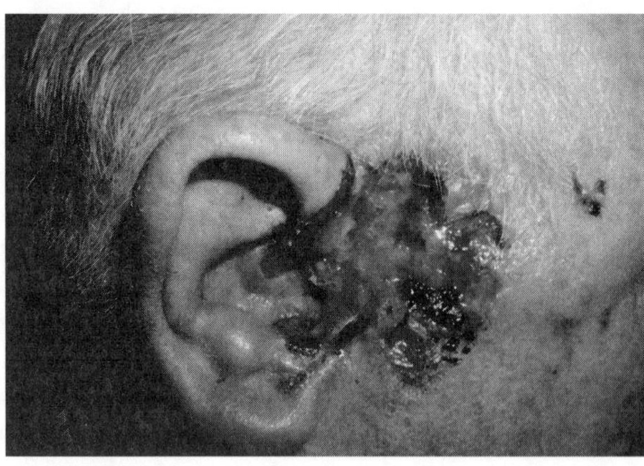

Figure 6.3 Basal cell carcinoma. This image can be found in color in the app.

Source: Courtesy of Klaus D. Peter.

Actinic Keratosis

Older to elderly fair-skinned adults complain of numerous dry, round, and red-colored lesions with a rough texture that do not heal. Lesions are slow growing. Most common locations are sun-exposed areas such as the cheeks, nose, face, neck, arms, and back. The risk is highest for those with light-colored skin, hair, and/or eyes. In some cases, a precancerous lesion of squamous cell carcinoma is a possibility. Patients with early-childhood history of severe sunburns are at higher risk for skin cancer (squamous cell carcinoma, BCC, melanoma).

Subungual Hematoma

Direct trauma to the nail bed results in pain and bleeding that is trapped between the nail bed and the finger/toenail. If the hematoma involves more than 25% of the area of the nail, there is a high risk of permanent ischemic damage to the nail matrix if the blood is not drained. One method of draining (trephination) a subungual hematoma is to straighten one end of a steel paperclip or to use an 18-gauge needle and heat it with a flame until it is very hot. The hot end is pushed down gently (90-degree angle) until a 3- to 4-mm hole is burned on the nail. The nail is pressed down gently until most or all of the blood is drained or suctioned with a smaller needle. Blood may continue draining for 24 to 36 hours.

Stevens–Johnson Syndrome (SJS) and Toxic Epidermal Necrolysis (TEN)

The classic lesions appear like a target (or a "bulls-eye"). Multiple lesions start erupting abruptly and can range from hives, blisters (bullae), petechiae, purpura, and necrosis and sloughing of the epidermis. Extensive mucosal surface involvement (eyes, nose, mouth, esophagus, and bronchial tree) is observed. There could be a prodrome of fever with flulike symptoms by 1 to 3 days before rashes appear. SJS is less severe (involves less than 10% body skin) compared with TEN (involves >30% of body skin). The most common triggers are medications such as allopurinol, anticonvulsants (lamotrigine, carbamazepine, phenobarbital), sulfonamides, and oxicam nonsteroidal anti-inflammatory drugs (NSAIDs). Mortality rate ranges from 10% (SJS) to 30% (TEN). Risk factors are HIV-infection (100-fold higher risk), infection, genetics, lupus, malignancies, and others. HIV infected patients have a 40-fold increased risk of SJS/TEN from trimethoprim–sulfamethoxazole compared with the general population.

NORMAL FINDINGS

Anatomy of the Skin

Three layers: Epidermis, dermis, and subcutaneous layer

- *Epidermis:* No blood vessels; gets nourishment from the dermis. Consists of two layers:
  - Top layer consists of keratinized cells (dead squamous epithelial cells).
  - Bottom layer is where melanocytes reside and vitamin D synthesis occurs.
- *Dermis:* Consists of blood vessels, sebaceous glands, and hair follicles.
- *Subcutaneous layer:* Is composed of fat, sweat glands, and hair follicles.

Skin Examination: Darker-Colored Skin

Urticaria and wheals can appear paler than surrounding skin (palpate for induration and warmth). Very dry dark skin can appear ashy to gray in color (check arms and legs). Skin conditions that are more common in people of African background are keloids, hyperpigmentation, and traction alopecia (due to chronic tight hair braiding).

Pseudofolliculitis barbae (barber's itch) affects up to 60% of African American men. It is caused by inflammation from the curly hair growing back into the skin. The "treatment" is to let the beard hair grow for 3 to 4 weeks. Advise patient to avoid shaving beard hair too short and too close to the skin.

Vitamin D Synthesis

People with darker skin require longer periods of sun exposure to produce vitamin D. A deficiency in pregnancy results in infantile rickets (brittle bones, skeletal abnormalities).

SKIN LESIONS

Screening for Melanoma

- The "A, B, C, D, E" of melanoma:
  - **A** (asymmetry)
  - **B** (border irregular)
  - **C** (color varies in the same region)
  - **D** (diameter >6 mm)
  - **E** (enlargement or change in size)
- Other symptoms to watch for include intermittent bleeding with mild trauma and new onset of itching.

Skin Cancer Statistics

Skin cancer is the most common cancer in the United States. Basal cell skin carcinoma is the most common type of skin cancer.

Skin Lesion Review

Primary Skin Lesions

- *Macule:* Flat nonpalpable lesion less than 1 cm diameter
  - *Example*: Freckles (ephelis), lentigo or lentigines (plural)
- *Papule:* Palpable solid lesion less than or equal to 0.5 cm in diameter
  - *Example*: Nevi (moles), acne, small cherry angiomas
- *Plaque:* Flattened elevated lesion with variable shape greater than 1 cm in diameter
  - *Example*: Psoriatic lesions

- *Bulla:* Elevated superficial blister filled with serous fluid and more than 1 cm in size
  - *Example:* Impetigo, second-degree burn with blisters, SJS lesions
- *Vesicle:* Elevated superficial skin lesion less than 1 cm in diameter and filled with serous fluid
  - *Example*: Herpetic lesions
- *Pustule:* Elevated superficial skin lesion less than 1 cm in diameter filled with purulent fluid
  - *Example*: Acne pustules

Secondary Skin Lesions

- Primary lesion that changes; complication of a primary lesion or injury
- *Lichenification*: Thickening of the epidermis with exaggeration of normal skin lines due to chronic itching (eczema)
- *Scale*: Flaking skin (psoriasis)
- *Crust*: Dried exudate, may be serous exudate (impetigo)
- *Ulceration*: Full-thickness loss of skin (decubiti or pressure injury)
- *Scar*: Permanent fibrotic changes following damage to the dermis (surgical scars)
- *Keloids/hypertrophic scar*: Overgrowth of scar tissue; more common in Blacks, Asians

DERMATOLOGY TERMS

- *Acral*: Distal portions of the limbs such as the hand or feet (acral melanoma)
- *Annular*: Ring-shaped (ringworm or tinea corporis)
- *Exanthem*: Another term for cutaneous rash
- *Flexural:* Skin flexures are body folds (eczema affects flexural folds)
- *Maculopapular rash*: Rash with color (usually pink to red) with small bumps that are raised above the skin (viral rashes)
- *Morbilliform:* Rash that resembles measles (pink rash with texture)
- *Nummular*: Coin-shaped, round (nummular eczema)
- *Purpura*: Bleeding into the skin; small bleeds are petechial (RMSF) and larger areas of bleeding are ecchymoses or purpura (meningococcemia)
- *Serpiginous*: Shaped like a snake (larva migrans)
- *Verrucous*: Wart-like

SKIN: CLINICAL FINDINGS

Urticaria (Hives)

Erythematous and raised skin lesions with discrete borders that are irregular, oval, or round. Lesions become more numerous and enlarge over minutes to hours, and then disappear. May occur as one episode or recurrent (usually daily) episodes that resolve in 24 hours and then recur. Skin that is compressed (e.g., with tight bra straps) may have lesions that assume a shape (such as linear-shaped lesions under bra strap). Urticaria is considered chronic if it lasts longer than 6 weeks. Most cases are self-limited. Urticaria has multiple etiologies (medications, viral/bacterial infections, insect bites, latex allergies, etc). If associated with angioedema or progresses to anaphylaxis, it can be life-threatening. See Figure 6.4.

Seborrheic Keratoses

Soft, wart-like, fleshy growths in the trunk that are located mostly on the back. Skin lesions look like they are "pasted" on the skin. Lesions on the same person can range in color from light tan to black. Start to appear during middle age (or later) and become more numerous as patient gets older. Painless.

Xanthelasma

Raised and yellow-colored soft plaques that are usually located under the brow or upper and/or lower lids of the eyes on the nasal side. If the patient is younger than 40 years of age, rule out hyperlipidemia. About 50% of patients with xanthelasma have hyperlipidemia. If the xanthomas are located on the fingers, it is pathognomic for familial hypercholesterolemia. Order a fasting (9 hours) lipid profile. Also known as *plane xanthomas*. See Figure 6.5.

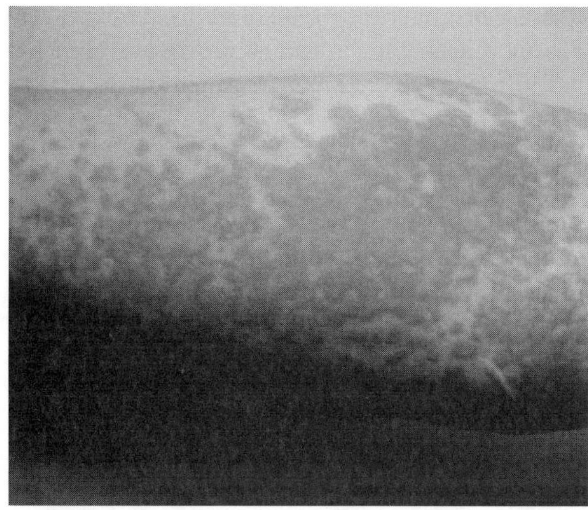

Figure 6.4 Urticaria. This image can be found in color in the app.

Source: Courtesy of James Heilman, MD.

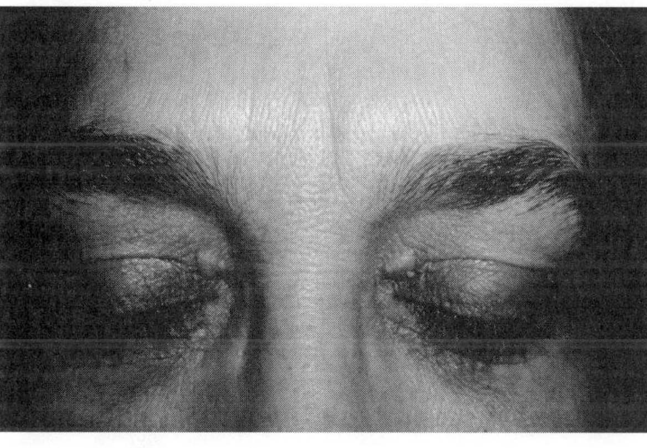

Figure 6.5 Xanthelasma. This image can be found in color in the app.

Source: Courtesy of Klaus D. Peter.

Melasma (Mask of Pregnancy)

Bilateral brown- to tan-colored stains located on the upper cheeks, malar area (cheeks and nose), forehead, and chin in some women who have been or are pregnant or on oral contraceptive pills (estrogen). The condition is more common in dark-skinned women. Stains are usually permanent but can lighten over time.

Vitiligo

White patches of skin (hypopigmentation) with irregular shapes that gradually develop and spread over time. It is chronic and progressive and it can be located anywhere on the body. Risk factors are presence of autoimmune disease (Graves' disease, Hashimoto's thyroiditis, rheumatoid arthritis [RA], psoriasis, pernicious anemia). Condition is more obvious and disfiguring in patients with darker skin. Refer to dermatologist for treatment options (topical steroids, light therapy, etc.). Advise patient to use sunscreen and avoid prolonged sun exposure (makes white patches more obvious). Psychic effects, such as low self-esteem, can occur.

Cherry Angioma

Benign small and smooth round papules that are a bright cherry-red color. Sizes range from 1 to 4 mm. Lesions are due to a nest of malformed arterioles in the skin. Always blanches with pressure. More common in middle-aged to older patients. No treatment is necessary. Benign.

Lipoma

Soft fatty cystic tumors that are usually painless and are located in the subcutaneous layer of the skin. Most are located on the neck, trunk, and arms. Most common type of benign soft tissue tumor. Tumors are round or oval shape and measure 1 to 10 cm or more, and they feel smooth with a discrete edge. They are asymptomatic unless they become too large or are irritated or ruptured. Surgical excision is an option.

Nevi (Moles)

Round macules to papules (junctional nevi) in colors ranging from light tan to dark brown. Their borders may be distinct or slightly irregular.

Xerosis

Inherited skin disorder that results in extremely dry skin and may involve mucosal surfaces such as the mouth (xerostomia) or the conjunctiva of the eye (xerophthalmia).

Acanthosis Nigricans

Diffuse velvety thickening of the skin that is usually located behind the neck and on the axilla. It is associated with diabetes, metabolic syndrome, obesity, and cancer of the GI tract.

Acrochordon (Skin Tags)

Painless and pedunculated outgrowths of skin are the same color as the patient's skin. Common locations are the neck and axillary area. When twisted or traumatized (i.e., gets caught on a necklace), it can become necrotic and drop off the skin. Up to 50% of adults have skin tags. More common in diabetics and the obese. See Figure 6.6.

TOPICAL STEROIDS

- Avoid steroids in case of suspected fungal etiology because it will worsen the infection. Steroids range in potency from class 1 (superpotent) to class 7 (least potent).
- Children and the face:
  - Do not use fluorinated topical steroids. Use class 7 (least potent) topical steroids such as 0.5% to 1% hydrocortisone. Class 6 (mild potency) steroids, such as fluocinolone acetonide (Synalar cream/solution), are prescription drugs. Next step if OTC hydrocortisone is not working.

- Topical steroids: Hypothalamic–pituitary–adrenal (HPA) axis suppression may occur with excessive or prolonged use (>2 weeks), especially in infants and children, or with use of potent to ultrapotent topical steroids. These agents can cause striae, skin atrophy, telangiectasia, acne, and hypopigmentation.

DISEASE REVIEW

Psoriasis

Inherited skin disorder in which squamous epithelial cells undergo rapid mitotic division and abnormal maturation. The rapid turnover of skin produces the classic psoriatic plaque. See Figure 6.7.

Special Findings

- *Koebner phenomenon:* New psoriatic plaques form over areas of skin trauma
- *Auspitz sign:* Pinpoint areas of bleeding in the skin when scales from a psoriatic plaque are removed

Classic Case

Patient complains of pruritic erythematous plaques covered with fine silvery-white scales along with pitted fingernails and toenails. The plaques are distributed in the scalp, elbows,

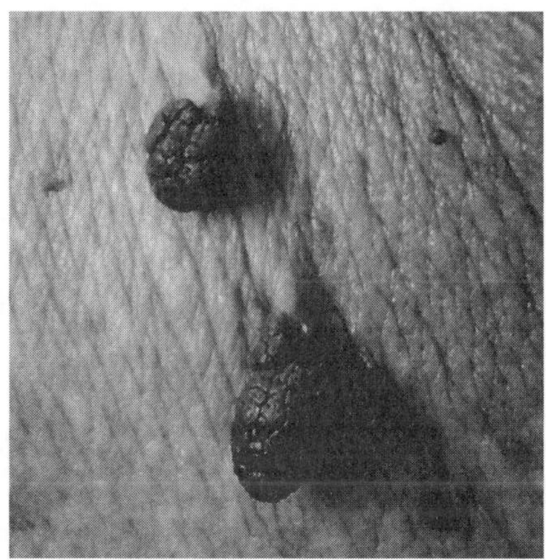

Figure 6.6 Skin tags (achrocordon). This image can be found in color in the app.

Source: Courtesy of Grook Da Oger.

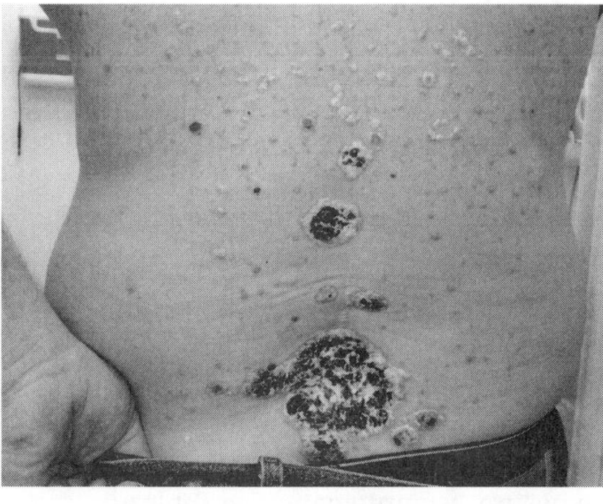

Figure 6.7 Psoriasis. This image can be found in color in the app.

Source: Lyons and Ousley (2015). Used with permission.

knees, sacrum, and the intergluteal folds. Partially resolving plaques are pink colored with minimal scaling. Patient with psoriatic arthritis will complain of painful red, warm, and swollen joints (migratory arthritis) in addition to the skin plaques.

Medications

- Topical steroids, topical retinoids (tazarotene), tar preparations (psoralen drug class)
- Severe disease: Methotrexate, cyclosporine, biologics (etanercept, adalimumab)

Black Box Warnings

Topical Tacrolimus

- Rare cases of malignancy (including skin and lymphoma); use sunblock; avoid if patient is immunocompromised
  - *Severe disease:* Antimetabolites (i.e., methotrexate), biologics/antitumor necrosis factor (TNF) agents

Biologics/Anti-TNF Agents

- Humira, Enbrel, and Remicade are associated with higher risk of serious/fatal infections, malignancy, tuberculosis (TB), fungal infections, sepsis, etc. (baseline purified protein derivative [PPD], CBC with differential).
- Goeckerman regimen (UVB light and tar-derived topicals) may induce remission in severe cases.

Complications

- *Guttate psoriasis (drop-shaped lesions)*: Severe form of psoriasis resulting from a beta-hemolytic *Streptococcus* group A infection (usually due to "strep" throat)

Actinic Keratoses

Precancerous precursor to squamous cell carcinoma. Older adults with fair skin, light-colored hair (blond, red), and blue eyes who are skin type I or II (white skin) and a history of chronic sun exposure (UV light) have highest incidence of skin cancer. A past history of blistering sunburns as a child increases risk of skin cancer, especially melanoma.

Classic Case

Older to elderly adult complains of numerous dry, round, and pink to red lesions with a rough and scaly texture that do not heal. Lesions are slow growing and become more numerous with age; most common locations are sun-exposed areas such as the cheeks, nose, face, neck, arms, and back. Early childhood history of frequent sunburns places person at higher risk.

Treatment Plan

Refer to dermatologist for biopsy (gold standard diagnosis). Treatment ranges from surgery and cryotherapy to topical medications (fluorouracil cream 5% [5-FU], imiquimod, etc.). If there are only a small number of lesions, they can be treated with cryotherapy. With larger numbers, 5-FU cream is used over several weeks. It selectively destroys sun-damaged cells in the skin. Treatment with 5-FU cream (Efudex) causes inflammation that appears as erythema (redness), oozing, crusting, scabs, and soreness, which disappears in a few weeks.

Tinea Versicolor

Superficial skin infection caused by yeasts *Pityrosporum orbiculare* or *Pityrosporum ovale*. See Figure 6.8.

Classic Case

Complains of multiple hypopigmented round macules on the chest, shoulders, and/or back that "appear" after skin becomes tan from sun exposure; asymptomatic. See Table 6.1.

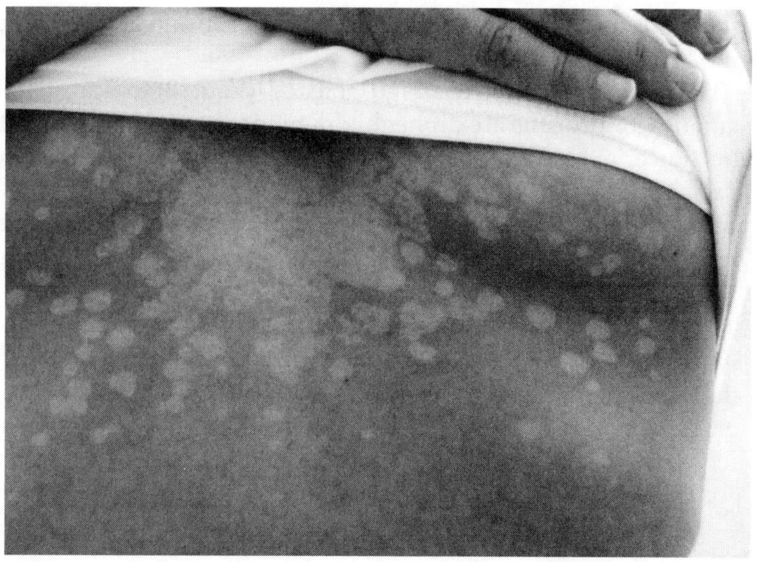

Figure 6.8 Tinea versicolor. This image can be found in color in the app.
Source: Courtesy of Sarahrosenau.

Labs

Potassium hydroxide (KOH) slide: Hyphae and spores ("spaghetti and meatballs")

Medications

Topical selenium sulfide and topical azole antifungals such as ketoconazole (Nizoral), terbinafine (Lamisil) cream BID × 2 weeks. Advise patient that hypopigmented spots will not spontaneously disappear after treatment (may take several months for pigment to fill in).

Atopic Dermatitis (Eczema)

Chronic inherited skin disorder marked by extremely pruritic rashes that are located on the hands, flexural folds, and neck (older child to adult). The rashes are exacerbated by stress and environmental factors (i.e., winter). The disorder is associated with atopic disorders such as asthma, allergic rhinitis, and multiple allergies (check for family history of atopy).

Classic Case

Infants up to 2 years of age have a larger area of rash distribution compared to teens and adults. The rashes are typically found on the cheeks, entire trunk, knees, and elbows.

Older children and adults have rashes on the hands, neck, and antecubital and popliteal space (flexural folds). The classic rash starts as multiple small vesicles that rupture, leaving painful, bright-red, weepy lesions. The lesions become lichenified from chronic itching and can persist for months. Fissures form that can be secondarily infected with bacteria.

Medications

- Topical steroids and emollients are first-line treatment.
  - *Mild disease:* Hydrocortisone 2.5% (low-potency, group 5)
  - *Moderate disease:* Triamcinolone acetonide (medium potency, group 4)

- Facial skin, skin folds (intertriginous area) are at higher for skin atrophy. Use hydrocortisone 1% (low potency, group 7).
- Halcinonide (Halog) is an example of a high-potency (group 2) topical steroid.
- Oral antihistamines for pruritus are diphenhydramine (Benadryl), hydroxyzine (Vistaril).
- Skin lubricants (Eucerin, Keri Lotion, baby oil): Avoid drying skin/xerosis because it will exacerbate eczema (i.e., no hot baths, harsh soaps, chemicals, wool clothing).
- Hydrating baths (avoid hot water/soaps) followed immediately by application of skin lubricants (Eucerin, Keri Lotion, Crisco, mineral oil). Do not wait until skin is dry before applying.

Contact Dermatitis

Inflammatory skin reaction caused by direct contact with an irritating external substance; can be a single lesion or generalized rash (i.e., sea-bather's itch). There are two types: irritant and allergic. Common offenders are poison ivy (Rhus dermatitis), nickel, latex rubber, chemicals, etc. Onset can occur within minutes to several hours after skin contact.

Classic Case

Acute onset of one to multiple bright-red and pruritic lesions that evolve into bullous or vesicular lesions; they easily rupture, leaving bright-red moist areas that are painful. May complain of burning or stinging. When rash dries, it becomes crusted; very pruritic and becomes lichenified from chronic itching. The shape may follow a pattern (i.e., a ring around a finger) or have asymmetric distribution.

Medications

- Stop exposure to substance. Topical steroids applied once to twice a day × 1 to 2 weeks. If skin is lichenified or does not involve face or flexural areas, use high-potency steroid (triamcinolone, Halog), Calamine lotion, oatmeal baths (Aveeno) PRN.
- Consider referral to allergist for patch testing.

Superficial Candidiasis

Superficial skin infection from the yeast *Candida albicans*. Environmental factors promoting overgrowth are increased warmth and humidity, friction, obesity, diabetes, and decreased immunity. It can infect skin, mucous membranes (thrush, vaginitis), and systemically. Intertrigo/intertriginous areas of the body (or apposed areas of skin that rub together) can be infected by either fungal (candidal intertrigo) and/or bacterial organisms.

Classic Case

External (Skin)

An obese adult complains of bright-red and shiny lesions that itch or burn, located on the intertriginous areas (under the breast in females, axillae, abdomen, groin, the web spaces between the toes). The rash may have satellite lesions (small red rashes around the main rash).

Thrush

Complains of a severe sore throat with white adherent plaques with a red base that are hard to dislodge on the pharynx. Thrush in "healthy adults" who are not on antibiotics may signal an immunodeficient condition.

Treatment Plan

- Nystatin powder and/or cream in skin folds (intertriginous areas) BID. OTC topical antifungals are miconazole, clotrimazole. Prescription needed for terconazole, ciclopirox.
- Keep skin dry and aerated.

- Administer clotrimazole troches (one troche dissolved in mouth slowly five times/day) or miconazole mucoadhesive buccal tablets.
- Another option is nystatin (Mycostatin) Oral suspension for oral thrush (swish and swallow) QID.
- "Magic mouthwash" (viscous lidocaine, diphenhydramine, Maalox) is compounded by pharmacists and is for severe sore throat (thrush, canker sores, mouth ulcers).
- HIV-seropositive patients: Oropharyngeal candida is the most common opportunistic infection. Moderate to severe cases (or recurrent disease): Oral fluconazole is preferred systemic antifungal.

Cellulitis

Acute skin infection of the deep dermis and underlying tissue, usually caused by gram-positive bacteria. There are two forms of cellulitis (purulent and nonpurulent). Points of entry are skin breaks, insect bites, abrasions, or preexisting skin infections (tinea pedis, impetigo). Community-acquired methicillin-resistant *Staphylococcus aureus* (MRSA) strain (USA300 MRSA) is a virulent strain that causes aggressive skin infections.

Orbital cellulitis and peritonsillar cellulitis: Refer to ED for parenteral antibiotics. Discussed in Chapter 5.

- *Purulent form of cellulitis: S. aureus* (gram positive). Community-acquired MRSA now common. Most cases are located on the lower leg (85%).
- *Nonpurulent form of cellulitis:* Usually due to streptococci (but may also be staphylococcal).
- *Dog and cat bites: Pasteurella multocida* (gram negative).
- *Puncture wounds (foot):* Contaminated with soft foam liner material or puncture wounds through sneakers. May be at risk for infection with *Pseudomonas aeruginosa.*
- *V. vulnificus*: Exposure of wound to brackish to saltwater (or eating raw oysters/clams) from the Gulf Coast or Chesapeake Bay can cause infection with this bacterium. Leading cause of shellfish-associated death in the United States.

Note

People with liver disease or immunocompromise or women who are pregnant should avoid eating raw or undercooked oysters or clams due to the possibility of *Vibrio vulnificus* infection. High mortality rate (50%) from *V. vulnificus* septicemia.

Classic Case

Acute onset of diffused pink to red-colored skin that is poorly demarcated with advancing margins. The lesion feels warm to touch, and it may become abscessed or it may be fluctuant (pointing) or draining pus. Abscess (boils) usually due to *Staphylococcus* or MRSA.

Infection may spread to lymph node chains (lymphangitis); this appears like red streaks radiating from the infected area. May involve lymphadenopathy. Patients may have systemic symptoms. Lower limb is most common location (85%).

Clenched-Fist Injuries

These injuries have a high risk of infection to joints (i.e., knuckles), fascia, nerves, and bones (osteomyelitis; especially if punched in the mouth or bitten by a human). Refer to ED for treatment. There may be a foreign body embedded, such as a tooth (x-ray needed) and/or a fracture.

Necrotizing Fasciitis ("Flesh-Eating" Bacteria)

Reddish to purple-colored lesion that increase rapidly in size. May have bullae. Infected area appears indurated ("woody" induration) with complaints of severe pain on affected site.

Folliculitis

Infection of hair follicle(s). May involve several follicles. Small (1-mm) round lesions filled with pus with erythema. Usually self-limiting. Avoid shaving or scrubbing area. Consider mupirocin (Bactroban) ointment or cream.

Furuncles (Boils)

An infected hair follicle that fills with pus (abscess). May have started out as folliculitis that worsened. It looks like a round red bump and is hot and tender to touch. When it is fluctuant, it can rupture and drain purulent green-colored discharge. Apply antibiotic ointment BID and cover with dressing until healed. See Figure 6.9.

- For small boils, use warm compress BID. If abscess is greater than 2 cm, incise and drain of abscess and/or empiric antibiotic treatment may be adequate.
- If located over a joint, refer to ED for plain radiograph (x-ray) of joint to rule out osteomyelitis. Best imaging method is MRI to detect bone infection.

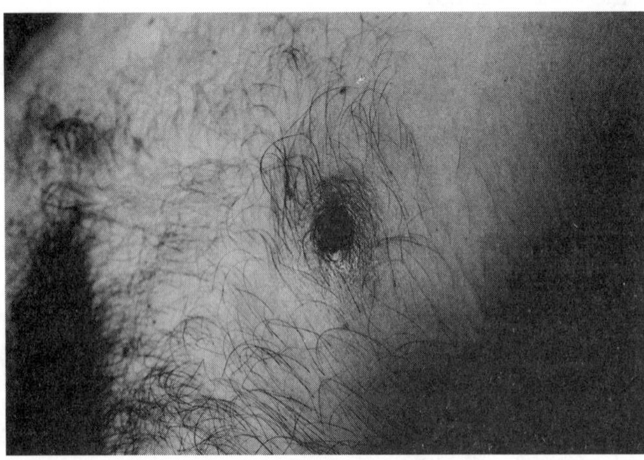

Figure 6.9 Furuncle or boil (caused by methicillin-resistant *Staphylococcus aureus*). This image can be found in color in the app.

Source: Courtesy of El Pantera.

Carbuncles (Multiple Abscesses)

Carbuncles are several boils that coalesce to form a large boil or abscess. Sometimes they may form several "heads." They are usually treated with systemic antibiotics.

Labs

- C&S advancing edge of lesion (if fluid or pus, vesicles, drainage)
- Lower-extremity cellulitis, also fungal culture for tinea pedis (swab interdigital spaces)
- CBC if fever or toxic or suspect necrotizing fasciitis (refer to ED)

Treatment Plan

This is for mild cases only. If toxic, rapid progression, immunocompromised, diabetic, joint involvement, suspect osteomyelitis and refer to ED for parenteral antibiotics.

- *Nonpurulent cellulitis (non-MRSA):* Dicloxacillin PO (orally) QID × 10 days (preferred due to high rate of beta-lactam resistance); cephalexin QID or clindamycin TID × 10 days
- *Penicillin allergic:* Azithromycin (Z Pack) × 5 days (macrolide)

- *Suspect MRSA:* Bactrim DS one tablet BID or doxycycline or minocycline PO BID × 10 days or clindamycin three to four times/day for 10 days (mild cases, duration of 5 days)
- *Td booster:* If last dose was more than 5 years ago
- Elevate affected limb

Follow-Up

Follow up with the patient within 48 hours. Patients treated with oral antibiotics usually start to show improvement in 48 to 72 hours. Refer cellulitis cases if:

- Systemic symptoms develop (i.e., fever, toxic) or worsen
- The cellulitis is not responding to treatment within 48 hours
- Cellulitis is spreading quickly or is a small lesion with black center (gangrene) associated with severe pain (necrotizing fasciitis)
- Patient is a diabetic, immunocompromised, or taking anti-TNF (rheumatoid arthritis)

Complications

- Osteomyelitis, septic arthritis, sepsis
- Tendon and fascial extension
- Rarely, death (high fatality rates for *V. vulnificus* infections)

Erysipelas

A subtype of cellulitis involving the upper dermis and superficial lymphatics that is usually caused by group A *Streptococcus*. See Figure 6.10.

Classic Case

Sudden onset of one large hot and indurated red skin lesion that has clear demarcated margins. It is usually located on the lower legs (the shins) or the cheeks. It is accompanied by fever and chills. Hospitalization may be needed for severe cases, infants, the elderly, and the immunocompromised.

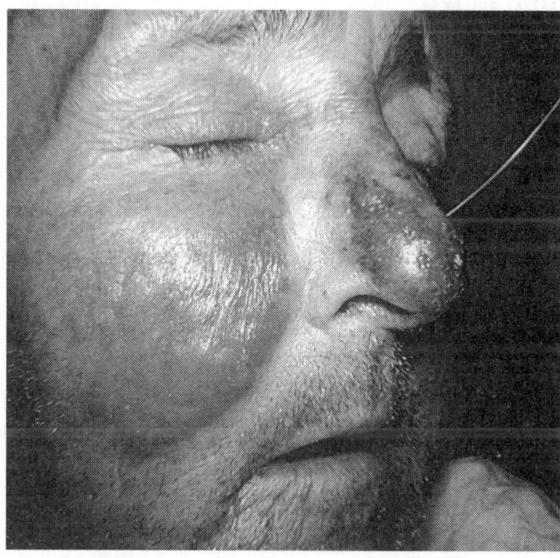

Figure 6.10 Erysipelas. This image can be found in color in the app.

Source: Courtesy of Dr. Thomas F. Sellers.

Bites: Human and Animal

Human Bites

The "dirtiest" bite of all. Watch for closed-fist injuries of the hands (may involve joint capsule and tendon damage). *Eikenella corrodens* and numerous bacteria may be involved.

Dog and Cat Bites

P. multocida (gram negative). Cat bites have a higher risk of infection than dog bites. Signs of infection are redness, swelling, and pain, and systemic symptoms may develop within 12 to 24 hours.

Treatment Plan (Both Human and Animal Bites)

- Amoxicillin–clavulanate (Augmentin) 875 mg/125 mg PO BID × 10 days. Penicillin allergy: Doxycycline BID, Bactrim DS BID *plus* coverage for anaerobes combine with metronidazole (Flagyl) BID or clindamycin TID
- Irrigate copiously with sterile saline. All bites and infected wounds need wound C&S
- Do not suture wounds at high risk for infection: Puncture wounds, wounds more than 12 hours old (24 hours on face), infected bite wounds, cat bites
- Cartilage injuries (cartilage does not regenerate); refer to plastic surgeon
- Tetanus prophylaxis (if last booster >5 years, needs booster)
- Follow up with patient within 24 to 48 hours after treatment

Referral of Wounds

- Closed-fist injuries or crush injuries: Refer to hand surgeon
- Cartilage damage or wounds with cosmetic effects: Refer to plastic surgeon
- Compromised hosts: Consider adult diabetics, absent/dysfunction of the spleen, immunocompromised

Rabies

- Consider bats, raccoons, skunks, foxes, coyotes (domestic animals can also have rabies).
- Rabies immune globulin plus rabies vaccine may be required. Call local health department for advice. Consider if wild animal acts tame, copious saliva, unprovoked attack, or animal looks ill.
- *Option:* Quarantine a domestic animal for 10 days (look for signs/symptoms of rabies).

Hidradenitis Suppurativa

Chronic and recurrent inflammatory disorder of the apocrine glands that results in painful nodules, abscesses, pustules in locations such as the axilla (most common location), mammary area, perianal, and the groin. More common in women (3:1 ratio). Important risk factors include smoking and obesity. No cure. See Figure 6.11.

Classic Case

Patient complains of recurrent episodes of painful, large, dark-red nodules, abscesses, and pustules. Ruptured lesions drain purulent green-colored discharge. Pain resolves when the abscess drains and heals. Lesions take from 10 to 30 days to heal. History of recurrent episodes on the same areas in the axilla results in sinus tracts, keloids, and multiple scars. Patient may be anxious and/or depressed.

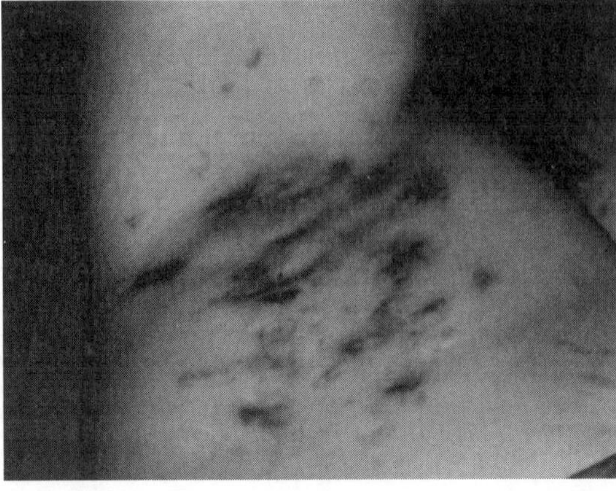

Figure 6.11 Hidradenitis suppurativa (mild). This image can be found in color in the app.

Source: Courtesy of BRI72783.

Treatment Plan

- Mild disease: Chlorhexidine (Hibiclens) 4% solution, or antibiotic soap
- Topical antibiotics (clindamycin 1% solution with/without benzoyl peroxide) × 12 weeks
- Warm compresses, sitz baths, topical and/or oral pain medication for pain
- Diet: Avoid high glycemic foods, dairy
- Smoking cessation. Weight loss if obese
- Oral antibiotics: Tetracycline 500 mg BID; doxycycline or minocycline BID for 7 to 10 days for mild disease
- Refer to dermatologist. Options include surgery, hormonal therapy, interlesional steroids, oral retinoids, metformin, biologics, laser therapy, and cryotherapy

Impetigo

Acute superficial skin infection caused by gram-positive bacteria (beta streptococcus or *S. aureus*). Most common bacterial skin infection in young children ages 2 to 5 years. More common in hot and humid environments (summer, subtropics, tropics). It can appear on normal skin or skin breaks (scratches, insect bites, acne, varicella lesions). If infection is due to beta *Streptococcus* (*Streptococcus pyogenes*), postglomerular nephritis can be a complication. There are two types: bullous (30%) and nonbullous (70%).

Classic Case

Acute onset of itchy pink-to-red lesions, which evolve into vesiculopustules that rupture. Bullous impetigo appear as large blisters that rupture easily. After rupture, red weeping shallow ulcers appear. When serous fluid dries up, it looks like lesions covered with honey-colored crusts. See Table 6.1. Can present with a few (two to three) to multiple lesions.

Labs

C&S of crusts/wound.

Treatment Plan

- Severe cases: Cephalexin (Keflex) QID, dicloxacillin QID × 10 days. *Penicillin allergic:* Azithromycin 250 mg × 5 days (macrolides), clindamycin × 10 days.
- If few lesions with no bullae, topical 2% mupirocin ointment (Bactroban) or fusidic acid 2% cream × 10 days may be useful.
- Clean lesions with antibacterial soap, Betadine, or chlorhexidine (Hibiclens); then apply topical antibacterial to lesions.
- Shower/bathe daily with antibacterial soap until healed. Do not share towels.
- Children in day care: Do not return to school until 48 to 72 hours after initiation of treatment.

Meningococcemia

A serious life-threatening infection caused by *Neisseria meningitides* (gram-negative diplococci) that are spread by respiratory droplets. Bacterial meningitis is a medical emergency. Mortality rate of 10% to 14%. Use droplet precautions.

- Do not delay treatment if high index of suspicion—refer to ED *stat*.

Classic Case

Described earlier under "Danger Signals."

Prophylaxis

- *Close contacts* (give as early as possible): Rifampin PO every 12 hours × 2 days
- Close contacts: Defined as being in close proximity to patient (<3 feet) who has had prolonged contact (>8 hours) or directly exposed to patient's oral secretions, going back to 7 days before onset of patient's symptoms until 24 hours after initiation of antibiotic

- Meningococcal vaccination: CDC recommends vaccination with meningococcal conjugate vaccine (MCV4 or Menactra) for freshman college students living in dormitories, military recruits, persons asplenia or a nonfunctioning spleen (i.e., sickle cell), patients on eculizumab (Soliris), others
- Routine meningococcal polysaccharide (MPSV 4 or Menomune) vaccine: Recommended for all preteens and teens (age 11 first dose with booster age 16 years)

Labs
- Lumbar punctures: Culture cerebrospinal fluid (CSF)
- Blood cultures, throat cultures, etc. (do not delay treatment to wait for lab results)
- CT or MRI of the brain

Treatment Plan
- Ceftriaxone (Rocephin) 2 g IV every 12 hours plus vancomycin IV every 8 to 12 hours
- Hospital, isolation precautions, supportive treatment

Complications
- Tissue infarction and necrosis (i.e., gangrene of the toes, foot, fingers, etc.) causing amputation
- Death

Early Lyme Disease
Erythema migrans is a skin lesion caused by the bite of an *Ixodes* tick infected with *Borrelia burgdorferi*. If untreated, infection becomes systemic and affects multiple organ systems. May only have rash or rash may be accompanied by flu-like symptoms.

Classic Case
Described earlier under "Danger Signals."

Labs
- Two-step (two-tier) testing recommended (designed to be done together)
  - First step is enzyme immunoassay (EIA); if negative, no further testing is recommended
  - If first test is positive (or equivocal/indeterminate), the second step test is the indirect immunofluorescence assay (IFA or immunoblot test or "western blot" test)
  - If both EIA and IFA tests are positive, person has Lyme infection
- Antibody tests may be false negative the first 4 to 6 weeks (infection present but no antibodies yet)

Treatment Plan
- Early Lyme only: Doxycycline BID (twice daily) × 10 days (first-line drug for both adults and children)
- Alternative: Amoxicillin 500 mg TID or cefuroxime axetil (Ceftin) 500 mg BID × 14 days

Complications
- Neuropathy (e.g., facial palsy), impaired memory
- Lyme arthritis, chronic fatigue

Rocky Mountain Spotted Fever
Caused by the bite of a dog tick (wood tick) that is infected with the parasite *Rickettsia rickettsii*. If high index of suspicion, do not delay treatment (do not wait for lab results). Treatment most effective if started within first 5 days of symptoms. Doxycycline is the first-line treatment for

all age groups (CDC, 2016). Check if resident of the southeastern or south-central states (NC, TN, OK, AK, and MO) or visitor to or vacationer in these states.

Classic Case

Described earlier under "Danger Signals." Diagnosis based on clinical signs and symptoms and can later be confirmed by confirmatory laboratory tests.

Labs

- Diagnostic: Antibody titers to *R. rickettsii* (by indirect fluorescent antibodies)
- Biopsy of skin lesion (3-mm punch biopsy), CBC, LFTs, CSF, others

Treatment Plan

First-line treatment (adults and children): Doxycycline BID × 7 to 14 days; refer *stat*

Complications

- Death
- Neurological sequelae (hearing loss, paraparesis, neuropathy, others)

How to Remove a Tick

1. Use fine-tipped tweezers to grasp the part of the tick closest to the skin.
2. Pull it upward with steady, even pressure. Do not twist or jerk (Figure 6.12).
3. After removing tick, clean bite area with rubbing alcohol, iodine scrub, or soap and water. Dispose tick by flushing it into toilet. Do not crush tick with bare fingers.

Not effective: Painting tick with nail polish or petroleum jelly or using heat to make the tick detach. The goal is to detach tick as quickly as possible after it is found.

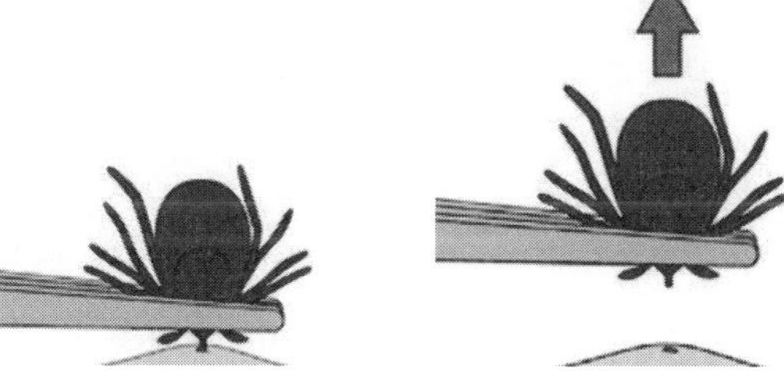

Figure 6.12 How to remove a tick. This image can be found in color in the app.

Source: CDC. Retrieved from https://www.cdc.gov/ticks/removing_a_tick.html

Varicella-Zoster Virus (VZV) Infections

Chickenpox (varicella) and herpes zoster (shingles) are both caused by the same virus. The primary infection is called *chickenpox* (varicella), and the reactivation of the infection is known as *shingles* (herpes zoster). After primary infection (chickenpox), the virus becomes latent within a dermatome (sensory ganglia) and is kept under control by an intact immune system.

- *Chickenpox:* Contagious from 1 to 2 days before the onset of the rash and until all of the lesions have crusted over (chickenpox and shingles). Duration of illness is 2 weeks.
- *Shingles:* Contagious with the onset of the rashes until all the lesions have crusted over.

Classic Case

Chickenpox/Varicella

Prodrome of fever, pharyngitis, and malaise that is followed within 24 hours by the eruption of pruritic vesicular lesions in different stages of development over a period of 4 days. The rashes start on the head and face and quickly spread to the trunk and extremities. It takes 1 to 2 weeks for the crusts to fall off and the skin to heal.

Shingles

Elderly or older adult reports acute onset of groups of papules and vesicles on a red base that rupture and become crusted. Crusted lesions follow a dermatomal pattern on one side of the body. Patient complains of pain, which can be quite severe. Some with prodrome may have severe pain/burning sensation at the site before the breakout. Shingles can last from 2 to 4 weeks. Immunocompromised and elderly patients are at higher risk for postherpetic neuralgia (PHN). Early treatment reduces risk. Treat within 48 to 72 hours after onset of breakout if patient is older than age 50 or immunocompromised. See Figure 6.13.

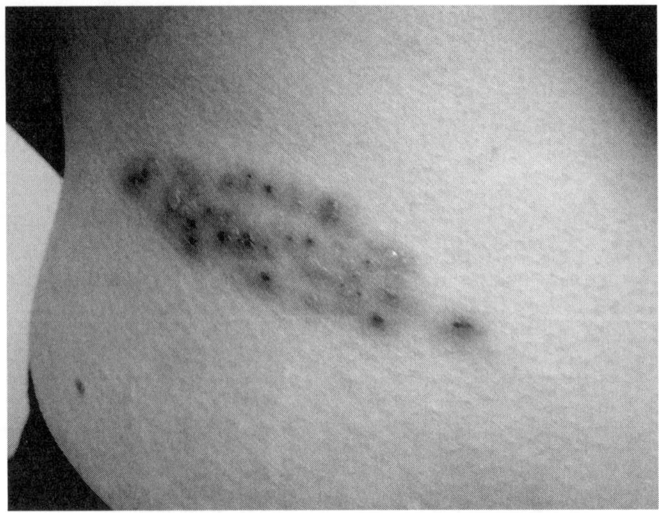

Figure 6.13 Shingles. This image can be found in color in the app.

Labs

Gold standard: Viral culture, polymerase chain reaction (PCR) for VZV

Medications

Acyclovir (Zovirax) five times per day or valacyclovir (Valtrex) BID × 10 days for initial breakouts and 7 days for flare-ups. Most effective when started within 48 to 72 hours after the appearance of the rash

Complications

- *PHN:* More common in elderly and immunocompromised patients. Treat PHN with tricyclic antidepressants (TCAs; i.e., low-dose amitriptyline), anticonvulsants (i.e., Depakote), or gabapentin TID. Apply lidocaine 5% patch (Lidoderm) to intact skin.

- *Herpes zoster ophthalmicus (CN V):* Can result in corneal blindness. Refer immediately to ophthalmologist or ED (described under "Danger Signals").
- *Others:* If Ramsay Hunt syndrome (herpes zoster oticus) triad of ipsilateral facial paralysis, ear pain, and vesicles in the ear canal and auricle, refer to neurologist.

Vaccines

- *Varicella vaccine (1995):* A person can still become infected with VZV but will have very mild disease with fewer lesions (compared with the unvaccinated). Advise reproductive-age women not to get pregnant within the next 1 month after vaccine administration.
- *Shingles/zoster vaccine (2006):* One dose is recommended for persons aged 60 years or older. A history of shingles or no history of chickenpox infection is not a contraindication to the shingles vaccine.
- *Contraindications:* People with AIDS, on chronic high-dose steroids, undergoing radiation or chemotherapy, and the immunocompromised should not get the vaccine.

CLINICAL PEARLS

- **A susceptible person (who has never had chickenpox or been vaccinated) can become infected from shingles, but that person's initial infection will manifest as chickenpox.**
- **Only a person who has had chickenpox (rarely the chickenpox vaccine) can get shingles.**

Herpetic Whitlow

Herpetic whitlow is a viral skin infection of the finger(s) caused by herpes simplex (type 1 or type 2) virus infection and results from direct contact with either a cold sore or genital herpes lesion. See Figure 6.14.

Classic Case

Patient complains of the acute onset of extremely painful red bumps and small blisters on the sides of the finger or the cuticle area or on the terminal phalanx of one or more fingers; may have recurrent outbreaks. Ask patient about coexisting symptoms of oral herpes or genital herpes.

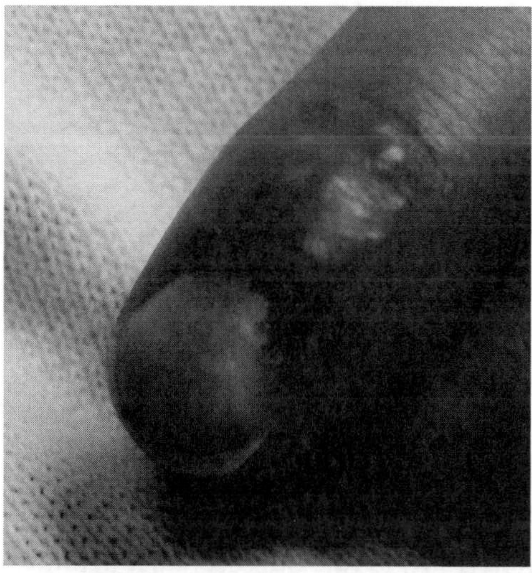

Figure 6.14 Herpetic whitlow. This image can be found in color in the app.

Source: Courtesy of James Heilman, MD.

Treatment Plan

Usually the symptoms are treated.

- *Self-limited infection:* Analgesics or NSAIDs for pain PRN
- *Severe infections:* Treat with acyclovir (Zovirax)

Patient Education

- Avoid sharing personal items, gloves, towels.
- Cover skin lesion completely with large adhesive bandage until the lesions heal.

Paronychia

Acute local bacterial skin infection of the proximal or lateral nail folds (cuticle) that resolves after the abscess drains. Causative bacteria are *S. aureus*, streptococci, or pseudomonas (gram negative). Chronic cases are associated with coexisting onychomycosis (fungal infection of nails). See Figure 6.15.

Classic Case

Complains of acute onset of a painful and red swollen area around the nail on a finger that eventually becomes abscessed. The most common locations are index finger and thumb. Reports a history of picking a hangnail, biting off hangnail, or of trimming of the cuticle during a manicure.

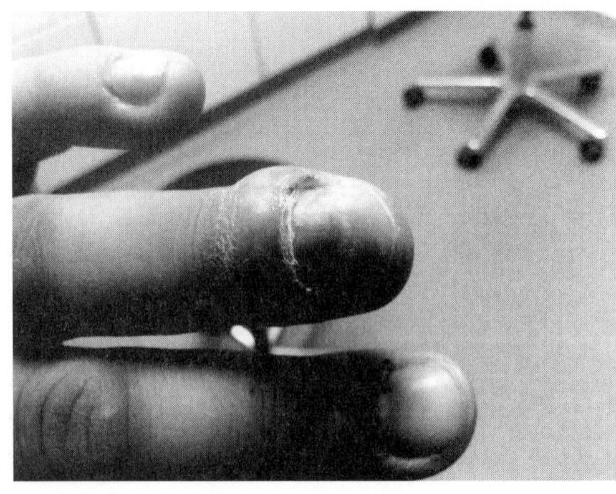

Figure 6.15 Paronychia. This image can be found in color in the app.

Source: Courtesy of C3f59.

Treatment Plan

- Soak affected finger or toe in warm water for 20 minutes three times a day.
- Apply topical antibiotic, such as triple antibiotic or mupirocin, to affected finger after soaking.
- *Abscess:* Incision and drainage (use no. 11 scalpel) or use the beveled edge of a large-gauge needle to gently separate the cuticle margin from the nail bed to drain the abscess.

Pityriasis Rosea

Self-limiting illness (6–8 weeks); this is a skin condition that may be caused by a viral infection.

Classic Case

Complains of oval lesions with fine scales that follow skin lines (cleavage lines) of the trunk or a "Christmas tree" pattern. See Table 6.1. Salmon-pink color in Whites. May be pruritic.

- *"Herald patch"*: This is the first lesion to appear and is largest in size; appears 2 weeks before full breakout.

Treatment Plan

- Advise patient that lesions will take about 4 weeks to resolve.
- If high risk of STDs, check rapid plasma reagent (RPR) to rule out secondary syphilis.

Scabies

Infestation of the skin by the *Sarcoptes scabiei* mite. The female mite burrows under the skin to lay her eggs; transmitted by close contact. May be asymptomatic the first 2 to 6 weeks. Even after treatment, the pruritus may persist for 2 to 4 weeks (sensitivity reaction to mites and their feces).

- *Norwegian scabies:* Lesions are covered with fine scales (looks like white plaques) and crusts; involves the nails (dystrophic nails), scalp, body; absent to mild pruritus; very contagious.

Classic Case

Complains of pruritic rashes located in the interdigital webs of the hands, axillae, breasts, buttock folds, waist, scrotum, and penis. Severe itching that is worse at nighttime and interferes with sleep. See Table 6.1. Other family members may also have the same symptoms.

Objective Findings

The rash appears as serpiginous (snake-like) or linear burrows. Lesions can be papular, vesicular, or crusted. Higher incidence in crowded conditions (i.e., nursing homes, etc.) and in the homeless.

Labs

Scrape burrow or scales with glass slide; use coverslip (wet mount). Look for mites or eggs.

Treatment Plan

- Permethrin 5% (Elimite): Apply cream from the neck to the feet and wash off after 8 to 14 hours. Repeat treatment in 7 days.
- Treat everyone in the same household at the same time. Any clothes/bedding used 3 days before and during treatment should be washed and dried using the hot settings.
- Pruritus usually improves in 48 hours but can last up to 2 to 4 weeks (even if mites are dead). Do not retreat (do wet mount to check for live mites). Treat itch with Benadryl and topical steroids.
- *Long-term care facility:* Treat all patients, staff, family members, and frequent visitors for scabies.

Tinea Infections (Dermatophytoses)

Infection of superficial keratinized tissue (skin, hair, nails) by tinea organisms. Tinea trichophyton, microsporum, and epidermophyton are classified as dermatophytes. Tinea infection is classified by location. Most cases of tinea can be treated with topical antifungal medication except for tinea capitis and moderate to severe onychomycosis or tinea unguium (toenails). See Figure 6.16.

Labs

- Fungal culture of scales/hair/nails or skin lesions
- KOH slide microscopy (low to medium power) reveals pseudohyphae and spores

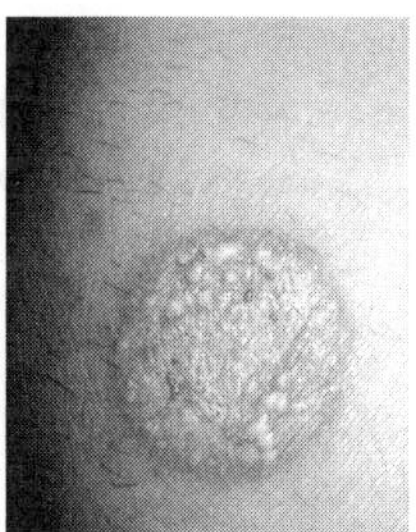
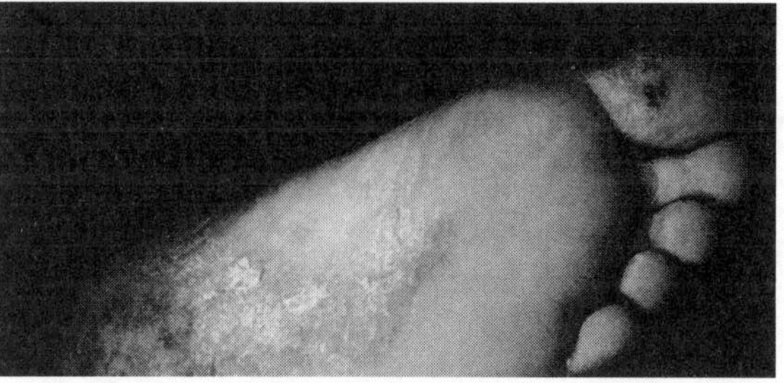
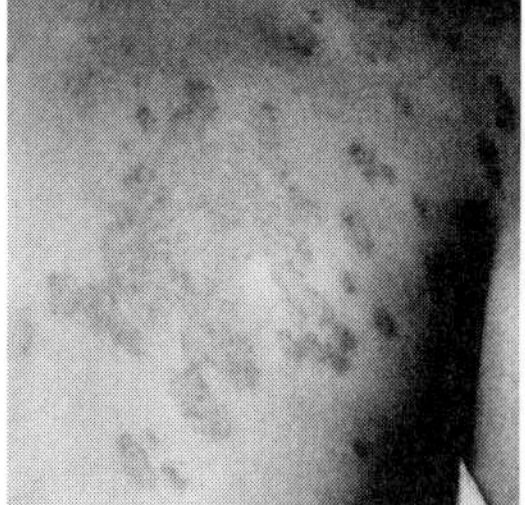

Figure 6.16 Tinea infections (ringworm).These images can be found in color in the app.

Sources: Courtesy of Corina G; Centers for Disease Control and Prevention; Dr. Lucille K. George/CDC.

Medications

- OTC topicals (creams, gels, sprays, solutions, powders)
  - *OTC azoles/imidazoles:* Clotrimazole (Lotrimin Ultra), naftifine (Naftin) once to BID, miconazole (Monistat) BID, ketoconazole (Nizoral) shampoo/cream once a day
  - *Prescription topical azole:* Terconazole (Terazol) BID
  - *OTC allylamines:* Terbinafine (Lamisil AT), butenafine (Lotrimin Ultra) once a day to BID
  - Tolnaftate (Tinactin) apply twice a day
- Avoid steroids unless severe inflammation (can reduce effectiveness antifungals)

Tinea Capitis (Ringworm of the Scalp)

Black dot tinea capitis (BDTC) is the most common type in the United States. African American children are at higher risk. Spread by close contact, fomites (shared hats, combs). Systemic treatment only (topicals are not effective).

Classic Case

School-aged child with asymptomatic scaly patch that gradually enlarges. The hairs inside the patch break off easily by the roots (looks like black dots) causing patchy alopecia.

Black dot sign: Broken hair shafts leave a dot-like pattern on scalp.

Treatment Plan

- Determine baseline LFTs and repeat 2 weeks after initiating systemic antifungal treatment. Monitor.
- *Gold standard:* Administer griseofulvin (microsize/ultramicrosize) daily to BID × 6 to 12 weeks.
- Avoid hepatotoxic substances (alcohol, statins, acetaminophen).

Complications

- Kerion: Inflammatory and indurated lesions that permanently damage hair follicles causing patchy alopecia (permanent).

Tinea Pedis (Athlete's Foot)

Two types: Scaly and dry form or moist type (strong odor). Dry type has scales. The scales can range from the entire sole, edges of the foot, or the toes only. Recurrences are common. Tinea pedis can spread to the fingernails of the dominant hand (from scratching feet).

Moist lesions occur between toe webs, lesions are white-colored with a strong unpleasant odor.

Tinea Corporis or Tinea Circinata (Ringworm of the Body)

Ringworm causes ring-like pruritic rashes with a collarette of fine scales that slowly enlarge with some central clearing. Most cases respond to topical antifungals. Severe cases with extensive skin involvement can be treated with oral antifungals (e.g., terbinafine, itraconazole, fluconazole).

Tinea Cruris ("Jock Itch")

Perineal and groin area has pruritic red rashes with fine scales; may be mistaken for candidal infection (bright-red rashes with satellite lesions) or intertrigo (bright-red diffused rash due to bacterial infection).

Tinea Manuum (Hands)

Pruritic round rashes with fine scales found on the hands. Usually infected from chronic scratching of foot that is also infected with tinea (athlete's foot).

Tinea Barbae (Beard Area)

Beard area is affected. Scaling occurs with pruritic red rashes.

Onychomycosis (Nails)

The nail becomes opaque, yellowed, and thickened with scaling under the nail [hyperkeratosis]. Also known as tinea unguium. It is usually caused by dermatophytes, but it can become infected with yeast and molds. The most common type is called distal subungual onychomycosis. Nail may separate from nail-bed (onycholysis). Great toe is the most common location. Treated with systemic antifungals, except for mild cases. If mild, a trial of topical treatment (Penlac "nail polish") is appropriate.

Labs

Fungal cultures of affected nails for confirmation of infection; KOH slide for microscopy

Medications

- Both pulse therapy and continuous therapy are acceptable. Baseline LFTs. Monitor periodically.
- Administer oral terbinafine (Lamisil) or itraconazole for 1 week per month for 2 to 3 months (pulse therapy).
- *Mild to moderate cases:* Topical antifungals such as efinaconazole (Jublia) and ciclopirox (Penlac). Apply Penlac nail lacquer × several weeks. Works best in mild cases on fingernails.
- Not all patients with onychomycosis need treatment.

Acne Vulgaris (Common Acne)

Acne is inflammation and infection of the pilosebaceous units. Has multifactorial causes such as high androgen levels, bacterial infection (*Propionibacterium acnes*), and genetic influences. Lesions are located mainly on the face, shoulders, chest, and back. Highest incidence during puberty and adolescence.

Mild Acne (Topicals Only)

Open comedones (blackheads), closed comedones (noninflammatory acne), with or without small papules are considered mild acne.

- *Prescription medications:* Tretinoin topical (Retin-A), benzoyl peroxide gel with erythromycin (Benzamycin) or with clindamycin topical (Cleocin)
- *Start at lowest dose:* Tretinoin topical (Retin-A) 0.25% cream every other day at bedtime × 2 to 3 weeks, then daily application at bedtime; alternative is azelaic acid or salicylic acid (OTC).

Retinoids also help decrease facial wrinkles and hyper/hypopigmentation. Advise patient that acne may worsen (first few weeks of use) with topical retinoids. In about 4 to 6 weeks, acne improves and clears up. The facial skin can become red and irritated (dryness, itch, peeling) in the first few weeks of use. Photosensitivity reaction is possible (use sunscreen). If no improvement in acne within 8 to 12 weeks, consider increasing Retin-A dose or adding benzoyl peroxide with erythromycin.

Moderate Acne (Topicals Plus Antibiotic)

Presence of papules and pustules (inflammatory lesions) with comedones is considered moderate acne.

Treatment Plan

- Continue with prescription topicals such as Retin-A, benzoyl peroxide combined with erythromycin (Benzamycin) or benzoyl peroxide gel with clindamycin.
- Add oral antibiotics: Administer tetracycline (500 mg BID or 250 mg TID) minocycline (Minocin), doxycycline, erythromycin, or clindamycin.

- Tetracyclines can be given for acne starting at about age 13 as growth of permanent teeth is finished except wisdom teeth (or third molars), which erupt between the ages of 17 and 25 years, tooth discoloration is not a consideration.
- *Tetracyclines* (Category D): Cause permanent discoloration of growing tooth enamel. Tetracyclines decrease effectiveness of oral contraceptives (use additional method). Not given during pregnancy or to children younger than age 13.
- *Others:* Certain oral contraceptives (Desogen, Yaz) are indicated for acne.
- Role of diet: Limited evidence that some types of dairy (i.e., skim milk) may affect acne.

Severe Cystic Acne

Consists of all of the preceding findings plus painful indurated nodules, cysts, abscesses, and pustules over face, shoulders, and chest.

Medications

- Isotretinoin (Accutane) is a category X drug (extremely teratogenic). It can only be prescribed by prescribers who are registered in the iPLEDGE program.
- Patients must use two forms of reliable contraception. Prescribe 1-month supply only. Monthly pregnancy testing with results shown to pharmacist is necessary before refills. Pregnancy test is needed 1 month after treatment is discontinued.
- Discontinue if the following are present: Severe depression, visual disturbance, hearing loss, tinnitus, GI pain, rectal bleeding, uncontrolled hypertriglyceridemia, pancreatitis, hepatitis.

Rosacea (Acne Rosacea)

Chronic and relapsing inflammatory skin disorder that is more common in people with light-colored skin. There are four subtypes of rosacea. First-line management is aimed at symptom control and avoidance of triggers that cause exacerbations (spicy foods, alcohol, sunlight, others). Patients with rosacea have sensitive skin, advise to avoid irritating skin products (toners, alpha hydroxyl acids, strong soaps). Apply skin moisturizer frequently.

Classic Case

Light-skinned adult to older patient with Celtic background (i.e., Irish, Scottish, English) complains of chronic and small acne-like papules and pustules around the nose, mouth, and chin. Telangiectasias may be present on the nasal area and cheeks. Patient blushes easily. Patient usually is blond or red haired and has light-colored eyes. Some have ocular symptoms such as red eyes, "dry eyes," or chronic blepharitis (ocular rosacea).

Medications

- Metronidazole (Metrogel) topical gel
- Azelaic acid (Azelex) topical gel
- Low-dose oral tetracycline or minocycline given over several weeks

Complications

- *Rhinophyma:* Hyperplasia of tissue at the tip of the nose from chronic severe disease
- *Ocular rosacea:* Blepharitis, conjunctival injection, lid margin telangiectasia

Molluscum Contagiosum

Dome-shaped papules (2- to 5-mm diameter) with central umbilication (white plug). Caused by skin infection with the poxvirus. Spread by skin-to-skin direct contact. More common in children. In immunocompetent host, it usually clears up by 6 to 12 months.

The CDC considers it an STD if lesions are located on the genitals in sexually active adolescents and adults. See Figure 6.17.

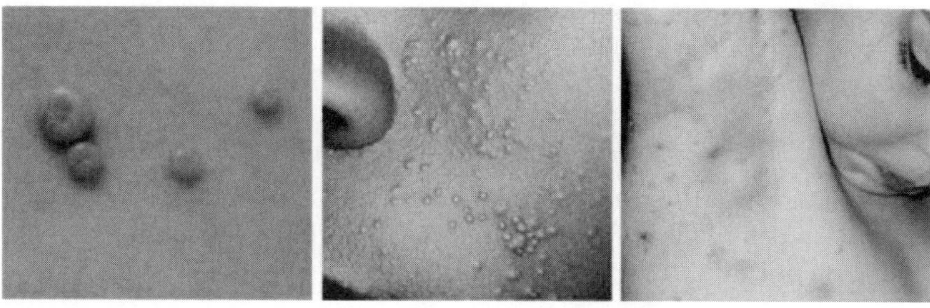

Figure 6.17 Molluscum contagiosum. These images can be found in color in the app.

Source: CDC. Retrieved from https://www.cdc.gov/poxvirus/molluscum-contagiosum/index.html

Burns (Thermal Burns)

Superficial Thickness (First Degree; Table 6.2)

- Erythema only (no blisters); painful (i.e., sunburns, mild scalds)
- Cleanse with mild soap and water (or saline): Cold packs for 24 to 48 hours
- Intact skin does not require topical antibiotics; apply a topical OTC anesthetics such as benzocaine if desired or aloe vera gel

Partial Thickness (Second Degree)

- Red-colored skin with superficial blisters (bullae); the burn is painful.
- Use water with mild soap or normal saline to clean broken skin (not hydrogen peroxide or full-strength Betadine). Do not rupture blisters. Treat with silver sulfadiazine cream (Silvadene) or triple antibiotic ointment such as Polysporin (bacitracin zinc and polymyxin B) and apply nonadherent dressings.
  - Sulfadiazine can damage the eyes (do not use near the eyes). Pregnant or breastfeeding women should not use this agent.
- Other: Apply biological dressings (i.e., DuoDERM), Tegaderm, others.
- Alternative medicine: Use a topical application of honey or aloe vera.

Full Thickness (Third Degree)

- *Initial assessment:* Rule out airway and breathing compromise. Smoke inhalation injury is a medical emergency. Third-degree burns are painless. Entire skin layer, subcutaneous area, and soft tissue fascia may be destroyed.
- *Refer:* Suspect inhalation injury if facial burns, electrical burns or burns on cartilaginous areas such as the nose and ears (cartilage will not regenerate). Also suspect if burns are on greater than 10% of body, circumferential (risk of compartment syndrome), and crosses major joints.

Total Percentage of Body Surface Area

Rule of Nines (Child):

- Body surface: 9% each arm
- Body surface: 14% each leg
- Body surface: 18% front trunk, 18% back of trunk

Rule of Nines (Adult):

- Body surface: 9% (each arm, head)
- Body surface: 18% (each leg, anterior trunk, or posterior trunk)

Example:

A 40-year-old chef suffers hot oil burns while cooking. He reports that he immediately went to the kitchen sink to cool off his burns. The nurse practitioner notes that the patient has bright-red skin on the right arm and the right thigh. The skin on the patient's chest and abdomen is bright red with several bullae on the surface.

What is this patient's diagnosis?

Answer:

Superficial-thickness burns (first-degree) on the right arm (9%) and right thigh (9% instead of 18% because it is on half of the leg) with partial-thickness burns (second-degree) on the chest and abdomen (anterior trunk 18%). The TBSA is 36%.

Criteria for Burn Center Referral

- Burns involving the face, hands, feet, genitals, major joints
- Electrical burns, lightning burns
- Partial-thickness burns greater than 10% TBSA
- Third-degree burn in any age group

Table 6.2 Minor Burn Criteria (American Burn Association)*

Burn Type	Description
Partial-thickness burns	<10% of TBSA in patients 10–50 years of age <5% of TBSA in patients younger than 10 or older than 50 years of age
Full-thickness burns	<2% of TBSA in any patient without other injury
Above criteria *plus*	May not involve face, hands, perineum, or feet May not cross major joints May not be circumferential No suspicion of inhalation injury No suspicion of high-voltage injury

*If meets above criteria, refer to ED or burn center.

TBSA, total body surface area.

BIOTERRORISM

Anthrax

Infection caused by *Bacillus anthracis* (gram-positive rods). There are three types of anthrax: cutaneous, GI, and pulmonary. Cutaneous anthrax lesion(s) begins as a papule that enlarges in 24 to 48 hours and develops eschar (necrosis) and ulceration. Usually lesions are located on the arms and the neck or face. Check for history of exposure or handling animals or hides, hair, or wool. Pulmonary anthrax (inhalational anthrax) is caused by inhaling aerosolized spores through (1) working with animals, wool, or animal hides/hair or (2) through bioterrorism. Fulminant inhalational anthrax causes death within days. Symptoms are flu-like and associated with cough, chest pain with cough, hemoptysis, dyspnea, hypoxia, and shock.

- Cutaneous anthrax (naturally acquired): Doxycycline BID, ciprofloxacin BID, levofloxacin BID for 7 to 10 days (if bioterrorism suspected, treat for 60 days)
- Without treatment, 20% of people with cutaneous anthrax may die
- Postexposure prophylaxis (bioterrorism suspected): Ciprofloxacin 500 mg PO BID × 60 days (alternate is doxycycline PO)
- Pathogens that have high mortality rates, are easily spread, and are airborne (i.e., aerosolized route) can be used for bioterrorism
- Highest-risk pathogens: Anthrax bacilli, smallpox virus

Smallpox (Variola Virus)

Infection targets respiratory and oropharyngeal mucosal surfaces. "Eliminated" in 1977. Incubation period of 2 weeks. Flu-like signs and symptoms. Numerous large nodules appear mostly in the center of the face and on the arms and legs. Treatment is symptomatic. Mortality rate is 20% to 50%.

Smallpox Vaccine

If vaccine is given within 3 to 4 days postexposure, can lessen severity of illness. Vaccinia immune globulin (for pregnant, immunosuppressed, etc.) is available from special clinics.

EXAM TIPS

- Most of the color photos on the American Nurses Credentialing Center (ANCC) exam are on skin disease and eye findings. As of December 2016, the American Academy of Nurse Practitioners Certification Board (AANPCB) exam does not include photos, but this may change in the future. Check my website for updates (www.npreview.com).
- Red spot-like rashes that start on the hands/palms and feet/soles accompanied by fever, headache, and myalgia indicate RMSF.
- Regarding tick removal, grasp part of tick closest to the skin (head) and apply steady upward pressure. Do not remove ticks by using nail polish, petroleum jelly, or heat.
- Identify skin diseases by photograph. Google images of the skin cancers, psoriasis, tinea versicolor, tinea corporis, and candida rash (satellite lesions).
- Melanoma does not have to be flat; it can present as a brown to dark-colored papule (resembling a mole but with irregular borders and other signs of melanoma).
- Differentiate between contact dermatitis and atopic dermatitis. The best clue is the unilateral location and the shape of the lesions in contact dermatitis.
- Rashes that are very pruritic at night and located on the interdigital webs and/or penis are scabies until proven otherwise.
- Preferred antibiotic for human, dog, and cat bites is amoxicillin–clavulanate (Augmentin).
- Do not confuse actinic keratosis (precursor to squamous cell cancer) with seborrheic keratoses (benign). Actinic keratosis is not physiological; it results from chronic UV exposure.
- MRSA infection: If patient is allergic to Bactrim, use doxycycline or minocycline or clindamycin.
- Know cutaneous anthrax and anthrax prophylaxis.
- Treatment for adult with recluse spider bite is antibiotic on wound, cold packs, NSAIDs.
- Know diagnosis and treatment of hidradenitis suppurativa.
- Be familiar with psoriasis and Koebner phenomenon, RMSF, meningococcemia, erythema migrans (Lyme disease), contact dermatitis, and rosacea.
- Know target rash of early Lyme disease and treatment for Lyme disease.
- Actinic keratosis is precancerous lesion for squamous cell skin cancer. If extensive, 5-FU (Efudex) topical cream is used (antimetabolite topical).
- An example of an antimetabolite or disease-modifying antirheumatic drug (DMARD) is methotrexate.
- Know how to treat mild and moderate acne. Mild acne is treated only with topicals.
- "Herald patch" or a "Christmas tree" pattern is found in pityriasis rosea.
- PHN prophylaxis: TCAs such as amitriptyline (Elavil)

- **Recognize erysipelas versus other types of cellulitis.**
- **Recognize herpetic whitlow, molluscum contagiosum, rosacea (treatment).**
- **Subungual hematoma can also be drained by trephination (straighten one end of a large paper clip or 18-gauge needle and heat it with a flame, then gently drill down nail until blood seeps out).**

CLINICAL PEARLS

- **The FDA recommends that health providers avoid prescribing oral ketoconazole (Nizoral PO) for fungal skin and nail infections because the harm (serious liver damage, etc.) outweighs the benefit. Topical ketoconazole shampoo is safe.**
- **Use ophthalmic-grade sterile cream and ointments for rashes near the eyes.**
- **Patients with scarlet fever are at higher risk for developing postglomerular nephritis (compared with "strep" throat).**
- **Recurrences of tinea pedis and tinea cruris infection are common (Goldstein & Goldstein, 2017).**
- **Patients on anti-TNF biologics are at higher risk for melanoma and squamous cell skin cancer.**

WOUNDS

A wound is a disruption or damage to the skin. There are four phases involved in wound healing. Some of the factors that impair the wound healing process are older/mature age, poor nutrition, impaired immune system, impaired mobility, stress (affects immune system), diabetes, certain medicines (drugs that impair clot formation, steroids), pressure loading, cigarette smoking, and secondary bacterial infection (Table 6.3).

Categories of Wound Healing

- *Primary healing (primary closure)*: Wound is closed within 24 hours by suturing or by application of tissue glue or butterfly strips (so that edges of wounds are well approximated). Causes the least amount of scarring.
- *Secondary intention*: Wound is left open with formation of granulation tissue and scarring. Wound heals from the bottom of the wound up. Wound edges are not well approximated. Causes more scarring than primary closure.
- *Tertiary intention (delayed primary closure)*: Wounds with heavy contamination or poor vascularity (crush injuries) are best left open to heal by secondary intention (granulation) and wound contraction. Then the wound edges are approximated in 3 to 4 days. Produces the most scar tissue.

Table 6.3 Phases of Wound Healing

Phase	Healing Event
Hemostasis	Constriction of local blood vessels, platelet aggregation, fibrin (clot) formation
Inflammation	Macrophages and lymphocytes proliferate, presence of inflammatory mediators such as cytokines and leukotrienes
Proliferation	Proliferation of basal and epithelial cells Angiogenesis
Remodeling	Remodeling of collagen, scar formation (cicatrix)

High-Risk Wounds That May Warrant Referral

- Infected wounds (pus is present, wound that is not healing, devitalized tissue, wound becomes hot and swollen)
- Closed-fist injuries: Refer to ED or urgent care clinic.
- Facial wounds with risk of cosmetic damage (e.g., large wound, bites, cartilage injury)
- Suspected foreign body or embedded object in wound that cannot be removed
- Injury to a joint capsule; if joint capsule penetrated, joint can become infected
- Electrical injuries
- Paint-gun or high-pressure wounds
- Chemical wounds (especially alkali-related damage) of the eyes or skin
- Suspected physical or child abuse
- Wounds with cosmetic concerns (cartilage wounds in the ears, nose); cartilage does not heal; refer to plastic surgeon or ED

Infected Wounds

1. Do not suture infected wounds (open greater than 24 hours). Wound will heal by secondary intention.
2. Infected wounds may have a mild case of cellulitis.
   - Without abscess: Treat with antibiotics such as cephalexin (Keflex) 250 mg QID or 500 mg BID, dicloxacillin (Dynapen) 500 mg every 6 hours for 10 days. If penicillin allergy, alternatives are azithromycin or clarithromycin (Biaxin).
   - With abscess, treat for MRSA: Administer trimethoprim–sulfamethoxazole (Bactrim DS) BID, doxycycline or minocycline BID × 10 days.
3. Infection can spread (cellulitis, lymphangitis). For severe cellulitis, hospitalize for treatment with systemic antibiotics.

Closed-Fist Injuries and Bite Wounds

1. Refer close-fist injuries to the ED or urgent care center. X-ray of the hand to rule out foreign body (i.e., teeth) and fracture. Sometimes, ultrasound is used to view foreign bodies that do not show up on x-rays.
2. Test distal pulses, skin color, range of motion (ROM), tendon damage, nerve damage, fracture.
3. Do not suture bite wounds or puncture wounds because of high risk of infection.
4. Antibiotic prophylaxis needed for animal and human bite wounds. First-line therapy is amoxicillin–clavulanic acid (Augmentin PO BID × 10 days).
5. Tetanus vaccine needed if last dose was more than 5 years ago. Use Tdap vaccine (tetanus, diphtheria, and acellular pertussis; if never had Tdap) in patients of age greater than 7 years.

Retained Foreign Bodies

1. Higher risk of infection. If unable to remove, refer to ER.
2. Plain x-ray is first-line imaging test. Ultrasound is used if suspected object or object does not show on x-rays (radiolucent).
3. May not be visible on x-rays:
   - Small glass splinters or particles
   - Splinters, thorns, fish bones
   - Plastics

Minor Burn (Superficial and Partial Thickness)

1. Wash area with water and mild soap.
2. Using sterile tongue blade, apply thin layer of 1% silver sulfadiazine (Silvadene) to burned area.

3. Cover burned area with nonstick gauze (e.g., Telfa). Secure with stretch-conforming gauze (e.g., Kerlix).
4. Apply Silvadene once to twice a day until the burn is healed. After skin is healed, consider using Desitin daily for 1 to 2 weeks to protect area from sunlight. Do not expose recently healed burned skin to sunlight (causes hyperpigmentation).
5. See previous "Burns" section for additional details.

Note

Silver sulfadiazine is contraindicated if patient has sulfa allergies. Do not apply it to the face (it will stain). If facial burns, use triple antibiotic or mupirocin (Bactroban) ointment.

Wound Care

1. During history, ask about mechanism of injury and other details about the incident.
2. Check for allergy to iodine, rubber, latex, lidocaine. If patient has rubber or latex allergy, do not use latex gloves. Use silicone-based disposable gloves.
3. Do not forget tetanus prophylaxis. If last dose was longer ago than 5 years, give Tdap booster.
4. Irrigate wound with normal saline (do not mix with Betadine, hydrogen peroxide, Hibiclens) and/or wash area with mild soap and water. Remove dirt.
5. Assess wound for neurovascular and tendon damage. Check distal pulses. Depending on injury, rule out foreign body.
6. Specific treatment depends on the type of wound and patient characteristics.

PRIMARY CARE PRACTICE: PROCEDURES

Local Anesthesia

There are two types of lidocaine 1% (plain or mixed with epinephrine). Do not use lidocaine with epinephrine on areas of the body at high risk of ischemia (tip of nose, ears, fingertips, toes, penis).

- *Drug*: Lidocaine 1% (plain) onset of action is from 2 to 5 minutes. Duration of action is from 30 minutes to 2 hours. Advise patient that he or she will feel a burning sensation at the start of the injection; this will disappear.
- *Contraindications to local anesthesia*: Do not administer if an infected injection site, allergy to anesthetic, or devascularized/ischemic tissue damage.
- *Adverse complications*: Complications may arise if patient has an allergic reaction, infection, if solution is injected directly into blood vessel, or there is injury to nerves and tendons in the area.
- *Example of anesthesia use*: Use anesthesia for wounds that need suturing, incisions (e.g., embedded splinter or paronychia), biopsy, others.

Digital Nerve Block (Fingers)

1. Clean web space on each side of the involved finger with alcohol or Betadine swab and allow to dry.
2. Draw up about 3 mL of plain lidocaine 1% from vial using a 5- to 10-mL syringe with an 18-gauge needle. Then change needle to smaller gauge (25- to 30-gauge, 1½ inches).
3. Place needle in perpendicular position above web space and insert into subcutaneous tissue space.

4. Before injecting, aspirate first to check for placement. If there is no blood, slowly inject the lidocaine into the web space (volar aspect). Inject slowly and use small amounts.
5. If blood is aspirated, withdraw needle slightly and reposition slightly (without removing the needle from the skin).
6. Reposition needle slightly and continue to infiltrate drug into the web space on each side of the injured finger.
7. Instruct patient that it may take 15 minutes for the anesthesia to become effective. Ask patient if area is numb (test by using tip of needle to test sensation) before suturing.

Infiltration Technique

1. Apply Betadine on intact skin around wound.
2. Slowly insert syringe (as directed above) into subcutaneous layer only and aspirate for blood.
3. Slowly infiltrate the edges of the wound, then withdraw slightly to move it to another area. The amount of lidocaine that is used varies based on the size of the wound and the location.

Suturing

General Rules

- Do not suture puncture wounds or human or animal bites.
- Do not suture heavily contaminated wounds.
- Lacerations that are more than 12 hours old are at higher risk for infection. Do not suture infected wounds.
- Do not suture wounds that have been open longer than 24 hours (high bacterial load).

Types of Sutures and Needles

- Example: Skin laceration
- Use nonabsorbable synthetic suture (i.e., nylon, Prolene)
- Preferred needle type to suture skin is a curved cutting needle.
- *Suture size*: The higher the number, the smaller the diameter (the same concept is used for needle size; size range is 00 to 10-0); the smallest diameter suture is 00 (about the size of human hair) and is used to repair small blood vessels; the preferred suture size is 3-0 to 5-0 (middle range)

Suture Placement

1. Evert the edges of the wound by inserting needle at 90-degree angle (ensures that wound edges are well approximated).
2. Use needle holder to hold needle. Use forceps to grab wound edges.
3. Usually, simple sutures are used on skin lacerations. Each suture is individually tied, then cut (simple interrupted sutures).
4. When cutting suture thread, do not cut too short. Leave a short tail (easier to remove).
5. Nonabsorbable synthetic sutures are preferred for lacerations/wounds of the skin.
6. If suturing scalp of a person with black hair, blue-colored suture thread is easier to visualize (for removal).

Suture Removal

Most sutures are removed within 7 to 10 days. Stitches that are left beyond 10 days may develop scars that resemble a "railroad track."

- Face: 5 to 7 days
- Scalp: 7 to 10 days
- Upper extremities: 7 to 10 days
- Lower extremities: 10 to 14 days

Use forceps and lift suture from the skin. Cut suture with scissors. Use forceps to grasp the knot and pull the suture gently out of the wound.

Skin Biopsy

Punch Biopsy

- Check for history of bleeding disorder and use of drugs that affect bleeding time (aspirin, warfarin). Patients with INR greater than 2.5 should not be biopsied. Check scar history (e.g., history of keloids or hypertrophic scarring).
- Refer to dermatologist for facial biopsies, biopsy of areas with cartilage, suspected melanoma, history of keloid/hypertrophic scarring, bleeding disorder, etc.
- Ask whether patient is allergic to lidocaine or rubber/latex (use silicone gloves).

Procedure

1. "Prep" skin site with alcohol wipes and allow to dry.
2. Using a tuberculin syringe, draw lidocaine 1% and epinephrine 1:100 (do not use with epinephrine if area is on the nose, ears, fingertips, toes, penis).
3. Inject slowly under the epidermis until a small bleb is formed. The color of the skin over the bleb area becomes paler due to the vasoconstricting effect of epinephrine.
4. Check site for numbness by using the point of the syringe and testing sensation on the bleb area. The skin will become numb within 5 to 10 minutes (lasts about 45–60 minutes).
5. Using a 3-mm skin punch, position instrument at 90 degrees (perpendicular to the skin).
6. Twist the punch instrument gently using a "drilling" motion until it has pierced the epidermis (there should be about ½ inch of the blade visible on top of the skin).
7. Remove from skin and lift plug gently with forceps (do not crush). Use a scalpel to cut the plug at the base. Immediately place it on the biopsy specimen container. Do not forget to label the specimen cup with the patient's name, location of the biopsy site, and the type of tissue obtained.
8. Cover area with sterile 2 × 2 gauze with tape (if bleeding) or with adhesive bandage if minimal bleeding. Instruct patient to change bandage once a day.
9. Instruct patient to keep the site dry. Instruct to avoid submerging site in water (avoid tub baths, swimming, hot tubs) until it is healed. Site will scab within a few days.

Note

The procedure descriptions provided in this chapter are designed for review purposes only. They are not intended for use in clinical practice.

7

Cardiovascular System Review

DANGER SIGNALS

Acute Myocardial Infarction (MI)

Also known as *ST elevation myocardial infarction (STEMI)* and *acute coronary syndrome (ACS)*. A middle-aged or older man complains of gradual onset of intense and steady chest discomfort or pain that is described as squeezing, tightness, crushing, heavy pressure ("an elephant sitting on my chest"), or band-like. The pain is provoked by physical exertion or eating a heavy meal. The pain or discomfort may radiate to the left side of the neck, jaw, and left arm (or both arms). Continues to have pain or discomfort at rest (angina relieved by rest and nitroglycerin). The patient may be diaphoretic with cool, clammy skin. Women and those who are elderly with MIs are more likely to present with nonspecific symptoms such as shortness of breath or dyspnea, weakness, nausea and vomiting, fatigue, and syncope. May complain of back pain instead of anterior chest pain.

Congestive Heart Failure (CHF)

Older patient complains of an acute (or gradual) onset of dyspnea, fatigue, dry cough, and swollen feet and ankles. The patient has a sudden (or gradual) increase in weight. Lung exam will reveal crackles on both the lung bases (bibasilar crackles) along with an S3 heart sound. History of preexisting coronary artery disease (CAD), angina, prior MI, or previous episode of CHF. Usually is taking diuretics and other antihypertensive medications.

Infective Endocarditis (IE)

Also known as *bacterial endocarditis*. Patient presents with fever, chills, and malaise that is associated with onset of a new murmur. Associated skin findings are found mostly on the fingers/hands and toes/feet. These are subungual hemorrhages (splinter hemorrhages on the nail bed), petechiae on the palate, painful violet-colored nodes on the fingers or feet (Osler nodes), and nontender red spots on the palms/soles (Janeway lesions). Funduscopic exam may show Roth spots or retinal hemorrhages. Usually fatal if not treated.

Dissecting Abdominal Aortic Aneurysm (AAA)

Elderly white male complains of sudden onset of severe, sharp, excruciating pain located in the abdomen, flank, and/or back. Accompanied by a distended abdomen and abnormal vital signs (hypotension). Older male patients who are smokers with hypertension (HTN) are at higher risk. Incidental finding on chest x-ray may show widened mediastinum, tracheal deviation, and obliteration of aortic knob (thoracic aortic dissection).

☑ NORMAL FINDINGS

Anatomy

Position of the Heart

The right ventricle is the chamber of the heart that lies closest to the sternum. The lower border of the left ventricle is where the apical impulse is generated. The heart is roughly the size of a large adult fist. The apex beat is caused by the left ventricle.

- *Apical impulse:* Located at the fifth intercostal space (ICS) by the midclavicular line on the left side of the chest

Displacement of the Point of Maximal Impulse (PMI)

- *Severe left ventricular hypertrophy (LVH) and cardiomyopathy:* The PMI is displaced laterally on the chest, is larger (more than 3 cm) in size, and is more prominent.
- *Pregnancy, third trimester:* As the uterus grows larger, it pushes up against the diaphragm and causes the heart to shift to the left of the chest anteriorly. The result is a displaced PMI that is located slightly upward on the left side of the chest. May hear S3 heart sound during pregnancy.

Deoxygenated Blood

- Enters the heart through the superior vena cava and inferior vena cava
- Right atrium → tricuspid valve → right ventricle → pulmonic valve → pulmonary artery → the lungs → alveoli (RBCs pick up oxygen and release carbon dioxide)

Oxygenated Blood

- Exits the lungs through the pulmonary veins and enters the heart
- Left atrium → mitral valve → left ventricle → aortic valve → aorta → general circulation

Systole and Diastole

The mnemonic to use is "motivated apples." These two words give you several clues. They will remind you of the names of the valves (which produce the sound) and the type of valve (atrioventricular [AV] or semilunar valve).

MOTIVATED	APPLES
M (mitral valve)	A (aortic valve)
T (tricuspid valve)	P (pulmonic valve)
AV (atrioventricular valves)	S (semilunar valves)

Heart Sounds

S1 (Systole): "Motivated" (M = mitral and T = tricuspid and AV = AV valves)

- The "lub" sound (of "lub-dub")
- Closure of the mitral and tricuspid valves
- AV valves

S2 (Diastole): "Apples" (A = aortic and P = pulmonic and S = semilunar valves)

- The "dub" sound (of "lub-dub")
- Closure of the aortic and pulmonic valves
- Semilunar valves

S3 Heart Sound

- Usually indicative of heart failure or CHF
- Occurs during early diastole (also called a "ventricular gallop" or an "S3 gallop")

- Sounds like "Kentucky"
- Always considered abnormal if it occurs after the age of 35 to 40 years
- This can be a normal finding in children, pregnant women, and some athletes (older than 35 years of age).

S4 Heart Sound
- Increased resistance due to a stiff left ventricle; usually indicates LVH
- Considered a normal finding in some elderly (slight stiffness of left ventricle)
- Occurs during late diastole (also called an "atrial gallop" or "atrial kick")
- Sounds like "Tennessee"
- Best heard at the apex or apical area (mitral area) using the bell of the stethoscope

Stethoscope Skills
Bell of Stethoscope
- Low tones such as the extra heart sounds (S3 or S4)
- Mitral stenosis

Diaphragm of the Stethoscope
- Mid- to high-pitched tones such as lung sounds
- Mitral regurgitation
- Aortic stenosis

Benign Variants
Physiologic S2
Best heard over the pulmonic area (or second ICS on the upper left side of sternum); due to splitting of the aortic and pulmonic components. A normal finding if it appears during inspiration and disappears at expiration.

S4 in the Elderly
Some healthy elderly patients have an S4 (late diastole) heart sound; also known as the "atrial kick" (the atria have to squeeze harder to overcome resistance of a stiff left ventricle). If there are no signs or symptoms of heart/valvular disease, it is considered a normal variant. Pathological S4 is associated with LVH due to increased resistance from the left ventricle.

SOLVING QUESTIONS: HEART MURMURS

To solve a murmur question correctly, only two pieces of information are needed.
- Look for the timing of the murmur (systole or diastole).
- Look for the location of the murmur (aortic, Erb's Point or mitral area).
  All the murmurs seen on the exams will fit into the following two mnemonics.

Timing
Systolic Murmurs
- Use the "MR. ASS" (Mitral regurgitation/aortic stenosis = systolic) mnemonic.

Diastolic Murmurs
- Use the "MS. ARD" (Mitral stenosis/aortic regurgitation = diastolic) mnemonic.

Location
Auscultatory Areas
It is necessary to memorize the locations of the auscultatory areas in order to correctly identify a heart murmur.

Mitral Area

- The mitral area is also known as the *apex* or the *apical area of the heart.*
- Fifth left ICS is about 8 to 9 cm from the midsternal line and slightly medial to the midclavicular line.
- PMI or the apical pulse is located in this area.

Aortic Area

- The aortic area is the second ICS to the right side of the upper border of the sternum.
- The location of the aortic area can also be described as the "second ICS by the right side of the sternum at the base of the heart." It can also be described as a murmur that is located on the right side of the upper sternum.

Erb's Point

- Erb's Point is located at the third to fourth ICS on the left sternal border.

Heart Murmurs: Mnemonics

MR. ASS (Use for Systolic Murmurs)

- Systolic murmurs are also described as occurring during S1, or as holosystolic, pansystolic, early systolic, late systolic, or midsystolic murmurs.
- Compared with diastolic murmurs, these murmurs are louder and can radiate to the neck or axillae.

MR (Mitral Regurgitation)

A pansystolic (or holosystolic) murmur:

- Heard best at the apex of the heart or the apical area
- Radiates to axilla
- Loud blowing and high-pitched murmur (use the diaphragm of the stethoscope)

AS (Aortic Stenosis)

A midsystolic ejection murmur:

- This murmur is best heard at the second ICS at the right side of the sternum.
- It radiates to the neck.
- A harsh and noisy murmur (use diaphragm of stethoscope). Patients with aortic stenosis should avoid physical overexertion, because there is increased risk of sudden death. Refer to cardiologist.
- Aortic stenosis is monitored by serial cardiac sonograms with Doppler flow studies. Surgical valve replacement needed if it worsens.

MS. ARD (Use for Diastolic Murmurs)

- Diastole is also known as the *S2 heart sound, early diastole, late diastole,* or *middiastole.*
- Diastolic murmurs are always indicative of heart disease (unlike systolic murmurs).

MS (Mitral Stenosis)

A low-pitched diastolic rumbling murmur:

- Heard best at the apex (or apical area) of the heart
- Also called an *opening snap* (use bell of the stethoscope)

AR (Aortic Regurgitation)

A high-pitched diastolic murmur (use diaphragm of the stethoscope):

- If AR is due to a diseased aortic valve, the murmur is located at the third ICS by the left sternal border (Erb's Point).

- If AR is due to an abnormal aortic root, the murmur is best heard at the right upper sternal border (aortic area).

Heart Murmurs: Grading System

- *Grade I:* A very soft murmur heard only under optimal conditions.
- *Grade II:* This is a mild to moderately loud murmur.
- *Grade III:* Loud murmur that is easily heard once the stethoscope is placed on the chest.
- *Grade IV:* A louder murmur. First time that a thrill is present. A thrill is like a "palpable murmur."
- *Grade V:* Very loud murmur heard with edge of stethoscope off chest. Thrill is more obvious.
- *Grade VI:* The murmur is so loud that it can be heard even with the stethoscope off the chest. The thrill is easily palpated.

ABNORMAL FINDINGS

Pathological Murmurs

- All diastolic murmurs are abnormal.
- All benign murmurs occur during systole (S2).
- Benign murmurs do not have a thrill; only very loud murmurs will produce a thrill.

EXAM TIPS

- There are usually two questions regarding heart murmurs on the exam.
- Learn to use the mnemonics "MR. ASS" and "MS. ARD."
- Memorize the locations of the mitral area as well as the aortic area.
- All murmurs with "mitral" in their names are only described as located:
  - On the apex of the heart or the apical area or
  - On the fifth ICS on the left side of the sternum medial to the midclavicular line
- If an apical/apex murmur occurs during S1, it is mitral regurgitation (MR. ASS). If an apical/apex murmur occurs during S2, it is mitral stenosis (MS. ARD).
- On the exam, only the systolic murmurs radiate (to the axilla in mitral regurgitation and to the neck with aortic stenosis).
- S3 is a sign of CHF; S4 is a sign of LVH.
- A split S2 is best heard at the pulmonic area (upper left sternum).
- Memorize the mnemonic "motivated apples" to help you remember the names of the valves that are responsible for producing S1 and S2.
- Grading murmurs: Be aware that the first time a thrill is palpated is at grade IV.
- Rule out AAA in an older male who has a pulsatile abdominal mass that is more than 3 cm in width. The next step is to order an abdominal ultrasound and CT.
- Learn the signs/symptoms of infective endocarditis (bacterial endocarditis).

DISEASE REVIEW

Cardiac Arrhythmias

Atrial Fibrillation (AF) and Atrial Flutter

AF is the most common cardiac arrhythmia in the United States. It is a major cause of stroke and classified as a supraventricular tachyarrhythmia. AF may be asymptomatic. If patient is hemodynamically unstable (chest pain/angina, hypotension, heart failure, cold clammy skin, acute kidney failure) with new onset of AF with severe symptoms, call 911. Risk of stroke/death is higher in elderly patients.

Risk Factors

- HTN, CAD, ACS, caffeine, nicotine, hyperthyroidism, alcohol intake ("holiday heart"), heart failure, LVH, pulmonary embolism (PE), chronic obstructive pulmonary disease (COPD), sleep apnea, other
- Paroxysmal AF (intermittent or self-terminating): Episodes terminate with 7 days or less (usually in less than 24 hours); it is usually asymptomatic

Classic Case

Patient reports the sudden onset of heart palpitations accompanied by feelings of weakness, dizziness, dyspnea/dyspnea on exertion, and reduction in exercise capacity. May complain of chest pain and feeling like passing out (presyncope to syncope). Rapid and irregular pulse may be more than 110 beats/min with hypotension. AF can be paroxysmal and stop spontaneously (within 7 days) or be persistent or long-standing.

Treatment Plan

- Search for underlying cause. Treatment depends on patient type and risk factors for stroke. Newer tool is the CHA_2DS_2-VASc score.
  - CHA_2DS_2-VASc scoring system (score of 0 is low risk): Score of 2 or more requires anticoagulation. C (CHF), H (HTN), A (age >75 years), D (diabetes), S_2 (stroke/TIA), V (vascular disease), A (age 65–74 years), S (sex: female gender is higher risk).
- Diagnostic test is the 12-lead EKG (does not show discrete P waves, irregularly irregular rhythm).
- *New onset:* EKG, TSH, electrolytes (calcium, potassium, magnesium, sodium), renal function, B-type natriuretic peptide (rule out heart failure), troponin.
- Consider 24-hour Holter monitor if paroxysmal AF. Digoxin level (if on digoxin).
- Order echocardiogram (rule out valvular pathology, which increases risk of stroke).
- *Lifestyle:* Avoid stimulants (caffeine, nicotine, decongestants) and alcohol (some patients).

Medications

- Patients are referred to cardiologists for medical management. An option for new-onset AF with stable patients is cardioversion (first 48 hours) or rate control.
- Management varies based on AF severity and symptoms.
- *Rate control:* Use beta-blockers, calcium channel blockers (CCBS), digoxin.
- Antiarrhythmics such as amiodarone (Cordarone). Amiodarone has a Food and Drug Administration (FDA) Black Box Warning of pulmonary and liver damage. Simvastatin with amiodarone can cause rhabdomyolysis.
- Warfarin (Coumadin; vitamin K antagonist) for anticoagulation remains the most prescribed therapy and the only recommended option for patients with severe or end-stage chronic kidney disease. Baseline INR, aPTT, CBC (check platelets), creatinine, LFTs.
  - Initial daily dose equal to or less than 5 mg, but frail, sensitive, or elderly patients older than 70 years of age should take lower dose (2.5 mg).

- Full effect takes from 2 to 3 days. Check INR every 2 to 3 days until therapeutic for two consecutive checks; then recheck weekly and so on until INR is stable at 2 to 3. Check every 4 weeks when stable.
- You may wish to check the institutional protocols or refer to anticoagulation clinic. If you do not have experience with anticoagulation, best to refer to cardiologist.

- If suspect a bleeding episode, check the INR with the PT and the PTT.
- Drug interactions for warfarin are given in Chapter 3.
- Antidote for warfarin is vitamin K.
- For nonvalvular AF, direct thrombin inhibitor dabigatran (Pradaxa) or the Factor Xa inhibitors rivaroxaban (Xarelto) and apixaban (Eliquis) do not require INR monitoring, have no major dietary restrictions, and have fewer drug interactions.
- Platelet inhibitors, such as clopidogrel (Plavix), either alone or in combination with other anticoagulants may be better tolerated but less effective than warfarin.

Complications

- Death caused by thromboembolic event (i.e., stroke, pulmonary embolism), CHF, angina, etc.
- Warfarin-associated intracerebral hemorrhage has very high mortality and causes 90% of warfarin deaths. It is a medical emergency. Call 911. Stop all anticoagulants, acetylsalicylic acid (ASA), nonsteroidal anti-inflammatory drugs (NSAIDs). Initiate vitamin K to reverse.
- Warfarin can be reversed, as can Pradaxa (Praxbind [reversal agent] is available in all 50 states)

Anticoagulation Guidelines (Table 7.1)

Atrial Fibrillation

- INR: 2.0 to 3.0

Synthetic/Prosthetic Valves

- INR: 2.5 to 3.5

Patient Education: Dietary Sources of Vitamin K

- Advise patients to be consistent with their day-to-day consumption of vitamin K foods.
- Give patient a list of foods with high levels of vitamin K ("greens" such as kale, collard, mustard, spinach, iceberg or romaine lettuce, brussels sprouts, potatoes).
- Only one serving per day is recommended for very high vitamin K foods.

Table 7.1 Elevated International Normalized Ratio (INR)

INR	Presence of Bleeding	Action
<5.0	None	Skip next dose and/or reduce slightly the maintenance dose. Check INR once or twice a week when adjusting dose. Do not give vitamin K.
5.0–9.0	None	Hold one or two doses; with or without administration of low-dosed vitamin K (1 to 2.5 mg). Monitor INR every 2 to 3 days until it is stable. Decrease the Coumadin maintenance dose.

INR, international normalized ratio.

Source: Adapted from Hull and Garcia (2017).

Paroxysmal Supraventricular Tachycardia (PSVT)

EKG shows tachycardia with peaked QRS complex with P waves present. May be seen in Wolff–Parkinson–White (WPW) syndrome, which is more common in children. Causes include digitalis toxicity, alcohol, hyperthyroidism, caffeine intake, alcohol, illegal drug use, etc.

Classic Case

Patient complains of the abrupt onset of palpitations, rapid pulse, lightheadedness, shortness of breath, and anxiety. Rapid heart rate can range from 150 to 250 beats/min.

Treatment Plan

- Check EKG. If shows WPW syndrome or is symptomatic, refer to cardiologist. If hemodynamically unstable, may require electrical cardioversion. Call 911.
- Vagal maneuvers: Carotid sinus massage (patient supine, monitor vital signs). Monitor with EKG. If a carotid sinus massage is needed, refer to a cardiologist. Contraindicated if history of transient ischemic attack or stroke in past 3 months or has carotid bruits.
- Holding one's breath and straining hard, or splashing ice cold water on the face may interrupt and stop this arrhythmia but is rarely used (elicits the diving reflex).

Pulsus Paradoxus

Also known as a *paradoxical pulse*. The paradox is that the apical pulse can still be heard even though the radial pulse is no longer palpable. It is measured by using the blood pressure cuff (sphygmomanometer) and a stethoscope. Certain pulmonary and cardiac conditions that compress the chambers of the heart (impair diastolic filling) can cause an exaggerated decrease of the systolic pressure of more than 10 mmHg (a drop of <10 mmHg is not pulsus paradoxus).

Pulmonary Cause

- Asthma, emphysema (increased positive pressure)

Cardiac Cause

- Tamponade, pericarditis, cardiac effusion (decreases movement of left ventricle)

EKG Interpretation

Because family nurse practitioners (NPs) function in the primary care area (not the CCU), they very well may be expected to diagnose complex rhythms. The important ones to memorize (EKG appearance) are AF (irregularly irregular rhythm with no p waves; see Figure 7.1),

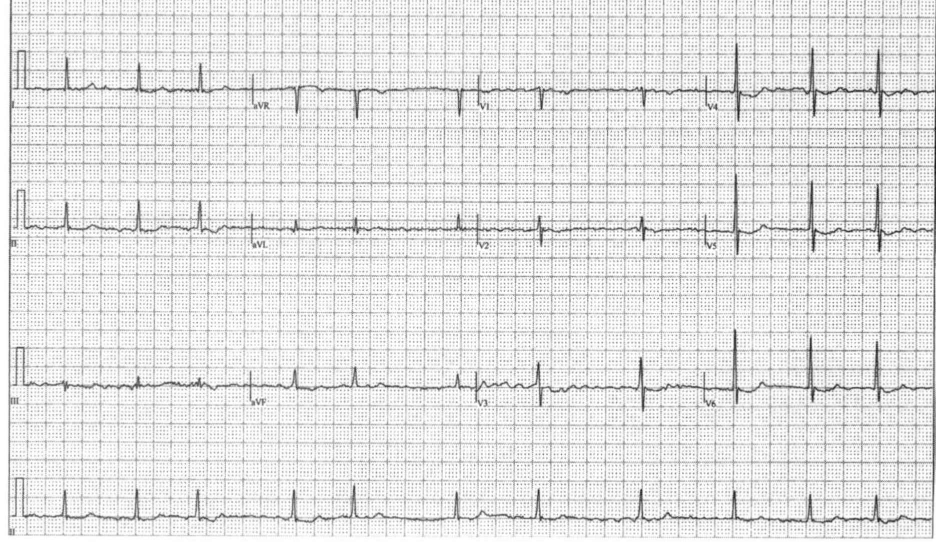

Figure 7.1 Atrial fibrillation.

ventricular tachycardia (jagged irregular QRS), and the norms such as sinus rhythm and sinus arrhythmia (see Figure 7.2).

Anterior wall MI (see Figure 7.3) or an anterior STEMI is the most common and serious type of MI. EKG changes include ST segment elevation (leads V2 to V4) and Q waves. Wide QRS complex resembles a "tombstone."

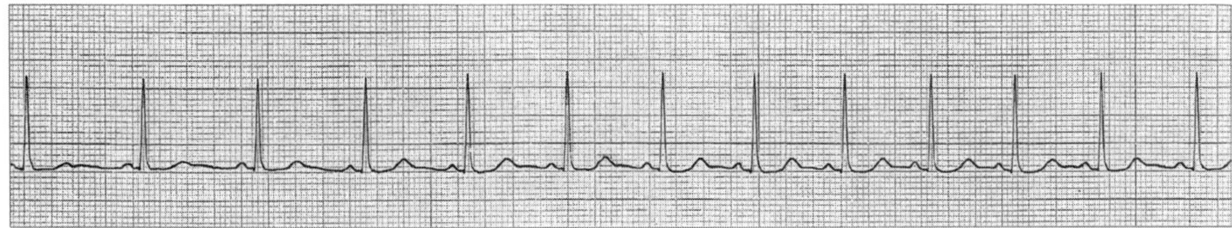

Figure 7.2 Sinus arrhythmia.

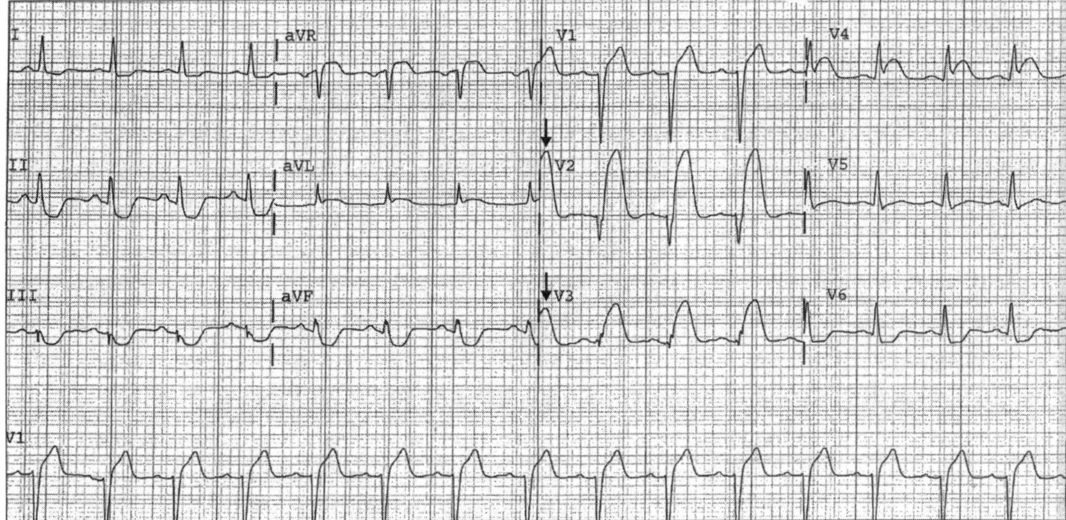

Figure 7.3 Anterior wall myocardial infarction.

EXAM TIPS

- One EKG strip may show up in the FNP or AGNP exam (ANCC or AANP exam).
- Memorize appearance of EKG with AF and anterior wall MI (tombstone-like pattern).
- AF: Goal is INR of 2 to 3.
- AF have many causes, such as alcohol intoxication; CAD, CHF, history of MI, older age, hypertension; stimulants (caffeine, decongestants, cocaine, amphetamines, etc.).
- Learn the proper procedure to check for pulsus paradoxus.
- If INR is between 4.01 to 4.99, hold one dose. Check Table 7.1. Do not give vitamin K.

CLINICAL PEARLS

- **Major bleeding episodes can occur even with a normal INR. Order an INR with the PT and the PTT if you suspect bleeding.**
- **It may take up to 3 days after changing the warfarin dose to see a change in the INR.**
- **Coumadin is an FDA category X drug.**

Hypertension

Correct BP Measurement

- Avoid smoking or caffeine intake 30 minutes before measurement. Instruct patient not to cross their legs (increases SBP).
- Begin BP measurement after at least 5 minutes of rest (mercury sphygmomanometer preferred over digital machines).
- Two or more readings separated by 2 minutes should be averaged per visit.
- Higher number determines BP stage (BP 140/100 is stage II instead of stage I; see Table 7.2).

Primary HTN

Previously known as *essential hypertension*. It is usually asymptomatic. Both the American Nurses Credentialing Center (ANCC) and the American Academy of Nurse Practitioners Certification Board (AANPCB) exams are now based on the JNC 8 Hypertension Guidelines (2014). The American College of Cardiology/American Heart Association 2017 guideline for high BP in adults has changed the BP classification and goals (BP <130/80). But as of May 2018, the JNC 8 is still the guideline that is followed on the exams. (Changes will be posted at www.npreview.com)

Peripheral Vascular Resistance × Cardiac Output

Any change in the PVR or CO results in a change in BP (increase/decrease). Examples:

- *Na+ (Sodium):*
  - Water retention increases vascular volume, increased CO (BP increases)

Table 7.2 Blood Pressure Stages

Stage	Systole	Diastole
Normal	<120 mmHg	<80 mmHg
Prehypertension	<120–139 mmHg	80–89 mmHg
Stage I	140–159 mmHg	90–99 mmHg
Stage II	>160 mmHg	>100 mmHg

- *Angiotensin I to Angiotensin II*:
  - Increased vasoconstriction will increase PVR (BP increases).
  - Younger patients have higher renin levels compared with the elderly.
- *Sympathetic System Stimulation*:
  - Epinephrine secretion causes tachycardia and vasoconstriction (BP increases).
- *Alpha-Blockers, Beta-Blockers, Calcium-Channel Blockers*:
  - Drugs decrease peripheral vascular resistance from vasodilation (BP decreases).
- *Pregnancy*:
  - Systemic vascular resistance is lowered due to hormones (systolic and diastolic BP decreases during the first and second trimesters).

Labs

- *Kidneys:* Creatinine, urinalysis
- *Endocrine:* TSH, fasting blood glucose
- *Electrolyte:* Potassium (K^+), sodium (Na^+), calcium (Ca^{2+})
- *Heart:* Cholesterol, HDL, LDL, triglycerides (complete lipid panel)
- *Anemia:* CBC
- Baseline EKG and chest x-ray (to rule out cardiomegaly)

Rule Out Target Organ Damage

Look for the following clinical findings:

Microvascular Damage

- Eyes
  - Silver and/or copper wire arterioles
  - Arteriovenous junction nicking (caused when an arteriole crosses on top of a vein)
  - Flame-shaped hemorrhages, papilledema
- Kidneys
  - Microalbuminuria and proteinuria
  - Elevated serum creatinine and abnormal eGFR (rule out kidney disease)
  - Peripheral or generalized edema

Macrovascular Damage

- Heart
  - S3 (CHF)
  - S4 (LVH)
  - Carotid bruits (narrowing due to plaque, increased risk of CAD)
  - CAD and acute MI
  - Decreased or absent peripheral pulses (peripheral arterial disease [PAD])
- Brain
  - Transient ischemic attacks (TIAs)
  - Hemorrhagic strokes

Secondary HTN

The causes of secondary HTN can be classified into three major groups:

1. Renal (renal artery stenosis, polycystic kidneys, chronic kidney disease)
2. Endocrine (hyperthyroidism, hyperaldosteronism, pheochromocytoma)
3. Other causes (obstructive sleep apnea, coarctation of the aorta)

Renal artery stenosis is more common in younger adults. Middle-aged adults are more likely to have endocrine-related disorders. Chronic kidney disease is more common in elderly patients.

Rule out secondary cause and maintain a high index of suspicion if the following:

- Age younger than 30 years
- Severe HTN or acute rise in BP (previously stable patient)
- Resistant HTN despite treatment with at least three antihypertensive agents
- Malignant HTN (severe HTN with end-organ damage such as retinal hemorrhages, papilledema, acute renal failure, and severe headache

Other causes include:

- Coarctation of the aorta
  - BP of the arms is higher than BP of the legs
  - Delayed or diminished femoral pulses (check both radial and femoral pulse at the same time)
- Sleep apnea
  - Sleep partner will report severe snoring with apneic episodes during sleep
  - Marked hypoxic episodes during sleep increases BP

Clinical Findings

Kidneys

- Bruit epigastric or flank area (renal artery stenosis); avoid angiotensin-converting enzyme inhibitors (ACEIs) and angiotensin receptor blockers (ARBs)
- Enlarged kidneys with cystic renal masses (polycystic kidney)
- Increased creatinine and decreased GFR (renal insufficiency to renal failure)

Endocrine

- Primary hyperaldosteronism
  - HTN with hypokalemia (low K+)
  - Normal to elevated sodium levels (high/normal Na+)
- Hyperthyroidism
  - Weight loss, tachycardia, fine tremor, moist skin, anxiety
  - New onset of AF (check EKG)
  - Check TSH
- Pheochromocytoma
  - Excessive secretion of catecholamines (severe HTN, arrhythmias)
  - Labile increase in BP accompanied by palpitations
  - Sudden onset of anxiety, sweating, severe headache

How to Diagnose HTN

Check BP (serial BP) and confirm diagnosis at another subsequent visit from 1 to 4 weeks (after initial visit). Check BP at home and keep diary. Does office BP correlate with home BP monitoring results? If home BP numbers lower, rule out white-coat hypertension.

JNC 8 treatment goals have been grouped by age, race, and disease (chronic kidney disease [CKD] and diabetes mellitus [DM]). In a nutshell, the goal is BP less than 140/90 mmHg for everyone. The exception is older patients (60 years of age or older) who *do not* have CKD and/or DM; the systolic BP can go up by 10 mmHg (<150/90 mmHg). See Tables 7.3, 7.4, and 7.5 for specific JNC guidelines.

Table 7.3 JNC 8 Hypertension Treatment Goal (by Age)

	BP Goal	Notes
Age 60 years or younger	<140/90 mmHg	Same BP goal for all (including DM/CKD)
Age 60 years or older	<150/90 mmHg	Systolic BP goal increased by 10 mm Hg *except* if DM and/or CKD

CKD, chronic kidney disease; DM, diabetes mellitus; JNC, Joint National Committee.

Source: Adapted from Eighth Joint National Committee on Prevention, Detection, Evaluation, and Treatment of High Blood Pressure (James et al., 2014).

Table 7.4 JNC 8 Hypertension Treatment Goal (by Race)

	BP Goal	Notes
Black*	<140/90 mmHg	Thiazide diuretics and CCBS (alone or combined with another drug class)
Non-Black*	<140/90 mmHg	Thiazide diuretics, ACEI, ARB, or CCB (alone or combined with another drug class)

**Except* if DM and/or CKD, choose ACEI or ARB alone or combined with other drug class.

ACEI, angiotensin-converting enzyme inhibitor; ARB, angiotensin receptor blocker; CCB, calcium channel blocker; CKD, chronic kidney disease; DM, diabetes mellitus; JNC, Joint National Committee.

Source: Adapted from Eighth Joint National Committee on Prevention, Detection, Evaluation, and Treatment of High Blood Pressure (James et al., 2014).

Table 7.5 JNC 8 Hypertension Treatment Goal (DM and/or CKD)

	BP Goal	Notes
Chronic kidney disease* (age 18 years or older)	<140/90	Initiate ACEI or ARB (alone or combined with another drug class)
Diabetes mellitus (age 18 years or older)	<140/90	Include ACEI or ARB (alone or combined with another drug class)

*Applies to all people with CKD regardless of race or DM status.

ACEI, angiotensin-converting enzyme inhibitor, ARB, angiotensin receptor blocker; JNC, Joint National Committee.

Source: Adapted from Eighth Joint National Committee on Prevention, Detection, Evaluation, and Treatment of High Blood Pressure (James et al., 2014).

"White Coat" Hypertension

Office BP readings are consistently elevated compared with home BP measurements. To rule out, have patient check his or her BP outside of the clinic a few times and compare with office BP.

Hypertensive Emergency

Diastolic BP greater than 120 mmHg (severe hypertension) with clinical findings of target organ damage such as nausea and vomiting (increased intracranial pressure [ICP]), CVA/TIA, subarachnoid hemorrhage, MI, acute PE, acute renal failure, retinopathy (flame-shaped hemorrhages), papilledema, acute severe low-back pain (dissecting aorta).

Isolated Systolic Hypertension in the Elderly

- Caused by loss of recoil in the arteries (atherosclerosis), which increases PVR.
- Pulse pressure (systolic BP – diastolic BP) increases in this disorder.
- For frail patients with severe orthostatic hypotension (falls, syncope) or if older than age 60 (without CKD or DM), it is now acceptable to have a systolic BP of up to 150 mmHg.

Treatment Plan

- Thiazide diuretics at low dose (chlorthalidone 12.5 to 25 mg/d)
- And/or can start with long-acting dihydropyridine CCB (amlodipine/Norvasc, nifedipine/Procardia XL) and/or ACEI or ARB

Orthostatic Hypotension

Elderly are at higher risk for orthostatic hypotension due to a less active autonomic nervous system and slower metabolism of drugs by the liver (prolongs half-life of drugs).

To Evaluate for Orthostatic Hypotension

- Check BP in both supine and standing positions, especially in the elderly, before and after treatment for HTN.
- Ask patient if dizzy or lightheaded with changes in position.

Lifestyle Recommendations

This is the first-line therapy for HTN, hyperlipidemia, and type 2 DM:

- Lose weight if overweight (body mass index [BMI] 25–29.9) or obese (BMI 30 or higher).
- Normal weight is a BMI of 18.5 to 24.9.
- Stop smoking. Reduce stress level.
- Reduce dietary sodium:
  - Less than 2.4 g per day (2,400 mg/d)
- Maintain adequate intake of potassium, calcium, and magnesium.
- Limit alcohol intake:
  - 1 ounce (30 mL) or less per day for men
  - 0.5 ounce or less per day for women
- Eat fatty cold-water fish (salmon, anchovy) three times a week.

DASH Diet (Dietary Approaches to Stop HTN)

Recommended for prehypertension, HTN, weight loss. Goal is to eat foods rich in potassium, magnesium, and calcium. Reduce red meat and processed foods. Eat more whole grains, legumes. Eat more fish and poultry.

- *Grains:* Seven to eight daily servings
- Fruits and vegetables: Four to five daily servings
- Nuts, seeds, and dry beans: Four to five servings per week
- Fats, oils, or fat-free dairy products: Two to three daily servings
- *Meat, poultry, and fish:* Two or fewer daily servings
- *Sweets:* Try to limit to fewer than five servings per week
- Avoid high-sodium foods:
  - Cold cuts, ready-made foods, any pickled foods (cucumbers, eggs, pork parts)

Dietary Sources of Minerals

- Calcium (low-fat dairy)
- Potassium (most fruits and vegetables)
- Magnesium (dried beans, whole grains, nuts)
- Omega-3 oils (anchovy, krill, salmon, flaxseed)

Exercise

Advise that aerobic physical activity will reduce LDL cholesterol and BP.

- Frequency: Three to four sessions per week
- Intensity: Moderate to vigorous (50%–80% of exercise capacity)
- Duration: 40 minutes average
- Modalities: Walking, treadmill, cycling, rowing, stair-climbing; include resistance exercises for 2 to 3 days (e.g., elastic bands, weight machines, dumbbells)

Medications

Under JNC 8, can initiate treatment with one to two antihypertensive medications (combination drug or two separate agents)

Diuretics: General

- All diuretics will decrease blood volume, venous pressure, and preload (cardiac filling).
- Effect is antagonized by NSAIDS. Monitor electrolytes, especially K+.

Thiazide Diuretics

- *Action:* Change the way that the kidney handles sodium, which increases urine output.
- Have a favorable effect with osteopenia/osteoporosis (slows down demineralization). All thiazides contain sulfa compounds. Avoid if patient has a sulfa allergy.

Side Effects

- "Hyper"
  - Hyperglycemia (be careful with diabetics)
  - Hyperuricemia (can precipitate a gout attack)
  - Hypertriglyceridemia and hypercholesteremia (check lipid profile)
- "Hypo"
  - Hypokalemia (potentiates digoxin toxicity, increases risk of arrhythmias)
  - Hyponatremia (hold diuretic, restrict water intake, replace K+ loss)
  - Hypomagnesemia

Contraindications

- Sensitivity to sulfa drugs and thiazides

Examples

- Hydrochlorothiazide 12.5 to 25 mg PO daily
- Chlorthalidone (Hygroton) 12.5 to 25 mg PO daily
- Indapamide (Lozol) PO daily

Loop Diuretics

Action: Inhibit the sodium–potassium–chloride pump of the kidney in the loop of Henle.

Side Effects

- Hypokalemia (potentiates digoxin toxicity, increases risk of arrhythmias)
- Hyponatremia (hold diuretic, restrict water intake, replace K+ loss)
- Hypomagnesemia
- Possibly altered excretion of lithium and salicylates

Contraindications

- Sensitivity to loop diuretics

Examples

- Furosemide (Lasix) PO BID
- Bumetanide (Bumex) PO BID

Sulfa Allergy and Diuretics

If people are allergic to sulfa, they may have cross-sensitivity to thiazides and loop diuretics. Other drugs with sulfa are sulfonylureas, sulfa antibiotics, sulfasalazine, some protease inhibitors (darunavir, fosamprenavir). May also be sensitive to topical sulfas (ophthalmic drops) or topical silver sulfadiazine (Silvadene).

Aldosterone Receptor Antagonist Diuretics

- *Action:* Antagonizes the action of aldosterone. Increases elimination of water in the kidneys and conserves potassium. Drug class also known as *mineralocorticoid receptor antagonists* or *antimineralcorticoid.*
- *Indications:* Administer for HTN, heart failure, hirsutism, precocious puberty.
- Avoid combining with potassium-sparing diuretics, ACEIS, or potassium supplements.

Side Effects

- Gynecomastia, galactorrhea
- Hyperkalemia
- GI (vomiting, diarrhea, stomach cramps), postmenopausal bleeding, erectile dysfunction

Contraindications

- Hyperkalemia (serum potassium greater than 5.5 mEq/L)
- Renal insufficiency (serum creatinine greater than 2.0 mg/dL in men or greater than 1.8 mg/dL for women)
- DM type 2 with microalbuminuria

Examples

- Spironolactone (Aldactone) daily
- Eplerenone (Inspra) daily

Beta-Blockers

- Avoid abrupt discontinuation after chronic use. Wean slowly. May precipitate severe rebound hypertension.
- *Action:* Decreases vasomotor activity, CO, inhibits renin and norepinephrine release.
- Blocks beta receptors on the heart and the peripheral vasculature. There are two types of beta-blocker receptors in the body: B1 (cardiac effects) and B2 (lungs and peripheral vasculature).

Contraindications

- Asthma, COPD, chronic bronchitis, emphysema (chronic lung disease)
- Second- and third-degree heart block (fine to use with first-degree block)
- Sinus bradycardia

Other Uses

- *Acute MI:* Reduces mortality during acute MI and post-MI
- *Migraine headache:* For prophylaxis only (not for acute attacks)
- *Glaucoma:* Reduces intraocular pressure (Betimol ophthalmic drops for open-angle glaucoma)
- *Resting tachycardia* (target heart rate <100 beats/min)
- *Angina pectoris:* Treats symptoms
- *Post-MI:* Decreases mortality
- *Hyperthyroidism and pheochromocytoma:* To control symptoms until primary disease treated
- *Beta-blockers:* Ends with "-olol":
  - Metoprolol (Lopressor) 100 mg QD to BID
  - Atenolol (Tenormin) 50 mg daily
  - Propranolol (long-acting Inderal) 40 mg BID
- Do not use propranolol (plain Inderal) to treat HTN (shorter half-life)

Calcium Channel Blockers (CCBS)

Action: Blocks voltage-gated calcium channels in cardiac smooth muscle and the blood vessels. Results in systemic vasodilation. The nondihydropyridines depress the muscles of the heart (inotropic effect). The dihydropyridines slow down heart rate (chronotropic effect).

Side Effects

- Headaches (due to vasodilation)
- Ankle edema (caused by vasodilation and considered benign)
- Heart block or bradycardia (depresses cardiac muscle and AV node)
- Reflex tachycardia (seen with dihydropyridines such as nifedipine)

Contraindications

- Second- and third-degree heart block (fine to use with first-degree block)
- Bradycardia
- CHF

Examples

Dihydropyridine CCBs ("-pine" ending):

- Nifedipine (Procardia XL) daily
- Amlodipine (Norvasc) daily
- Felodipine (Plendil) daily

Nondihydropyridine CCBs:

- Verapamil (Calan SR) daily to BID
- Diltiazem (Cardizem CD) daily

ACEIs and ARBs

- Blocks conversion of angiotensin I to II (more potent vasoconstrictor)
- DM and/or CKD: Drugs of choice (protect kidneys)

Pregnancy Category C (First Trimester) and Category D (Second and Third Trimesters)

- Fetal kidney malformations and fetal hypotension

Side Effects

- Dry hacking cough (up to 10% with ACEIs; less with ARBs)
- Hyperkalemia, angioedema (rare but may be life-threatening)

Contraindications

- Moderate to severe kidney disease
- Renal artery stenosis
  - Precipitates acute renal failure if given ACEI or ARB
  - Hyperkalemia (this is also a side effect of ACEIs and ARBs; will have additive effect)

Examples

- ACEIs
  - Ramipril (Altace) once a day in one to two divided doses
  - Benazepril (Lotensin) once a day initially
  - Enalapril (Vasotec) once a day in one to two divided doses

- ARBs
  - Losartan (Cozaar) once a day in one to two divided doses
  - Candesartan (Atacand) once a day in one to two divided doses
  - Olmesartan (Benicar) once a day in one to two divided doses

Alpha-1 Blockers/Antagonists

Also known as *alpha-adrenergic blockers*. Suffix of "zosin." Potent vasodilators. Common side effects are dizziness and hypotension. Give at bedtime at very low doses and slowly titrate up.

Side Effects

- "First-dose orthostatic hypotension" is common (warn patient).
- Side effects are dizziness and postural hypotension (common side effect).
- May cause severe hypotension and reflex tachycardia.
- Give at bedtime. Start at very low doses and titrate up slowly until good BP control. Advise patient to get out of bed slowly to prevent postural hypotension.
- Not a first-line choice for HTN except for men with both HTN and benign prostatic hyperplasia (BPH). Alpha-blockers relax smooth muscle found on the bladder neck and the prostate gland and relieves obstructive voiding symptoms such as weak urinary stream, urgency, and nocturia.

Examples

- Terazosin (Hytrin): Used for both HTN and BPH (starting dose 1 mg PO at bedtime)
- Doxazosin (Cardura): Used for both HTN and BPH
- Tamsulosin (Flomax): Used for BPH only

*Sample Case Scenarios (JNC 8)**

Can initiate with one to two antihypertensive medications (combined or two separate agents).

- *Stable heart failure*: ACEI or ARB as first line, plus BB plus diuretic and others
- *DM*: ACEI or ARB as first line; if African American, can start with CCB or thiazide
- *CKD*: ARB or ACEI as first line; can add CCB or thiazides
- *Stroke history*: ACEI or ARB as first-line drugs; add CCB or thiazide as second-line drugs
- *African Americans* (including people with DM): Thiazides or CCBs

EXAM TIPS

- **Follow JNC 8 guidelines for both ANCC and AANPCB exams.**
- ***Eye findings:* Learn to distinguish the findings in hypertensive retinopathy (copper and silver wire arterioles, arteriovenous nicking) from those in diabetic retinopathy (neovascularization, cotton wall spots, microaneurysms). Arteriovenous nicking occurs when a retinal vein is compressed by an arteriole that causes the venule to collapse.**
- **Isolated systolic HTN in the elderly: Preferred medications are low-dose thiazide diuretic or CCB (long-acting dihydropyridine).**
- **To assess orthostatic hypotension, measure both, the supine first, then standing BP.**
- **Memorize the side effects of thiazide diuretics.**
- **Side effect of spironolactone is gynecomastia**
- ***ACEIs or ARBs:* Use for DM, CKD, and heart failure. It may cause a dry cough (10%).**
- **Careful when combining ACEIs with potassium-sparing diuretics (i.e., triamterene, spironolactone) because of increased risk of hyperkalemia.**
- **Bilateral renal artery stenosis: ACEIs or ARBs will precipitate acute renal failure.**
- **Alpha-blockers are not first-line drugs for HTN except if patient has preexisting BPH.**

**Source:* Joint National Committee (2014).

- **Women with HTN and osteopenia/osteoporosis should receive thiazides. Thiazides help bone loss by slowing down calcium loss (from the bone) and stimulating osteoclasts.**

CLINICAL PEARLS

- **Hypertensive patients who are less than 20/10 mmHg above goal can initially be treated with monotherapy (Mann, 2017).**
- **Per JNC 8, consider chlorthalidone or indapamide (instead of hydrochlorothiazide); better evidence and longer half-life.**

Heart Failure

Numerous causes and precipitating factors such as an acute MI, CAD, HTN, fluid retention, valvular abnormalities, arrhythmias, and so on. Ejection fraction (EF) less than 40% is also known as *systolic heart failure* (or heart failure with reduced ejection fraction/HFrEF). If EF more than 40%, also known as *diastolic failure* (or heart failure with preserved ejection fraction/HFpEF).

Left Ventricular Failure

- Crackles, bibasilar rales (rales on lower lobes of the lungs), cough, dyspnea, decreased breath sounds, dullness to percussion
- Paroxysmal nocturnal dyspnea, orthopnea, nocturnal nonproductive cough, wheezing (cardiac asthma), hypertension, and fatigue are symptoms of both left and right heart failure

Right Ventricular Failure

- Jugular venous distention (JVD): Normal JVD is 4 cm or less
- Enlarged spleen, enlarged liver causes anorexia, nausea, and abdominal pain
- Lower extremity edema with cool skin

Other PE Findings

- Presence of S3 gallop, which can be accompanied by anasarca (severe generalized edema due to effusion of fluid into the extracellular space)

Labs

- Chest x-ray result will show increased heart size, interstitial and alveolar edema, Kerley B lines, and other signs of pulmonary edema
- EKG, CPK, cardiac troponins, B-type natriuretic peptide
- BUN and creatinine, electrolytes, CBC, liver function tests
- Echocardiogram with Doppler flow study
- Weight should be checked daily to detect fluid accumulation

Treatment Plan

- If acute decompensated heart failure: Refer to ED (IV furosemide, oxygen, vasodilators, others).
- Stable HF (HFrEF) with hypertension: Start on ACEI or ARB, then add a beta-blocker, aldosterone-receptor antagonist (spironolactone), and other medications as needed (Colucci, 2018; Ferri, 2016).
- Limit sodium intake.
- Patients with HF are best managed by cardiologists or at a heart clinic.
- Use beta-blocker if heart failure with reduced EF (carvedilol, bisoprolol, extended- release metoprolol succinate); start with very low dose; careful with initial dosing, can worsen; consult or refer to experienced heart clinic

- Use New York Heart Association (NYHA) system to classify patient's degree of cardiac disability (Table 7.6)
- Refer to cardiologist; if in distress, refer to ED

Table 7.6 New York Heart Association Functional Capacity Ratings

Classification	Degree of Disability
Class I	No limitations on physical activity
Class II	Ordinary physical activity results in fatigue, exertional dyspnea
Class III	Marked limitation in physical activity
Class IV	Symptoms are present at rest, with or without physical activity

Source: American Heart Association (2011).

Lifestyle Modification for Heart Failure

- Restrict or abstain from alcohol. Smoking cessation if smoker; weight loss
- Restrict sodium to 2 to 3 g/d
- Fluid restriction (1.5–2 L/d) may help some patients

Note

Here is an easy way to remember whether a sign or symptom is from the left or right side of the heart:

- Both *left* and *lung* start with the letter L. Symptoms are lung related, such as dyspnea, orthopnea, and paroxysmal nocturnal dyspnea.
- Right-sided heart failure symptoms are GI related (anorexia, nausea, and right upper quadrant abdominal pain)

Deep Vein Thrombosis (DVT)

Thrombi develop inside the deep venous system of the legs or pelvis secondary to stasis, trauma to vessel walls, inflammation, or increased coagulation. Pulmonary embolus is considered another manifestation of this thromboembolic disorder.

Etiology (three categories):

1. *Stasis:* Prolonged travel/inactivity (more than 3 hours), bed rest, CHF
2. *Inherited coagulation disorders:* Factor C deficiency, Leiden, and so forth
3. *Increased coagulation due to external factors:* Oral contraceptive use, pregnancy, bone fractures especially of the long bones, trauma, recent surgery, malignancy

Classic Case

A patient with risk factors for DVT complains of gradual onset of swelling on a lower extremity after a history of travel (more than 3 hours) or prolonged sitting. The patient complains of a painful and swollen lower extremity that is red and warm. If patient has PE, it may be accompanied by abrupt onset of chest pain, dyspnea, dizziness, or syncope. Many patients are asymptomatic.

Treatment Plan

- *Homan's sign:* Lower leg pain on dorsiflexion of the foot (low sensitivity)
- CBC, platelets, clotting time (PT/PTT, INR), D-dimer level, chest x-ray, EKG
- Ultrasonography (whole leg or proximal leg)
- Hospital admission, heparin IV then warfarin PO (Coumadin) for 3 to 6 months (first episode) or longer
- For recurrent DVT or elderly, antithrombotic treatment may last a lifetime

Complications

- Pulmonary emboli
- Stroke and other embolic episodes

EXAM TIPS

- **Memorize goal for atrial fibrillation is an INR of 2.0 to 3.0.**
- **Learn how to manage elevated INR (see Table 7.1).**
- **Memorize presentation of a patient with NYHA class II heart disease.**
- **First line medication for stable HF is an ACEI or ARB.**
- **The S3 heart sound is a sign of HF, although it can also be heard in pregnant women and children/young adults.**
- **Learn DVT risk factors.**

Superficial Thrombophlebitis

Inflammation of a superficial vein due to local trauma. Higher risk if indwelling catheters, intravenous drugs (e.g., potassium), secondary bacterial infection (*S. aureus*). Some patients may have coexistent DVT.

Classic Case

Adult patient complains of an acute onset of an indurated vein (localized redness, swelling, and tenderness). Usually located on the extremities. The patient is afebrile with normal vital signs.

Objective Findings

- Indurated cord-like vein that is warm and tender to touch with a surrounding area of erythema.
- There should be no swelling or edema of the entire limb (think of DVT).

Treatment Plan

- Administer NSAIDs, such as ibuprofen or naproxen sodium (Anaprox DS), BID.
- Warm compresses. Elevate limb.
- If septic cause, admit to hospital.

Peripheral Arterial Disease (PAD)

Gradual (decades) narrowing and/or occlusion of medium to large arteries in the lower extremities. Blood flow to the extremities gradually decreases over time, resulting in permanent ischemic damage (gangrene of the toes/foot). Higher risk with HTN, smoking, diabetes, and hyperlipidemia. Previously known as peripheral vascular disease.

Classic Case

Older patient who has a history of smoking and hyperlipidemia complains of worsening pain on ambulation (intermittent claudication) that is instantly relieved by rest. Over time, symptoms worsen until the patient's walking distance is greatly limited. Atrophic skin changes. Some have gangrene on one or more toes.

Ankle-Brachial Index (ABI)

ABI score equal or less than 0.9 is diagnostic for PAD. ABI score of 0.91 to 1.3 is normal.

Procedure

- Systolic BP of the ankle and the arm (brachial) is checked after in a supine position for 10 minutes by using a BP cuff and ultrasound probe.
- An ABI score is done for each leg.
- To calculate ABI, the SBP of each foot is divided by the SBP of both arms.

Objective Findings

- *Skin:* Atrophic changes (shiny and hyperpigmented ankles that are hairless and cool to touch); gangrene of the toe(s)
- *Cardiovascular:* Decreased to absent dorsal pedal pulse (may include popliteal and posterior tibial pulse), increased capillary refill time (less than 2 seconds), and bruits over partially blocked arteries

Treatment Plan

- Initial method (low tech): Check pedal and posterior tibial pulses.
- Ankle-Brachial index (ABI) Score: Used to evaluate severity of PAD; done by checking systolic BP of ankles and upper arm; score of 0.9 or less is diagnostic of PAD.
- Encourage smoking cessation (smoking causes vasoconstriction) and daily ambulation exercises
- Pentoxifylline (Trental) if indicated, but effect is marginal (compared with cilostazol)
- Cilostazol (Pletal) is a phosphodiesterase inhibitor (direct vasodilator); can be taken with aspirin or clopidogrel. Grapefruit juice, diltiazem, and omeprazole can increase serum concentration if taken together. Percutaneous angioplasty or surgery for severe cases

Complications

- Gangrene of foot and/or lower limb with amputation
- Increased risk of CAD
- Increased risk of carotid plaquing (check for carotid bruits)

Raynaud's Phenomenon

Reversible vasospasm of the peripheral arterioles on the fingers and toes. Cause is unknown. Associated with an increased risk of autoimmune disorders (e.g., thyroid disorder, pernicious anemia, rheumatoid arthritis). Most patients are females (60% to 90%), with a gender ratio of 8:1. Patients with no underlying disease have "primary" Raynaud's phenomenon. Up to 95% of patients with scleroderma have "secondary" Raynaud's phenomenon.

Classic Case

A middle-aged woman complains of chronic and recurrent episodes of color changes on her fingertips in a symmetric pattern (both hands and both feet). The colors range from white (pallor) and blue (cyanosis) to red (reperfusion). Complains of numbness and tingling. Attacks last for several hours. Hands and feet become numb with very cold temperatures. Ischemic changes may be present after a severe episode such as shallow ulcers (that eventually heal) on some of the fingertips.

Treatment Plan

- Avoid touching cold objects, cold weather; avoid stimulants (e.g., caffeine)
- Smoking cessation is important; nifedipine (Adalat) or amlodipine (Norvasc)
- *Evaluate:* Check distal pulses, ischemic signs (ischemic ulcers at the fingers/toes)
- Do not use any vasoconstricting drugs (e.g., Imitrex, ergots, pseudoephedrine/decongestants, amphetamines); avoid nonselective beta-blockers

Complications

- Small ulcers in the fingertips and toes

EXAM TIPS

- ***Raynaud's phenomenon:*** **Think of the colors of the American flag as a reminder for this disorder.**
- **Medicines for Raynaud's phenomenon include CCBs (nifedipine, amlodipine).**

Bacterial Endocarditis

Presentation ranges from full-blown disease to subacute endocarditis. Bacterial pathogens are gram positive (i.e., viridans streptococcus, *S. aureus*, etc.). Also known as IE. Parenteral antibacterial treatment for native valve endocarditis can range from 4 to 6 weeks.

Classic Case

A middle-aged male presents with fever, chills, and malaise that are associated with subungual hemorrhages (splinter hemorrhages on nail bed) and tender violet-colored nodules on the fingers and/or on the toes (Osler's nodes). Palms and soles may have tender red spots on the skin (Janeway lesions). Some patients may have a heart murmur.

Treatment Plan

- Refer to cardiologist or ED for hospitalization and intravenous antibiotics
- Blood cultures × three (first 24 hours)
- CBC (elevated WBCs) and sedimentation rate greater than 20 mm per hour (elevated)

Complications

- Valvular destruction, myocardial abscess, emboli, etc.

Endocarditis Prophylaxis (Table 7.7)

- Antibiotic prophylaxis is *no longer recommended* for:
  - Mitral valve prolapse
  - Genitourinary or GI incisions/invasive procedures (except if there is an existing infection present such as a urinary tract infection [UTI] before a cystoscopy)
- Standard regimen: Give 1 hour before procedure:
  - Amoxicillin 2 g PO × 1 dose (adults)
  - Amoxicillin 50 mg/kg 1 hour before procedure × one dose (children)

Table 7.7 Endocarditis Prophylaxis

High Risk Condition	Invasive Procedures
Previous history of bacterial endocarditis	Dental procedures that traumatize oral mucosa, gingiva, or the periapical area of the teeth
Prosthetic valves	Invasive procedures on the respiratory tract (especially if tissue is infected)
Certain types of congenital heart disease	
Cardiac transplant with valvulopathy	

Source: Adapted from Wilson et al. (2007).

Penicillin Allergy

- Clindamycin 600 mg or clarithromycin (Biaxin) 500 mg or cephalexin (Keflex) 2 g

Mitral Valve Prolapse (MVP)

The classic finding is an S_2 "click" followed by a systolic murmur. Some patients with MVP are at higher risk of thromboemboli, TIAs, AF, and ruptured chordae tendineae. Diagnosed by cardiac echocardiogram with Doppler flow study.

Classic Case

Tall and thin adult female patient complains of fatigue, palpitations, and lightheadedness (orthostatic hypotension) that is aggravated by heavy exertion. May be asymptomatic. Associated with pectus excavatum, hypermobility of the joints, arm span greater than height (rule out Marfan's syndrome).

Treatment Plan

- Asymptomatic MVP does not need treatment.
- MVP with palpitations is treated with beta-blockers, avoidance of caffeine, alcohol, and cigarettes.
- Holter monitoring is useful in detecting significant arrhythmias.

Hyperlipidemia

The treatment guidelines and type of statin and intensity (low, moderate, or high dose) are from the 2014 updated American College of Cardiology (ACC) and American Heart Association (AHA) Guideline on the Treatment of Blood Cholesterol to Reduce Atherosclerotic Cardiovascular Disease Risk. See the ACC web address for tool (http://tools.acc.org/ascvd-risk-estimator).

To determine the risk of atherosclerotic cardiovascular disease (ASCVD), use the ACC's new "ASCVD Risk Estimator" tool (or the Pooled Cohort Equations for ASCVD risk prediction). The free app is available and can be accessed directly online (see previous paragraph).

Screening Guidelines

- Complete lipid profile (fasting) starting at age 20 (then every 5 years)
- Older than age 40 years, screen every 2 to 3 years
- Preexisting hyperlipidemia: Screen annually or more frequently

Total Cholesterol

- *Normal:* Less than 200 mg/dL
- *Borderline:* Between 200 and 239 mg/dL
- *High:* Greater than 240 mg/dL

HDL Cholesterol (HDL-C)

- Men: Greater than 40 mg/dL
- Women: Greater than 50 mg/dL
- If less than 40 mg/dL, associated with increased risk of CAD even if normal LDL or cholesterol
- High carbohydrate and low-fat diets and smoking are associated with low HDL
- Lifestyle modifications: Do regular moderate cardiovascular/aerobic exercises most days of the week, lose weight, eat healthy fats (salmon, tuna, nuts), eliminate trans fats, stop smoking

LDL cholesterol (LDL-C)

- *Optimal:* Less than 100 mg/dL
- *LDL:* Less than 130 mg/dL for low-risk patients with fewer than two risk factors
- *Very high:* Greater than 190 mg/dL
- *Heart disease or diabetes:* Less than 100 mg/dL

Triglycerides

- *Normal:* Less than 150 mg/dL
- High risk of acute pancreatitis: 1000 mg/dL or higher
- If triglycerides >500 mg/dL or higher:
    - Treat triglycerides first. Give fibrate such as fenofibrate (Tricor), niacin (Niaspan), OTC niacin, or high-dose fish oil (EPA/DHA). Prescription fish oil: Lovaza 4 g/d; when triglycerides are under control, switch target to lowering LDL
- Possible causes: Metabolic syndrome, DM, familial hypertriglyceridemia, alcohol abuse, hyperthyroidism, kidney disease, medications (anabolic steroids, Accutane, etc.)

- Lifestyle modifications: Decrease sugar and simple carbohydrates (junk food), avoid alcoholic drinks, follow low-fat diet, eat fish with omega-3 (salmon, sardines) twice a week, lose weight and increase aerobic type physical activity.

Risk Factors: Heart Disease

- HTN
- Family history of premature heart disease (women with MI before age 65 years or men with MI before age 55 years)
- DM (considered a CHD risk equivalent even if patient has no history of preexisting heart disease)
- Dyslipidemia
- Low HDL-C (<40 mg/dL)
- Age (men older than 45 or women older than 55)
- Cigarette smoking
- Obesity (BMI ≥30 kg/m^2)
- Microalbuminuria
- Carotid artery disease
- PVD

Treatment Plan: Hyperlipidemia

- First-line treatment is lifestyle changes (weight loss, exercise most days of the week, better diet low in saturated fat, smoking cessation), but the presence of ASCVD and other factors, initiate statin therapy with lifestyle changes.
- Reduce dietary salt intake and learn about the DASH diet (low salt, low saturated fat <30%).
- Encourage use of soluble fiber in diet (e.g., inulin, guar gum, fruit, vegetables) to enhance lowering of LDL (lowers LDL by blocking absorption in GI tract up to 10%).
- Target goal is to lower LDL first (except if very high triglyceride levels). If high triglycerides (500 mg/dL or higher), treat hypertriglyceridemia first because patients are at high risk for acute pancreatitis.
- Low HDL alone (even if normal LDL and cholesterol) is a risk factor for heart disease.

ACC and AHA Updated Guidelines

The 2013 ACC and AHA updated guidelines have no recommendations for or against specific target levels for LDL or HDL in the primary or secondary prevention of ASCVD. The expert panel did not find evidence to support use of specific LDL-C or HDL-C target levels. Previously, the goal for secondary prevention was LDL of 70 mg/dL and for primary prevention LDL of less than 100 mg/dL.

The ACC and AHA Guideline on the Treatment of Blood Cholesterol to Reduce ASCVD Risk (2014) list four statin benefit groups, which are discussed in terms of type of prevention (secondary or primary). These are outlined here and summarized in Table 7.8. Table 7.9 categorizes statin drugs by level of intensity of treatment.

A. Secondary Prevention (ASCVD):
   1. Patients with any form of ASCVD (history of MI, CAD, angina, stroke/TIA, PAD, coronary revascularization)
      - Younger than 75 years: High-intensity statin
      - Older than 75 years (or not candidate for high-intensity statin): Moderate-intensity statin

B. Primary Prevention (No ASCVD)
   2. LDL-C 190 mg/dL or higher: High-intensity statin
   3. DM (aged 40–75 years) with LDL 70 to 189 mg/dL: Moderate-intensity statin
   4. Without DM or ASCVD (aged 40–75 years) with an estimated 10-year ASCVD risk of 7.5% or higher: Moderate-intensity to high-intensity statin

Note

Lack of ASCVD but 10-year ASCVD risk (5% to less than 7.5%): First-line therapy is a heart-healthy lifestyle.

Table 7.8 ACC/AHA Updated Guideline on the Treatment of Blood Cholesterol (2014)

Characteristics	Statin Intensity
21–75 years with ASCVD	High intensity
21 years or older (low-density lipoprotein of 190 mg/dL or higher) *but* without ASCVD	High intensity
Older than 75 years with ASCVD (or not a candidate for high-intensity statin)	Moderate intensity
Estimated 10-year ASCVD risk 7.5% or higher (without DM or ASCVD)	Moderate to high intensity
*DM (40–75 years) with LDL 70–189 mg/dL	Moderate intensity

ACC, American College of Cardiology; AHA, American Heart Association; ASCVD, atherosclerotic cardiovascular disease; DM, diabetes mellitus; LDL, low-density lipoprotein.

Table 7.9 Statin Intensity Dosages

High Intensity Statins	Moderate Intensity Statins	Low Intensity Statins
Lower LDL ≥50%	Lower LDL 30%–50%	Lower LDL <30%
Atorvastatin (Lipitor) 40–80 mg/d*	Atorvastatin 10–20 mg/d	
Rosuvastatin (Crestor) 20–40 mg/d	Rosuvastatin (Crestor) 5–10 mg/d	
	Simvastatin (Zocor) 20–40 mg/d	Simvastatin 10 mg/d
	Pravastatin (Pravachol) 40–80 mg/d	Pravastatin 10–20 mg/d
	Lovastatin (Mevacor) 40 mg/d	Lovastatin 20 mg/d
		Fluvastatin 20–40 mg/d

*Initiation at 80 mg/d is not recommended by Food and Drug Administration; increases risk of myopathy/rhabdomyolysis. Start at lower dose and titrate up 80-mg dose (if tolerated).

LDL, low-density lipoprotein.

Lipid-Lowering Medications

HMG COA reductase inhibitors (statins) are best at lowering LDL, and some can moderately increase HDL. Under 2014 ACC/AHA guidelines, only two high-intensity statins are recommended: atorvastatin (Lipitor; 40–80 mg/d) and rosuvastatin (Crestor; 20–40 mg/d; see Table 7.9.) But in "real life," start at lower doses and titrate dose slowly until correct dose reached.

If high-intensity statin candidate, start at lower doses and titrate up slowly. Some patients may not tolerate high-intensity statins (muscle pains, weakness, etc.) but can tolerate moderate-intensity statins. If not effective after a few months, consider low- to moderate-intensity statin dosing.

- Pravastatin (Pravachol), lovastatin (Mevacor), simvastatin (Zocor)
- Simvastatin and lovastatin drug interactions (high risk of rhabdomyolysis):
  - Avoid grapefruit juice
  - Fibrates
  - Antifungals (itraconazole, ketoconazole)
  - Macrolides (erythromycin, clarithromycin, telithromycin)
  - Amiodarone (Cordarone), some CCBs (diltiazem, amlodipine, verapamil)
- Combination regimens (especially in high doses) of statins, fibrates, niacin, and/or ezetimibe increase the risk of rhabdomyolysis and drug-induced hepatitis and are now discouraged

Nicotinic Acid and Fibrates

- *Nicotinic acid:* Niacin (OTC) daily to TID, Niaspan (slow-release niacin) daily. Avoid combining niacin with statins (higher risk of liver damage).
- *Fibrates:* Gemfibrozil (Lopid), fenofibrate (Tricor). Do not use with severe renal disease.
- *Action:* Reduces production of triglycerides by the liver and increases production of HDL.
- Very good agents for lowering triglycerides and elevating HDL level. Less effective at lowering LDLs compared with the statins.
- *Side effects of niacin:* Flushing, itching, tingling, hepatotoxicity; GI effects. Take ASA (aspirin) with niacin after a meal. Divide niacin and take half (or less) of the tablet until higher dose tolerated.
- *Side effects of fibrates:* Dyspepsia, gallstones, are side effects; myopathy

Bile Acid Sequestrants

- Cholestyramine (Questran Light), colestipol (Colestid), colesevelam (Welchol)
  - *Action:* Work locally in the small intestine; interfere with fat absorption, including fat-soluble vitamins (vitamins A, D, E, and K)
- Alternative drug for patients who cannot tolerate statins, fibrates, and niacin
- Used alone, it is not as effective as statins in lowering LDL; no hepatotoxicity
  - *Side effects:* Bloating, flatulence, abdominal pain; start at low doses and titrate up slowly
  - Side effects mainly from the GI tract; advise patient to take multivitamin tablets daily

Other Lipid-Lowering Drugs

- Ezetimibe (Zetia) and combination of simvastatin and ezetimibe (Vytorin)
  - Can be taken alone or combined with a statin; can also cause rhabdomyolysis (rare)
  - *Side effects:* Diarrhea, joint pains, tiredness
- Prescribe fish oil omega-3 DHA/EPA Lovaza 4 g/d (for high triglycerides)

Lab Tests

- Avoid combination regimen (especially in high doses) of statins, fibrates, niacin, ezetimibe, and drugs that affect the CYP450 system; increases risk of rhabdomyolysis and drug-induced hepatitis.
- Test baseline LFTs and periodic testing as clinically indicated.

Rhabdomyolysis

Acute breakdown of skeletal muscle (myoglobins) will cause acute renal failure. Triad of muscle pain, weakness, and dark urine. Look for muscle pain and aches that persist (not associated with muscular exertion). Higher doses or combination therapy have higher risk.

- *Labs:* Order creatine kinase if markedly elevated (at least five times the upper limit of normal from 1,500 to >100,000 IU/L).
- *Urine:* Reddish-brown color (myoglobinuria) and proteinuria in up to 45% LFTs (will be elevated). Other labs are UA, BUN, creatinine, potassium/electrolytes, EKG, others.

Acute Drug-Induced Hepatitis

Anorexia, nausea, dark-colored urine, jaundice, fatigue, flu-like symptoms

- *Labs:* Elevated ALT and AST

Patient Education

- Minimize alcohol intake or other hepatotoxic substances while on statins.
- Avoid prescribing to alcoholics.
- Advise patient to report symptoms of hepatitis or rhabdomyolysis. If present, tell patient to stop the drug and to call or go to ED.

EXAM TIPS

- First-line treatment for hypertension (or prehypertension) is lifestyle and dietary changes.
- First-line treatment for hyperlipidemia is lifestyle, but presence of ASCVD or equivalents, need drug therapy, too.
- You must memorize some values. These are (list is not all inclusive):
  - An adult (21–75 years) with any type of ASCVD (CAD, PAD, stroke, TIA, etc.) is given high-intensity statins such as atorvastatin 40 to 80 mg or rosuvastatin 20 to 40 mg.
  - An adult with LDL greater than 190 mg/dL (without ASCVD or DM) is a candidate for high-intensity statin dosing.
  - If 10-year estimated ASCVD risk (for up to 75 years of age) is 7.5% or higher, high-intensity statin dosing is recommended. But if risk is less (5%–7.5%), try lifestyle first.
- If patient has markedly high triglycerides (500 mg/dL or higher), lower triglyceride first (niacin or fibrate) before treating the high cholesterol and LDL levels. High triglycerides increase risk of acute pancreatitis.
  - Educate to avoid alcohol, acetaminophen (hepatotoxic) use.
  - Obese patients: Encourage weight loss and reduce simple carbohydrates, sugars, junk foods. Treat first before treating high LDL.
  - Advise patient to reduce intake of simple carbohydrates, "junk" foods, and fried foods.
- Niacin and fibrates are best agents for lowering triglycerides.
- Become familiar with dietary sources of magnesium, potassium, and calcium.
- Bacterial endocarditis prophylaxis drug and dose, splinter hemorrhages on nails, Janeway lesions (red macules palms/soles not painful), Osler's nodes (painful violaceous nodes found mostly on pads of the fingers and toes, thenar eminence).

CLINICAL PEARLS

- Statins may cause memory loss, confusion, etc. (cognitive effects), which are reversible upon discontinuation of statin therapy.
- Patients on simvastatin and lovastatin should avoid grapefruit juice. Also, they should not mix these two statins with macrolides.
- Muscle pain (mild to severe) from rhabdomyolysis is usually located on the calves, thighs, lower back, and/or shoulders. Urine will be darker than normal (reddish-brown color). Rule out rhabdomyolysis if patient on a statin complains of muscular pain with dark-colored urine.

Obesity

All obese and overweight patients should have their BMI and abdominal obesity calculated (Table 7.10). Evaluate for metabolic syndrome and DM type 2. In the United States, more than one third (36.5%) of adults are obese (Centers for Disease Control and Prevention, 2016). Non-Hispanic Blacks have the highest rates of obesity (48.1%), followed by Hispanics (42.5%) and non-Hispanic Whites (34.5%). Among the obese, 40.2% are middle-aged adults (age 40–59 years).

Table 7.10 Body Mass Index (BMI)

Classification	BMI
Underweight	<18.5
Normal weight	18.5–24.9
Overweight	25–29.9
Obese	30–39.9
Grossly obese	>40.0

Abdominal Obesity

The "apple-shaped" body type is considered more dangerous for health compared with the "pear-shaped" body type.

Waist Circumference

- *Males:* Greater than 40 inches or 102 cm
- *Females:* Greater than 35 inches or 88 cm

Waist-to-Hip Ratio

- Waist-to-hip ratio: 1.0 or higher (males)
- Waist-to-hip ratio: 0.8 or higher (females)

Metabolic Syndrome

Metabolic syndrome is a metabolic disorder with a cluster of symptoms. These patients are at higher risk for type 2 DM and cardiovascular disease.

Criteria for Metabolic Syndrome (Adult Treatment Panel III)

At least three characteristics must be present to diagnose metabolic syndrome:

1. Abdominal obesity (greater than 40 inches in men and greater than 35 inches in women)
2. HTN
3. Hyperlipidemia
   - Fasting plasma glucose (>100 mg/dL)
   - Elevated triglycerides (>150 mg/dL)
   - Decreased HDL (<40 mg/dL)

Labs

- Fasting (from 9 to 12 hours) lipid profile (especially triglycerides and HDL)
- Fasting blood glucose

Nonalcoholic Fatty Liver Disease (NAFLD)

Nonalcoholic fatty liver disease (NAFLD) is caused by triglyceride fat deposits in the hepatocytes of the liver. Most are asymptomatic.

- *Risk factors:* Obesity, diabetes, metabolic syndrome, HTN, certain drugs

Classic Case

Usually asymptomatic. Some patients may have hepatomegaly. Annual physical exam labs will show mild to moderate elevations of ALT and AST. If symptomatic, complains of fatigue and malaise with vague right upper quadrant pain. Associated with obesity, metabolic syndrome, DM, and hyperlipidemia.

Labs

- Liver function tests. ALT and AST may be slightly elevated.
- Order hepatitis A, B, and C profile.
- Refer to GI specialist for management and a liver biopsy (*gold standard*).

Treatment Plan

- Lose weight. Exercise and watch diet.
- Discontinue alcohol intake permanently.
- Avoid hepatotoxic drugs (i.e., acetaminophen, isoniazid, statins).
- Recommend vaccination for hepatitis A and B. Recommend annual flu vaccine.
- Refer to GI specialist for liver biopsy.

Calculating BMI

The BMI is a measure of the ratio of weight to height. Muscular patients can have falsely elevated BMIs (higher muscle mass).

Formula for BMI calculation: Weight (kilograms)/Height (meters)^2

Patient Education

- All obese and overweight patients should be advised to lose weight (especially diabetics).
- Lifestyle changes are important (diet, nutrition, exercise, portion control).
- Daily aerobic exercise (walking, swimming, biking, etc.) for 30 to 45 minutes is recommended.
  - Weight Watchers: Some patients like the support and education (tertiary prevention).

EXAM TIPS

- **Know metabolic syndrome criteria (abdominal obesity, HTN, hyperlipidemia or elevated triglycerides and low HDL, elevated fasting glucose >100 mg/dL) caused by hyperinsulinemia and peripheral insulin resistance.**
- **Nonalcoholic fatty liver disease (NAFLD) is associated with metabolic syndrome and/or obesity. Look for slight elevation of ALT and AST (not related to alcohol or medications) and negative hepatitis A, B, and C.**
- **Abdominal obesity in males (>40 inches), females (>35 inches).**
- **Do not confuse BMI formula with the PEF (peak expiratory flow). PEF is calculated using the height, age, gender (mnemonic is "HAG").**
- **A person with a BMI of 27 is overweight (initiate lifestyle education).**

8

Pulmonary System Review

DANGER SIGNALS

Pulmonary Emboli

An older adult complains of sudden onset of dyspnea and coughing. Cough may be productive of pink-tinged frothy sputum. Other symptoms are tachycardia, pallor, and feelings of impending doom. Any condition that increases risk of blood clots will increase risk of pulmonary embolism (PE). These patients have a history of atrial fibrillation, estrogen therapy, smoking, surgery, cancer, pregnancy, long bone fractures, and prolonged inactivity.

Impending Respiratory Failure (Asthmatic Exacerbation)

An asthmatic patient presents with tachypnea (>20 breaths/min), tachycardia or bradycardia, cyanosis, and anxiety. The patient appears exhausted, fatigued, diaphoretic, and uses accessory muscles to help with breathing. Physical exam reveals cyanosis and "quiet" lungs with no wheezing or breath sounds audible. When speaking, the patient may speak only one to two words (cannot form complete sentence because needs to breathe).

Treatment Plan

Adrenaline injection *stat*. Call 911. Oxygen at 4 to 5 L/min; albuterol nebulizer treatments; parenteral steroids, antihistamines (diphenhydramine), and H2 blocker (cimetidine).

After treatment, a good sign is if breath sounds and wheezing are present (a sign that bronchi are becoming more open). Usually discharge with oral steroids for several days (e.g., Medrol Dose Pack).

NORMAL FINDINGS

- *Lower lobes:* Vesicular breath sounds (soft and low)
- *Upper lobes:* Bronchial breath sounds (louder)

Egophony

- *Normal:* Will hear "eee" clearly instead of "bah"
- *Abnormal:* Will hear "bah" sound
- *Normal:* The "eee" sound is louder over the large bronchi because larger airways are better at transmitting sounds; lower lobes have a softer sounding "eee"

Tactile Fremitus

- Instruct patient to say "99" or "one, two, three"; use finger pads to palpate lungs and feel for vibrations

- *Normal:* Stronger vibrations are palpable on the upper lobes and softer vibrations on lower lobes
- *Abnormal:* The findings are reversed; may palpate stronger vibrations on one lower lobe (i.e., consolidation); asymmetrical findings are always abnormal

Whispered Pectoriloquy

- Instruct patient to whisper "99" or "one, two, three." Compare both lungs. If there is lung consolidation, the whispered words are easily heard on the lower lobes of the lungs.
- *Normal:* Voice louder and easy to understand in the upper lobes. Voice sounds are muffled on the lower lobes.
- *Abnormal:* Clear voice sounds in the lower lobes or muffled sounds on the upper lobes.

Percussion

- Use middle or index finger as the pleximeter finger on one hand. The finger on the other hand is the hammer.
- *Normal:* Resonance is heard over normal lung tissue.
- *Tympany or hyperresonance:* Occurs with chronic obstructive pulmonary disease (COPD), emphysema (overinflating). If empty, the stomach area may be tympanic.
- *Dull tone:* Bacterial pneumonia with lobar consolidation, pleural effusion (fluid or tumor). A solid organ, such as the liver, sounds dull.

Pulmonary Function Tests

Measures Severity of Obstructive or Restrictive Pulmonary Dysfunction

- Obstructive dysfunction (reduction in airflow rates)
  - Asthma, COPD (chronic bronchitis and emphysema), bronchiectasis, others
- Restrictive dysfunction (reduction of lung volume due to decreased lung compliance)
  - Pulmonary fibrosis, pleural disease, diaphragm obstruction, others

DISEASE REVIEW

Chronic Obstructive Pulmonary Disease (COPD)

COPD includes both emphysema and chronic bronchitis. Some patients may also have an asthma component (chronic obstructive asthma). Most patients have a mixture; one or the other may predominate. The disease is characterized by the loss of elastic recoil of the lungs and alveolar damage that takes decades. The most common risk factors are chronic cigarette smoking and older age. Chronic lung disease is the third leading cause of death in the United States.

Chronic Bronchitis

This is defined as coughing with excessive mucus production for at least 3 or more months for a minimum of 2 or more consecutive years.

Emphysema

Permanent alveolar damage and loss of elastic recoil result in chronic hyperinflation of the lungs. Expiratory respiratory phase is markedly prolonged.

Risk Factors

- Chronic smoking (etiology in up to 90% of cases of COPD), older age (>40 years)
- Occupational exposure (coal dust, grain dust)

- Alpha-1 trypsin deficiency (rare condition); patients have severe lung damage at earlier ages; alpha-1 trypsin protects lungs from oxidative and environmental damage

Classic Case

An elderly man with a history of many years of cigarette smoking complains of getting short of breath upon physical exertion that worsens over time; accompanied by a chronic cough that is productive of large amounts of white to light-yellow sputum (chronic bronchitis) or progressive dyspnea with minimal cough, barrel chest, and weight loss (emphysema).

Objective Findings

- *Emphysema component:* Increased anterior–posterior diameter, decreased breath and heart sounds, use of accessory muscles, pursed-lip breathing, and weight loss
- *Percussion:* Hyperresonance
- Tactile fremitus and egophony: decreased
- *CXR:* Flattened diaphragms with hyperinflation; bullae sometimes present
- *Chronic bronchitis component:* Productive cough, wheezing, and coarse crackles

Treatment Plan

- 2017 Global Initiative for Chronic Obstructive Lung Disease (GOLD) treatment guidelines are listed in Table 8.1.

Safety Issues

- *Short-acting beta-agonists (SABAs; albuterol, levalbuterol, or metaproterenol):* May cause adverse cardiac side effects (palpitations, tachycardia). Use with caution if patient has hypertension, angina, and/or hyperthyroidism. Avoid combining with caffeinated drinks.
- *Anticholinergics (Atrovent, Spiriva):* Avoid if patient has narrow-angle glaucoma, benign prostatic hyperplasia (BPH), or bladder neck obstruction.

General Treatment of COPD

- Smoking cessation is ***very important;*** options include nicotine patches or gum, bupropion (Zyban) or varenicline (Chantix), patient education, and behavioral counseling
- Annual influenza vaccination; give pneumococcal vaccine (PPSV23/Pneumovax) and PCV13/Prevnar); administer 12 months apart

Table 8.1 Treatment of COPD: GOLD Guidelines (2017)

Patient Group (Category)	Recommendations
Category A (GOLD 1–2) Minimally symptomatic COPD (low risk of exacerbation)	Short-acting B2 agonist (SABA) PRN alone or in combination SABA with short-acting anticholinergic (more effective).
Category B (GOLD 1–2) More symptomatic (low risk of exacerbation)	Long-acting B2 agonist (LABA) or long-acting anticholinergic (newer name is long-acting muscarinic agent (LAMA). May use SABA for rescue PRN.
Category C (GOLD 3–4) Minimally symptomatic (but high risk of exacerbation)	LAMA is first line. If poor control, use combination LABA and LAMA. Alternative is LABA with inhaled glucocorticoid, methylxanthines (theophylline).
Category D (GOLD 3–4) High risk	High-risk; refer to pulmonologist.

COPD, chronic obstructive pulmonary disease; GOLD, Global Initiative for Chronic Obstructive Lung Disease; PRN, as needed.

Source: 2017 Global Initiative for Chronic Obstructive Lung Disease (GOLD) (2017).

- Pulmonary hygiene (postural drainage, etc.) or pulmonary rehabilitation
- Treat lung infections aggressively

Management of Stable COPD

Once COPD has been diagnosed, effective management should be based on an individualized assessment of current symptoms and future risks.

- Reduce symptoms
- Relieve symptoms:
  - Improve exercise tolerance
  - Improve health status *and* prevent disease progression, prevent and treat exacerbations, and reduce mortality

Nonpharmacological Treatment

Nonpharmacological management of COPD should be in accordance with the individualized assessment of symptoms and exacerbation risk:

- Smoking cessation (can include pharmacological treatment)
- Physical activity
- Influenza vaccination
- Pneumococcal vaccination
- Pulmonary rehabilitation

Pharmacological Treatment

Treatment Tips

- For all COPD patients (or category A patients), prescribe a SABA to be used "as needed" for dypsnea; it can be used alone or combined with a short-acting anticholinergic or a LAMA
- If patient has poor symptom relief and is at low risk of exacerbation (category B), regular use of a LABA (with short-acting anticholinergic, as needed) or regular use of a LAMA (with a SABA as needed) are acceptable. GOLD categories and treatment options are listed in Table 8.1 (Ferguson & Make, 2017).
- Bronchodilators:
  - Short-acting beta-agonists (SABA): Albuterol, levalbuterol (use PRN as rescue drug)
  - Long-acting beta-agonists (LABA): Salmeterol, formoterol, vilanterol
  - Short-acting anticholinergics: Ipratropium (Atrovent)
  - Long-acting anticholinergics/long-acting muscarinic agent (LAMA): Tiotropium (Spiriva), umeclidinium powder (Ellipta) long-acting formulations are preferred over short-acting formulations
  - Combined use of SABAs or LABAs and short-acting anticholinergics or LAMAs may be considered if symptoms are not improved with single agents
  - Inhaled bronchodilators are preferred over oral bronchodilators
  - Treatment with theophylline is not recommended
- Corticosteroids and phosphodiesterase-4 inhibitors
  - Long-term therapy with ICS plus LABA is recommended for patients with severe airflow limitation (GOLD 3–4 category) with frequent exacerbations; refer to specialist
  - Long-term monotherapy with oral corticosteroids is not recommended
  - The phosphodiesterase-4 inhibitor roflumilast (Daliresp) is used for severe COPD. This may increase the risk of suicide. Could be multiple serious drug interactions (dexamethasone, carbamazepine, rifampin, St. John's wort, others).

Management of Exacerbations

- Patients with characteristics of a moderate to severe exacerbation should be hospitalized, as they are at higher risk of death.
- An exacerbation of COPD is defined as an acute event characterized by a worsening of the patient's respiratory symptoms that is beyond normal day-to-day variations and leads to a change in medication.
- The most common cause appears to be respiratory tract infections (viral or bacterial).
- Chest radiographs are useful in excluding alternative diagnoses.
- An EKG may aid in the diagnosis of coexisting cardiac problems.
- Spirometry tests are not recommended during an exacerbation because they can be difficult to perform and measurements are not accurate enough.
- At higher risk for *Haemophilus influenzae* pneumonia, suspect secondary bacterial infection if acute onset of fever, purulent sputum, increased wheezing, and dyspnea.
- *Treatment options:* Bactrim DS, doxycycline, or Ceftin BID for 10 days; for severe infection, Augmentin or respiratory quinolones (Avelox, Levaquin) for 3 to 7 days; Medrol Dose Pack PRN.
- Health care providers should strongly enforce stringent measures against active cigarette smoking. Patients hospitalized because of exacerbations of COPD are at increased risk for deep vein thrombosis and PE; thromboprophylactic measures should be enhanced.

Referral

- Moderate to severe COPD
- Severe exacerbations or rapid progression
- Age younger than 40
- Weight loss

EXAM TIPS

- First-line treatment for mild COPD (2017 guidelines) is either a SABA or a short-acting anticholinergic. If poor relief on single agent, add a second agent. If on SABA, add short-acting anticholinergic (Atrovent).
- If short-acting meds are not controlling symptoms, next step is to start patient on a LABA (or a LAMA). Continue using short-acting SABA as needed. See Table 8.1 for more details.
- If poor control, switch to an LABA (salmeterol, formoterol) or long-acting anticholinergic/long-acting muscarinic (tiotropium).
- Ipratropium (Atrovent) is a short-acting anticholinergic.
- Salmeterol and formoterol are LABAs.
- Do not use LABAs (salmeterol, formoterol) for rescue treatment.
- The only drugs for rescue treatment are in the SABA class.

CLINICAL PEARLS

- Long-term use of oral corticosteroids increases the risk of pneumonia.
- When you are treating a COPD patient, pick an antibiotic that has coverage against *Streptococcus pneumoniae* and *H. influenzae* (gram negative).

COMMON LUNG INFECTIONS (TABLE 8.2)

Community-Acquired Bacterial Pneumonia (CAP)

Bacterial lung infection results in inflammatory changes and damage to the lungs. The bacterium causing the most deaths in outpatients is *Streptococcus pneumoniae* (gram positive).

Table 8.2 Common Lung Infections

Disease	Signs and Symptoms
Acute bacterial pneumonia (CAP)	Acute onset. High fever and chills. Productive cough and large amount of green to rust-colored sputum. Pleuritic chest pain with cough.
No.1 *Streptococcus pneumoniae* (gram positive)	Crackles; decreased breath sounds, dull CBC: Leukocytosis; elevated neutrophils. Band forms may be seen.
Atypical pneumonia No.1 *Mycoplasma pneumoniae*	CXR reveals lobar infiltrates. Gradual onset. Low-grade fever. Headache, sore throat. Cough. Wheezing. Sometimes, rash. CXR: Interstitial to patchy infiltrates.
Viral pneumonia Influenza, RSV	Fever. Cough. Pleurisy. Shortness of breath. Scanty sputum production. Myalgias. Breath sounds: Decreased breath sounds, rales.
Acute bronchitis	Paroxysms of dry and severe cough that interrupts sleep. Cough dry to productive. Light-colored sputum. Can last up to 4–6 weeks. No antibiotics. Treat symptoms.

CAP, community-acquired pneumonia; CBC, complete blood count; CXR, chest x-ray; RSV, respiratory syncytial virus.

Organisms

- The most common pathogens are *S. pneumoniae* or pneumococcus (gram positive), atypical bacteria (*Mycoplasma pneumoniae*), and respiratory viruses (e.g., influenza, parainfluenza, respiratory syncytial virus)
- *Haemophilus influenzae*: More common in smokers, COPD (gram negative)
- Cystic fibrosis (CF): Number one bacteria is *Pseudomonas aeruginosa* (gram negative)

Classic Case

An older adult presents with sudden onset of a high fever (>100.4°F) with chills that is accompanied by a productive cough with purulent sputum (rust-colored sputum seen with streptococcal pneumonia). The patient complains of pleuritic chest pain with coughing and dyspnea.

Elderly patients may have atypical symptoms (afebrile or low-grade fever, no cough or mild cough, weakness, confusion, etc.).

Objective Findings

- *Auscultation:* Rhonchi, crackles, and wheezing
- *Percussion:* Dullness over affected lobe
- Tactile fremitus and egophony: Increased
- Abnormal whispered pectoriloquy (whispered words louder)

Labs

- CXR is the gold standard (definitive test) for diagnosing CAP, not sputum culture; repeat within 6 weeks to document clearing
- CXR result shows lobar consolidation in classic bacterial pneumonia
- Order a posttreatment CXR to ensure clearing of infection

- Order CBC: Leukocytosis (>10.5 ×10^9/L) with a possible "shift to the left" (increased band forms)
- Routine diagnostic tests (sputum culture and sensitivity [C&S]) to identify etiologic diagnosis are an option for outpatients with CAP

Treatment Plan

Infectious Diseases Society of America and American Thoracic Society Guidelines for Outpatient CAP*

No comorbidity (previously healthy and no risk factors for drug-resistant *S. pneumoniae* infection):

- Macrolides are preferred.
  - Azithromycin (Z-Pack) daily × 5 days
  - Clarithromycin (Biaxin) BID × 7 days
- If patient had an antibiotic in previous 3 months or macrolide-resistance (>25%):
  - Doxycycline 100 mg BID × 5 to 7 days
  - Levofloxacin (Levaquin) 750 mg × 5 days
  - Azithromycin or clarithromycin plus amoxicillin or Augmentin

With comorbidity (i.e., alcoholism; congestive heart failure [CHF]; chronic heart, lung, liver or kidney disease; antibiotics in previous 3 months; diabetes; splenectomy/asplenia; others) or high rates (>25%) of macrolide-resistant *S. pneumoniae*:

- Respiratory fluoroquinolone as *one*-drug therapy (duration 5–7 days)
  - Moxifloxacin (Avelox) 400 mg PO once a day
  - Levofloxacin (Levaquin) 750 mg daily (minimum dose 750 mg/d)
  - Gemifloxacin (Factive) 400 mg PO once a day *or*
- Beta-lactam plus macrolide (duration 7 days)
  - Amoxicillin clavulanate (Augmentin) 1,000/62.5 mg PO BID × 7 days *or*
  - Cefdinir (Omnicef) 300 mg PO every 12 hours × 7 days plus azithromycin or clarithromycin
- *Poor prognosis* (refer for hospitalization):
  - Elderly: Age 60 years or older, acute mental status changes, CHF
  - Multiple lobar involvement
  - Acute mental status change
  - Alcoholics (aspiration pneumonia)
  - Patient meets the "CURB-65" criterion for hospital admission. "CURB-65" is a tool to assess whether a patient needs hospitalization (each factor is worth 1 point). If score >1, patient should be hospitalized (Lim, et al., 2003).
    C (*c*onfusion)
    U (blood *u*rea nitrogen >19.6 mg/dL)
    R (*r*espiration >30 breaths/min)
    B (*b*lood pressure <90/60 mmHg)
  - 65 years of age or older

Prevention

- Influenza vaccine for all persons older than 50 years or if contact with persons who are at higher risk for death from pneumonia, health care workers, others
- Pneumococcal polysaccharide vaccine (Pneumovax) if older than 65 years or with high-risk condition

---

*Adapted from Mandell et al. (2007).

Pneumococcal Vaccine (Adults)

- PCV13 (pneumococcal conjugate vaccine: Prevnar 13)
- PPSV23 (pneumococcal polysaccharide vaccine: Pneumovax 23, Pnu-Imune 23)

Recommended Pneumococcal Vaccines for All Adults 65 Years or Older

- Dose of PCV13 first, followed by a dose of PPSV23, at least 1 year later.
- For patients having received any doses of PPSV23, the dose of PCV13 should be given at least 1 year after receipt of the most recent PPSV23 dose.
- For patients having received a dose of PCV13 at a younger age, another dose of PCV13 is not recommended. But with PPSV23, another dose is recommended within 5 years (do not confuse them with each other).

Healthy Patients

- Single dosages usually sufficient at age 65 years (lifetime)
- 60% to 70% effective

Underlying Disease

- 50% effective

Severely Immunocompromised

- Only 10% effective

Recommended for:

- Persons aged 65 years or older
- Impaired immunity
  - Splenectomy, asplenia, or diseased spleen
  - Alcoholics/cirrhosis of the liver
  - HIV infection
  - Chronic renal failure
- Preexisting heart and lung disease
  - Asthma, congenital heart disease, emphysema, others
- Blood disorders
  - Sickle cell anemia
  - Hodgkin's lymphoma, multiple myeloma

High-Risk Patients

- Repeat vaccine in 5 to 7 years (boosts antibodies):
  - If first dose was given before age of 65 years
  - Asplenia, chronic renal failure (give at 19 years of age if asplenia, chronic renal disease)
  - Immunocompromised states
  - Blood cancers: Lymphoma, Hodgkin's disease, leukemia

Atypical Pneumonia

An infection of the lungs by atypical bacteria. More common in children and young adults. Seasonal outbreaks (summer/fall). Highly contagious. Also known as *walking pneumonia*.

Organisms

- *Mycoplasma pneumoniae* (atypical bacteria)
- *Chlamydia pneumoniae* (atypical bacteria)
- *Legionella pneumoniae* (atypical bacteria): Found in areas with moisture such as air conditioners (hospitalize, more severe with higher mortality)

Classic Case

A young adult complains of several weeks of fatigue that is accompanied by severe paroxysmal coughing that is mostly nonproductive. Gradual onset of symptoms. Illness may have started with cold-like symptoms (sore throat, clear rhinitis, and low-grade fever). Patient continues to go to work/school despite symptoms; may have coworkers with same symptoms.

Objective Findings

- *Auscultation:* Wheezing and diffused crackles/rales
- *Nose:* Clear mucus (may have rhinitis of clear mucus)
- *Throat:* Erythematous without pus or exudate
- *CXR:* Diffuse interstitial infiltrates (up to 20% have pleural effusion)
- *CBC:* May have normal results

Medications

- Macrolides:
  - Doxycycline 100 mg BID × 7 to 10 days
  - Alternatives:
    - Azithromycin (Z-Pack) × 5 days
    - Levofloxacin (Levaquin) 750 mg × 5 days
- Antitussives (dextromethorphan, Tessalon Perles) PRN
- Increase fluids and rest

Acute Bronchitis

Acute viral (sometimes bacterial) infection of the bronchi causes inflammatory changes in the trachea, bronchi, and bronchioles, which results in increased reactivity of the upper airways. Usually self-limited. Also known as *tracheobronchitis*. Caused by adenovirus, influenza (winter/spring), coronavirus, respiratory syncytial virus, others.

Classic Case

A young adult complains of the sudden new onset of a cough that is keeping him awake at night. Cough is mainly dry, but it may become productive later with small amounts of sputum. The patient may have frequent paroxysms of coughing; may have low-grade fever, mild wheezing, and/or chest pain with cough.

Objective Findings

- *Lungs:* Ranges from clear to severe wheezing (prolonged expiratory phase), rhonchi
- *Percussion:* Resonant
- *CXR:* Normal
- Afebrile to low-grade fever

Treatment Plan

- Treatment is symptomatic. Increase fluids and rest; stop smoking (if smoker)
- Administer dextromethorphan BID to QID, Tessalon Perles (benzonatate) TID PRN (antitussives)
- Administer guaifenesin PRN (expectorant/mucolytic)
- For wheezing, use albuterol inhaler (Ventolin) QID or nebulized treatment PRN
- For severe wheezing, consider short-term oral steroid (Medrol Dose Pack)

Complications

- Exacerbation of asthma (increased risk of status asthmaticus)
- Pneumonia from secondary bacterial infection (pneumococcus, mycoplasma, others)

Pertussis

Also known as *whooping cough*. Caused by *Bordetella pertussis* bacteria (gram negative). A coughing illness of at least 14 days' duration with one of the following findings: paroxysmal coughing, inspiratory whooping (or posttussive vomiting) without apparent cause. Illness can last from a few weeks to months. Unvaccinated children and adults with expired vaccinations are risk factors for pertusssis. Pertussis has three stages (catarrhal, paroxysmal, and convalescent). Most infectious period is early in the disease (catarrhal stage) up to 21 days of cough (if not treated with appropriate antibiotic).

Classic Case

Suspect pertussis in previously "healthy" patient with a severe hacking cough of greater than 2 weeks' duration. Initial symptoms are low-grade fever and rhinorrhea with a mild cough (catarrhal stage). Cough becomes severe with inspiratory "whooping" sound. The patient may vomit afterward (paroxysmal stage). Cough becomes less severe and less frequent and finally resolves (convalescent stage).

Labs

- Nasopharyngeal swab for culture and polymerase chain reaction (PCR)
- Pertussis antibodies by enzyme-linked immunosorbent assay (ELISA)
- *CBC:* Elevated white blood cells (WBCs) and marked lymphocytosis (up to 80% lymphocytes in WBC differential); CXR should be negative; if positive, due to secondary bacterial infection

Treatment Plan (Adolescents to Adults)

- First line: Macrolides
  - Azithromycin (Z-Pack) 500 mg on day 1, then 250 mg daily from days 2 to 5
  - Erythromycin 500 mg QID × 14 days
  - *Alternative:* Clarithromycin (Biaxin) BID × 7 days
- Chemoprophylaxis for close contacts; respiratory droplet precautions needed
- Antitussives, mucolytics, rest, and hydration; frequent small meals

Tdap Booster

- Aged 11 to 18 years (and 18 years to adulthood): Centers for Disease Control and Prevention (CDC) recommends using Tdap (instead of Td).

Complications

- Sinusitis, otitis media, pneumonia, fainting, rib fractures, and others

EXAM TIPS

- **Recognize presentation of bacterial pneumonia versus atypical pneumonia.**
- **The top two bacteria in CAP are:**
  - ***S. pneumoniae***
  - ***H. influenzae***
- **The top two bacteria in atypical pneumonia are:**
  - ***Mycoplasma pneumoniae***
  - ***Chlamydia pneumoniae***
- **Phlegm is rust-colored or blood-tinged.**
- **COPD/smoker with pneumonia: More likely to have *H. influenzae* bacteria.**
- **Know presentation and treatment of pertussis (whooping cough).**
- **Symptomatic treatment for acute bronchitis. Do not pick antibiotics as a treatment option for acute bronchitis.**
- **Outpatient CAP: Diagnosis is based on presentation, signs and symptoms, and CXR. Do not order phlegm for C&S; instead, order CXR. CBC is not required for diagnosis.**

CLINICAL PEARLS

- **Depending on the stage of the disease and hydration status, the CXR result may be "normal" during the early phase of bacterial pneumonia (lobar pneumonia).**
- **Suspect pertussis in a "healthy" adult with no fever who has been coughing for more than 2 to 3 weeks, especially if previously treated with an antibiotic (that was not a macrolide) and is getting worse (rule out pneumonia first).**
- **Emphasize importance of adequate fluid intake (best mucolytic, thins out mucus).**
- **Lung cancer can present as recurrent pneumonia (due to mass blocking bronchioles).**
- **If *S. pneumoniae* macrolide resistance greater than 25%, do not use macrolide monotherapy. See CAP treatment guidelines notes.**

Common Cold (Viral Upper Respiratory Infection)

Self-limiting infection (range of 4–10 days). Most contagious from days 2 to 3. More common in crowded areas and in small children. Transmission is by respiratory droplets and fomites. Highly contagious. Most cases occur in the winter months.

Classic Case

A patient has acute onset of fever, sore throat, frequent sneezing in early phase accompanied by nasal congestion, runny eyes, and rhinorrhea of clear mucus (coryza). The patient may complain of headache.

Objective Findings

- *Nasal turbinates:* Swollen with clear mucus (may also have blocked tympanic membrane)
- Anterior pharynx: Reddened
- *Cervical nodes:* Smooth, mobile, and small or "shotty" nodes (0.5 cm size or less) in the submandibular and anterior cervical chain
- *Lungs:* Clear

Treatment Plan

- Treat symptoms; increase fluids and rest; wash hands frequently
- Analgesics (acetaminophen) or nonsteroidal anti-inflammatory drugs (NSAIDs) (ibuprofen) for fever and aches PRN
- Oral decongestants (i.e., pseudoephedrine/Sudafed) PRN
- Topical nasal decongestants (i.e., Afrin) can be used BID up to 3 days PRN only; do not use for more than 3 days due to risk of rebound nasal congestion (rhinitis medicamentosa)
- Antitussives (i.e., dextromethorphan/Robitussin) PRN
- Antihistamines (i.e., diphenhydramine/Benadryl) for nasal congestion PRN

Complications

- Acute sinusitis
- Acute otitis media

Tuberculosis (TB)

An infection caused by *Mycobacterium tuberculosis* bacteria. Most common site of infection is the lungs (85%). Other sites include the kidneys, brain, lymph nodes, adrenals, and bone.

Most contagious forms are pulmonary TB, pleural TB, and laryngeal TB (coughing spreads aerosol droplets). CXR (reactivated TB) will show cavitations and adenopathy and granulomas on the hila of the lungs.

High-Risk Populations

Immigrants (from high-prevalence countries), migrant farm workers, illegal drug users, homeless, inmates of jails, nursing home and adult living facility residents, HIV-infected, immunocompromised

Latent TB Infection (LTBI)

An intact immune system causes macrophages to sequester the bacteria in the lymph nodes (mediastinum) in the form of granulomas. Not infectious.

Prior Bacillus Calmette-Guerin (BCG) Vaccine*

- May cause false-positive reaction to TB skin test
- TB blood tests are preferred method of TB testing for people who received the BCG vaccine
- TB blood tests: Use QuantiFERON-TB Gold in-tube test (QFT-GIT), T-Spot TB test

Miliary TB

Also known as *disseminated TB disease.* Infects multiple organ systems. More common in younger children (<5 years) and the elderly. CXR will show classic "milia seed" pattern.

Multidrug-Resistant TB (or Extensively Drug-Resistant TB)

Bacteria resistant to at least two of the best anti-TB drugs, isoniazid (INH) and rifampin (these drugs are considered first-line drugs).

Reactivated TB Infection or Active TB Disease (Infectious)

Latent bacteria become reactivated due to depressed immune system. Most TB cases (90%) of active disease in the United States are reactivated infections.

Classic Case

An adult patient (from high-risk population) complains of fever, anorexia, fatigue, and night sweats along with a mild nonproductive cough (early phase). Aggressive infections (later sign) will have productive cough with blood-stained sputum (hemoptysis) along with weight loss (late sign).

Treatment Plan

- Report TB to local health department for contact tracing ASAP. TB is a reportable disease.
- All active TB patients should be tested for HIV infection.
- Initial regimen for suspected TB before C&S results are available. Use four drugs: INH, rifampin, ethambutol, and pyrazinamide. Duration is 2 months of intensive treatment and 18 weeks of continuation phase treatment.
- Narrow down number of medications after C&S results reveal most effective drugs.
- Several treatment regimens are available. Check TB website (www.cdc.gov/TB).

Directly Observed Treatment (DOT)

Mandatory for noncompliant patients. Success is dependent on medication compliance.

- *How:* Patient is observed by a nurse when he or she takes the medications. Mouth, cheek, and area under the tongue are checked to make sure the pill was swallowed adequately.

Warning

Ethambutol causes optic neuritis. Avoid if patient has abnormal vision (i.e., blindness, retinal vein occlusion, and so forth).

---

*Adapted from Centers for Disease Control and Prevention (2017).

Recent Mantoux Test (PPD) Converters and Chemoprophylaxis for Latent TB infection (LTBI)

Recent PPD converter is defined as a person with history of negative PPD results who then converts to a positive PPD. Higher risk of active TB disease (up to 10%) within first 1 to 2 years after seroconversion.

- Assess for signs and symptoms of TB (cough, night sweats, weight loss)
- Order CXR (make sure has no upper lobe cavitations and mediastinal adenopathy)
- HIV-negative: Prescribe INH 300 mg/d for 9 months
- HIV-positive: Prescribe INH 300 mg/d for at least 12 months
- Check baseline liver function tests and monitor

Generally, preventive treatment for LTBI is encouraged for those younger than 35 years of age. After age of 35 years, much higher risk of liver damage from INH chemoprophylaxis. Assess risk versus benefits and discuss with the patient.

TB Skin Test (Mantoux Test) (Table 8.3)

Look for an induration (feels harder). The red color is not as important. If a PPD result is a bright-red color but is not indurated (skin feels soft), it is a negative result.

- Induration of 5 mm or greater:
  - HIV (+)
  - Recent contact with infectious TB cases
  - CXR with fibrotic changes consistent with previous TB disease
  - Any child who had close contact with an infected person or TB symptoms (before age of 5 years)
  - Immunocompromised (i.e., organ transplant, bone marrow transplant, renal failure, patients on biologic drugs, others)
- Induration of 10 mm or greater:
  - Recent immigrants (within the past 5 years) from high-prevalence countries (Latin America, Asia, Africa, India, Pacific islands)
  - Child younger than 4 years of age or children/adolescents exposed to high-risk adult
  - Intravenous drug user, health care worker, homeless
  - Employees or residents from high-risk congregate settings (jails, nursing homes)
- Induration of 15 mm or greater:
  - Persons with no known risk factors for TB

Labs

TB Skin Test (TST)

- *Mantoux test/TST:* Inject 0.1 mL of 5TU-PPD subdermally. Do not use the tine test (has not been used for many years).

Blood Tests for TB

- *QuantiFERON-TB Gold in-tube test or the T-SPOT TB test* (also known as *interferon-gamma release assays [IGRAs]*): Blood tests that measure gamma-interferon (from lymphocytes).
- *IGRA test results:* Available within 24 hours (only one visit required). If history of previous BCG vaccination, IGRA blood tests preferred.

Sputum Tests for TB

- Early morning deep cough specimen; collect for 3 consecutive days
- Sputum nucleic acid amplification test (NAAT) is a rapid test (1–3 days)

Table 8.3 TB Skin Test Results (Mantoux or the PPD)

Size	Test Results
≥5mm	HIV (+)
	Recent contact with infectious TB cases
	CXR with fibrotic changes consistent with previous TB disease
	Any child who had close contact or has TB symptoms (before age of 5 years)
	Immunocompromised (i.e., organ transplant, bone marrow transplant, renal failure, patients on biologic drugs, others)
≥10mm	Recent immigrants (within past 5 years) from high-prevalence countries (Latin America, Asia, Africa, India, Pacific islands)
	Child younger than 4 years of age or children/adolescents exposed to high-risk adult Intravenous drug user, health care worker, homeless
	Employees or residents from high-risk congregate settings (jails, nursing homes)
≥15mm	Persons with no risk factors for TB

CXR, chest x-ray; PPD, purified protein derivative; TB, tuberculosis.

- Sputum for C&S is gold standard for diagnosing pulmonary TB infection; can take <8 weeks to grow
- Acid fast bacilli (AFB) smear: Positive AFB is not diagnostic, but it is suggestive of TB infection
- Order sputum for NAAT, C&S, and AFB smear if suspect active TB infection

Booster Phenomenon (LTBI)

A person with LTBI can have a false negative reaction to the tuberculin skin test (TST) or the PPD if they have not been tested for many years.

- Two-step tuberculin skin testing is recommended by the CDC.

Explanation

- When the TST/PPD is done the first time, there is no reaction (false negative). The first TB skin test "jogs the memory" of the immune system.
- If PPD repeated (1–3 weeks later), a positive reaction (boosted reaction) means that the patient has latent TB infection.
- Follow up with chest x-ray and inquire about signs/symptoms of TB infection. Offer LTBI prophylaxis.
- If the second PPD is negative, it means the person probably does not have a TB infection (CDC, 2014).

EXAM TIPS

- **A PPD result may be listed as 9.5 mm. If the patient falls under the 10-mm group, then it is negative (by definition) unless the patient has the signs/symptoms and/or CXR findings suggestive of TB.**
- **Memorize the criteria for the 5-mm and 10-mm results.**
- **You may be asked to identify a photograph of a CXR (radiography) of a patient with pulmonary TB or bacterial pneumonia (usually right middle-lobe pneumonia). An example of a TB chest film photograph appears in Figure 8.1 at the end of this chapter.**

- **Memorize the appearance of a posterior–anterior CXR of a person with healed pulmonary TB. The classic findings are pulmonary nodules and/or cavitations (round black holes) on the upper lobes with or without fibrotic changes (scars).**
- **With right middle-lobe pneumonia, look for consolidation (white-colored area) on the right middle lobe, which is located at about the same level as the right breast on the front of the chest.**

CLINICAL PEARLS

- **The QuantiFERON-TB Gold in-tube and the T-SPOT TB tests are available at public health clinics.**
- **They only require one visit for the patient to be tested (one vial of blood).**
- **Never treat TB with fewer than three drugs.**
- **According to the CDC, on the average, about 10 contacts are listed for each index person with infectious TB.**
- **Persons with HIV infection with CD4 fewer than 500 or patients who are taking tumor necrosis factor antagonists (or biologics) are at very high risk for active TB disease after initial exposure (primary TB).**
- **The tuberculin skin test is considered both valid and safe to use throughout pregnancy.**
- **Younger children are more likely than older children to develop life-threatening forms of TB disease.**

Asthma

Reversible airway obstruction caused by chronic inflammation of the bronchial tree. Results in increased airway responsiveness to stimuli (internal or external). Genetic predisposition with positive family history of allergies, eczema, and allergic rhinitis (atopy or atopic history). Exacerbations can be life-threatening (status asthmaticus). Rule out allergic asthma (refer allergy testing), gastroesophageal reflux disease (GERD), rhinitis, sinusitis, stress.

Treatment Goals (All Asthmatics)

- Can perform usual "normal" activities with no limitations (can attend school full time, play "normally," go to work full time, no job absence due to asthmatic symptoms)
- Minimal to no exacerbations (daytime and nighttime)
- Minimal use of rescue medicine (<2 days a week albuterol use)
- Avoid emergency department (ED) visits/hospitalization
- Maintain near normal pulmonary function (reduce permanent lung damage)

Classic Case

A young-adult patient with asthma complains of worsening symptoms after a recent bout of a viral upper respiratory infection (URI). The patient is using her albuterol inhaler more than normal (about three times/day or more) to treat the symptoms; complains of shortness of breath, wheezing, and chest tightness that is sometimes accompanied by a dry cough in the night and early morning (e.g., 3 a.m.) that awakens her from sleep.

Objective Findings

- *Lungs:* Wheezing with prolonged expiratory phase. As asthma worsens, the wheezing occurs during both inspiration and expiration. With severe bronchoconstriction, breath sounds are faint or inaudible.
- *Cardiovascular:* Tachycardia, rapid pulse, is seen.

Trigger Factors for Asthma

- Viral URIs, airborne allergens
- Airborne allergens: Dust mites, mold, cockroaches
- Food allergies: Sulfites, red and yellow dye, seafood
- Cold air or cold weather and fumes from chemicals or smoke
- Emotional stress and exercise (exercise-induced asthma)
- GERD (reflux of acidic gastric contents irritates airways)
- Acetylsalicylic acid (ASA) or NSAIDs (patients with nasal polyps are more sensitive to ASA and NSAIDs)

Treatment Plan

Nebulizer treatments: Give up to three treatments every 20 minutes as needed. Short course of oral corticosteroids may be needed for exacerbations. If low-dose ICSs, add LABAs (or increase dose to medium-dose ICSs only).

Asthma Medications

"Rescue" Medicine

Only one drug class used for rescue: SABAs

- SABAs in metered-dose inhalers (MDI) or by nebulizer
  - Albuterol (Ventolin HFA) or pirbuterol (Maxair) two inhalations every 4 to 6 hours PRN
  - Levalbuterol (Xopenex HFA): Two inhalations every 4 to 6 hours PRN; less likely to cause cardiac stimulation (fewer palpitations, less tachycardia)
- Quick onset (15–30 min) and lasts about 4 to 6 hours
  - Used for quick relief (of wheezing) but does not treat underlying inflammation
  - With nebulizer, give up to three treatments every 20 minutes as needed; short course of oral corticosteroids may be needed for exacerbations (Medrol Dose Pack)

Long-Term Control Medications for Asthma (Table 8.4)

- ICSs alone or with LABAs must be taken every day to be effective.
- LABAs are *not* rescue drugs. Must be taken BID.
- LABAs (used alone) increase the risk of death from asthma. Combination of LABA and ICS is safer.
  - Example: Fluticasone with salmeterol (Advair), budesonide with formoterol (Symbicort)

Sustained-Release Theophylline (Theo-24)

- *Drug class:* Methylxanthine. Used as an adjunct drug. Acts as a bronchodilator.
- Monitor levels to reduce risk of toxicity. The drug has multiple drug interactions such as the following:
  - Macrolides, quinolones
  - Cimetidine
  - Anticonvulsants such as phenytoin, carbamazepine (Tigerton)
  - Check blood levels: Normal is 12 to 15 mg/dL

Spacers or Chambers

Use of a "spacer" or "chamber" (AeroChamber) is encouraged. It will increase delivery of the aerosolized drug to the lungs and minimize oral thrush (for inhaled steroids).

Table 8.4 Asthma: Long-Term Control Medications

Drug Class	Brand Name	Side Effects/Adverse Effects
Inhaled corticosteroids	Triamcinolone (Azmacort) BID Budesonide (Pulmicort) BID	Oral thrush (gargle or drink water after use); HPA axis suppression, glaucoma, others
	Fluticasone (Flovent) BID	
LABA	Salmeterol (Serevent) BID Formoterol (Foradil) BID	Warn patients of increased risk of asthma deaths; not to be used as rescue drug
Combination of LABA with corticosteroid	Salmeterol + fluticasone (Advair) BID Budesonide with formoterol (Symbicort)	LABA combined with corticosteroid safer
Leukotriene inhibitors	Montelukast (Singular) daily Zafirlukast (Accolate) BID	Neuropsychological effects (agitation, aggression, depression, others)
	Zileuton (Silo) daily	Monitor liver function tests (zileuton)
Mast cell stabilizers (Cromoglycates)	Cromolyn sodium (Intal) QID Nedocromil sodium (Tilade) QID	Cromolyn (Intal) and nedocromil (Tilade) inhalers have both been discontinued in the United States; cromolyn for nebulization still available
Methylxanthines	Theophylline (not used often) daily	Sympathomimetic. Avoid with seizures, hypertension, stroke
	Starting dose 300 mg/day BID	Several drug interactions
Anti-immunoglobulin E antibodies (IgE)	Omalizumab (Xolair)	Anaphylaxis can occur with first dose or after long-term use. Be equipped and prepared to treat anaphylaxis when starting this drug

BID, twice a day; HPA, hypothalamic-pituitary-adrenal; LABA, long-acting beta-antagonist; LFT, liver function test; QID, four times a day.

*Asthma Classification, Stepwise Approach, and Treatment Guidelines (12 Years or Older)**

Step 1

- Intermittent asthma (FEV1 >80% predicted)
  - Daytime symptoms less than 2 days/week; nighttime awakenings less than two per month
  - SABA: Albuterol (Ventolin) metered-dose inhaler as needed

Step 2

- Mild persistent asthma (FEV1 >80% predicted). Daytime symptoms more than 2 days/week but not daily. Nighttime awakenings three to four per month.
  - Albuterol (Ventolin) metered-dose inhaler as needed
- Plus
  - Preferred treatment: Low-dose ICS
  - Alternative: Cromolyn/nedocromil, leukotriene receptor antagonist, or theophylline

Step 3

- Moderate persistent asthma (FEV1 60%–80% of predicted daily symptoms): Nighttime awakenings more than one per week (but not nightly)
  - Albuterol metered dose inhaler as needed

*National Heart, Lung, and Blood Institute, National Asthma Education and Prevention Program, Expert Panel Report 3: Guidelines for the Diagnosis and Management of Asthma, Full Report 2007).

- Plus
  - Preferred treatment: Low-dose ICS plus LABA or medium-dose ICS
  - Example: Fluticasone with salmeterol (Advair) or budesonide with formoterol (Symbicort) *or* medium-dose ICS alone (budesonide [Pulmicort], fluticasone [Flovent])

Step 4

- Severe persistent asthma (FEV1 <60% predicted): Symptoms of asthma throughout the day; nocturnal awakenings nightly
- Albuterol metered dose inhaler as needed
- Plus
  - Preferred treatment: Medium-dose ICS plus LABA
  - Example: Fluticasone with salmeterol (Advair), budesonide with formoterol (Symbicort)
- For steps 3 to 4, alternative treatment is medium-dose ICS plus LTRA (montelukast, zafirlukast), theophylline, or zileuton
  Note: Steps 5 and 6 are not discussed (not needed for exam)

Lab Monitoring

- Theophylline requires serum concentration monitoring
- Zileuton (Zyflo); must monitor liver function

Patient Education

- Review inhaler technique (use spacer if patient has problems)
- Teach about rescue medications and long-term controller medications
- Develop a written asthma action plan; partner with patient and family
- Control and limit exposure to allergens if allergic asthma; consider immunotherapy with allergist
- Teach how to use spirometer; recognize worsening

Exercise-Induced Asthma (Exercise-Induced Bronchospasm)

Premedicate 10 to 15 minutes before the activity with two puffs of a SABA (albuterol/Ventolin, levalbuterol/Xopenex, pirbuterol/Maxair). Effect will last up to 4 hours.

SUMMARY: ASTHMA TREATMENT

- Every asthma patient should be on an SABA (albuterol) PRN.
- Next step is ICS (preferred drug). Dose depends on asthma severity.
- If ICS is not enough, add an LABA (use combination medications Advair, Symbicort) *or* increased ICS dose (low to medium dose).
- *Alternatives:* Use leukotriene inhibitors, sustained-release theophylline, or mast cell stabilizer.

Asthmatic Exacerbation

- Respiratory distress: Tachypnea, using accessory muscles (intercostals, abdominal) to breathe, talks in brief/fragmented sentences, severe diaphoresis, fatigue, agitation.
- Lungs: Minimal to no breath sounds audible during lung auscultation. Peak expiratory flow (PEF) less than 40%. Lips/skin blue-tinged (cyanosis). Check O_2 saturation. Use supplemental oxygen.
- Give nebulizer treatment: Albuterol or levalbuterol/saline solution by nebulizer. May repeat every 20 minutes (for three doses). If unable to use inhaled bronchodilators, give epinephrine IM.

- After nebulizer treatment(s):
  - Listen for breath sounds. If inspiratory and expiratory wheezing is present, this is a good sign (signals opening up of airways). If there is a lack of breath sounds or wheezing after a nebulizer treatment, this is a bad sign (patient is not responding). Call 911.
- Discharge:
  - For moderate to severe exacerbations: Medrol Dose Pack or prednisone tabs 40 mg/day × 4 days (no weaning necessary if 4 days or less and not steroid dependent). Continue medications and increase dose (or add another controller drug).
- Refer to ED (call 911):
  - If poor to no response to nebulizer treatment (PEF <40% of expected), call 911.
  - If no response to nebulizer treatment, impending respiratory arrest: Give Epi-Pen *stat*. Call 911.

Peak Expiratory Flow Rate: PEFR or PEF

Measures effectiveness of treatment, worsening symptoms, and exacerbations. During expiration, patient is instructed to blow hard using the spirometer (three times). The highest value is recorded (personal best).

- PEF is based on height (H), age (A), and gender (G), or HAG
- Mnemonic: HAG (height, age, gender)

Spirometer Parameters

- *Green Zone:* 80% to 100% of expected volume
  - Maintain or reduce medications.
- *Yellow Zone:* 50% to 80% of expected volume
  - Maintenance therapy needs to be increased or patient is having an acute exacerbation.
- *Red Zone:* Below 50% of expected
  - If after treatment patient's PEFR is still 50% below expected value, call 911. If in respiratory distress, give epinephrine injection. Call 911.

CHEST RADIOGRAPH (CXR) INTERPRETATION

You may see one CXR film on the exam. Here are some basics. "X-rays" are radiation (gamma rays) that pass through the human body and hit a metal target (the film). Depending on the type of tissue, they are absorbed differently. Posterior–anterior (PA) view is when the x-ray goes through the back. Anterior–posterior (AP) view is when the x-ray goes through the front of the chest. Lateral view is the view from the side of the chest.

Appearance

- *Air:* Appears as black color (low density so less absorption) over lung field
- *Bones:* Appears as white
- *Metals:* Bright white (high absorption)
- *Tissue:* Different grayish shades (medium absorption)
- *Fluid:* Grayish to whitish
- *Tissues visible:* Trachea, bronchus, aorta, heart, lungs, pulmonary arteries, diaphragm, gastric bubble, ribs

Abnormal Conditions

- Emphysema: Black color in the hilum (above the clavicles), a lot of black color in hyperinflated lungs, blunted costovertebral angle (CVA; diaphragm flat instead of dome-shaped)
- Lobar pneumonia/bacterial pneumonia: Grayish to white areas on a lobe or lobes of lung (consolidation) from purulent fluid
- TB: Upper lobe with cavitation (black round holes), fibrosis (scarring), and pulmonary infiltrates (fluid) in active TB disease (Figure 8.1)
- Left ventricular hypertrophy (LVH)/cardiomyopathy: Heart occupies more than 50% of the chest diameter; it is enlarged

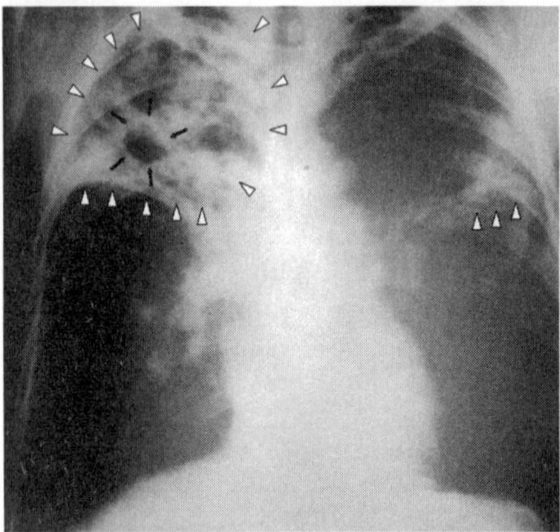

Figure 8.1 Chest radiograph: Tuberculosis.

Source: Adapted from the Centers for Disease Control and Prevention.

EXAM TIPS

- **Expect questions about asthma (diagnosis, treatment). Memorize an asthma stage because you may get "numbers" and have to figure out the asthma severity of a patient. Suggest memorizing Step 3 (i.e., FEV1 of 60%–80%, etc.).**
  - **If FEV1 is greater than 80%, it is either intermittent or mild persistent asthma. Check night awakenings. If they occur less than two times per month, it is intermittent asthma.**
  - **If patient on low-dose ICS and has poor control (Step 2), add cromolyn or leukotriene receptor antagonists (LTRAs; montelukast, zafirlukast). If Step 3, should be on low-dose ICS plus LABA (i.e., Advair).**
- **Memorize factors needed to figure out PEF (use HAG mnemonic).**
- **Do not confuse asthma "rescue" drugs with "long-term controller" drugs.**
- **Remember that all asthmatics need an SABA (i.e., albuterol).**
- **Chronic use of high-dose inhaled steroids can cause osteoporosis, growth failure in children, glaucoma, cataracts, immune suppression, hypothalamic–pituitary–adrenal suppression, and other effects.**
- **Recognize respiratory failure. Severe respiratory distress: Tachypnea, disappearance of or lack of wheezing, accessory muscle use, diaphoresis, and exhaustion.**

- During a severe asthmatic exacerbation, it is hard to hear breath sounds. After SABA treatment, expect to hear inspiratory and expiratory wheezing.
- First-line treatment for severe asthmatic exacerbation or respiratory distress is an adrenaline injection.

CLINICAL PEARLS

- If you suspect that the patient has allergic asthma, check serum immunoglobulin G allergy panels (mold allergy, grass allergy panels, others). Refer to allergist for scratch testing and treatment.
- Consider supplementing with calcium with vitamin D 1,200 mg tabs QD for menopausal women and other high-risk patients (for osteoporosis) such as males who are on medium- to high-dose inhaled steroids long term.
- Consider bone density testing (in males or females) who are on chronic steroids to rule out osteopenia or osteoporosis
- Annual eye exams if on long-term steroids since higher risk of cataracts and glaucoma.
- Exercise-induced bronchospasm is a marker for inadequate asthma control.

9

Endocrine System Review

⚠ DANGER SIGNALS

Hypoglycemia

Hypoglycemia refers to blood glucose that is less than 50 mg/dL. Complains of weakness, feels like "passing out," hand tremors, and anxiety. Difficulty concentrating. More common in people with type 1 diabetes mellitus (DM; only 5%–10% of DM is type 1, average of two episodes per week). If severe hypoglycemia is uncorrected, it will progress to coma.

Nondiabetic hypoglycemia is rare and is either reactive (diet related) or fasting (disease related). For diabetic individuals, the American Diabetes Association defines level 1 hypoglycemia (glucose alert) as fasting blood sugar (FBS) 70 mg/dl or less. Level 2 hypoglycemia is blood glucose of 54 ml/dl or less. A blood glucose of this level is sufficiently low to indicate serious, clinically important hypoglycemia. Symptoms of hypoglycemia can range from difficulty concentrating, weakness, and "hand tremors" to anxiety and irritability. Left uncorrected severe hypoglycemia can lead to coma or death.

Type 1 DM

School-aged child with recent onset of persistent thirst (polydipsia) with frequent urination (polyuria) and weight loss. Feeling of hunger even though eating increased amount of food; weight loss. May be accompanied by blurred vision (osmotic effect on the lens). Breath has a "fruity" odor. Large amount of ketones in urine. Children may present with diabetic ketoacidosis (DKA); with neurological symptoms, such as drowsiness and lethargy, which can progress to coma. May report a recent viral-like illness before the onset of symptoms. Diagnosis peaks from ages 4 to 6 years and again from ages 10 to 14 years.

Thyroid Cancer

A single thyroid nodule, usually located on the upper half of one lobe in a patient, which may be accompanied by enlarged cervical lymph node lump, swelling, or pain. May complain of hoarseness and problems with swallowing (dysphagia, dyspnea, or cough). Higher incidence in the Asian race. Radiation therapy during childhood for certain cancers (Wilms' tumor, lymphoma, neuroblastoma) and/or a low-iodine diet increases risk. Higher prevalence in women (3:1). Highest incidence from age 20 to 55 years. Positive family history of thyroid cancer. Metastasis is by lymph route.

Pheochromocytoma

A pheochromocytoma is a rare hormone-releasing adrenal tumor. It generally occurs in ages 20 to 50, but can be at any age. Random episodes of headache (can be mild to severe), diaphoresis, and tachycardia accompanied by hypertension. Episodes resolve spontaneously. In between attacks, patient's vital signs are normal. Triggers include physical exertion, anxiety, stress, surgery, anesthesia, changes in body position, or labor and delivery. Foods high in tyramine (some cheeses, beers, wines, chocolates, dried or smoked meats), as well as monoamine oxidase inhibitors (MAOIs) and stimulant drugs are other triggers.

Hyperprolactinemia

Can be a sign of a pituitary adenoma. Slow onset. Women may present with amenorrhea. Galactorrhea in both males and females. Serum prolactin is elevated. When tumor is large enough to cause a mass effect, the patient will complain of headaches and vision changes.

NORMAL FINDINGS

- The endocrine system works as a "negative feedback" system. If a low level of "active" hormone occurs, it stimulates production. Inversely, high levels of hormones stop production.
- The hypothalamus stimulates the anterior pituitary gland into producing the "stimulating hormones" (such as follicle-stimulating hormone [FSH], luteinizing hormone [LH], thyroid-stimulating hormone [TSH]).
- These "stimulating hormones" tell the target organs (ovaries, thyroid, etc.) to produce "active" hormones (estrogen, thyroid hormone, etc.).
- High levels of these "active" hormones work in reverse. The hypothalamus directs the anterior pituitary into stopping production of the stimulating hormones (TSH, LH, FSH, etc).

ENDOCRINE GLANDS (FIGURE 9.1)

These glands interact to form the hypothalamic–pituitary–adrenal (HPA) axis.

Hypothalamus

Coordinates the nervous and endocrine system by sending signals via the pituitary gland. The gland interacts to form the HPA axis. Produces neurohormones that stimulate or stop production of pituitary hormones.

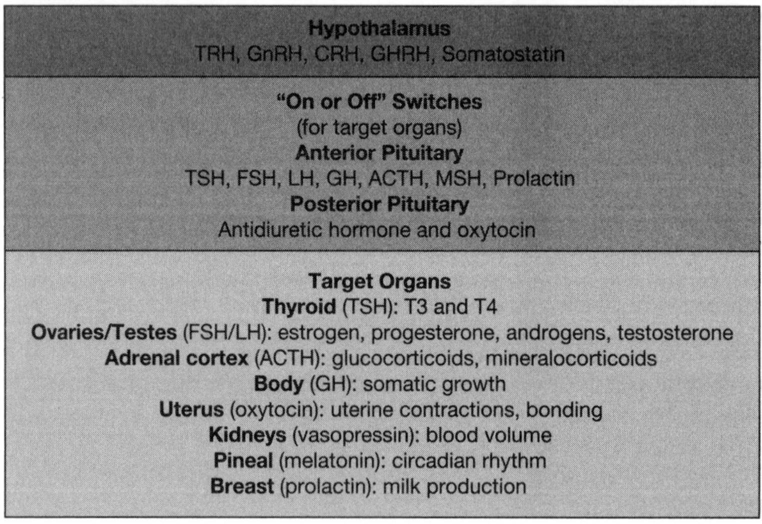

Figure 9.1 The endocrine system.

ACTH, adrenocorticotropin hormone; CRH, corticotropin-releasing hormone; FSH, follicle-stimulating hormone; GH, growth hormone; GHRH, growth hormone–releasing hormone; GnRH, gonadotropin-releasing hormone; LH, luteinizing hormone; MSH, melanocyte-stimulating hormone; TRH, thyroid-releasing hormone; TSH, thyroid-stimulating hormone.

Pituitary Gland

Located at the sella turcica (base of the brain). Stimulated by the hypothalamus into producing the "stimulating hormones" such as FSH, LH, TSH, adrenocorticotropic hormone (ACTH), and growth hormone (GH).

Anterior Pituitary Gland (Adenohypophysis)

The pituitary gland is located at the base of the brain (sella turcica). It has two lobes (anterior and posterior). It produces hormones that directly regulate the target organs (ovary, testes, thyroid, adrenals, etc.).

- FSH (follicle-stimulating hormone)
  - Stimulates the ovaries enabling growth of follicles (or eggs)
  - Production of estrogen
- LH (luteinizing hormone)
  - Stimulates the ovaries to ovulate
  - Production of progesterone (by corpus luteum)
  - In males, LH stimulates the testicles (Leydig cells) to produce testosterone
- TSH (thyroid-stimulating hormone)
  - Stimulates thyroid gland
  - Production of triiodothyronine (T3) and thyroxine (T4)
- GH (growth hormone)
  - Stimulates somatic growth of the body
- ACTH (adrenocorticotropic hormone)
  - Stimulates the adrenal glands (two portions of gland—medulla and cortex)
  - Production of glucocorticoids (cortisol) and mineralocorticoids (aldosterone)
- Prolactin
  - Affects lactation and milk production
- Melanocyte-stimulating hormone
  - Production of melatonin in response to UV light; highest levels at night between 11 p.m. and 3 a.m.

Posterior Pituitary Gland

Secretes antidiuretic hormone (vasopressin) and oxytocin, which are made by the hypothalamus but stored and secreted by the posterior pituitary.

Thyroid Gland

A butterfly-shaped organ (two lobes) located below the prominence of the thyroid cartilage (Adam's apple). It is 2 inches long, and the lobes are connected by the isthmus. Uses iodine to produce T3 and T4.

Parathyroid Glands

Located behind the thyroid glands (two glands behind each lobe). Produces parathyroid hormone (PTH), which is responsible for the calcium balance of the body by regulating the calcium loss or gain from the bones, kidneys, and GI tract (calcium absorption).

Pineal Gland

Pea-sized gland located inside the brain that produces melatonin. Melatonin regulates the sleep–wake cycle. Darkness stimulates melatonin production and light suppresses it.

DISEASE REVIEW

Primary Hyperthyroidism (Thyrotoxicosis)

The classic finding is a very low (or undetectable) TSH with elevations in both serum free T4 and T3 levels. The most common cause for hyperthyroidism (70%–80%) in the United States is a chronic autoimmune disorder called *Graves' disease*.

Graves' Disease

Graves' disease accounts for 60% to 80% of all types of hyperthyroidism. An autoimmune disorder causing hyperfunction and production of excess thyroid hormones (T3 and T4). Higher incidence in women (7:1 ratio). These women are also at higher risk for other autoimmune diseases such as rheumatoid arthritis (RA) and pernicious anemia (PA) and for osteopenia/osteoporosis due to increased metabolism.

Classic Case

Middle-aged woman loses a large amount of weight rapidly with anxiety and insomnia. Cardiac symptoms (due to overstimulation) are palpitations, hypertension, atrial fibrillation, or premature atrial contractions. Warm and moist skin with increased perspiration. May present with ophthalmopathy and lid lag (Graves' ophthalmopathy). More frequent bowel movements (looser stools). Amenorrhea and heat intolerance. Enlarged thyroid (goiter) and/or thyroid nodules present. May be accompanied by pretibial myxedema (thickening of the skin usually located in the shins giving an orange-peel appearance).

Objective Findings

- *Thyroid*: Diffusely enlarged gland (goiter), toxic adenoma, or multinodular goiter. May be tender to palpation or asymptomatic
- *Extremities:* Fine tremors on both hands, sweaty palms, pretibial myxedema
- *Eyes:* Lid lag. Exophthalmos in one or both eyes
- *Cardiac:* Tachycardia, atrial fibrillation, congestive heart failure, cardiomyopathy
- *Integumentary:* Fine hair, warm skin
- *Neurological*: Brisk deep tendon reflexes

Labs

- Look for very low TSH (<0.5 mU/L) with elevated serum free T4 and T3. If Graves' disease, will have positive thyrotropin receptor antibodies (TRAb), which is also known as the *thyroid-stimulating immunoglobulin (TSI)*. The thyroid peroxidase antibody (TPO) is positive with Graves' disease as well as in Hashimoto's disease.
- *Workup as follows:* Check TSH. If low, order thyroid panel. Look for very low TSH (<0.5 mU/L) with elevated serum free T4 and elevated T3. (In some patients with very low TSH, only either the serum T4 or the serum T3 will be elevated.) Next step is to order antibody tests to confirm whether Graves' disease is present (TRAb and TPO or TSI).
- If thyroid has a single palpable mass/nodule, order thyroid ultrasound. Refer to endocrinologist for management.
- *Imaging studies:* Thyroid ultrasound, 24-hour radioactive iodine uptake (RAIU) shows diffuse uptake (goiter). If solitary toxic nodule, shows warm or "hot" nodule or "cold" nodule. Absolute contraindications for this test are pregnancy and breastfeeding.

Medications (Thionamides)

- *Propylthiouracil (PTU):* Shrinks thyroid gland/decreases hormone production
- *Methimazole (Tapazole):* Shrinks thyroid gland/decreases hormone production
- *Side effects:* Skin rash, granulocytopenia/aplastic anemia, thrombocytopenia (check CBC with platelets), hepatic necrosis (monitor CBC, LFTs)

Adjunctive Treatment

Given before thyroid under control to alleviate the symptoms of hyperstimulation (i.e., anxiety, tachycardia, palpitations). Beta-blockers are effective (i.e., propranolol, metoprolol, atenolol).

Radioactive Iodine

Contraindicated during pregnancy or lactation. Permanent destruction of thyroid gland results in hypothyroidism for life (needs thyroid supplementation for life).

- *Pregnancy:* (hyperthyroidism): PTU is preferred treatment, if needed. High-risk pregnancy, refer to obstetrician.
- PTU is preferred treatment for moderate to severe hyperthyroidism (can cause liver failure).

Complications

Thyroid storm (thyrotoxicosis): During the thyroid storm, an individual's heart rate, blood pressure, and body temperature can soar to dangerously high levels. Acute worsening of symptoms due to stress or infection. Look for decreased level of consciousness (LOC), fever, abdominal pain. Life-threatening. Immediate hospitalization needed.

Thyroid Gland Tests

- *Thyroid gland ultrasound:* Used to detect goiter (generalized enlargement of gland), multinodular goiter, single nodule, and solid versus cystic masses
- *Fine-needle biopsy:* Used as a diagnostic test for thyroid cancer
- *Thyroid scan* (24-hour thyroid scan with RAIU): Shows metabolic activity of thyroid gland
  - *Cold spot:* Not metabolically active (more worrisome; rule out thyroid cancer); fine needle aspiration biopsy
  - *Hot spot:* Metabolically active nodule with homogeneous uptake; usually benign; helpful in diagnosing recurrent disease

Laboratory Findings of Thyroid Disease

- TSH (thyroid-stimulating hormone or thyrotropin):
  - *Normal range:* TSH of 0.5 to 5.0 mU/L (third-generation test) has normal range.
  - TSH is used for both screening and monitoring response to treatment.
    - Recheck TSH every 6 to 8 weeks. Dose of levothyroxine (Synthroid) is based on the TSH level. Goal is a TSH less than 5.0 mU/L.
    - When TSH is stable, recheck every 6 to 12 months.

Treatment

- Alternative/natural medication (controversial): Armour thyroid is produced from desiccated (dried) pig thyroid glands (contains both T3 and T4).
- Drug-induced thyroid disease: Lithium, amiodarone, high doses of iodine, interferon-alfa, dopamine. Monitor TSH.

Primary Hypothyroidism

The classic lab finding for hypothyroidism is a high TSH with low free T4 levels (do not confuse with total T4). Diagnosis is based on the lab findings.

Some of the most common causes are Hashimoto's thyroiditis, postpartum thyroiditis, and thyroid ablation with radioactive iodine (to treat hyperthyroidism). Hashimoto's thyroiditis is the most common cause of hypothyroidism in the United States.

Hashimoto's Thyroiditis

A chronic autoimmune disorder of the thyroid gland. There is generally no pain with this thyroid swelling. The body produces destructive antibodies (TPO) against the thyroid gland that gradually destroys it. Almost all patients (90%) with Hashimoto's thyroiditis have elevated TPOs. Most patients have developed a goiter. More common in women with ratio of 8:1 (women:men).

Classic Case

A middle-aged-to-older woman who is overweight complains of fatigue, weight gain, cold intolerance, constipation, and menstrual abnormalities. May have alopecia on the outer one third on both eyebrows. Serum cholesterol is elevated. May have a history of another autoimmune disorder (RA, PA, etc.).

Severe hypothyroidism (myxedema) is an endocrine emergency that is now rare (mortality 30%–40%). Patients presents with cognitive symptoms such as slowed thinking, poor short-term memory, depression (or dementia), hypotension, and hypothermia.

Labs (Table 9.1)

- Order TSH first (TSH >5.0 mU/L). If elevated, order TSH again with free T4 (free thyroxine). If TSH is high and serum free T4 is low, diagnosis of hypothyroidism.
- Next step is to order TPOs to confirm Hashimoto's thyroiditis (most common cause of hypothyroidism).
- TPOs: If elevated, confirms Hashimoto's thyroiditis (gold standard test for diagnosing Hashimoto's thyroiditis).

Subclinical Hypothyroidism (Nonpregnant Adults)

If TSH is greater than 5 mU/L (elevated), but serum free T4 is within normal range, diagnosis is subclinical hypothyroidism (asymptomatic to mild symptoms of hypothyroidism). Decision to treat with Synthroid should be individualized. Some choose not to treat, but recheck same labs again in 12 months.

Treatment Plan

- Starting dose of levothyroxine (Synthroid) ranges from 25 to 50 mcg/day.
- Start with lowest dose for elderly or patients with history of heart disease (watch for angina, acute myocardial infarction [MI], atrial fibrillation).
- Increase Synthroid dose every few weeks until TSH is normalized (<5.0 mU/L).
- Recheck TSH every 6 to 8 weeks until TSH is normalized (TSH <5.0 mU/L). When under control, check TSH every 12 months.
- Advise patient to report if palpitations, nervousness, or tremors because this means that Synthroid dose is too high (decrease dose until symptoms are gone and TSH in normal range).

Table 9.1 Laboratory Results in Thyroid Disease

Condition	TSH	Free T4	T3
Hypothyroidism	>5.0 mU/L	Low	Low
Subclinical hypothyroidism	>5.0 mU/L	Normal	Normal
Hyperthyroidism	<0.5 mU/L	High	High
Subclinical hyperthyroidism	<0.5 mU/L	Normal	Normal

T3, triiodothyronine; T4, thyroxine; TSH, thyroid-stimulating hormone.

EXAM TIPS

- **Learn to diagnose subclinical hypothyroidism (TSH elevated with normal free T4).**
- **If patient has elevated TSH (TSH >5.0 mU/L), workup needed for hypothyroidism (order TSH, free T4, etc.).**

- Start elderly patients at low dose of Synthroid (12.5–25 mcg/d) and gradually increase to avoid adverse cardiac effects from overstimulation (palpitations, angina, MI).
- Patient with normal free T4 but with elevated TSH—do not treat (subclinical hypothyroidism). Recheck TSH in about 6 months.
- Check TSH every 6 to 8 weeks (do not order earlier than 6 weeks) to monitor treatment response. If TSH is 0.5 to 5.0 mU/L, it is within normal limits and the patient is at the right dose (Synthroid).
- Radioactive iodine treatment results in hypothyroidism for life. Supplement with thyroid hormone for life.
- If TSH is suppressed (e.g., TSH 0.1 mU/L), workup needed for hyperthyroidism.
- Chronic amenorrhea and hypermetabolism result in osteoporosis. Supplement with calcium with vitamin D 1,200 mg; engage in weight-bearing exercises.

CLINICAL PEARLS

- Many patients with subclinical hypothyroidism will eventually develop overt hypothyroidism.
- Advise patient to crush Synthroid tablets with teeth inside mouth before swallowing with water for better absorption. These tablets are synthetic T4 (levothyroxine).
- Alternative medicine practitioners are more likely to prescribe Armour thyroid tablets (desiccated thyroid glands from pigs), which contain natural T3 and T4 for hypothyroidism.
- All hyperthyroid patients should be referred to an endocrinologist as soon as possible.

DIABETES MELLITUS

A chronic metabolic disorder affecting the body's metabolism of carbohydrates and fat. The result is microvascular and macrovascular damage, neuropathy, and immune system effects.

- *Microvascular damage:* Retinopathy, nephropathy, and neuropathy
- *Macrovascular damage:* Atherosclerosis, heart disease (coronary artery disease, MI)
- *Target organs:* Eyes, kidneys, heart/vascular system, peripheral nerves, especially in the feet; DM is the most common reason for chronic renal failure requiring dialysis and lower limb amputations in the United States

Type 1 DM

The massive destruction of B-cells in the islets of Langerhans results in an abrupt cessation of insulin production. If uncorrected, body fat will be used for fuel. Ketones, the metabolic product of fat breakdown, build up in the body until the result is diabetic ketotic acidosis (ketoacidosis) and coma. Most patients are juveniles; occasionally occurs in adults (maturity onset diabetes of the young [MODY]). The CDC reports 5% to 10% of U.S. cases.

Type 2 DM

Progressive decreased secretion of insulin (with peripheral insulin resistance) resulting in a chronic state of hyperglycemia and hyperinsulinemia. Has strong genetic component.

Type 2 DM represents 90% to 95% of U.S. cases. Obesity epidemic is increasing rates of type 2 DM in younger patients.

Risk Factors for Type 2 DM (Screen These Patients)

- Overweight or obese (body mass index [BMI] 25 or greater)
- Abdominal obesity; sedentary lifestyle

- Metabolic syndrome
- Hispanic, African American, Asian, Pacific Islander, or American Indian ancestry, or positive family history
- History of gestational diabetes or infant weighing greater than 9 lbs at birth
- Impaired fasting blood sugar/glucose (IFG) or impaired glucose tolerance (IGT) is considered at higher risk for type 2 DM (prediabetes)

Metabolic Syndrome

- Presence of any three of the following four traits:
  - Obesity, abdominal obesity. Waist:
    - In men, greater than 40 inches/102 cm
    - In women, greater than 35 inches/88 cm
  - Hypertension or BP of more than 130/85 mmHg
  - Dyslipidemia: Triglycerides greater than 150 mg/dL, HDL less than 40 (males) or less than 50 (females)
  - Hyperglycemia: Fasting plasma glucose (FPG) greater than 100 mg/dL or type 2 DM
- Other names are *insulin-resistance syndrome* or *syndrome X*
- Affected people have higher risk of type 2 DM and cardiovascular disease

Increased Risk of DM (Prediabetes)

- Glycosylated hemoglobin (A1C) between 5.7% and 6.4%

  or
- Fasting glucose of 100 to 125 mg/dL (impaired FPG)

  or
- 2-hour oral glucose tolerance test (OGTT; 75 g load) of 140 to 199 mg/dL

Diagnostic Criteria for DM

- A1C equal to or greater than 6.5%

  or
- FPG equal to or greater than 126 mg/dL (fasting is no caloric intake for at least 8 hours)

  or
- Symptoms of hyperglycemia (polyuria, polydipsia, polyphagia) plus random blood glucose equal to or greater than 200 mg/dL

  or
- Two-hour plasma glucose greater than or equal to 200 mg/dL during an OGTT with a 75-g glucose load

Serum Blood Glucose Norms (Nondiabetic Adults; Table 9.2)

- FPG: 70 to 100 mg/dL
- Peak postprandial plasma glucose: Less than 180 mg/dL
- Glycosylated hemoglobin (A1C: <6.0%)
  - Defined as the average blood glucose levels over previous 3 months; no fasting required; test measures excess glucose that attaches to the hemoglobin of the red blood cells
- If able to tolerate A1C goal of 6% (especially younger diabetics), continue with the same goal
- Less stringent goals are acceptable for some (frail elderly, history of severe hypoglycemia, extensive comorbidity, limited life expectancy)
  - A1C goal of up to 8% is acceptable

Labs

- Newly diagnosed diabetics: Check A1C every 3 months until blood glucose controlled or when changing therapy, then check twice a year (every 6 months)
- Lipid profile at least once a year with 9- to 12-hour fasting

Table 9.2 Recommendations for Nonpregnant Adult Diabetics

Test	Goal
Blood pressure	<140/80 mmHg
LDL cholesterol	<100 mg/dL
A1C	<7% (exceptions exist)
Preprandial capillary plasma glucose (fasting)	70 to 130 mg/dL
Peak postprandial capillary plasma glucose (2 hours after meal)	<180 mg/dL

LDL, low-density lipoprotein.
Source: American Diabetes Association (2017).

- Random or "on spot" urine for microalbuminuria at least once a year
  - Urine albumin-to-creatinine ratio better than microalbumin test (spot urine sample) for evaluating microalbumin (the earliest sign of diabetic renal disease)
  - If positive, order 24-hour urine for protein and creatinine
- Angiotensin-converting enzyme inhibitors (ACEIs) or angiotensin receptor blockers (ARBs) with tighter control of blood glucose/A1C may help renal disease
- Check electrolytes (potassium, magnesium, sodium), liver function panel, and TSH

Treatment Plan

- *Every visit:* Check BP, feet, weight and BMI, blood sugar.
- Check feet:
  - Check for vibration sense (128-Hz tuning fork): Place on bony prominence of the big toe (metatarsophalangeal [MTP] joint); if unable to sense vibration or asymmetry, patient has peripheral neuropathy
  - Light and deep touch, numbness: Place at right angle on plantar surface, push into skin until it buckles slightly (monofilament tool)
  - Check pedal pulses, ankle reflexes, and skin are examined for acanthosis nigricans, insulin injection or insertion sites, lipodystrophy

Recommendations: Preventive Care

- CDC recommends adults older than 50 be given SHINGRIX in two doses, 2 to 6 months apart.
- Influenza immunization every year
- Pneumococcal polysaccharide vaccine: If vaccinated before 65 years of age, give one-time revaccination in 5 years; if age 65 years, give one dose of the vaccine only
- Prescribe aspirin 81 mg if high risk for MI, stroke (if younger than 30 years of age, not recommended)
- *Ophthalmologist:* Yearly dilated eye exam needed: If type 2: eye exam at diagnosis; if type 1 DM, first eye exam needed 5 years after diagnosis
- *Podiatrist:* Refer to once to twice a year, especially with older diabetics
- *BP goal:* Goal is 130/80 mmHg
- *Dental/tooth care:* Important (poor oral health associated with heart disease)

Dietary and Nutrition Recommendations (or Macronutrients)

- Alcohol: Advise females not to exceed one drink per day and for males two drinks per day
- Monitor carbohydrate intake (i.e., carbohydrate counting)
- Saturated fat (animal fats, beef fat) intake should be less than 7% of total calories

- Reduce intake of trans fats (will lower LDL and increase HDL), such as most fried foods and "junk foods"
- Refer patient to a dietician at least once or more often if problems with diet
- Routine vitamin supplementation of antioxidants is not yet advised

Hypoglycemia

- *High risk:* Level 1 hypoglycemia (glucose alert): FBS 70 mg/dL or less; level 2 hypoglycemia: blood glucose 54 mg/dL or less
- *Look for:* Sweaty palms, tiredness, dizziness, rapid pulse, strange behavior, confusion, and weakness; if patient on beta-blockers, the hypoglycemic response can be blunted or blocked

Treatment Plan

- Glucose (15–20 g) is preferred treatment for conscious patients. Other options are 4 oz of orange juice, regular soft drink, hard candy. Recheck blood glucose 15 minutes after treatment. When blood glucose is normalized, eat a meal or snack afterward (complex carbohydrates, protein).
- Glucagon: Prescribe for patients at significant risk for severe hypoglycemia.
- Severe hypoglycemia is defined as blood glucose less than 54 mg/dL.

Illness and Surgery

- Do not stop taking antidiabetic medicine. Keep taking insulin or oral medications as scheduled unless fasting blood glucose (FBG) is lower than normal.
- Requires frequent self-monitoring of blood glucose.
- Eat small amounts of food every 3 to 4 hours to keep FBG as normal as possible.
- *Contact health care provider if:* Dehydrated, vomiting, or diarrhea for several hours, blood glucose is greater than 300 mg/dL, changes in LOC (feel sleepier than normal/cannot think clearly).

Exercise

- Increases glucose utilization by the muscles. Patients may need to reduce their usual dose of medicine (or eat snacks before the activity and afterward to compensate).
- If patient does not compensate (reducing the dose of insulin, increasing caloric intake, snacking before and after), there is an increased risk of hypoglycemia within a few hours.
- *Example:* If patient exercises in the afternoon, high risk of hypoglycemia at night/bedtime if he or she does not compensate by eating snacks, eating more food at dinner, or lowering insulin dose.

Snacks for Exercise

- Eat simple carbohydrates (candy, juices) before or during exercise.
- Eat complex carbohydrates (granola bars) after exercise (avoids postexercise hypoglycemia).

Other Diabetic Issues

Dawn Phenomenon

This is a normal physiological event; a hormonal surge in all people causing an elevation in the FBG occurs daily, early in the morning between 4:00 and 8:00 a.m. Without normal insulin responses, diabetics experience rising FBG levels. Healthy people can make the insulin to combat this phenomenon.

Somogyi Effect (Rebound Hyperglycemia)

Severe nocturnal hypoglycemia stimulates counterregulatory hormones, such as glucagon, to be released from the liver. The high levels of glucagon in the systemic circulation result in high fasting blood glucose by 7:00 a.m. The condition is due to overtreatment with the evening and/or bedtime insulin (dose is too high). More common in people with type 1 DM.

- *Diagnosis:* Check blood glucose very early in the morning (3:00 a.m.) for 1 to 2 weeks.
- *Treatment:* Eat a snack before bedtime, or eliminate dinnertime intermediate-acting insulin (NPH) dose or lower the bedtime dose for both NPH and regular insulin.

Diabetic Retinopathy

Neovascularization (new growth of fragile arterioles in retina), microaneurysms (dot and blot hemorrhages due to neovascularization), cotton-wool spots or soft exudates (nerve fiber layer infarcts), and hard exudates.

- Patients with type 1 DM: Screen after age 10 years.
- Patients with type 2 diabetes: Refer to ophthalmologist shortly after diagnosis; then eye exam needed every 6 to 12 months.

Diabetic Foot Care

Patients with peripheral neuropathy should avoid excessive running or walking to minimize the risk of foot injury.

- Patients with type 2 diabetes: Refer to podiatrist at least once a year.
- Wear shoes that fit properly. Never go barefoot.
- Check feet daily, especially the soles of the feet (use mirror).
- Trim nails squarely (not rounded) to prevent ingrown toenails.
- Report redness, skin breakdown, or trauma to health care provider immediately (main cause of lower leg amputations in the United States).

Charcot's Foot and Ankle (Neuropathic Arthropathy)

Deformity of the foot that is caused by joint and bone dislocation and fractures due to neuropathy and loss of sensation to the foot and ankle. May affect only one foot or both feet. If severe, foot deformity includes collapse of midfoot arch (rocker bottom foot).

Diabetic Medications

Biguanides

- First line: Metformin (Glucophage):
  - Decreases gluconeogenesis and decreases peripheral insulin resistance. Very rarely may cause hypoglycemia. Prescribe in addition to diet and exercise (lifestyle).
- Metformin is preferred for obese patients. According to the 2018 position statement and by the American Diabetes Association it is reported that metformin is neutral for weight change and has a potential for a modest weight loss. Metformin may cause gastrointestinal side effects, such as diarrhea and nausea.
- For decreased vitamin B_{12} levels (7%), consider vitamin supplementation.
- **Contraindications**:
  - Do not use if renal disease, hepatic disease acidosis, alcoholics, hypoxia.
  - *Labs*: Monitor renal function (serum creatinine, GFR, UA) and LFTs.
- Increased risk of lactic acidosis (pH <7.25):
  - Occurs during hypoxia, hypoperfusion, renal insufficiency.
- *IV contrast dye testing:* Hold metformin on day of procedure and 48 hours after.
  - Check baseline creatinine and recheck after procedure. If serum creatinine remains elevated after the procedure, do not restart metformin. Serum creatinine must be normalized before drug can be resumed.

Sulfonylureas

- Stimulates the beta cells of the pancreas to secrete more insulin.
- *First generation:* Administer chlorpropamide (Diabinese) daily or BID.
  - Long half-life (12 hours). Not commonly used because of high risk of severe hypoglycemia.

- *Second generation:* Administer glipizide (Glucotrol, Glucotrol XL) maximum dose of 40 mg/d, glyburide (DiaBeta) maximum dose of 20 mg/d, glimepiride (Amaryl) maximum dose of 8 mg/d

Adverse Effects

- The Food and Drug Administration (FDA) has a special warning on increased risk of cardiovascular mortality based on studies of an older sulfonylurea (tolbutamide).
- Hypoglycemia (diaphoresis, pallor, sweating, tremor); increased risk of photosensitivity (use sunscreen)
- Blood dyscrasias (monitor CBC)
- Avoid if impaired hepatic or renal function (monitor LFTs, creatinine, UA)
- Causes weight gain (monitor weight and BMI)

Thiazolidinediones (TZDs)

- Pioglitazone (Actos):
  - Enhances insulin sensitivity in muscle tissue (decreases peripheral tissue resistance) and reduces hepatic glucagon production (gluconeogenesis). Take daily with meal at breakfast.
- Can be combined with metformin, sulfonylureas, glucagonlike peptide 1 (GLP-1), sodium-glucose cotransporter-2 (SGLT2) inhibitors, dipeptidyl peptidase-4 (DPP-4) inhibitors, insulins
- **Contraindications:**
  - FDA Black Box warning: DO NOT USE with NYHA class III and class IV heart disease, symptomatic heart failure (congestive heart failure [CHF]).
  - Causes water retention and edema (aggravates or will precipitate heart failure [CHF]).
  - Avoid if bladder cancer or history of bladder cancer (UA, urine cytology), active liver disease, type 1 DM, pregnancy.
  - Causes weight gain (monitor weight and BMI).
- *Labs:* Check LFTs.

Bile-Acid Sequestrants

- Cholestyramine (Questran), colesevelam (Welchol), colestipol (Colestid)
- Reduces hepatic glucose production and may reduce intestinal absorption of glucose
- Take with meals; lowers LDL
  - Side effects are GI related, such as nausea, bloating, constipation, increased triglycerides
  - Side effects are a common reason for noncompliance; start patient on a low dose and titrate up slowly
  - Kidney and liver effects (check serum creatinine, GFR, LFTs)

Meglitinide (Glinides)

- Repaglinide (Prandin), nateglinide (Starlix)
- Stimulates pancreatic secretion of insulin; indicated for type 2 diabetics with postprandial hyperglycemia
- Weight-neutral; may cause hypoglycemia
  - Rapid-acting with a very short half-life (<1 hour)
  - Take before meals or up to 30 minutes after a meal
  - Hold dose if skipping a meal
  - Side effects are bloating, abdominal cramps, diarrhea, flatulence

Diabetic Medications: Subcutaneous Route

This is not an inclusive list. For specific information about types of insulin, see Table 9.3.

Table 9.3 Types of Insulin

Insulin Type	Onset (Starts at)	Peak	Duration (Mean)*
Rapid-acting analogs Insulin lispro/aspart/glulisine	15 minutes	30 minutes to 2½ hours	About 4½ hours
Short-acting regular human insulin	30 minutes	1–5 hours	6–8 hours
Intermediate NPH Human NPH	1 hour	6–14 hours	18–24 hours
Basal insulin analogs Insulin glargine (Lantus) Insulin detemir (Levemir)	1 hour	None	24 hours Insulin detemir usually BID
Premixed Humulin 70/30 (NPH/reg.) Humulin 50/50 Other types available	30 minutes	4.4 hours	About 24 hours

*Times are based on broad estimates and are designed for use only for the nurse practitioner certification exams. Do not use for clinical practice. All insulins cause hypoglycemia and weight gain.
BID, twice a day; NPH, neutral protamine Hagedorn.

Rapid-Acting Insulin

- Humalog (insulin lispro)

Short-Acting Insulin (Regular)

- Humulin R

NPH

Considered a "basal insulin" (has no "peaks")

- Humulin N
- Lantus (insulin glargine), Levemir (insulin detemir)
  - Give once a day at the same time

Insulin Mixtures

- Humulin 70/30 (70% NPH insulin, 30% regular insulin)
- If mixing NPH and regular insulin, use the mixture immediately
- Rapid-acting insulin can be mixed with NPH, but it should be used 15 minutes before a meal

Insulin Pumps

Insulin pumps require intensive training; the insulin pumps are expensive. Can be used for both type 1 or type 2 diabetics. Patients should remove pump when swimming or showering.

Other Medications for Diabetes

Alpha-Glucosidase Inhibitor

- Slows intestinal carbohydrate digestion and absorption; a nonsystemic oral drug
- Does not cause hypoglycemia; modest effect on A1C level
- GI side effects are flatulence, diarrhea

Incretin Mimetics or Glucagonlike Peptide (GLP-1) Mimetics

- Exenatide (Byetta) BID or liraglutide (Victoza) once-a-day injections (SC)
- Stimulate GLP-1, causing an increase in insulin production and inhibits postprandial glucagon release (will decrease postprandial hyperglycemia); increases satiety

- Causes weight loss, suppress appetite, does not cause hypoglycemia
- May cause pancreatitis (monitor amylase, lipase), medullary thyroid tumors in animals, and C-cell hyperplasia
- Warning: Contraindicated if personal or family history of medullary thyroid carcinoma, multiple endocrine neoplasia syndrome type 2 (MEN-2)

Sodium-Glucose Cotransporter-2 (GLT2) Inhibitors

- Canagliflozin (Invokana), dapagliflozin (Farxiga), empagliflozin (Jardiance)
- Blocks glucose reabsorption by the kidney (proximal nephron) and increases glucosuria
- Effective in all stages of type 2 DM; no hypoglycemia
- FDA warning: May lead to DKA; symptoms: difficulty breathing, nausea, vomiting, abdominal pain, confusion, and unusual fatigue or sleepiness
- Causes weight loss, hypotension (volume depletion)
- Renal signs and symptoms: Polyuria, increased creatinine; increase in UTIs and pyelonephritis (urosepsis)
- Warning: Increased risk of leg and foot amputations

Dipeptidyl Peptidase-4 (DPP-4) Inhibitors

- Sitagliptin (Januvia), saxagliptin (Onglyza), linagliptin (Tradjenta), others
- Inhibit DPP-4 activity; increase active incretin concentrations
- Increase insulin secretion and decrease glucagon; no hypoglycemia
- FDA warning: May cause joint pain that can be severe and disabling (may occur on day 1 or years later)
- May cause angioedema/urticaria, acute pancreatitis

> **Note**
>
> Do not combine incretin mimetics (Byetta, Victoza) with any incretin enhancers (Januvia, Onglyza). Both act on incretin.

Amylin Mimetic/Analog (Symlin)

- Decreases glucagon secretion; slows gastric emptying; leads to feeling satiety early; causes weight loss
- Route: Injectable; frequent dosing; requires patient training
- Causes hypoglycemia if used with insulin (decrease insulin dose)

SOLVING AN INSULIN-RELATED QUESTION

The nurse practitioner certification exams are based on the primary care model of care. In general, it is not necessary to memorize specific doses. Keep in mind some broad concepts such as the peak and duration of each type of insulin. For example:

- Rapid-acting insulin covers "one meal at a time"
- Regular insulin lasts "from meal to meal"
- NPH insulin lasts "from breakfast to dinner"
- Lantus is "once a day"

Case Scenario

A patient with type 1 diabetes is on regular insulin and NPH insulin (not premixed, but separate) injected twice a day. The first dose is injected before breakfast and the second dose is injected at bedtime. The blood sugar results from the patient's diary (fasting, before lunch, dinner, and bedtime) show that the lunchtime values are higher than normal. *Which insulin dose should be increased or decreased?*

In this case, the NPH component of the morning dose should be increased. Regular insulin peaks between breakfast and lunch (most of it is gone by lunchtime). In contrast, NPH insulin peaks between 6 and 14 hours. Therefore, it will cover the postprandial spike after lunch.

CLINICAL INFORMATION

- Rapid-acting insulins (insulin lispro) are used mostly by type 1 diabetics before each meal.
- Intermediate-acting insulin (NPH) can be used once to twice a day.

Summary of Prescribing Medications for Type 2 Diabetics

- Try lifestyle changes (weight loss) for 3 to 6 months if mild A1C elevation.
- In addition to lifestyle, metformin is first-line treatment for most type 2 diabetics. Start on metformin 500 mg daily (maximum dose is 2,000 mg/dL or 2 g).
  - If metformin dose is at maximum (and blood sugar or A1C is still high), add a sulfonylurea (e.g., Glucotrol XL 20 mg/d).
    or
  - If patient is on a sulfonylurea at the maximum dose (e.g., Glucotrol XL 40 mg/d) and blood sugar/A1C is still elevated, then add metformin.
- Choice of second or third agent are any of other drug classes used to treat type 2 DM.
  - If on maximal metformin dose (2 g), other choices to add are DPP-4 inhibitors (Januvia, Onglyza), incretin mimetics (Byetta), and/or TZDs (Actos), others.
  - Do not combine insulins with meglitinides (severe hypoglycemia).
- If blood sugar or A1C is still elevated and patient is on both metformin and sulfonylurea, consider starting patient on a basal insulin (Lantus SC once a day).
- If patient refuses insulin, other options are thioglitazones (Actos), Byetta, others. Keep in mind the contraindications for each drug class.

Antidiabetic Medications: Effect on Weight

- *Causes weight loss:* Metformin, incretin mimetic, GLT-2 inhibitors
- *Causes weight gain:* Insulins, Sulfonylureas, TZDs (Actos)
- *Weight-neutral:* Meglitinides (Starlix, Prandin), bile-acid sequestrants (Welchol), alpha-glucosidase inhibitors

DM: Management

- Refer to dietician to learn about carbohydrate counting. The American Diabetes Association (2017) recommends including fat and protein counting. Lifestyle changes are first-line treatment.
- Weight loss improves metabolic control in type 2 diabetics.
- Eating more fiber and whole grains (brown rice, whole wheat) may help.
- Exercise increases cellular glucose uptake in the body.
- Type 2 diabetics not well controlled on multiple oral agents, diet, and lifestyle changes are good candidates for basal insulin therapy.

DM: Possible Complications

- *Eyes:* Cataracts, diabetic retinopathy, blindness
- *Cardiovascular:* Hyperlipidemia, coronary artery disease, MI, hypertension
- *Kidneys:* Renal disease, renal failure
- *Feet:* Foot ulcers, skin infections, peripheral neuropathy, amputation
- *Gynecological/genitourinary:* Balanitis (candidal infection of the glans penis), candidal vaginitis

Primary Prevention

For individuals at high risk of type 2 DM: Encourage weight loss (7% of body weight) and regular physical activity (150 min/week). Increase dietary fiber and foods with whole grains.

EXAM TIPS

- First-line medication for type 2 DM is metformin (Glucophage).
  - If patient on metformin 500 mg daily and A1C is high (>7%), raise dose to metformin 500 mg BID. If A1C is still high (>7%) and on metformin 500 mg BID, increase dose to metformin 1,000 mg BID (or 1 g BID).
  - If taking maximum dose of metformin (1 g BID), can use several drug classes with it such as a sulfonylurea like glipizide (Glucotrol XL) 5 mg PO daily (do not exceed maximum dose of glipizide 20 mg/d), DPP-4 inhibitor (Januvia, Onglyza), TZD (Actos), others.
- If a patient's A1C is 9 or higher, start on basal insulin. Or if on two oral drugs and A1C is 9 or higher, start on basal insulin.
- Photographs of fundi appear on the exam. Search for photographs online of diabetic retinopathy. Findings are cotton wool spots (soft exudates), neovascularization, microaneurysms with dot and blot hemorrhages.
  - Learn what cotton wool spots (or soft exudates) look like.
- Hypertensive retinopathy findings are silver wire/copper wire arterioles, arteriovenous nicking.
- Hemoglobin A1C is the average blood glucose level in previous 3 months (12 weeks).
- Actos can cause water retention, which may precipitate CHF. Contraindicated if history of heart failure or NYHA class III or IV (moderate to severe heart failure).
- Tell patient to disconnect insulin pump if swimming, bathing, or showering. Certain sports (e.g., wrestling) require that an insulin pump be disconnected during activity.
  - Microvascular complications of diabetes are retinopathy, nephropathy, or neuropathy.
  - Macrovascular complications are coronary artery disease, peripheral arterial disease, or stroke.
- Charcot's foot and ankle is more common in diabetics.
- Lid lag is a symptom of Graves' opthalmopathy (hyperthyroidism).
- Alopecia of outer one third of eyebrow and myxedema are symptoms of hypothyroidism.

CLINICAL PEARLS

- People with subclinical and overt hyperthyroidism are at higher risk of bone (osteopenia/osteoporosis) and cardiac (atrial fibrillation) complications.
- New-onset atrial fibrillation, check TSH.
  - Keep TSH between 1.0 and 4.0 mU/L as goal for thyroid hormone supplementation.
- Diabetics are at higher risk for cataracts and glaucoma.
- In morbidly obese patients, bariatric surgery can result in remission of type 2 diabetes.

10

Gastrointestinal System Review

⚠ DANGER SIGNALS

Acute Appendicitis

Patient who is a young adult complains of an acute onset of periumbilical pain that is steadily getting worse. Over a period of 12 to 24 hours, the pain starts to localize at McBurney's point. The patient has no appetite (anorexia). Classic exam findings include low-grade fever and right lower quadrant (RLQ) pain (McBurney's point) with rebound and guarding. The psoas and obturator signs are positive.

When the appendix ruptures, clinical signs of acute abdomen occur, such as involuntary guarding, rebound, and a board-like abdomen.

Acute Cholecystitis

Overweight female patient complains of severe right upper quadrant (RUQ) or epigastric pain that occurs within 1 hour (or more) after eating a fatty meal. Pain may radiate to the right shoulder. Accompanied by nausea/vomiting and anorexia. If left untreated, may develop gangrene of the gallbladder (20%). May require hospitalization.

Acute Diverticulitis

Elderly patient with acute onset of high fever, anorexia, nausea/vomiting, and left lower quadrant (LLQ) abdominal pain. Risk factors for acute diverticulitis include increased age, constipation, low dietary fiber intake, obesity, lack of exercise, and frequent nonsteroidal anti-inflammatory drug (NSAID) use. Signs of acute abdomen are rebound, positive Rovsing's sign, and board-like abdomen. CBC will show leukocytosis with neutrophilia and shift to the left. The presence of band forms signals severe bacterial infection (bands are immature neutrophils). Complications include abscess, sepsis, ileus, small bowel obstruction, hemorrhage, perforation, fistula, and phlegmon stricture. May be life-threatening.

Acute Pancreatitis

Adult patient complains of the acute onset of fever, nausea, and vomiting that is associated with rapid onset of abdominal pain that radiates to the midback ("boring") located in the epigastric region. Frequent causes include drugs (approximately 90% of cases of acute pancreatitis), biliary factors, and alcohol abuse. Abdominal exam reveals guarding and tenderness over the epigastric area or the upper abdomen. Positive Cullen's sign (blue discoloration around umbilicus) and Grey–Turner's sign (blue discoloration on the flanks). The patient may have an ileus, may show signs and symptoms of shock. Refer to ED.

Clostridium difficile Colitis

Severe watery diarrhea from 10 to 15 stools a day that is accompanied by lower abdominal pain with cramping and fever. Symptoms usually appear within 5 to 10 days after initiation of antibiotics. Antibiotics, such as clindamycin (Cleocin), fluoroquinolones, cephalosporins, and penicillins, have been implicated as more likely to cause *C. difficile* infection. Most cases occur in patients in hospitals as well as in those residing in nursing facilities.

Colon Cancer

Very gradual (years) with vague GI symptoms. Tumor may bleed intermittently and patient may have iron-deficiency anemia. Changes in bowel habits, stool, or bloody stool. Heme-positive stool, dark tarry stool, mass on abdominal palpation. Older patient (older than 50 years of age), especially with history of multiple polyps or inflammatory bowel disease such as Crohn's disease (CD) or ulcerative colitis (UC).

Crohn's Disease (CD)

Inflammatory bowel disease that may affect any part(s) of GI tract from mouth (canker sores), small to large intestine, rectum, and anus. If ileum involved, there is watery diarrhea without blood or mucus. If colon involved, there is bloody diarrhea with mucus. During relapses, fever, anorexia, weight loss, dehydration, fatigue with periumbilical to RLQ abdominal pain occur. Fistula formation and anal disease only occur with CD (not UC). May palpate tender abdominal mass. Remissions and relapses are common. Higher risk of toxic megacolon and colon cancer. Risk of development of lymphoma is also increased, especially for patients treated with azathioprine. More common in Ashkenazi Jews.

Ulcerative Colitis

Inflammatory bowel disease that affects the colon/rectum. Bloody diarrhea with mucus (hematochezia) more common with UC than with CD. Severe "squeezing" cramping pain located on the left side of the abdomen with bloating and gas that is exacerbated by food. Relapses characterized by fever, anorexia, weight loss, and fatigue. Accompanied by arthralgias and arthritis (15%–40%) that affect large joints, sacrum, and ankylosing spondylitis. May have iron deficiency anemia or anemia of chronic disease. Disease has remissions and relapses. Increased risk of colon cancer. Risk of toxic megacolon.

Zollinger–Ellison Syndrome

A gastrinoma located on the pancreas or the stomach; secretes gastrin, which stimulates high levels of acid production in the stomach. The end result is the development of multiple and severe ulcers in the stomach and duodenum. Complaints of epigastric to midabdominal pain. Stools may be a tarry color. Screening by serum fasting gastrin level.

☑ NORMAL FINDINGS

Route of Food or Drink From the Mouth

Esophagus → stomach (hydrochloric acid, intrinsic factor) → duodenum (bile, amylase, lipase) → jejunum → ileum → colon → cecum → rectum → anus

Abdominal Contents

- *Right upper quadrant (RUQ):* Liver, gallbladder, ascending colon, kidney (right), pancreas (small portion); right kidney is lower than the left because of displacement by the liver
- *Left upper quadrant (LUQ):* Stomach, pancreas, descending colon, kidney (left)
- *Right lower quadrant (RLQ):* Appendix, ileum, cecum, ovary (right)
- *Left lower quadrant (LLQ):* Sigmoid colon, ovary (left)
- *Suprapubic area:* Bladder, uterus, rectum

ABDOMINAL MANEUVERS

Acute Abdomen or Peritonitis

Psoas/Iliopsoas

- Positive finding if right lower quadrant (RLQ) abdominal pain occurs during maneuver. Indicates irritation to the iliopsoas group of hip flexors in the abdomen. A positive finding suggests peritoneal irritation.
- With patient in supine position, have patient raise right leg against the pressure of the professional's hand resistance
- With patient on left side, extend the right leg from the hip

Obturator Sign (Supine Position)

Positive if inward rotation of the hip causes RLQ abdominal pain. Rotate right hip through full range of motion. Positive sign is pain with the movement or flexion of the hip.

Rovsing's Sign (Supine Position)

Deep palpation of the left lower quadrant of the abdomen results in referred pain to the RLQ, which is a positive Rovsing's sign.

McBurney's Point

Area located between the superior iliac crest and umbilicus in the RLQ. Tenderness or pain is a sign of possible acute appendicitis.

Markle Test (Heel Jar)

Instruct patient to raise heels and then drop them suddenly. An alternative is to ask the patient to jump in place. Positive if pain is elicited or if patient refuses to perform because of pain.

Involuntary Guarding

With abdominal palpation, the abdominal muscles reflexively become tense or board-like.

Rebound Tenderness

Patient complains of worsening abdominal pain when hand is released after palpation of abdomen compared to the pain felt during deep palpation.

Murphy's Maneuver (Figure 10.1)

Press deeply on the RUQ under the costal border during inspiration. Midinspiratory arrest is a positive finding (Murphy's sign).

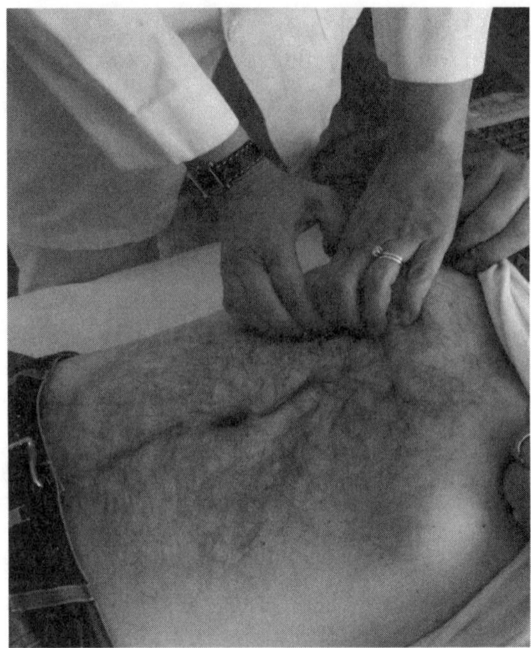

Figure 10.1 Murphy's sign.

DISEASE REVIEW

Gastroesophageal Reflux Disease (GERD)

Forty percent of U.S. adults have GERD. Acidic gastric contents regurgitate from the stomach into the esophagus due to inappropriate relaxation of the lower esophageal sphincter. Chronic GERD causes damage to squamous epithelium of the esophagus and in about 10% of GERD patients may result in Barrett's esophagus (a precancer), which increases risk of squamous cell cancer (cancer of the esophagus).

Classic Case

Middle-aged to older adult complains of chronic heartburn of many years' duration. Symptoms associated with large and/or fatty meals that worsen when supine. Long-term history of self-medication with over-the-counter (OTC) antacids and H2-blockers. Risk factors may include the chronic use of NSAIDs, aspirin, or alcohol.

Objective Findings

- Acidic or sour odor to breath
- Reflux of sour acidic stomach contents, especially with overeating
- Thinning tooth enamel (rear molars) due to increased hydrochloric acid
- Chronic sore red throat (not associated with a cold)
- Chronic coughing

Treatment Plan

First-line (mild/intermittent GERD) treatment is lifestyle changes. Avoid large and/or high-fat meals, especially 3 to 4 hours before bedtime; lose weight; avoid mints, chocolate, and alcohol (relaxes gastric sphincter); and avoid aspirin, NSAIDs, caffeine, carbonated beverages, and other aggravating foods. Cease smoking. Smoking increases stomach acid and lowers esophageal sphincter pressure. Ask whether on medications with a GERD side effect such as beta-blockers, calcium channel blockers, and alpha-1 or alpha-2 adrenergic receptor agonists.

Can combine lifestyle changes with antacids and/or H2-blockers (low-dose H2-receptor antagonists) as needed. If poor response, next step is to prescribe medications.

Medications

- H2-blockers: Ranitidine (Zantac), nizatidine (Axid), famotidine (Pepcid)
- Proton-pump inhibitors (PPIs): Omeprazole (Prilosec), esomeprazole (Nexium), lansoprazole (Prevacid), pantoprazole (Protonix)
  - Long-term therapy associated with hip fractures, pneumonia, and *C. difficile* infection. Do not discontinue PPIs abruptly because doing so can cause rebound symptoms (worsens symptoms); taper dose to wean.
- Antacids (mild symptoms): Aluminum-magnesium-simethicone (Mylanta, Maalox), calcium carbonate (Tums, Caltrate), aluminum-magnesium (Gaviscon); minerals can bind with certain medications such as tetracycline and levothyroxine (Synthroid)
- If no relief after 4 to 8 weeks therapy, high risk for Barrett's esophagus (long-term GERD, White male older than 50 years) or worrisome symptoms, refer to GI specialist for upper endoscopy/biopsy (gold standard)
- *Worrisome symptoms:* Progressive dysphagia (difficulty swallowing that is worsening), iron-deficiency anemia (blood loss), weight loss, Hemoccult positive

Complications

- Barrett's esophagus (a precancer for esophageal cancer)
- Esophageal cancer

EXAM TIPS

- Barrett's esophagus is a precancer (esophageal cancer). Diagnosed by upper endoscopy with biopsy.
- Know lifestyle factors to teach patient (no mints, avoid caffeine, etc.)
- Know Cullen's sign (edema and bruising of the subcutaneous tissue around the umbilicus) and Grey–Turner's sign (bruising/bluish discoloration of the flank area that may indicate retroperitoneal hemorrhage).
- Classic pain of acute pancreatitis is severe midepigastric pain that radiates to midback.
- Know Rovsing's sign.
- Be aware of presentation of acute appendicitis.
- Psoas and obturator signs are positive for acute appendicitis.
- Know how to perform psoas maneuver.

CLINICAL PEARLS

- Any patient with at least a decade or more history of chronic heartburn should be referred to a gastroenterologist for an endoscopy to rule out Barrett's esophagus.
- Patients with Barrett's esophagus have up to 30 times higher risk of cancer of the esophagus (adenocarcinoma type).

Irritable Bowel Syndrome (IBS)

A chronic functional disorder of the colon (normal colonic tissue) marked by exacerbations and remissions (spontaneous). Commonly exacerbated by excess stress. It may be classified as diarrhea predominant or constipation predominant. In some cases, it may alternate between the two.

Classic Case

Young adult to middle-aged female complains of intermittent episodes of moderate to severe cramping pain in the lower abdomen, especially in the LLQ. Bloating with flatulence. Relief obtained after defecation. Stools range from diarrhea to constipation or both types with increased frequency of bowel movements.

Objective Findings

- A complete physical exam should be performed to exclude other causes.
- Vital signs are typically normal.
- *Abdominal exam:* Tenderness in lower quadrants during an exacerbation. Otherwise the exam is normal.
- *Rectal exam:* Stool is normal with no blood or pus.
  - Stools are heme negative.

Treatment Plan

- Increase dietary fiber. Supplement fiber with psyllium (Metamucil or Konsyl), methylcellulose (Citrucel), wheat dextrin (Benefiber). Start at low dose (causes gas).
- Avoid gas-producing foods: Beans, onions, cabbage, high-fructose corn syrup. If poor response, use a trial diet of lactose avoidance or gluten avoidance.
- Antispasmodics for abdominal pain: Administer dicyclomine (Bentyl) or hyoscyamine as needed.
  - IBS with constipation: Begin a trial of fiber supplements, polyethylene glycol (osmotic laxative). If severe constipation: Prescribe lubiprostone or linaclotide (contraindicated in pediatric patients younger than 6 years, has caused death from dehydration).
  - IBS with diarrhea: Take loperamide (Imodium) before regularly scheduled meals.
  - Severe diarrhea–predominant IBS: Administer alosetron (warning: ischemic colitis, which can be fatal).
- Decrease life stress. Address anxiety/stress with patient and offer treatment strategies.
- *Rule out:* Amoebic, parasitic, or bacterial infections; inflammatory disease of the GI tract; and so forth. Check stool for ova and parasites (especially diarrheal stools) with culture.

PEPTIC ULCER DISEASE (PUD)

Gastric Ulcer and Duodenal Ulcer Disease

Duodenal ulcers are more common than gastric ulcers. Gastric ulcers have higher risk of malignancy (up to 10%) compared with duodenal ulcers, which are mostly benign. *Helicobacter pylori* is a common cause of both duodenal and gastric ulcers.

Etiology

- *H. pylori* (gram-negative bacteria)
- Chronic NSAID use, which disrupts prostaglandin production; results in reduction of GI blood flow with reduction of protective mucus layer
- Tobacco and/or alcohol use; stress after acute illness, ventilator support, extensive burns, or head injury

- Bisphosphonates (Fosamax, Actonel)
- *Worrisome symptoms:* Early satiety, anorexia, anemia (bleeding), recurrent vomiting, hematemesis, weight loss

Classic Case

Middle-aged to older adult complains of episodic epigastric pain, burning/gnawing pain, or ache (80%). Pain relieved by food and/or antacids (50%) with recurrence 2 to 4 hours after a meal. Pain also recurs when hungry or stomach is empty. Self-medicating with OTC antacids. May be taking NSAIDs or aspirin. Black or tarry stools (melena), red/maroon blood in stool (hematochezia), coffee-ground emesis, or iron-deficiency anemia indicates GI bleeding.

Objective Findings

- *Abdominal exam:* Normal or mildly tender epigastric area during flare-ups
- Hemoccult can be positive if actively bleeding

Labs

- CBC (iron-deficiency anemia means bleeding) and fecal occult blood test (FOBT) are needed.
- All patients diagnosed with PUD should be tested for *H. pylori* infection.
- If positive, refer to gastroenterologist.
  - *Serology (titers): H. pylori* immunoglobulin (IgG) levels elevated. Do not use document eradication (use urea breath test or stool antigen test).
  - *Urea breath test:* Indicative of active *H. pylori* infection and is commonly used to document eradication of *H. pylori* after treatment.
  - *Stool antigen*: Can be used for screening and posttreatment to document eradication.
    - Urea breath test and stool/fecal antigen test are more sensitive for active infection than serology/titers.
  - *Gold standard:* Upper endoscopy and biopsy of gastric and/or duodenal tissue are gold-standard tests.
  - *Multiple severe ulcers:* Use fasting gastrin levels to rule out Zollinger–Ellison syndrome as needed.

Treatment Plan

Treatment for H. pylori-Negative Ulcers

- Stop use of NSAIDs. If a patient needs long-term NSAIDs, ulcer formation risk can be decreased if combined with a PPI or misoprostol.
- Encourage smoking cessation.
- Combine lifestyle changes with PPIs or H2-blockers. Duration of therapy is from 4 to 8 weeks. Treat with H2-blockers or with PPIs. If recurrent ulcers, poor response after 4 to 8 weeks of therapy, suspect bleeding ulcer, refer to GI.
- H2-blockers (or H2-antagonists):
  - Ranitidine (Zantac) 150 mg BID or 300 mg at bedtime
  - Nizatidine (Axid) 150 mg BID or 300 mg at bedtime
  - Famotidine (Pepcid) 40 mg at bedtime
- PPIs:
  - Omeprazole (Prilosec) 20 mg daily
  - Esomeprazole (Nexium) 40 mg daily
  - Lansoprazole (Prevacid 15–30 mg daily

Treatment for H. pylori-Positive Ulcers

- Triple therapy
  - Clarithromycin (Biaxin) 500 mg BID *plus* amoxicillin 1 g BID *or* metronidazole (Flagyl) 500 mg BID if allergic to amoxicillin × 14 days *plus*
  - PPI for 4 to 8 weeks to allow ulcer to heal
- Quadruple therapy
  - Bismuth subsalicylate tab 600 mg QID *plus*
  - Metronidazole tab 250 mg QID *plus*
  - Tetracycline cap 500 mg QID × 2 weeks *plus*
  - PPI for 4 to 8 weeks to allow ulcer to heal
- Sequential therapy and other "new" treatment regimens for *H. pylori* are available for clinical use, but not necessary information for the exam

EXAM TIPS

- **Determine whether question is about H. pylori-negative ulcers or H. pylori-positive ulcers. H. pylori-positive ulcers require antibiotics for 14 days.**
- **Barrett's esophagus is a precursor for esophageal cancer.**
- **Worrisome symptoms for esophageal cancer include pain on swallowing, early satiety, and weight loss.**
- **Treatment is the same as for acute diverticulitis.**
- **IBS: Increase fiber intake.**
- **Recognize UC versus CD (see discussion earlier in chapter).**
- **If patient needs treatment for GERD, start with H2-blockers; if poor relief, step up to PPIs.**
- **Know how to perform Rovsing's and Markle maneuvers. Positive tests mean acute abdomen.**
- **Positive psoas or obturator signs are caused by appendicitis.**

CLINICAL PEARLS

- **High rates of clarithromycin resistance (42%) in the United States. Avoid using clarithromycin therapy if there is high resistance in your area. Eradication rates in the United States using traditional triple therapy are now less than 80%.**
- **PPIs cure ulcers faster than H2-blockers.**

Diverticulitis

- Diverticula are small pouch-like herniations on the external surface of the colon secondary to a chronic lack of dietary fiber; higher incidence in Western societies
- Diverticulitis occurs when diverticula; high risk of rupture and bleeding; can be life-threatening
- *Hospitalize if*: Patient is elderly, has high fever, leukocytosis, comorbidities, or is immunocompromised

Classic Case

Elderly patient presents with acute onset of fever with LLQ abdominal pain with anorexia, nausea, and/or vomiting. Abdominal palpation reveals tenderness on the left lower quadrant. Hematochezia (bloody stool) and anemia if hemorrhaging.

Objective Findings

- *Acute diverticulitis:* If acute abdomen, positive for rebound, positive Rovsing's sign, and board-like abdomen, refer to ED
- *Diverticulosis:* Physical exam is normal; no palpable mass; no tenderness

Labs

- CBC with leukocytosis, neutrophilia greater than 70% and shift to the left (band forms); the presence of band forms signals severe bacterial infection; bands are immature neutrophils; refer to ED
- FOBT positive if bleeding
- Reticulocytosis if acute bleeding and low hemoglobin/hematocrit

Treatment Plan

Uncomplicated cases of diverticulitis can usually be treated in the outpatient setting. While the routine use of antibiotics in uncomplicated diverticulitis is controversial, one recommendation would be to cover for anaerobes and gram-negative organisms.

- Ciprofloxacin 500 mg BID *plus* metronidazole (Flagyl) 500 mg TID × 10 to 14 days
- Opiates should be avoided during the acute phase because they make increased intraluminal pressure and promote an ileus
- Increasing fiber intake is not recommended in the acute management of diverticulitis
- Probiotics have been used to prevent recurrences with mixed success
- Close follow-up: If no response in 48 to 72 hours or symptoms worsen (high fever, toxic), refer to ED; moderate to severe cases: hospitalize

Chronic Therapy for Diverticulosis

- High-fiber diet with fiber supplementation such as psyllium (Metamucil) or methylcellulose (Citrucel); avoiding nuts, seeds, and popcorn is not evidence based

Complications

- Abscess, perforation with peritonitis
- Ileus, sepsis, death

Acute Pancreatitis

- Acute inflammation of the pancreas secondary to many factors such as alcohol abuse, gallstones (cholelithiasis), elevated triglyceride levels, infections
- Pancreatic enzymes become activated inside pancreas, causing autodigestion
- Varies in severity from mild to life-threatening/death
- Elevated triglycerides (>800 mg/dL) at very high risk for acute pancreatitis

Classic Case

Adult patient complains of the acute onset of fever, nausea, and vomiting that is associated with rapid onset of abdominal pain that radiates to the midback, located in the epigastric region. Abdominal exam reveals guarding and tenderness over the epigastric area or the upper abdomen. Positive Cullen's and Grey–Turner's sign. May have ileus, signs and symptoms of shock. Refer patient to ED.

Objective Findings

- *Cullen's sign:* Bluish discoloration around umbilicus (hemorrhagic pancreatitis)
- *Grey–Turner's sign:* Bluish discoloration on the flank area (hemorrhagic pancreatitis)
- Hypoactive bowel sounds (ileus), jaundice, guarding, and board-like upper abdomen if peritonitis

Labs
- Elevated pancreatic enzymes such as serum amylase, lipase, and trypsin
- Elevated AST, ALT, gamma glutamyl transferase (GGT), bilirubin, leukocytosis, and other values
- Abdominal ultrasound and CT

Complications
- Multiple serious complications such as ileus, sepsis, shock, multiorgan failure, death
- May cause diabetes

Clostridium difficile Colitis
C. difficile infection is a gram-positive, spore-forming anaerobic bacillus that releases toxins that produce clinical disease. The classic symptom is watery diarrhea a few days after starting antibiotic treatment due to changes in intestinal flora caused by antibiotics. Antibiotics such as clindamycin (Cleocin), fluoroquinolones, cephalosporins, and penicillins are more likely to cause *C. difficile* infection. *C. difficile* is a gram-negative anaerobic bacteria. Most cases occur in hospitalized patients; may also occur in institutionalized patients (nursing facilities). It is spread by fecal oral contact. Alcohol-based hand sanitizer's are ineffective against *C. difficile.*

Classic Case
Severe watery diarrhea from 10 to 15 stools a day accompanied by lower abdominal pain with cramping and fever. Patient is currently on antibiotics or recently completed a course of antibiotics. Symptoms usually appear within 5 to 10 days after initiation of antibiotics.

Labs
- Polymerase chain reaction (PCR)-based testing is preferred for identification of *C. difficile*. It is rapid, highly sensitive, and highly specific.
- CBC with leukocytosis (>15,000 cells/µL)
- Stool assay (by enzyme-linked immunosorbent assay) for *C. difficile* toxins
- Repeat testing during this same episode of diarrhea is not recommended because infective agents, such as parasites, can persist for 3 to 6 weeks after treatment. Testing and treatment of asymptomatic patients is not recommended.

Treatment (for nonsevere disease)
- Metronidazole (Flagyl) TID for 10 to 14 days
- Avoid antimotility agents (loperamide) or opiates because they can worsen and prolong disorder
- Probiotic use is controversial
- Increase fluid intake; eat food as tolerated

HEPATITIS

Hepatitis Serology

IgG Anti-HAV (Hepatitis A Antibody IgG Type)-Positive
- Antibodies present (immune)
- No virus present and not infectious
- *How:* History of native hepatitis A infection or vaccination with hepatitis A vaccine (Havrix)

IgM Anti-HAV (Hepatitis A Antibody IgM Type)-Positive

- Acute infection; patient is contagious
- Hepatitis A virus still present (infectious); no immunity yet

HBsAg (Hepatitis B Surface Antigen)

- Screening test for hepatitis B
- If positive, patient has the virus and is infectious
- *How:* Presence of antigen means either an acute infection or chronic hepatitis B infection

Anti-HBs (Hepatitis B Surface Antibody)-Positive

- Antibodies present and is immune
- Presence may be due to either a past infection or vaccination with hepatitis B vaccine

HbeAg (Hepatitis B "e" Antigen)

- Indicates active viral replication; may be highly infectious
- Persistence of the "e" antigen indicates chronic hepatitis B

Chronic Hepatitis Infection: Two Types

- Chronic infection with mildly elevated LFTs
- Chronic and active infection with elevated LFTs (active viral replication)
- Patient is at higher risk for cirrhosis, liver failure, and liver cancer

Anti-HCV (Antibody Hepatitis C Virus)

- Screening test for hepatitis C
- Up to 85% of cases become carriers
- Unlike hepatitis A and B, a positive anti-HCV (antibody) does not always mean that the patient has recovered from the infection and has developed immunity; it may instead indicate current infection because up to 85% of cases become carriers
- If this test is positive:
  - Order HCV RNA or HCV polymerase chain reaction (PCR) to rule out chronic infection
  - If positive, then patient has hepatitis C; refer to GI specialist for liver biopsy/treatment

Hepatitis D (Delta Virus)

- Requires the presence of hepatitis B to get the infection; can be an acute or a chronic infection
- Infection with both hepatitis B and hepatitis D increases the risk of fulminant hepatitis, cirrhosis, and severe liver damage; low prevalence in the United States

Liver Function Tests (LFTs)

Aspartate Aminotransferase (AST)

- Also known as *serum glutamic oxaloacetic transaminase (SGOT)*
- *Normal:* 0 to 45 mg/dL
- Present in the liver, heart muscle, skeletal muscle, kidney, and lung
- Not specific for liver injury because it is elevated in other conditions (e.g., acute myocardial infarction)

Alanine Aminotransferase (ALT)

- Also known as *serum glutamic pyruvic transaminase (SGPT)*
- *Normal:* 0 to 40 mg/dL
- Found mainly in the liver; a positive finding indicates liver inflammation
- More specific for hepatic inflammation than AST

AST/ALT Ratio (or SGOT/SGPT Ratio)

- A ratio of 2.0 or higher may be indicative of alcohol abuse

Serum GGT

- Sensitive indicator of alcohol abuse. May be a "lone" elevation
- Level is elevated in liver disease and acute pancreatitis

Alkaline Phosphatase

- Enzyme derived from bone, liver, gallbladder, kidneys, GI tract, and placenta
- Higher levels seen during growth spurts (bones) in children and teens
- Also may be elevated with healing fractures, osteomalacia, bone malignancy, vitamin D deficiency, and others

Viral Hepatitis

Hepatitis A, B, and C

Hepatitis A

- No chronic or carrier state exists for hepatitis A
- *Transmission:* Transmitted via fecal and oral route from contaminated food or drink
- Self-limiting infection; treatment is symptomatic; vaccine available (Havrix) and recommended for travelers to areas where hepatitis A is endemic
- Hepatitis A is reportable to the public health department
- Advise patients to avoid use of oral contraceptive pills and hormone replacement therapy to avoid cholestasis; avoid alcohol use
- Avoid working in food-related jobs for 1 week after onset of infection

Hepatitis B

- *Transmission:* Transmitted via sexual activity (semen, vaginal secretions, and saliva), blood, blood products, organs
- Vertical transmission occurs from mother to infant; hepatitis B can either be acute and self-limiting or it can be a chronic infection
- *Treatment:* First-line agents for treatment of hepatitis B include pegylated interferon alfa (PEG-IFN-a), entecavir (ETV), and tenofovir disoproxil fumarate (TDF)

Hepatitis C

- *Transmission:* Transmitted via sharing needles, blood transfusions before 1992, mother to infant (vertical transmission), needle-stick injuries in health care settings. Less common, spread by sexual contact, sharing personal items (razors or toothbrushes).
- Approximately 75% to 85% of people who become infected with hepatitis C will develop chronic infection. The disease is the most common cause of liver cancer and liver transplantation in the United States.
- *High-risk groups:* Intravenous drug users, hemophiliacs, or anyone with history of frequent transfusions, or persons born between 1945 and 1965 are at risk.
  - The Centers for Disease Control and Prevention (CDC) recommends screening (at least once) adults born from 1945 through 1965.

- Hepatitis C has the highest risk of chronic hepatitis infection and cirrhosis (30%). Cirrhosis markedly increases the risk of liver cancer or liver failure. Refer to GI for management.
- Advise patient not to share razors, toothbrushes, and nail clippers and to cover cuts and sores.
- Report acute cases of hepatitis C to the health department.
- *Treatment:* Administer antivirals such as ledipasvir-sofosbuvir (Harvoni), ribavirin, and pegylated interferon alpha-2a/2b. Use liver biopsy to stage disease.

Acute Hepatitis

An acute liver inflammation with multiple causes. Examples include viral infection, hepatotoxic drugs (i.e., statins), excessive alcohol intake, and toxins.

Classic Case

Sexually active adult complains of a new onset of fatigue, nausea, and dark-colored urine for several days. New sexual partner (<3 months).

Objective Findings

- Skin and sclera have a yellow tinge (jaundiced or icteric)
- *Liver:* Tenderness over the liver occurs with percussion and deep palpation

Labs

- *ALT and AST:* Levels are elevated up to 10× normal during the acute phase of the illness
- Other LFTs, such as the serum bilirubin and gamma glutamyl transpeptidase (GGT); these may be elevated

Treatment Plan

Remove and treat the cause (if possible). Avoid hepatotoxic agents such as alcoholic drinks, acetaminophen, and statins (e.g., pravastatin or Pravachol). Treatment is supportive.

Case Studies for Viral Hepatitis

Patient A

- HBsAg: negative
- Anti-HBs: positive
- HBeAg: negative
- *Results:* Patient A indicative of either:
  - History of old hepatitis B infection; has antibodies for hepatitis B (anti-HBs positive) or history of vaccination against hepatitis B
  - Not a carrier of hepatitis B (HBeAg negative, HBsAg negative)

Patient B

- HBsAg: positive
- HBeAg: positive
- Anti-HBs: negative
- Anti-HAV: positive
- Anti-HCV: negative
- *Results:* Patient B indicative of:
  - Current hepatitis B infection (HBsAg positive)
  - Chronic carrier of hepatitis B (both HBsAg and HBeAg are positive)

  - Presence of antibodies to hepatitis A (anti-HAV); patient either had a previous hepatitis A infection or received the hepatitis A vaccine
- This patient is a carrier of the hepatitis B virus; if the HBeAg is positive, it means that the patient is highly contagious

EXAM TIPS

- There will be a serology question (as just shown). You will have to figure out what type of viral hepatitis the patient has (A, B, or C). It is usually hepatitis B. HBsAg-positive status always means an infected patient (new infection or chronic).
- PCR tests are not antibody tests. They test for presence of viral RNA. A positive result means that the virus is present. This test can be performed for diagnosing disease such as hepatitis C or HIV.
- Hepatitis C has highest risk of cirrhosis and liver cancer.
- Screening test for hepatitis C virus is called the HCV antibody (HCV Ab). If positive, next step is to order HCV RNA test. If positive, patient has hepatitis C.
- GGT is elevated in liver disease and biliary obstruction. A "lone" elevation in the GGT is a sensitive indicator of possible alcoholism.
- Alkaline phosphatase (ALP) is normally elevated during the teen years due to bone growth. The ALP may also be elevated in bone disorders such as vitamin D deficiency, Paget's disease, and bone cancer. A GGT, which would be elevated with liver disease, may be drawn to differentiate between liver disease and bone disorders.
- A person must have hepatitis B to become infected with hepatitis D. Hepatitis D requires the hepatitis B helper cells to replicate and become active. There is no vaccine for hepatitis D, but hepatitis B vaccination will prevent acquisition of hepatitis D.
- ALT is more sensitive to liver damage than AST. AST is also found in other organs such as the heart and skeletal system. AST and ALT may be elevated and may reflect acute liver injury or inflammation. However, these levels may be normal in chronic liver disease, such as cirrhosis.
- Be aware of GERD management and treatment.
- Acute pancreatitis symptoms: Amylase and lipase are sensitive tests used for pancreatic inflammation (pancreatitis).

11

Renal System Review

DANGER SIGNALS

Acute Pyelonephritis

Patient presents with acute onset of high fever, chills, nausea/vomiting, dysuria, frequency, and unilateral flank pain. The flank pain is described as a deep ache. May complain of nausea (with/without vomiting). May have recent history of urinary tract infection (UTI). Indications for hospitalization include inability to maintain oral hydration, persistently high fever (>101 F/ >38.4 C), toxic appearance, immune-compromised, or suspect noncompliance to treatment.

Acute Kidney Injury (Acute Renal Failure)

Patient presents with the abrupt onset of oliguria, edema, and weight gain (fluid retention). Complains of lethargy, nausea, and loss of appetite.

Rapid decrease in renal function. Elevated serum creatinine. During the early stages, the serum creatinine and the estimated glomerular filtration rate (eGFR) may not accurately reflect true renal function. Most cases of acute kidney injury (acute decline of GFR) are usually reversible.

Bladder Cancer

Elderly male patient (median age at diagnosis: 73 years), a smoker, presents with painless hematuria. The hematuria can be microscopic or gross (urine pink to reddish color). Some patients only notice a problem after they see a blood-tinged stain on underwear (males, menopausal females). The hematuria may only appear at the end of voiding. May have irritative voiding symptoms (dysuria, frequency, nocturia) that are not related to a UTI. Order a UA, urine C&S, and urine for cytology. Patients who have advanced disease with metastases may complain of lower abdominal or pelvic pain, perineal pain, low-back pain, or bone pain.

NORMAL FINDINGS

Kidneys

The kidneys are located in the retroperitoneal area. The right kidney is lower than the left kidney because of displacement by the liver. The basic functional units of the kidney are the nephrons, which contain the glomeruli.

Function

Kidneys are the body's regulators of electrolytes and fluids. Water is reabsorbed back into the body by the action of antidiuretic hormone and aldosterone. Kidneys excrete water-soluble waste products of metabolism (i.e., creatinine, urea, uric acid) into the urine. They also produce the hormone erythropoietin, which stimulates bone marrow into producing more RBCs. The average daily urine output is 1,500 mL. *Oliguria* is defined as a urinary output of less than 400 mL per day (adults). Kidneys also secrete several hormones such as erythropoietin (RBC production), renin and bradykinin (blood pressure), prostaglandins (renal perfusion), and calcitriol/vitamin D_3 (bone).

LABORATORY TESTING

Serum Creatinine

- *Male:* 0.7 to 1.3 mg/dL
- *Female:* 0.6 to 1.1 mg/dL

When renal function decreases, the creatinine level will increase. Creatinine is the end-product of creatine metabolism, which comes mostly from muscle. Serum creatinine may be falsely decreased in people with low muscle volume (elderly). Elevated values are seen with renal damage or failure, nephrotoxic drugs, etc. Factors that affect the serum creatinine are gender (males have higher levels), race (African Americans have more muscle mass), and muscle mass.

Creatinine Clearance (24-Hour Urine)

When renal function decreases, the creatinine clearance also decreases. This test is ordered to evaluate patients with proteinuria, albuminuria, and microalbuminuria. It is a more sensitive test than the serum creatinine alone because it reflects the renal function within a 24-hour period. Creatinine clearance is relatively constant and is not affected by fluid status, diet, or exercise. Creatinine clearance is doubled for every 50% reduction of the GFR. Exercise should be avoided immediately prior to and during the period of specimen collection.

Estimated Glomerular Filtration Rate (eGFR)

- *Normal:* eGFR greater than 90 mL/min
- *Renal failure:* eGFR less than 15 mL/min (stage 5 chronic kidney disease)

The eGFR is the number derived by using the serum creatinine in a prediction equation (i.e., Cockcroft–Gault). The more damaged the kidneys, the lower the eGFR value. The GFR is the amount of fluid filtered by the glomerulus within a certain unit of time. It is used to evaluate renal function and to stage chronic kidney disease.

- Best if patient does not eat cooked meat 12 hours before the blood test
- GFR is less reliable (interpret with care): Drastic increase/reduction muscle mass (bodybuilders, amputees, wasting disorders), pregnancy, and acute renal failure

Blood Urea Nitrogen (BUN)

Among patients with heart failure, lower GFR with higher BUN is associated with higher mortality. The BUN is not as sensitive as the serum creatinine or the GFR. A high BUN may be caused by acute renal failure, high-protein diet, hemolysis, congestive heart failure, or drugs. Low BUN can be caused by liver damage or liver disease. If a patient has an abnormal BUN level, check the eGFR. If the eGFR is normal, the renal function is probably normal. The BUN is a measure of the kidney's ability to excrete urea (waste product of protein metabolism).

BUN-to-Creatinine Ratio

The ratio between the BUN and serum creatinine (BUN:Cr). It is used to help evaluate dehydration, hypovolemia, acute renal failure, and it is useful for classifying the type of renal failure (renal, infrarenal, or postrenal).

Urinalysis (UA)

Epithelial Cells

- Large amounts of squamous epithelial cells in a urine sample indicate contamination.
- A few epithelial cells are considered normal. (Squamous epithelial cells are associated with the external urethra and transitional epithelial cells, the bladder.)

Leukocytes

- Normal WBCs in urine: less than or equal to 10 WBCs/mL
- Called *leukocyte esterase test* with dipstick strips
- Presence of leukocytes in urine (pyuria) is always abnormal in males (infection)
- UA is a more sensitive test for infection in males than females

Urine for Culture and Sensitivity

- Greater than or equal to 10^5 colony-forming units (CFU)/mL of bacteria of one dominant bacteria (usually *Escherichia coli*) are indicative of a UTI
- If multiple bacteria are present, it is considered a contaminated sample
- Lower values are indicative of bacteriuria

Red Blood Cells

- Few RBCs (<5 cells) is considered normal
- Hematuria is seen with kidney stones, pyelonephritis, and sometimes in cystitis
- Can be contaminated by menses or hemorrhoids

Protein

- Indicates kidney damage (chronic kidney disease)
- May be present in acute pyelonephritis (resolves after treatment)
- Urine dipsticks detect only albumin, not microalbumin (Bence-Jones proteins)
- Order 24-hour urine for protein and creatinine clearance

Nitrites

- Indicative of probable infection with *E. coli*
- Due to breakdown of nitrates to nitrites by certain bacteria (*E. coli, Klebsiella, Proteus, Enterobacter, Citrobacter, Pseudomonas*).

Casts

- Casts are shaped like cylinders because they are formed in the renal tubules
- Hyaline casts are "normal" and may be seen in concentrated urine and after strenuous exercise
- WBC cast may be seen with infections (UTI, pyelonephritis)
- RBC casts and proteinuria are diagnostic of glomerulonephritis

Ph

- (4.6–8.0 reference range) Useful in the evaluation of kidney stones and infections. Citrus and low carbohydrate diet are associated with lower acidity and high protein diet is associated with higher acidity.

DISEASE REVIEW

Hematuria

Microscopic hematuria is revealed by a positive urine dipstick for heme or by microscopic UA (presence of three to five RBCs or more per high-power field). It can be transient or persistent. Suspect gross (or visible) hematuria if color of urine is pink, red, or brown or blood clots are present. If dipstick is heme positive, next step is to order a microscopic UA. If infection is suspected, order urine for C&S. If malignancy is suspected, send urine for cytology. Risk factors for urothelial or renal malignancy are age older than 50 years, male, smoker, and gross hematuria.

Asymptomatic Bacteriuria

No antibiotic treatment is recommended for patients with Foley catheters, suprapubic, or condom catheters (chronic or intermittent), the elderly (institutionalized), and those with spinal cord injury. Defined as urine culture growth of 100,000 CFU/mL or more. Symptomatic bacteriuria (leukocytosis, fever, chills, malaise) is treated as a UTI. Always treat pregnant women with antibiotics (up to 30% risk of pyelonephritis).

Urinary Tract Infections

Cystitis (urinary bladder inflammation) can be uncomplicated, recurrent, a reinfection, or relapse. The majority of infections are caused by *E. coli* (75%–95%). Other causal agents are *Staphylococcus saprophyticus, Proteus mirabilis*, and *Klebsiella pneumoniae*. UTIs in children younger than age 3 and pregnant women (20%–40% chance) are more likely to progress to pyelonephritis.

- *Infancy*: UTIs are common in boys (usually due to anatomical abnormality)
- *Children*: UTIs in children need further evaluation. May indicate vesicoureteral reflux or even possible sexual abuse.
- *Females:* Highest incidence is during the reproductive-age years

Risk Factors

- Female gender; pregnancy
- History of a recent UTI or history of recurrent infections
- Diabetes mellitus (or immunocompromised status)
- Failure to void after sex or increased sexual intercourse (i.e., honeymoon bladder)
- Spermicide use within past year (alone or with diaphragm)
- Other risk factors: Infected renal calculi, low fluid intake, poor hygiene, catheterization

Classic Case

A sexually active female complains of new onset of dysuria, frequency, frequent urge to urinate, and nocturia. May also complain of suprapubic discomfort. Not associated with fever. Urine dipstick will show a moderate to large number of leukocytes and will be positive for nitrites. May show a few RBCs (due to inflammation), and be negative for ketones (unless fasting), and protein.

Labs

- UA dipstick (midstream sample): Leukocyte positive (WBCs ≥10/mcL)
- Nitrites: Negative or positive (*E. coli* converts urinary nitrate to nitrite)
- Sometimes: Hematuria (>5 RBCs) and/or a few WBC casts
- Urine C&S: Definitions
  - *UTI infection*: 100,000 CFU/mL (or 10^5 CFU/mL) with pyuria
  - *Multiple bacteria*: Contaminated sample
  - *Bacteriuria* (with or without indwelling catheter): More than 100,000 CFU/mL
- Urinary casts (tubular-shaped structures)
  - *RBC casts*: Microscopic bleeding in the glomeruli; suspect glomerulonephritis (accompanied by edema, weight gain, dark cola-colored urine or hypertension)
  - *WBC casts*: Due to inflammation; rule out pyelonephritis, interstitial nephritis

Medications

Uncomplicated UTIs

- Healthy female patients aged 18 years to 65 years can have the "3-day" treatment regimen (these agents are used for 5–7 days for complicated UTIs). Routine urine C&S before and after treatment is not recommended for this population.
  - Trimethoprim–sulfamethoxazole (Bactrim, Septra) BID × 3 days
  - Bacterial resistance greater than 20% or sulfa-allergic: Nitrofurantoin BID × 5 days, or Fosfomycin 3 g × one dose or Augmentin 875/125 mg BID × 5 to 7 days
  - Alternatives: Ciprofloxacin (Cipro) BID or levofloxacin (Levaquin) daily (age 18 years or older) × 3 days
  - Phenazopyridine (Pyridium) by mouth BID × 2 days PRN (as Uristat, AZO); pyridium will turn urine an orange/yellow color; will stain contact lenses; avoid if liver or renal disease, glucose-6-phosphate dehydrogenase (G6PD) anemia
  - Increase fluid intake to more than 2.5 L/d (except if heart failure); restrict dietary oxalate; high oxalate foods are beans, spinach, beets, potato chips, french fries, nuts, tea

Note

If clinical symptoms persist 48 to 72 hours after initiating antibiotics, order urine C&S and UA. Rule out pyelonephritis. Switch to another antibiotic drug class and treat for 7 to 10 days.

Complicated UTIs

- Must treat these patients for a minimum of 7 days or longer
  - Males
  - Poorly controlled diabetes
  - Pregnant women
  - Children or elderly
  - Immunocompromised (chronic high-dosed steroids, biologics, HIV infection)
  - Recurrent UTIs or reinfections
  - Anatomical abnormalities (including kidney stones, reflux, obstruction)
- Treatment regimens
  - Ciprofloxacin (Cipro) 500 mg BID or levofloxacin 750 mg once a day for 7 to 10 days
  - Trimethoprim–sulfamethoxazole (Bactrim, Septra) BID or cefixime (Suprax) 400 mg BID for 7 to 10 days
  - *Postcoital UTIs*: Bactrim or Bactrim DS one tablet after sex (or low-dose nitrofurantoin, Cipro, Keflex); increase fluids before and after sex
  - Antimicrobial prophylaxis (recurrent UTI): Bactrim one tablet at HS
  - *Sulfa allergy*: Cephalexin (Keflex), Ceclor, Cipro (older than 18 years); consider prophylactic antibiotics for 6 months or longer (after ruling out pathology)

Labs

- UA and urine C&S before and after treatment (to document resolution)
- *UTIs*: Special categories

Males

- UTIs are never "normal" in males. Rule out ureteral stricture, infected kidney stones, anatomical abnormality, acute prostatitis, sexually transmitted diseases, and so forth. Must be evaluated further. Refer to urologist.

Recurrent UTIs (in Women)

- Three or more UTIs in 1 year or two infections within 6 months; never normal in males
- *Rule out urological abnormality*: Infected stones, reflux, fistulas, ureteral stenosis, and so forth are abnormalities

Note

Long-term use of nitrofurantoin is associated with lung problems, chronic hepatitis, and neuropathy. Nitrofurantoin is contraindicated with renal insufficiency. Baseline chest x-ray, liver function tests, and neurological exam should be obtained and patients monitored closely.

Acute Pyelonephritis

Acute bacterial infection of the kidney(s) is most commonly due to gram-negative bacteria such as *E. coli* (75%–95%), *P. mirabilis*, and *K. pneumoniae* (gram-negative anaerobe). Outpatient treatment is only for milder cases that are uncomplicated (immunocompetent adult female with normal urinary/renal systems without comorbidities) and for compliant patients.

Classic Case

Adult patient presents with acute onset of high fever, chills, nausea/vomiting, and one-sided flank pain. Some patients may also have symptoms of cystitis such as dysuria, frequency, and urgency.

Physical Exam

- Temperature equal or greater than 38°C (100.4°F)
- Costovertebral angle tenderness on one kidney
- *UA*: Large amount of leukocytes, hematuria, WBC casts, and mild proteinuria
- *Urine C&S*: Presence of 10^5 CFU/mL of one organism
- *CBC*: Leukocytosis (WBC >11,000/mcL), neutrophilia (>80%) with shift to the left
- *Shift to the left*: Presence of bands or stabs (immature neutrophils) means serious infection
- Chemistry profile (serum creatinine, others)

Treatment Plan

- May treat mild uncomplicated cases as outpatients with close follow-up (or refer to urology). For moderate to severe (or complicated) cases, hospitalization is required.
- Outpatient treatment for young, healthy adults may include a fluoroquinolone.
- Ceftriaxone (Rocephin) 1 g intramuscular injection (one dose) during office visit may be given if fluoroquinolone resistance suspected (>10%), or susceptibility unknown.
- Treat with ciprofloxacin (Cipro) BID × 7 days or levofloxacin (Levaquin) daily × 7 days.
- Second-line treatment: Use amoxicillin–clavulanate (Augmentin) BID × 14 days. Trimethoprim–sulfamethoxazole (Bactrim, Septra) BID × 14 days (use only if bacteria is known to be susceptible).
- Close follow-up needed for 12 to 24 hours
- Coexisting condition that compromises immune system or is toxic: Refer or hospitalize.
- *Refer*: Pregnant women, children/elderly, anatomical abnormalities, diabetics, others should be referred to a physician for treatment.
  - Fluoroquinolones and aminoglycosides are contraindicated in pregnancy.
- *Complications*: Gram-negative septicemia, shock, renal failure are complications of pyelonephritis.

Nephrolithiasis (Urolithiasis)

The majority of kidney stones are made up of calcium oxalate (70%–80%). The location and the size of the stone determine the pain. For example, stones located in the upper urethra or renal pelvis cause flank pain and tenderness, whereas stones on the lower urethra cause pain that radiates to the testicle or the labia of the vagina. Both can cause abdominal pain.

Risk Factors

- Family history of stones, low fluid intake, gout
- Bariatric surgery (excrete higher levels of oxalate)

Classic Case

Adult with acute onset of severe colicky flank pain on one side that comes in waves. When the pain is most severe, the patient cannot stay still and may stand and walk. The pain builds in intensity, then lessens and disappears (until the stone moves again). Painful episodes may last from 20 to 60 minutes. For some, the pain can be extreme and associated with nausea and vomiting. Majority have gross or microscopic hematuria. Majority (50%) will pass stone within 48 hours. Patient should be asked about history of previous episodes, high-protein diet, gout, gastric bypass, high-dose vitamin C.

Labs

- Instruct patient to strain urine for several days and to bring kidney stone to office (if passed) for analysis by laboratory
- Order renal ultrasound to determine location and stone size
- UA needed until the episode resolves
- Refer to urology: Large stone, inability to pass stone, acute renal failure
- Refer to ED: High fever (possible urosepsis), extreme pain, acute renal failure
- Pregnant women who present with abdominal pain should be evaluated for an ectopic pregnancy, abruptio placentae, preterm labor, cholilithiasis, and kidney stones

Diet

- Increase fluid intake up to 2 L/d (if tolerated); if calcium oxalate stones, dietary modifications should be advised
- Avoid high-oxalate foods such as rhubarb, spinach, beets, chocolate, tea, and meats

EXAM TIPS

- **Memorize definition of UTI (>100,000 CFU/mL of one organism).**
- **Recognize classic case of UTI and acute pyelonephritis, and be able to distinguish between the two.**
- **Healthy women diagnosed with uncomplicated UTIs may be treated using a 3-day treatment plan.**
- **Become familiar with UA results of UTIs.**
- **Pyelonephritis may be treated with a shortened 7-day course of antibiotics when using fluoroquinolones such as ciprofloxacin (Cipro) and levofloxacin (Levaquin).**
- **WBC casts with proteinuria are associated with pyelonephritis.**
- **Serum creatinine is a better measure of renal function than the BUN or BUN:Cr ratio. But the eGFR is considered the best measure of renal function in primary care.**
- **Right kidney sits lower than the left kidney because of displacement by the liver.**
- **Large numbers of squamous epithelial cells in the urine sample mean contamination.**
- **Memorize the normal WBC count (10.5) and the neutrophil or segs (segmented neutrophils; >80%).**

- Neutrophils make up from 50% to 75% of all the WBCs in a sample.
- Presence of band or stabs (immature WBCs) in CBC is indicative of a serious bacterial infection.
- Use of spermicides can increase the risk of UTIs in females.

CLINICAL PEARLS

- A study showed that some women with the classic symptoms of acute UTI may have lower counts of bacteria (<10,000 CFU/mL). Of these women, 88% had a UTI.
- Avoid long-term use of nitrofurantoin, if possible (associated with lung problems, chronic hepatitis, and neuropathy).
- Serum potassium should be monitored upon initiation of angiotensin-converting enzyme inhibitor or angiotensin receptor blocker therapy if the patient has kidney disease. Potassium levels may initially rise and then taper off in 2 to 3 months. Continued monitoring of serum potassium is recommended.
- Patients with preexisting kidney disease and/or diabetes are at higher risk of kidney damage from contrast media. CT, MRI, and angiogram contrast media may damage kidneys (2%) or cause nephrogenic systemic fibrosis.
- Imaging test with the highest sensitivity/specificity for kidney stones is noncontrast CT scan (initial imaging is renal ultrasonography).

12

Nervous System Review

DISEASE REVIEW

Dangerous Headaches

- Abrupt onset of severe headache ("thunderclap" headache)
- "Worst headache of my life"
- First onset of headache at age 50 years
- Sudden onset of headache after coughing, exertion, straining, or sex (exertional headache)
- Sudden change in level of consciousness
- Focal neurological signs (such as unequal pupil size)
- Headache with papilledema (increased intracranial pressure [ICP] secondary to any of those listed here)
- "Worse-case" scenario of headaches (rule out) includes the following:
    - Subarachnoid hemorrhage or acute subdural hemorrhage
    - Leaking aneurysm
    - Bacterial meningitis
    - Increased ICP
    - Brain abscess
    - Brain tumor

Acute Bacterial Meningitis

Acute onset of high fever, severe headache, and stiff neck and meningismus. Meningococcal disease (discussed in "Danger Signals" section in Chapter 6). Classic purple-colored petechial rashes appear. Accompanied by nausea, vomiting, and photophobia. Rapid worsening of symptoms progressing to lethargy, confusion, and finally coma. If not treated, fatal. Bacterial meningitis is a reportable disease.

Temporal Arteritis (Giant Cell Arteritis)

Acute onset of headache that is located on one temple on an older patient. The affected temple has an indurated, reddened, and cord-like temporal artery (tender to touch) that is accompanied by scalp tenderness. Abrupt onset of visual disturbances and/or transient blindness of affected eye (amaurosis fugax). Some may complain of jaw pain or jaw claudication (caused by artery obstruction). Markedly elevated sedimentation rate (ESR) and C-reactive protein (CRP). Patients with polymyalgia rheumatica are at very high risk of developing temporal arteritis (up to 30%). If untreated, temporal arteritis will lead to blindness.

Acute/Narrow Angle-Closure Glaucoma

Acute onset of headaches behind an eye or around one eye accompanied by eye pain, blurred vision (like looking through a steamed window), and nausea and/or vomiting. The cornea looks hazy and the affected pupil is dilated midway. More common in older adults. Refer to emergency department (ED).

Stroke (Cerebrovascular Accident; CVA)

Classified as either embolic (80%) or hemorrhagic (20%). A patient who has risk factor(s) for embolization (i.e., atrial fibrillation, prolonged immobilization) presents with acute onset of stuttering/speech disturbance, one-sided facial weakness, and weakness of the arms and/or legs (hemiparesis). Patients who have hemorrhagic stroke often have poorly controlled hypertension and present with the abrupt onset of a severe headache, nausea/vomiting, and nuchal rigidity (subarachnoid bleed). Call 911.

Chronic Subdural Hematoma (SDH)

Chronic SDH presents gradually and symptoms may not show until a few weeks after the injury. Patient with a history of head trauma (falls, accidents) presents with a history of headaches and gradual cognitive impairment (apathy, somnolence, confusion). More common in alcoholics, the elderly, and those who are on anticoagulation or aspirin therapy. The area of bleeding is between the dura and subarachnoid membranes of the brain.

Subarachnoid Hemorrhage (SAH)

Sudden onset of severe headache described as "the worst headache of my life" accompanied by photophobia, nausea/vomiting, meningeal irritation (stiff neck, positive Brudzinski and Kernig signs) with a rapid decline in level of consciousness. Patient may have a period of brief lucidity followed by coma (sometimes referred to as a "talk and die" bleed). In the elderly, the most common cause is head trauma during a fall; among younger patients, it is motor vehicle accidents. Some suffer a "sentinel headache" or the sudden onset of a severe headache (caused by a minor leak) that resolves before the major hemorrhage happens. Sentinel headaches can occur from a few days up to 20 days before the event. Call 911.

NEUROLOGICAL TESTING

Neurological Exam

Mental Status (Frontal Lobes)

- Mini-Mental State Exam (MMSE)
- Cranial nerve exam

MMSE

- Orientation (name, age, address, job, time/date/season)
- Registration (Recite three unrelated words. Distract patient for 5 minutes, then ask the patient to repeat the words.)
- Attention and calculation
- Spell "world" backward or indicate serial 7s (subtract 7 starting at 100)
- Language
- While speaking to patient, look for aphasia (impairment in language resulting in difficulty speaking)

Cerebellar System

- *Romberg test*: Tell patient to stand with arms/hands straight on each side and with the feet together, then instruct patient to close both eyes while standing in the same position and observe
  - *Positive:* Test is positive if excessive swaying, patient falls down, keeps feet far apart to maintain balance
  - Next tell patient to hold arms straight forward and close eyes, then observe
- *Tandem gait*: Tell patient to walk a straight line in normal gait, then instruct patient to walk in a straight line with one foot in front of the other
  - *Positive:* Test is positive if patient is unable to perform tandem walking, loses balance, and falls

Cerebellar Testing

Coordination (Diadochokinesia)

- *Rapid alternative movements:* Tell patient to place lower arms on top of each thigh and to move them by alternating between supination and pronation positions.
- *Heel-to-shin testing:* Patient is in a supine position with extended legs. Tell patient to place the left heel on the right knee and then move it down the shin (repeat with right heel on left knee).

Sensory System (Tell Patient to Close Eyes for These Tests)

- *Vibration sense*: Use 128-Hz tuning fork and tap lightly, then place one end into the distal joint of each thumb. Patient should have eyes closed.
- *Sharp–dull touch*: Use the sharp end of a safety pin for sharp touch and the other end for dull.
- *Temperature*: Test the ability to differentiate hot or cold.

Stereognosis (Ability to Recognize Familiar Object Through Sense of Touch Only)

- Place a familiar object (i.e., coin, key, pen) on the patient's palm and tell the patient to identify the object with the eyes closed.

Graphesthesia (Ability to Identify Figures "Written" on Skin)

- "Write" a large letter or number on the patient's palms using fingers (patient's eyes are closed).

Motor Exam

- *Gait*: Observe the patient's "normal gait." Check quadriceps and other leg muscles for atrophy.
- Pronator drift test:
  - Have patient stretch out the arms with palms facing up, then close eyes.
  - Wait for 5 to 10 seconds. Test is positive if one arm goes downward or drifts.
- Gross (legs) and fine motor movements (hands). Test walking, using hands for manipulation/pincer grasp, jumping, and so forth.

Reflexes

- Both sides should be compared to each other and should be equal.

Grading Reflexes

0	No response
1+	Low response
2+	Normal or average response
3+	Brisker than average
4+	Very brisk response (sustained clonus)

Reflex Testing

Quadriceps Reflex (Knee-Jerk Response)

- Reflex center at L2 to L4. Tap patellar tendon briskly on each side.

Achilles Reflex (Ankle-Jerk Response)

- Reflex center at L5 to S2 (tibial nerve). With patient's legs dangling off the exam table, hold the foot in slight dorsiflexion and briskly tap the Achilles tendon.

Plantar Reflex (Babinski's Sign)

- Reflex center L4 to S2. Stroke plantar surface of foot on the lateral border from heel toward the big toe (plantar flexion is normal response). Babinski's sign is positive if toes spread like a fan. Adults should have a negative Babinski sign.

NEUROLOGICAL MANEUVERS

These tests are used to assess for meningeal irritation. All of these tests are done with the patient in a supine position. In general, these are more sensitive tests in children compared with adults.

Kernig's Sign

- Flex patient's hips one at a time, then attempt to straighten the leg while keeping the hip flexed at 90 degrees.
- *Positive*: There is resistance to leg straightening because of painful hamstrings (due to inflammation on lumbar nerve roots) and/or complaints of back pain.

Brudzinski's Sign (Figure 12.1)

- Passively flex/bend the patient's neck toward the chest.
- *Positive*: Patient reflexively flexes the hips and knee to relieve pressure and pain (due to inflammation of lumbar nerve roots).

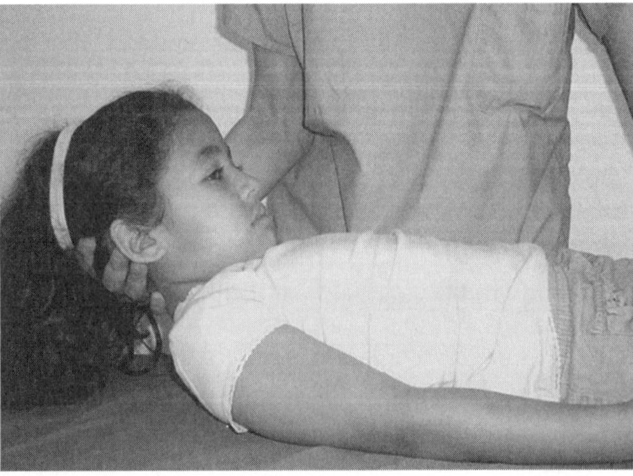

Figure 12.1 Brudzinski's test.

Nuchal Rigidity

- Tell patient to touch chest with the chin. Inability to touch the chest secondary to pain is a positive finding.

Cranial Nerve (CN) Testing

- *Mnemonic*: "On Old Olympus Towering Tops, A Finn and German Viewed Some Hops." The first letter stands for the name of the cranial nerve. The word order corresponds to the sequential numbering of the cranial nerves.
  CN I: On (olfactory)
  CN II: Old (optic)
  CN III: Olympus (oculomotor)
  CN IV: Towering (trochlear)
  CN V: Tops (trigeminal)
  CN VI: A (abducens)
  CN VII: Finn (facial)
  CN VIII: And (acoustic)
  CN IX: German (glossopharyngeal)
  CN X: Viewed (vagus)
  CN XI: Some (spinal accessory)
  CN XII: Hops (hypoglossal)

EXAM TIPS

- Memorization tips on cranial nerves:
  CN I: You have one nose.
  CN II: You have two eyes.
  CN VIII: The number 8 stands for two ears sitting on top of each other.
  CN XI: The number reminds you of the shoulders shrugging together.
- Because cranial nerves are listed only by number on the test (not by name), the correct chronological order is important. Memorize the mnemonic to guide you.
- Herpes zoster infection (shingles) of CN V ophthalmic branch can result in corneal blindness.
- Rash at tip of nose and the temple area: Rule out shingles infection of the trigeminal nerve.
- CNs are listed by number only.

DISEASE REVIEW

Acute Bacterial Meningitis

- A serious acute bacterial infection of the leptomeninges that cover the brain and the spinal cord.
- The most common pathogens in adults are *Streptococcus pneumoniae, Neisseria meningitides,* and *Haemophilus influenzae* (the latter two are gram negative).
- Bacterial meningitis is a reportable disease (local health department).

Classic Case

Acute onset of high fever, severe headache, stiff neck (nuchal rigidity), and rapid changes in mental status and level of consciousness (LOC). Up to 78% of patients have mental status changes (confusion, lethargy, stupor). Other symptoms include photophobia and nausea/vomiting. Some patients may not present with all three symptoms (triad of fever, nuchal rigidity, and change in LOC).

Labs

- Lumbar puncture: CSF contains large numbers of WBCs (CSF cloudy). Definitive diagnosis made from bacteria isolated from the CSF, with presence of elevated protein and low glucose levels in the CSF.
- Elevated opening pressure. Obtain CT or MRI scan.
- Lab tests: Obtain CBC with differential, metabolic panel, coagulation profile, platelet counts, and blood cultures × 2.
- Gram stain and C&S of the CSF fluid and the blood are needed (before antibiotics are begun).

Medications (IV)

- *Infants*: Ampicillin or third-generation cephalosporin
- *Adults*: Third-generation cephalosporin plus chloramphenicol
- *Older than age 50*: Amoxicillin plus third-generation cephalosporin
- Prophylaxis of close contacts with rifampin or ceftriaxone
- Immunization with the pneumococcal vaccination shown to decrease incidence

Complications

- Patients who recover usually have permanent neurologic sequelae.
- Elderly patients have a higher mortality rate due to the presence of comorbid conditions.

Migraine Headaches (With or Without Aura)

Migraine headache with aura (precedes the migraine headache) may present as scotomas (blind spots on visual field) or flashing lights that precede the headache. A positive family history and being female puts one at higher risk (3:1). In children, migraine headaches can present as abdominal pain.

Classic Case

An adult woman complains of the gradual onset of a bad throbbing headache behind one eye that gradually worsened over several hours. Reports sensitivity to bright light (photophobia) and to noise (phonophobia). Frequently accompanied by nausea and/or vomiting, which can be severe. Migraines can last from 2 to 3 days and may become bilateral if it is not treated (Table 12.1).

Treatment Plan

- Neurological exam will be normal.
- Rest in a quiet and darkened room with an ice pack to forehead.
- *Nausea*: Drink ginger ale or chew dry toast.
- Avoid heavy fatty meals.
- Avoid precipitating foods or activities such as:
  - Monosodium glutamate (MSG) in Chinese food; chocolate; nitrates/nitrites found in hot dogs, luncheon meat, and sausage
  - Red wines, beer, caffeine
  - Sleep changes, stress, barometric weather changes

- Odor trigger such as tobacco smoke, perfumes, and strong odors
- Visual triggers such as strobe lights, sunlight, glares

Abortive Treatment

- 5-HT-1 agonists: Sumatriptan (Imitrex):
  - First, rule out cardiovascular disease. Do not use if history or signs of ischemic heart disease (MI, angina), CVA, transient ischemic attacks (TIAs), uncontrolled hypertension, or hemiplegic migraine.
  - Warn patient of possible flushing, tingling, chest/neck/sinus/jaw discomfort, etc.
  - Supervise first dose, especially if patient has risk factors for cardiovascular disease (diabetics, obese, males >40 years, high lipids, etc.). Give first dose in office (theoretical risk of an acute MI).
  - Consider EKG monitoring if patient is at high risk for heart disease.
  - Higher risk of serotonin syndrome if combined with selective serotonin reuptake inhibitors (SSRIs) or selective norepinephrine reuptake inhibitors (SNRIs; duloxetine/Cymbalta, venlafaxine/Effexor). Do not start within 2 weeks of monoamine oxidase inhibitor (MAOI) use.
  - Do not combine with ergots or within 24 hours of ergot use (i.e., ergotamine/caffeine or Cafergot).
- Nonsteroidal anti-inflammatory drugs (NSAIDs), analgesics (e.g., Extra-Strength Tylenol), or narcotics (e.g., codeine, hydrocodone).

Table 12.1 Classic Signs and Symptoms: Headaches

Headache	Symptoms	Aggravating Factors
Migraine without aura	Throbbing pain behind one eye Photophobia, phonophobia Nausea/vomiting	Red wine, MSG, aspartame, menstruation, stress, etc.
Migraine with aura	Preceding symptoms plus scotoma, scintillating lights, halos, etc.	Foods high in triptans Teenage to middle-age females
Trigeminal neuralgia (CN V)	Intense and very brief; sharp stabbing pain; one cheek (2nd branch CN V)	Cold food, cold air, talking, touch, chewing Older adults and elderly
Cluster	Severe "ice-pick" piercing pain behind one eye and temple; with tearing, rhinorrhea, ptosis, and miosis on one side (Horner's syndrome)	Occurs at same time daily in clusters for weeks to months Middle-aged males
Temporal arteritis (also known as *giant cell arteritis*)	Unilateral pain, temporal area with scalp tenderness; skin over artery is indurated, tender, warm, and reddened; amaurosis fugax (temporary blindness) may occur	Medical urgency Polymyalgia rheumatica common in these patients (up to 50%) Older adults and elderly
Muscle tension	Bilateral "band-like" pain, continuous dull pain, may last day; may be accompanied by spasms of the trapezius muscles	Stress Adults

CN, cranial nerve; MSG, monosodium glutamate.

- Ergotamine/caffeine (Cafergot):
  - Ergot alkaloids are potent vasoconstrictors
  - Do not mix with other vasoconstrictors (triptans, decongestants, etc.)
  - Common side effect is nausea
  - Ergots and triptans should not be given within 14 days of an MAOI
- Antiemetics:
  - Trimethobenzamide (Tigan) is administered via IM, suppository, PO
  - Metoclopramide (Reglan) increases peristalsis in the duodenum and jejunum

Prophylactic Treatment

- *Beta-blockers*: Propranolol (Inderal) daily or BID (other beta-blockers can also be used)
- *Tricyclic antidepressants (TCAs)*: Amitriptyline (Elavil) at bedtime (HS)
- *Other TCAs*: Desipramine (Norpramin), imipramine (Tofranil), nortriptyline (Pamelor)
- *Other drug classes*: Anticonvulsants (valproate, topiramate), gabapentin (Neurontin); topiramate should not be prescribed, or it should be discontinued, if the patient has a history of kidney stones

Contraindications (Vasoconstricting Drugs)

- Suspected or known cardiovascular disease (angina, MI, peripheral arterial disease)
- Suspected or known CVA and/or TIAs
- Hyperlipidemia, males older than 40 years of age, menopausal females
- Uncontrolled hypertension
- Complex migraine (i.e., basilar/hemiplegic migraine)

Basilar or Hemiplegic Migraines

Focal neurological findings (i.e., CN exam) with stroke-like signs and symptoms. Resembles a TIA. These patients are at higher risk of stroke. Avoid giving estrogens or any agents promoting clot formation.

EXAM TIPS

- **Distinguish the drugs used for abortive treatment versus chronic prophylaxis.**
- **Answer options may list the drug class instead of the generic name.**

Temporal Arteritis (Giant Cell Arteritis)

Acute onset of a unilateral headache that is located on the temple and is associated with temporal artery inflammation. A systemic inflammatory disorder (vasculitis) of the medium and large arteries of the body. Mean age of diagnosis is 72 years of age. Visual loss is not uncommon and occurs in 15% to 20% of patients (despite availability of steroids).

Classic Case

An older man complains of headache on his temple along with marked scalp tenderness on the same side. Presence of an indurated cord-like temporal artery that is warm and tender. Sometimes accompanied by jaw claudication (pain with chewing that is relieved when he stops chewing).

Complains of visual symptoms such as amaurosis fugax (transient monocular loss of vision or partial visual field defect) or blindness. Can be accompanied by systemic symptoms such as low-grade fever and fatigue. Sedimentation rate is markedly elevated (see Table 12.1).

Labs

- Check ESR/sedimentation rate (often reaches 100 mm/hr or more)
- Normal range is between 0 to 22 mm/hr (men) and 0 to 29 mm/hr (women)
- Check the CRP, which will be elevated

Treatment Plan

- Refer to ophthalmologist, rheumatologist, or refer to ED *stat*
- Temporal artery biopsy is definitive test (gold standard) and is done by an ophthalmologist or surgeon
- High-dosed steroids are part of first-line treatment (prednisone 40–60 mg PO daily)

Complications

- Permanent blindness may occur if not diagnosed early (ischemic optic neuropathy)

EXAM TIPS

- **Temporal arteritis is treated with high-dosed prednisone for several weeks. Referral to rheumatology specialist for management.**
- **Sedimentation rate is screening test for temporal arteritis (elevated).**

Polymyalgia Rheumatica (PMR)

- PMR patients are at very high risk (up to 40%–50%) of developing temporal arteritis. Educate patients diagnosed with PMR on how to recognize symptoms of temporal arteritis.
- *Signs/symptoms*: Bilateral joint stiffness and aching (lasting 30 minutes or longer, commonly in the morning hours) located in the shoulders, neck, hips, and torso (difficulty putting on clothes/bra, having difficulty getting up out of bed or a chair). Females 50 years of age or older are commonly affected. Symptoms usually respond quickly to oral steroids (i.e., prednisone daily).

CLINICAL PEARLS

- **If history and physical exam are suggestive, treat with oral steroids as soon as possible.**
- **Order sedimentation rate and CRP. Both will be elevated.**
- **Serial labs (ESR, CRP) should be ordered until symptoms improve and should be monitored frequently.**

Trigeminal Neuralgia (Tic Douloureux)

The trigeminal nerve (CN V) has three divisions: the ophthalmic (V1), maxillary (V2), and the mandibular (V3) branches. Most cases are caused by compression of the nerve root by an artery or tumor, causing a unilateral facial pain that follows one of the branches of the trigeminal nerve. The pain is usually located close to the nasal border and the cheeks. There are two types. Type 1 involves extreme, shock-like facial pain, lasting from seconds to 2 minutes per episode, which may last up to 2 hours at a time. Type 2 is constant, aching, burning facial pain of lower intensity. May also occur together. More common in women and peaks in their 60s (see Table 12.1).

Classic Case

An older woman complains of the sudden onset of severe and sharp shooting pains on one side of her face or around the nose that are triggered by chewing, eating cold foods, and cold air. The severe lacerating pain (piercing knife-like pain) lasts a few seconds. The patient may stop chewing or speaking momentarily (few seconds) if it causes the pain.

Treatment Plan

- Administer high doses of anticonvulsants such as carbamazepine (Tegretol) or phenytoin (Dilantin).
- Muscle relaxants (baclofen, Robaxin, Norflex, or Flexeril) are effective when used with an anticonvulsant. Oxcarbazepine (Trileptal) most recently used as first-line drug with fewer side effects. Gabapentin and topiramate also used effectively.
- Obtain MRI or CT scan to rule out a tumor/artery pressing on a nerve or multiple sclerosis (MS).

Bell's Palsy

Abrupt onset of unilateral facial paralysis due to dysfunction of the motor branch of the facial nerve (CN VII). Facial paralysis can progress rapidly within 24 hours. Skin sensation remains intact, but tear production on the affected side may stop. Most cases resolve spontaneously. Etiology ranges from viral infection, an autoimmune process, or pressure from a tumor or blood vessel.

Classic Case

An older adult reports waking up that morning with one side of his face paralyzed. Complains of difficulty chewing and swallowing food on the same side. Unable to fully close eyelids.

Treatment Plan

- Rule out stroke, TIA, mastoid infections, bone fracture, Lyme disease, and tumor
- Administer corticosteroids at high doses × 10 days (wean)
- Administer acyclovir (Zovirax) if herpes simplex suspected
- Protect cornea from drying and ulceration with applications of an eye lubricant (a.m.) and lubricating ointment at bedtime; patch eye if patient is unable to fully close the eyelid to protect the eye from injury

Complications

Can cause corneal ulceration. Prolonged cases (several weeks) may leave permanent neurological sequelae, such as permanent facial weakness, in up to 10% of patients.

Cluster Headache

An idiopathic and severe one-sided headache that is marked by recurrent episodes of brief "ice-pick" (lacerating pain) located behind one eye that is accompanied by tearing and clear rhinitis (see Table 12.1).

- Abrupt onset; may get agitated during a headache episode
- The attacks happen several times a day (cluster)
- Resolves spontaneously, but may return in the future in some patients
- More common in adult males in their 30s to 40s

Classic Case

A 35-year-old man complains of the abrupt onset of recurrent episodes of brief "ice-pick" (lacerating pain) headaches behind one eye that are accompanied by autonomic symptoms such as tearing and clear nasal discharge (rhinitis). Some may have drooping eyelid (ptosis).

Treatment Plan

- Acute treatment:
  - High-dose oxygen may relieve headache (100% oxygen at least 12 L/min by mask); continue oxygen treatment for 15 minutes. Do not use this treatment if a patient has chronic obstructive pulmonary disease (COPD).
  - Administer sumatriptan (Imitrex) by injection or intranasal route
- *Prophylaxis:* If chronic, verapamil PO daily is effective for use as prophylaxis

Complications

- Higher risk of suicide (males) compared with the other types of chronic headaches

Muscle Tension Headache

Emotional/psychic stress in some people causes the muscles of the scalp and the neck to become chronically tense (or in contraction). This is a bilateral headache.

Classic Case

An adult patient complains of a headache that is "band-like" and feels like "someone is squeezing my head." The pain is described as dull and constant. Often accompanied by tensing of the neck muscles (see Table 12.1). The headache may last several days. Patient reports recent increased life stressor(s).

Treatment Plan

- NSAIDs, such as naproxen sodium (Anaprox DS), BID or ibuprofen 800 mg (Motrin) PO QID or analgesics (acetaminophen QID) or aspirin PRN
- Narcotics and butalbital are habit forming and increase the risk of rebound headaches
- Combination over-the-counter (OTC) medications of analgesics/aspirin plus caffeine (Anacin, Excedrin, others); use with caution due to increased risk of addictive use of these medications
- Stress reduction and relaxation: Try yoga, tai chi; exercise several times per week; gradually reduce and stop caffeine intake; follow a regular eating/sleep schedule; pursue counseling with therapist

Rebound Headache

Patient complains of daily headaches (or almost daily headaches). May be accompanied by irritability, depression, and insomnia. Caused by overuse of abortive medicines such as analgesics, NSAIDs, aspirin, or narcotics. Treatment is to discontinue the medicine immediately (if not contraindicated) or to gradually taper the dose and/or reduce frequency.

Transient Ischemic Attack (TIA)

A TIA is a transient episode of neurological dysfunction caused by focal ischemia (brain, spinal cord, or retinal ischemia) without acute infarction of the brain as seen in stroke. The timing for resolution (24 hours, included in previous definition) has been removed. It is now known that permanent neurological damage can occur with TIAs (as seen in cerebrovascular accidents [CVAs], or strokes). TIA is also known as a "mini-stroke" or "minor stroke." These patients are at very high risk for severe stroke in the future.

Depending on severity of the TIA, the signs and symptoms can be subtle to severe. The longer the episode of the TIA, the higher the risk of ischemic brain damage. The TIA can progress into a full-blown stroke. Signs and symptoms of CVA or stroke can be insidious and start a few days before the major episode occurs.

Note

Up to 20% of patients with TIA will have a stroke within 90 days, and from 25% to 50% of these strokes occur within the first 48 hours.

Classic Case

Adult to elderly male patient reports acute onset of one-sided weakness of the right arm and right leg accompanied by dizziness, vertigo, and poor balance. The patient is difficult to understand because his speech is slurred (dysphasia). When instructed to smile and grimace, the right side of his face has no movement and is lopsided. Patient is accompanied by a spouse who reports that he has a history of hypertension, atrial fibrillation, hyperlipidemia, and type 2 diabetes. If symptoms progress to stroke, one-sided weakness worsens and level of consciousness ranges from confusion, stupor, to coma. If a TIA episode, the signs and symptoms eventually resolve, but patient remains at higher risk of future stroke.

"FAST" Mnemonic for Recognizing Stroke

F Face drooping (Instruct patient to smile. Is face lopsided?)
A Arm weakness (Instruct patient to raise both arms. Does one arm drift downward?)
S Speech difficulty (Instruct patient to say, "The sky is blue.")
T Time to call 911 (Even if symptoms go away, call 911.)
(Do not delay; American Heart Association/American Stroke Association, n.d.)

Hospitalization Criteria

Consider hospitalization within first 24 to 48 hours if:

- Patient's first TIA or duration of TIA is 1 hour or longer
- High risk for cardiac emboli (e.g., atrial fibrillation)
- Symptomatic internal carotid stenosis greater than 50%
- Hypercoagulable state
- Crescendo TIAs (two or more TIAs in 1 week)
- High ABCD2 score (Table 12.2; higher scores are associated with higher risk of stroke at 2, 7, 30, and 90 days after TIA)

Treatment Plan

- Refer patient to ED for further evaluation. Find out cause of TIA (or stroke) such as atrial fibrillation, carotid/vertebral atherosclerosis, hypercoagulable state, cocaine use, hypertension, etc. Perform workup to find the extent of brain damage.
- Schedule CT and/or MRI scan as soon as possible (within first 24 hours of the episode). The diffusion-weighted MRI is the preferred imaging method.
- Rule out intracranial hemorrhage before starting aspirin (50–325 mg/d), plus extended-release dipyridamole or clopidogrel.
- Maintain blood pressure below 140/90 mmHg.

Table 12.2 ABCD2 Score

Risk Factor	Points	Score
Age >65 years	1	
BP: Systolic 140 mmHg or diastolic 90 mmHg	1	
Clinical features of TIA (choose one only) Unilateral weakness with/without speech impairment Speech impairment without unilateral weakness	2 1	
Duration TIA duration >60 minutes TIA duration 10–59 minutes	 2 1	
Diabetes	1	
Total ABCD2 score	(0–7)	

BP, blood pressure; TIA, transient ischemic attack.

Scores: Four to 5 points (hospitalization justified in most situations); 6 to 7 points (hospitalization observation worthwhile).

Cerebrovascular Accident (CVA) or Stroke

A stroke can be caused either by emboli/thrombosis or by hemorrhage. In both, permanent neurological damage results from ischemia to the affected brain tissues. The most common risk factors for stroke are atrial fibrillation and hypertension. Other risk factors include aneurysms, trauma, bleeding abnormalities and use of anticoagulants (e.g., warfarin [Coumadin]), use of stimulants (cocaine/illicit drugs), sickle cell disease, diabetes, oral contraceptive use, smoking, and thrompophilia. Blacks, Hispanics, and American Indian/Alaskan Natives have a higher prevalence of stroke. The sources of bleeding can be intracerebral hemorrhage (ICH) or subarachnoid hemorrhage (SAH). An ischemic stroke is due to emboli that broke off from thrombus formation in the body; common locations are the lower extremities and the heart (atrial fibrillation).

Classic Case

A patient with embolic stroke presents with the abrupt onset of difficulty speaking, unilateral hemiparesis, and weakness of the arms or legs (or both). Patients with hemorrhagic stroke often initially present with severe headache, nausea/vomiting, photophobia, and nuchal rigidity that is accompanied by hemiparesis and difficulty speaking.

Hemorrhagic Stroke

- SAH or ICH: Sudden onset of severe "thunderclap" headache that is described as "the worst headache of my life." The pain from the headache may radiate to the neck or back. Rapid decrease in level of consciousness (coma, death). SAH usually begins abruptly compared to more gradual ICH.
- Vomiting is more common in hemorrhagic strokes (compared with embolic strokes). Usually caused by a ruptured aneurysm or vascular malformations.
- "Sentinel headache" may be seen in SAH. About 30% of patients have minor hemorrhagic episodes that present with sudden severe headache as the only symptom.

Acute Ischemic Stroke

- Signs and symptoms are dependent on artery involved. For example:
  - Left middle cerebral artery: Right side of face, right arm, right leg with aphasia (expressive, receptive, or both)
  - Right middle cerebral artery: Left side of face, left arm, left leg with hemineglect and possible hemianopsia

Treatment Plan

- Call 911
- Assess the "ABCs" as soon as possible; check for airway patency, chest movement, breath sounds from both lungs, and circulation
- Check vital signs and neuro status

Emergency Department Management

- Assess the ABCs and stabilize patient
- Initial imaging study in the ED is CT scan (without contrast), then an MRI study; decide whether patient is a candidate for antithrombolytic therapy, interventional radiological procedures, and so on

Labs

- PT, PTT, INR
- CBC with differential and platelet count
- Serum blood glucose

- Total lipid profile (cholesterol, LDL, HDL, triglycerides)
- EKG (rule out acute MI)
- Electrolytes, creatinine, urea nitrogen

Screening for Visual Field Loss

- Homonymous hemianopsia: Visual field loss involving either the two left halves (or the two right halves) of the visual field; most common cause is stroke; there are many types of hemianopsia.
- Perform screening test: Visual fields by confrontation

Example: Left-Sided Homonymous Hemianopsia

The diagram at right shows the intact and missing visual fields of a person who has left-sided homonymous hemianopsia. The "x" signifies the missing visual fields and the equal signs "==" are the intact visual field.

Left Eye	*Right Eye*
xxxxx====	xxxx====
xxxxx====	xxxx====
xxxxx====	xxxx====

Examples of Brain Damage: Temporal Lobe

- *Apraxia*: Patient has difficulty performing purposeful movements.
- *Broca's aphasia*: Also known as "nonfluent aphasia." Patient comprehends speech relatively well (and can read), but has extreme difficulty with the motor aspects of speech. Speech length is usually less than four words.
- *Wernicke's aphasia*: Also known as "fluent aphasia." Patient has difficulty with comprehension, but has no problem with producing speech. Reading and writing can be markedly impaired.
- *Frontal lobe damage*: The frontal lobes are the areas where intelligence, executive skills, logic, and personality reside. Damage will cause dementia, memory loss/difficulties, inability to learn, etc.

Long-Term Management

- Remove or treat the cause of the emboli (e.g., atrial fibrillation; control hypertension)
- For embolic strokes: Anticoagulation therapy; statin therapy; keep INR between 2.0 and 3.0
- For hemorrhagic strokes: Avoid heparin, warfarin, aspirin
- Rehabilitation: Physical therapy, occupational therapy, speech therapy
- Patient should be in the care of a neurologist after stroke
- Primary care NPs do not start anticoagulation for stroke; needs physician or AGAC-NP

Common Drugs: Headache Treatment (Table 12.3)

Acute Treatment (PRN Only)

NSAIDs

- Naproxen sodium (Naprosyn, Aleve) BID or ibuprofen (Advil, Motrin) TID to QID
- *Side effects:* GI pain/bleeding/ulceration, renal damage, increased BP in hypertension

Triptans

- Administer sumatriptan (Imitrex) injection, inhalant, PO tablets, or sublingual tablets
- *Side effects:* Nausea, acute MI, etc.
- Use with caution in patients with cardiovascular comorbidities
- Triptans should not be given within 24 hours of an ergot
- Do not give within 14 days of an MAOI

Table 12.3 Treatment of Headaches

Headache	Acute Treatment	Prophylaxis/Other
Migraine	Ice pack on forehead; rest in quiet and darkened room	TCAs Episodic migraine (<14 headache days per month)
	Triptans (Imitrex), Tigan suppositories (for nausea)	Beta-blockers (propranolol, metoprolol, timolol)
	Ultram, NSAIDs, analgesics, narcotics	
Temporal arteritis	Refer to ED or ophthalmologist *stat.* Lab: ESR ↑ (sed rate) (screening lab test)	Permanent blindness can result; temporal artery biopsy is the gold standard diagnosis
	High-dose steroids	
Cluster	100% oxygen at 12 L/min; use mask; intranasal 4% lidocaine	May become suicidal Spontaneous resolution; can recur
Trigeminal neuralgia	Carbamazepine (Tegretol) or phenytoin (Dilantin); check serum levels	Tegretol or Dilantin for several weeks to months; watch for drug interactions
Muscle tension	NSAIDs, Tylenol, hot bath/shower, massage, etc.	Stress reduction, yoga, massage, biofeedback

ED, emergency department; ESR, erythrocyte sedimentation rate; NSAIDs, nonsteroidal anti-inflammatory drugs; TCAs, tricyclic antidepressants.

Analgesics

- Acetaminophen (Tylenol) QID PRN
- *Side effects:* Hepatic damage, etc.
- Prophylaxis (must be taken daily to work)

Prophylaxis

Tricyclic Antidepressants (TCAs)

- Amitriptyline (Elavil) at half-strength or imipramine (Tofranil) at half-strength
- *Side effects:* Sedation, dry mouth, confusion in elderly, etc.

Beta-Blockers

- Propranolol (Inderal LA) or atenolol (Tenormin) daily
- *Contraindications:* Second- or third-degree atrioventricular (AV) block, asthma, COPD, bradycardia, etc.

Antiseizure Medications

- Topiramate (Topamax) BID
- Requires titration to maximum dose of 100 mg/24 hr
- Should not be prescribed in patients with a history of kidney stones

Carpal Tunnel Syndrome (CTS)

Commonly caused by activities that require repetitive wrist/hand motion. Both hands affected in 50% of patients. Median nerve (Figure 12.2) compression due to swelling of the carpal tunnel. Other factors that increase risk are hypothyroidism, pregnancy, and obesity.

Classic Case

An adult patient who uses his hands frequently for his job (i.e., computer typing) complains of gradual onset (over weeks to months) of numbness and tingling (paresthesias) on the thumb, index finger, and middle finger areas. Hand grip of affected hand(s) is weaker. May complain of problems lifting heavy objects with the affected hand. Chronic severe cases involve atrophy of the thenar eminence (the group of muscles on the palm of the hand at the base of the thumb), which is a late sign. History of an occupation or hobby that involves frequent wrist/hand movements.

Tinel's Sign (Figure 12.3)

- Tap anterior wrist briskly
- *Positive finding*: "Pins and needles" sensation of the median nerve over the hand after lightly percussing the wrist

Phalen's Sign (Figure 12.4)

- Engage in full flexion of wrist for 60 seconds
- *Positive finding*: Tingling sensation of the median nerve over the hand evoked by passive flexion of the wrist for 1 minute

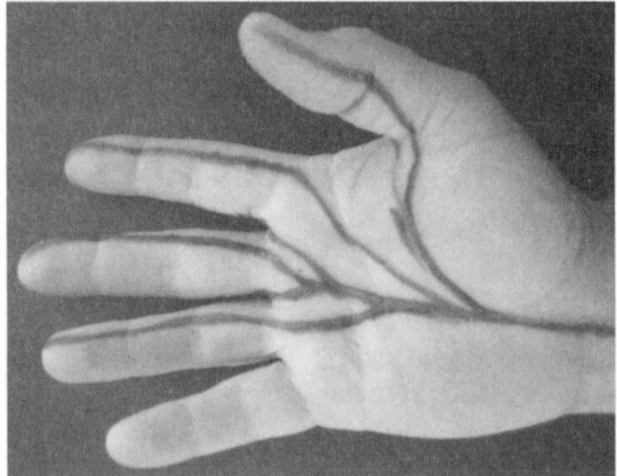

Figure 12.2 Median nerve.

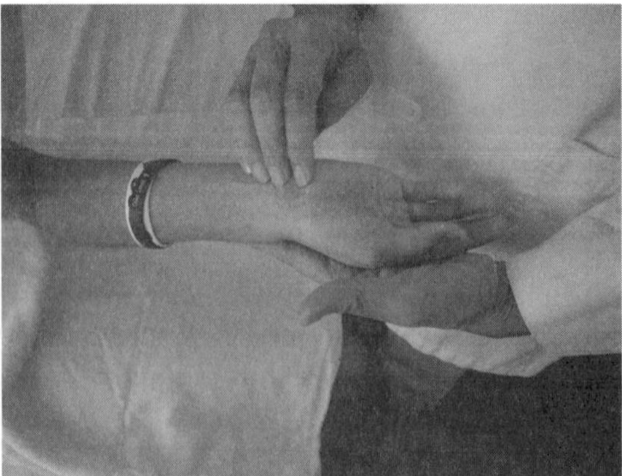

Figure 12.3 Tinel's sign.

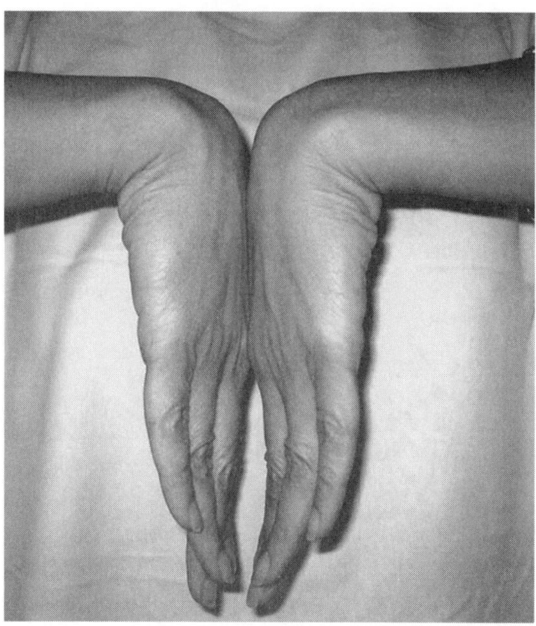

Figure 12.4 Phalen's sign.

EXAM TIPS

- Recognize both Tinel's and Phalen's signs (tests for carpal tunnel syndrome).
- Learn classic presentation of CTS (inflammation of the median nerve).
- Alternative headache remedy is an herb called butterburr.
- With the exception of muscle tension headaches, which are bilateral, all of the headaches seen on the exam (and notes) are unilateral.
- Muscle tension: Causes band-like head pain; may last for days.
- Migraine: Presents with throbbing, nausea, photophobia, phonophobia.
- Cluster: Only headache accompanied by tearing and nasal congestion; severe pain is behind one eye/one side of head. Occurs several times a day. Spontaneously resolves. Seen more in middle-aged males. Treated with high-dose oxygen (contraindicated in COPD).
- Trigeminal neuralgia (tic douloureux): Pain on one side of face/cheek is precipitated by talking, chewing, cold food, or cold air on affected area.
- Temporal arteritis: Indurated temporal artery, pain felt behind eye/scalp. Treated with high dose steroids or other anti-inflammatory medication. Untreated may lead to blindness.
- Always order cerebral imaging for patients with a change in their usual headache pattern (change in frequency, duration, severity, location, etc.).

13

Hematological System Review

DANGER SIGNALS

Acute Hemorrhage

Blood loss of 15% or higher results in orthostatic hypotension (systolic BP drop of >20 mmHg). Look for signs and symptoms of shock. When checking the CBC, be aware that the initial hemoglobin and hematocrit (during active bleeding) may be in the normal range. The correct hemoglobin value will not show up until about 24 hours after onset of the hemorrhage. The normal bone marrow will respond to blood loss by releasing immature RBCs (reticulocytosis).

Neutropenia

- Individuals with neutropenia have frequent infections (especially bacterial) with symptoms of fever, sore throat, oral thrush, and so forth.
- *Neutropenia* is defined as an absolute neutrophil count (ANC) of less than 1,500/mm^3.
- African Americans may have a lower ANC count that is "benign" (bone marrow aspirate normal).

Vitamin B_{12} Deficiency

Gradual onset of symmetrical peripheral neuropathy starting in the feet and/or arms. Other neurological signs are numbness, ataxia (positive Romberg test), loss of vibration and position sense, impaired memory, and dementia (severe cases). Peripheral smear shows macro-ovalocytes, some megaloblasts, and multisegmented neutrophils (more than five to six lobes).

Hodgkin's Lymphoma

A cancer of the beta lymphocytes (B cells). Night sweats, fevers, and pain with ingestion of alcoholic drinks. Generalized pruritus with painless enlarged lymph nodes (neck). Anorexia and weight loss. Higher incidence among young adults (20–40 years) or older adults (>60 years), males, and Whites. Identified by the presence of Reed-Sternberg cells.

Non-Hodgkin's Lymphoma

A cancer of the lymphocytes (usually B cells) and killer cells. Usually occurs in the older adult (>65 years) and presents with night sweats, fever, weight loss, generalized lymphadenopathy (painless). The prognosis is poor.

Multiple Myeloma

A cancer of the plasma cells. Symptoms of fatigue, weakness, and bone pain that is usually located in the back or chest. Causes proteinuria with Bence-Jones proteins, hypercalcemia, normocytic anemia. More common in older adults.

Thrombocytopenia

Thrombocytopenia is defined as a platelet count of less than 150,000/µL. Symptoms usually do not show until the platelet count is less than 100,000/µL. Look for easy bruising (ecchymosis, petechiae), bleeding gums, spontaneous nosebleeds, hematuria, etc.

- *Normal platelet count*: Range is from 150,000–450,000/µL.

Easy Bruising

Bruising on the distal lower and upper extremities is usually related to physical activities. Children commonly have bruises on the anterior shin area. The presence of petechiae and/or purpura, large hematomas (from mild trauma) not accompanied by other symptoms (fever, headaches, infection) is suspicious. Check medications (acetylsalicylic acid [ASA], NSAIDs, heparin, warfarin, selective serotonin reuptake inhibitors [SSRIs], steroids, etc.). Evaluate patient for a possible coagulation disorder (von Willebrand disease, vitamin C deficiency or scurvy, etc.). Initial labs to order are CBC, PT, and PTT. Platelet count greater than 150,000/µL is normal (rules out thrombocytopenia).

LABORATORY TESTING

Laboratory Norms

Hemoglobin

- *Males*: 14.0 to 18.0 g/dL
- *Females*: 12.0 to 16.0 g/dL
- Long-term high-altitude (mountain) exposure/chronic hypoxia: Elevated (secondary polycythemia)

Hematocrit

- The proportion of RBCs in 1 mL of plasma
- *Males*: 42% to 52%
- *Females*: 37% to 47%

Mean Corpuscular Volume (MCV)

- *Normal:* 80 to 100 fL (femtoliter)
- A measure of the average size of the RBCs in a sample of blood
  - MCV less than 80 fL with microcytic anemia
  - MCV between 80 and 100 fL with normocytic anemia
  - MCV more than 100 fL with macrocytic anemia

Mean Corpuscular Hgb Concentration (MCHC)

- A measure of the average color of the RBCs in a sample of blood
- Decreased in iron-deficiency anemia and thalassemia (hypochromic); normal in macrocytic and normocytic anemias
- *Normal*: 31.0 to 37.0 g/dL

Mean Corpuscular Hemoglobin (MCH)

- Indirect measure of the color of RBCs. Decreased values mean pale or hypochromic RBCs. MCH is decreased in iron-deficiency anemia and thalassemia. Normal with the macrocytic anemias.
- *Normal*: Range is 25.0 to 35.0 pg/cell.

Total Iron-Binding Capacity (TIBC)

- A measure of available transferrin that is left unbound (to iron). Transferrin is used to transport iron in the body. Elevated if there is not enough iron to transport (as seen with iron-deficiency anemia). Normal TIBC is seen with thalassemia, vitamin B_{12} deficiency, and folate-deficiency anemia (because iron levels are normal).

- *Normal*: Range is 250 to 410 mcg/dL.

Serum Ferritin

- Serum ferritin is the stored form of iron. Produced in the intestines. Stored in body tissue such as the spleen, liver, and bone marrow. Correlates with iron storage status in a healthy adult. Most sensitive test for iron-deficiency anemia.
- *Iron-deficiency anemia*: Serum ferritin is markedly decreased.
- *Thalassemia trait*: Levels are normal to high. May be high if patient was misdiagnosed with iron-deficiency anemia and erroneously given iron supplementation. Avoid iron supplements before testing serum ferritin level.
- *Normal*: Range is 20 to 400 ng/mL.

Serum Iron

- Decreased in iron-deficiency anemia. Normal to high in thalassemia and the macrocytic anemias. Not as sensitive as ferritin. Affected by recent blood transfusions.
- *Normal*: Range is 50 to 175 mcg/dL.

Red Cell Distribution Width (RDW)

- A measure of the variability of the size of RBCs in a given sample. Elevated in iron-deficiency anemia and thalassemia.

Reticulocytes

- Immature RBCs that still have their nuclei. Reticulocytes are slightly larger in size than a RBC. After 24 hours in circulation, reticulocytes lose their nuclei and mature into RBCs (no nuclei). The bone marrow normally will release small amounts to replace damaged RBCs. RBCs survive 120 days before being sequestered by the spleen and broken down by the liver into iron and globulin (recycled) and bilirubin (bile).
- *Normal*: Range is 0.5% to 2.5% (of total RBC count).

Reticulocytosis (More Than 2.5% of Total RBC Count)

- An elevation of reticulocytes is seen when the bone marrow is stimulated into producing RBCs. It is elevated with supplementation of iron, folate, or vitamin B_{12} (after deficiency), after acute bleeding episodes, hemolysis, leukemia, and with erythropoietin (EPO) treatment. Chronic bleeding does not cause elevation of the reticulocytes due to compensation.
- If no reticulocytosis after an acute bleeding episode (after 3 to 4 days), hemolysis, or after appropriate supplementation of deficient mineral (iron, folate, or vitamin B_{12}), or with EPO, rule out bone marrow failure (i.e., aplastic anemia). Diagnosed by bone marrow biopsy.

Poikilocytosis (Peripheral Smear)

- Seen with severe iron-deficiency anemia. RBCs abnormal with variable shapes seen in the peripheral smear. May be accompanied by anisocytosis (variable sizes of RBCs).

Serum Folate and Vitamin B_{12}

- Low values if deficiency exists. Deficiency will cause a macrocytic anemia.
- *Normal folate level*: Range is 3.1 to 17.5 ng/mL.
- *Normal vitamin B_{12} level*: More than 250 pg/mL is normal.

White Blood Cells With Differential

- *White cell differential*: Percentage of each type of leukocyte in a sample of blood. The differential for each type of WBC should add up to a total of 100%.
- Normal WBC count (child older than 2 years to adults) is 5.0 to 10.0 × 10^9 (5,000 to 10,000/10 mm^3).
    - *Neutrophils or segs (segmented neutrophils):* 55% to 70%
    - *Band forms or stabs (immature neutrophils):* 0% to 5%
    - *Lymphocytes:* 20% to 40%
    - *Monocytes:* 2% to 8%
    - *Eosinophils:* 1% to 4%
    - *Basophils:* 0.5% to 1%

HEMOGLOBIN

Hemoglobin Electrophoresis

The gold-standard (definitive) test to diagnose hemoglobinopathies such as sickle cell anemia, the thalassemias, and many others. Normal hemoglobin contains two alpha and two beta chains.

- *Adult norms*: Hemoglobin A (HbA) 97% and hemoglobin A2 (HbA2) 2.5%. An extremely small amount (<1%) of total hemoglobin is fetal hemoglobin (HbF), which is a normal finding.

Secondary Polycythemia

Chronic smokers, individuals with long-term chronic obstructive pulmonary disease (COPD), long-term residence at high altitudes, or EPO treatment have a higher incidence of secondary polycythemia (as opposed to primary polycythemia vera).

- Polycythemia is defined as:
    - Hematocrit in adults of more than 48% (women) and more than 52% (men)
    - Hemoglobin in adults of more than 16.5% (women) and more than 18.5% (men)

High-Altitude Stress

Lower barometric pressure causes a reduction in the arterial PO_2. Patients with coronary artery disease (CAD), congestive heart failure (CHF), or sickle cell anemia are at higher risk of complications.

DISEASE REVIEW

ANEMIAS

Anemia is simply defined as a decrease in the hemoglobin/hematocrit value below the norm for the patient's age and gender. See Table 13.1 for laboratory characteristics.

Iron-Deficiency Anemia

Microcytic and hypochromic anemia (small and pale RBCs) are caused by iron deficiency. Iron-deficiency anemia is the most common type of anemia in the world for all races, ages, and gender.

Classic Case

Pallor of the skin, conjunctiva, and nail beds. Complaints of daily fatigue and exertional dyspnea. May have glossitis (sore and shiny red tongue) and angular cheilitis (irritated skin or fissures at the corners of the mouth). Cravings for nonfood items such as ice or dirt (pica). Severe anemia will cause spoon-shaped nails (koilonychia), systolic murmurs, tachycardia, or heart failure.

Etiology

Most common cause is blood loss (overt or occult). Reproductive-aged females (heavy periods, pregnancy), poor diet, GI blood loss, postgastrectomy, and increased physiologic requirement are risk factors.

Infants: Rule out chronic intake of cow's milk before 12 months of age (causes GI bleeding) in anemic infants.

Labs

Decreased

- Hemoglobin and hematocrit
- MCV less than 80 fL
- MCHC (paler color)
- Ferritin and iron level

Increased

- TIBC

Peripheral Smear

- Anisocytosis (variations in size) and poikilocytosis (variations in shape)

Table 13.1 Laboratory Findings: Anemia

Type of Anemia	Diagnostic Tests	Red Blood Cell Changes
Iron deficiency	**Ferritin/serum iron ↓**	MCV <80 fL (microcytic)
	TIBC ↑	MCHC ↓ (hypochromic)
	RDW ↑	Poikilocytosis (variable shapes)
		Anisocytosis (variable sizes)
Thalassemia minor	**Hemoglobin electrophoresis**	Abnormal if beta-thalassemia
		Normal if alpha-thalassemia
		MCV <80 fL (microcytic)
		MCHC ↓ (hypochromic)
Pernicious anemia	**Antiparietal antibodies ↑**	MCV >100 fL (macrocytic)
	Most common cause of vitamin B_{12}-deficiency anemia	Megaloblastic RBCs
		Normal color (normochromic)
Folate deficiency	**Folate level ↓**	MCV >100 fL (macrocytic)
	Homocysteine ↑	Megaloblastic RBCs
		Normal color (normochromic)
Vitamin B_{12} deficiency	**B_{12} level ↓**	MCV >100 fL (macrocytic) paresthesias, numbness
	Hypersegmented neutrophils	Megaloblastic RBCs
	(more than 5–6 lobes)	Normal color (normochromic)
Normocytic anemia	**MCV 80–100 fL**	MCV 80–100 fL (normal-sized RBCs)
	History of chronic disease or inflammatory disease such as rheumatoid arthritis	Normochromic RBCs

(continued)

Table 13.1 Laboratory Findings: Anemia *(continued)*

Type of Anemia	Diagnostic Tests	Red Blood Cell Changes
Sickle cell anemia	**Hemoglobin electrophoresis**	Sickle-shaped RBCs with shortened life span of 10 to 20 days (norm is 120 days)
	HbS and HbF both elevated	
	Reticulocytosis	
	A hemolytic anemia	Howell–Jolly bodies and target cells (peripheral smear)
		Normocytic/normochromic

Note: Boldfaced lab tests are diagnostic or the gold standard for the exams.
HbF, fetal hemoglobin; HbS, hemoglobin S; MCHC, mean corpuscular hemoglobin concentration; MCV, mean corpuscular volume; RBC, red blood cell; RDW, red cell distribution width; TIBC, total iron-binding capacity.

Treatment Plan

- Identify cause of anemia and correct cause (if possible). Rule out GI malignancy.
- Ferrous sulfate 325 mg PO TID between meals (take with vitamin C or orange juice for better absorption). Treat iron-deficiency anemia from 3 to 6 months to restore ferritin stores. Use of cast-iron cookware also provides additional iron.
- Increase fiber and fluids. Consider fiber supplements (psyllium, guar gum) for constipation.
- Iron-rich foods are red meat, some beans (e.g., black beans), and green leafy vegetables.
- *Common side effects of iron*: Constipation, black-colored stools, stomach upset may occur.
- *Interactions*: Avoid taking iron supplement at the same time as antacids, dairy products, quinolones, or tetracyclines (inactivates iron).
- Check the reticulocyte count and CBC approximately 2 weeks after starting supplementation to check for treatment response (elevated reticulocytes, hemoglobin/hematocrit will increase).

Thalassemia Minor (or Trait)

A genetic disorder in which the bone marrow produces abnormal hemoglobin (defective alpha- or beta-globin chains). Normal hemoglobin contains two alpha and two beta chains. Results in a microcytic/hypochromic anemia.

- *Ethnic groups*: Occurs in people from the Mediterranean, North Africa, Middle East, and Southeast Asia.
- Alpha thalassemia is more common in Southeast Asians (Chinese, Cambodians, Filipinos, Thai people).

Classic Case

Vast majority of individuals are asymptomatic. Discovered incidentally because of abnormal CBC results, which reveal microcytic and hypochromic RBCs. Total RBC count may be mildly elevated. Ethnic background is either Mediterranean or Asian.

Treatment Plan

- *Gold-standard diagnostic test*: Hemoglobin electrophoresis
  - In beta-thalassemia, abnormal (elevated hemoglobin, HbA2, HgF)
  - In iron-deficiency anemia, normal
- *Blood smear*: Microcytosis, anisocytosis, and poikilocytosis
- Serum ferritin and iron level: Normal (but low in iron-deficiency anemia)

- Genetic counseling: Educate about the possibility of having a child with the disease if partner also has trait (25% chance, or one in four, of their children)
- Thalassemia minor/trait does not need treatment (asymptomatic genetic disease)

Anemia of Chronic Kidney Disease (CKD)

Anemia of CKD is a hypoproliferative, normocytic, and normochromic anemia.

- Defined as hemoglobin less than 11 g/dL in pregnant women, less than 12 g/dL in nonpregnant women, and less than 13 g/dL in men.
- Occurs due to the decrease in renal EPO production secondary to the CKD, which reduces the production of reticulocyte and RBC production and causes worsening anemia. In addition, patients may also have functional iron deficiency and/or acute and chronic inflammatory conditions.
- *Initial testing*: Obtain CBC, serum ferritin, serum transferrin saturation, vitamin B_{12}, folate, and reticulocyte count.

Treatment Plan

- The anemia should be treated using conventional methods. If not improving, then erythropoiesis-stimulating agents should be used. Iron therapy (PO or IV) may also be used. PO iron may be used for patients not treated with dialysis.
- IV iron is used for hemodialysis patients and/or other patients with severe iron deficiency.

EXAM TIPS

- The screening test for all anemias is the CBC (hemoglobin/hematocrit).
- The diagnostic test for thalassemia and sickle cell anemia is the hemoglobin electrophoresis.
- Learn to differentiate the lab results of thalassemia from iron-deficiency anemia.
- If the ferritin level is low, the patient has iron-deficiency anemia.
- If the ferritin level is normal to high, the patient has thalassemia minor/trait.
- The ethnic background may not be "revealed" in a question about thalassemia.
- Patients with chronic illness and/or autoimmune disease have higher risk of normocytic anemia.

CLINICAL PEARLS

- Best absorbed form of iron supplementation (and cheapest) is ferrous sulfate (available over the counter [OTC]).
- If patient took an antacid, wait about 4 hours before taking iron pill (minimizes binding).
- Iron interacts with tetracycline antibiotics, levothyroxine, and bisphosphonates (decreases effectiveness). To avoid, take iron 2 hours before or after antibiotic.
- Failure to respond (if treatment compliant) may be a sign of continuing blood loss, misdiagnosis (has thalassemia instead of iron-deficiency anemia), malabsorption (i.e., celiac disease).
- Iron poisoning in children (especially if age <6 years) may cause death. Advise patient to store iron supplements in an area that is not accessible to children (or to grandchildren).
- Medications reported to lower hemoglobin levels and worsen anemia include angiotensin receptor blockers (ARBs) and angiotensin-converting enzyme inhibitors (ACEIs) in patients of chronic diseases (CKD, diabetes, chronic HF, hypertension).

Aplastic Anemia

Aplastic anemia is caused by destruction of the pluripotent stem cells inside the bone marrow and has multiple causes (radiation, adverse effect of a drug, viral infection, others). Bone marrow production slows or stops—all cell lines are affected. The result is pancytopenia (leukopenia, anemia, thrombocytopenia).

Classic Case

Patient with severe case of anemia presents with fatigue and weakness. Skin and mucosa are a pale color. Tachycardia and systolic flow murmur are present. Neutropenia results in bacterial and fungal infections. Thrombocytopenia results in large bruises from trauma and bleeding. Signs and symptoms depend on the severity of the aplastic anemia.

Labs

- CBC with differential
- Platelet count
- Gold standard is the bone marrow biopsy

Treatment Plan

- Refer to hematologist as soon as possible. If septic, refer to the emergency department.

Macrocytic/Megaloblastic Anemias

Vitamin B_{12}-Deficiency Anemia

Caused by a deficiency in vitamin B_{12}, which is necessary for the health of the neurons and the brain, and for normal DNA production of RBCs. Total body supply of vitamin B_{12} lasts from 3 to 4 years. Common causes of vitamin B_{12}-deficiency anemia include malabsorption (due to pernicious anemia, gastric disease/infections or medications such as antacids, H2-receptor antagonists, proton-pump inhibitors and metformin). Chronic vitamin B_{12} deficiency causes nerve damage (i.e., peripheral neuropathy, paraplegia) and brain damage (dementia if severe). Neurologic damage may not be reversible. Highest incidence in older women. Most common cause is pernicious anemia.

Pernicious Anemia

An autoimmune disorder caused by the destruction of parietal cells in the fundus (by antiparietal antibodies) resulting in cessation of intrinsic factor production. Intrinsic factor is necessary in order to absorb vitamin B_{12} from the small intestine.

Cobalamin (vitamin B_{12}) deficiency may result from dietary insufficiency of vitamin B_{12}. May occur in patients with stomach, small bowel, and pancreatic disorders; infections; and severe dietary deficiencies of meats and milk, as seen in strict vegetarians. Dietary deficiency may take more than 5 years to occur. Iron deficiency commonly coexists with pernicious anemia. Patients with pernicious anemia have a two- to threefold increase in incidence of gastric carcinoma.

- *Other causes of vitamin B_{12} deficiency*: Alterations in gastric anatomy (i.e., bariatric surgery, gastrectomy), strict vegans, alcoholics, small bowel disease
- *Vitamin B_{12} sources*: All foods of animal origin (meat, poultry, eggs, milk, cheese)

Classic Case

Older to elderly woman complains of gradual onset of paresthesias on her feet and/or hands that is slowly getting more severe. She has pallor, pale conjunctiva, glossitis, and other signs of anemia.

Neuropathic symptoms may include any of the following:

- Tingling/numbness of hands and feet
- Neuropathy starts in peripheral nerves and migrates centrally

- Difficulty walking (gross motor)
- Difficulty in performing fine motor skills (hands)

Objective Findings

Decreased reflexes in affected extremity. If the legs are involved, the ankle jerk (Achilles reflex) will be reduced ("+1" is sluggish and "0" is none). Normal reflex is grade "+2."

- *Motor tests*: Weak hand grip, decreased vibration sense, abnormal Romberg, and so forth.
- Inflamed tongue, or glossitis (not a specific finding because it is found in other disorders) are seen.

Warning

Always check both serum B_{12} and serum folate levels in macrocytic anemia. A patient can be deficient in both B_{12} and folate. The hemoglobin and hematocrit will go up with folate supplementation only (even if still deficient in B_{12}). Untreated B_{12} deficiency anemia results in permanent neurologic sequelae (neuropathy, brain damage).

Treatment Plan

Check for both vitamin B_{12} level and folate level (both levels must always be checked together).

- Decreased vitamin B_{12} level (<150 pg/mL)
- *Antibody tests*: Antiparietal and anti-intrinsic factor (IF) antibody
- *24-hour urine test for methylmalonic acid (MMA):* elevated
- *Homocysteine level*: Elevated in vitamin B_{12} (and folate) deficiency
- *Schilling test*: Not commonly used now; positive if vitamin B_{12} (radioactive) excretion is normal after administration of intrinsic factor (but has poor excretion when given vitamin B_{12} alone)
- *Peripheral blood smear*: Macrocytosis, hypersegmented neutrophils (more than 5 to 6 lobes), evidence of defective erythropoiesis
- Check the reticulocyte count and CBC approximately 2 weeks after starting supplementation to check for treatment response (elevated reticulocytes, hemoglobin/ hematocrit will increase).

Medications

- *Pernicious anemia*: Initially, give B_{12} injections 1,000 mcg (1 mg) per week for 4 weeks; then monthly B_{12} injections for lifetime. Alternative is very high oral doses of B_{12} (1,000–2,000 mcg) PO daily. Oral vitamin B_{12} replacement may be as effective as parenteral vitamin B_{12}. Parenteral replacement should be used for patients with neurologic changes and/or concerns regarding gastric absorption of vitamin B_{12}.

EXAM TIPS

- **Pernicious anemia results in:**
  - **Vitamin B_{12}-deficiency anemia**
  - **Macrocytic/megaloblastic normochromic anemia**
  - **Neurologic symptoms**
- **A cheap screening test for sickle cell is the Sickledex, but the gold standard is hemoglobin electrophoresis.**
- **Every state in the United States, the District of Columbia, and the U.S. territories requires that every newborn be tested for sickle cell disease as part of the newborn screening test after birth.**
- **If the parietal antibody test (antiparietal antibody) and/or the intrinsic factor antibody test (anti-IF) are elevated, the patient has pernicious anemia.**

CLINICAL PEARLS

- **In a person with normal bone marrow, supplementing the deficient substance (iron, B_{12}, folate) will cause the hemoglobin/hematocrit to increase starting at 1 to 2 weeks; the hemoglogin/hematocrit will be back to normal within 4 to 8 weeks.**
- **Serum vitamin B_{12} levels may be normal in up to 5% of patients with vitamin B_{12} deficiency. Do not rely on vitamin B_{12} levels alone. Also check antibodies, urine MMA, etc.**
- **Missing a diagnosis of vitamin B_{12} deficiency can result in irreversible neurological damage.**
- **Any patient complaining of neuropathy or who has dementia should have vitamin B_{12} levels checked.**
- **Almost one out of every 500 African Americans in the United States has sickle cell anemia.**

Folic Acid-Deficiency Anemia

Deficiency in folate results in damage to the DNA of RBCs, which causes macrocytosis (MCV >100 fL). The body's supply of folate lasts 2 to 3 months. Does not cause neurologic damage.

- *Most common cause*: Inadequate dietary intake (elderly, infants, alcoholics, overcooking vegetables, low citrus intake). Chronic alcoholism and poor nutrition contribute to a decrease in the amount of vitamin B_{12} released from dietary proteins.
- *Other causes*: Increased physiologic need (pregnancy), malabsorption (gluten enteropathy) cause folic acid-deficiency anemia.
- *Drugs (long term)* that interfere with folate absorption: Phenytoin (Dilantin), trimethoprim-sulfa, metformin, methotrexate, sulfasalazine, zidovudine (Retrovir, azidothymidine), others.

Classic Case

Elderly patient and/or alcoholic older man complains of anemia signs/symptoms (tiredness, fatigue, pallor, and a reddened and sore tongue, or glossitis). No neurological complaints. If anemia is severe (applies to all anemias), may have tachycardia, palpitations, angina, or HF.

Treatment Plan

- *CBC*: Decreased hemoglobin and hematocrit, increased MCV
- *Peripheral smear*: Macro-ovalocytes, hypersegmented neutrophils (more than 5 to 6 lobes)
- *Folate level*: Low (if more than 4 ng/mL, rules out folate deficiency)
- *Food sources*: Leafy green vegetables (kale, collard greens), grains, beans, liver

Medications

- Correct primary cause. Improve diet. Stop overcooking vegetables.
- Administer folic acid PO 1 to 5 mg/d. Treat until RBC indicators and anemia are normal.
- Women of childbearing age: It is recommended that all women who may become pregnant take a folic acid supplement, 400 mcg daily, at least 1 month (or longer) prior to conception to enhance normal fetal development and decrease the incidence of neural tube defects. Women who have had a previous child born with a neural tube defect require higher doses of folic acid, 4 mg daily.

Sickle Cell Anemia

Sickle cell anemia is a genetic hemolytic anemia (autosomal recessive). It takes many forms, ranging from sickle cell trait to various forms of full-blown disease. Persons with sickle cell anemia have an increased resistance to malarial infection (*Plasmodium falciparum* from mosquito bite). Higher risk of death from infection with encapsulated bacteria (i.e., *Streptococcus pneumoniae, Haemophilus influenzae*, etc.) due to hyposplenia. Patients with splenectomy (for other causes) are also at higher risk of death.

In the United States, it is most commonly found in African Americans (one in 500 have the disease and more than 2 million carry the trait). Higher prevalence in people from Africa, the Mediterranean, the Middle East, and some areas of India. Mean hemoglobin of about 8 g/dL and a shortened RBC life span (17 vs. 120 days).

- Sickledex is the screening test and hemoglobin electrophoresis is the diagnostic test
- *Hemoglobin electrophoresis:* 80% to 100% HbS, elevated HbF (no HbA)

Classic Case

Most patients with sickle cell trait are asymptomatic. Patients who have the full-blown sickle cell disease are extremely anemic, have frequent sickling episodes, and have painful crises (of affected organ systems). Signs and symptoms include ischemic necrosis of bones or skin, renal and/or liver dysfunction. priapism, hemolytic episodes, hyposplenism, frequent infections, others.

Labs

- CBC is the screening test
- Gold-standard test is the hemoglobin electrophoresis (HbS)

Treatment Plan

- Refer patients with disease to hematologist.
- As of 2008, screening for sickle cell disease is mandatory for all states in the United States (Vinchinsky & Mahoney, 2016).
- Sickle cell is an autosomal recessive pattern genetic disease. Genetic counseling needed if both partners are at risk. If each parent has the sickle cell trait, one child out of four will have the disease. Prenatal screening is available as early as 8 to 10 weeks gestation via chorionic villus sampling or amniocentesis.

EXAM TIPS

- **If patient has anemia with MCV 76, the next step is to order TIBC, ferritin, serum iron. If ferritin/iron levels are low, patient has iron deficiency, but if these tests are normal, patient probably has thallassemia trait.**
- **Order both vitamin B_{12} and folate levels when evaluating MCV greater than 100 fL (even if no neurological symptoms).**
- **Pernicious anemia results in vitamin B_{12} deficiency.**
- **Pernicious anemia is a macrocytic anemia.**
- **Learn food groups for both folate and vitamin B_{12}.**
- **RBC size is described in many ways, such as:**
  - **MCV <80 fL: Microcytic and hypochromic RBCs, small and pale RBCs**
  - **MCV >100 fL: Macrocytes or macroovalocytes, larger than normal RBCs, or RBCs with enlarged cytoplasms**
- **Ethnic background may not be mentioned in a thalassemia problem, or it may be a distractor.**
- **Only vitamin B_{12}-deficiency anemia has neurologic symptoms (tingling, numbness).**

SUMMARY: MICROCYTIC ANEMIAS

Iron-Deficiency Anemia Versus Thalassemia Trait

Ferritin Level

- Low in iron deficiency
- Normal to high in thalassemia

Serum Iron

- Decreased in iron deficiency
- Normal to high in thalassemia

TIBC

- Elevated in iron deficiency
- Normal or borderline thalassemia

MCHC

- A measure of RBC color
- Decreased in iron deficiency
- Normal in thalassemia

Hemoglobin Electrophoresis

- Normal in iron deficiency
- Abnormal in thalassemia

Ethnic Background

- Ethnicity or age does not matter in iron-deficiency anemia
- Iron-deficiency anemia is the most common anemia overall in any age group, gender, or ethnicity
- Thalassemia is seen in people from Southeast Asia (e.g., China), the Mediterranean (e.g., Italy), North Africa (e.g., Morocco), the Middle East (e.g., Libya), and Asia (e.g., India)
- Alpha thalassemia is more common in Asians

14

Musculoskeletal System Review

DANGER SIGNALS

Navicular Fracture (Scaphoid Bone Fracture; Figure 14.1)

Wrist pain on palpation of the anatomic snuffbox. Pain on axial loading of the thumb. History of falling forward with outstretched hand (hyperextension of the wrist) to break the fall. Initial x-ray of the wrist may be normal, but a repeat x-ray in 2 weeks will show the scaphoid fracture (due to callus bone formation). High risk of avascular necrosis and nonunion. Splint wrist (thumb spica splint) and refer to a hand surgeon.

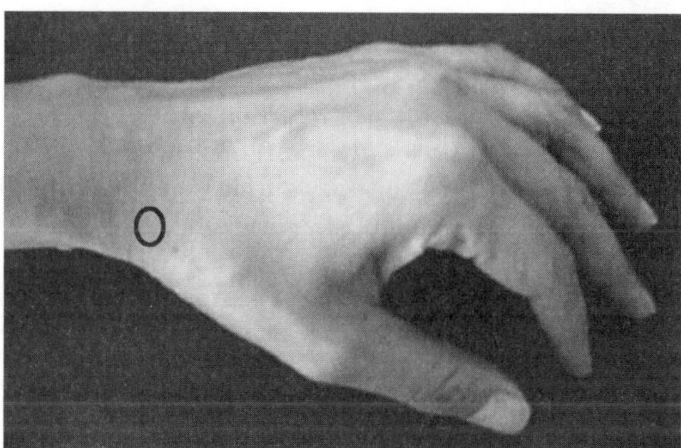

Figure 14.1 Navicular space.

Colles Fracture

Fracture of the distal radius (with or without ulnar fracture) of the forearm along with dorsal displacement of wrist. History of falling forward with outstretched hand (as in navicular fracture). This fracture is also known as the "dinner fork" fracture due to the appearance of arm and wrist after the fracture. It is the most common type of wrist fracture.

Hip Fracture

Patient has a history of slipping or falling. Sudden onset of one-sided hip pain. Unable to walk and bear weight on affected hip. If mild fracture, may bear weight on affected hip. If displaced fracture, presence of severe hip pain with external rotation of the hip/leg (abduction) and leg shortening. More common in elderly. Elderly have a 1-year mortality rate from 12% to 37%, related to complications of immobility such as pneumonia and deep vein thrombophlebitis.

Pelvic Fracture

History of significant or high-energy trauma such as a motor vehicle or motorcycle accident. Signs and symptoms depend on degree of injury to the pelvic bones and other pelvic structures such as nerves, blood vessels, and pelvic organs. Look for ecchymosis and swelling in the lower abdomen, the hips, groin, and/or scrotum. May have bladder and/or fecal incontinence, vaginal or rectal bleeding, hematuria, numbness, etc. May cause internal hemorrhage, which can be life-threatening. Check airway, breathing, and circulation first (the ABCs).

Cauda Equina Syndrome

Acute onset of saddle anesthesia, bladder incontinence (or retention of urine), and fecal incontinence. Accompanied by bilateral leg numbness and weakness. Pressure (most common cause is a bulging disk) on a sacral nerve root results in inflammatory and ischemic changes to the nerves. A surgical emergency. Needs spinal decompression. Refer to ED.

Low-Back Pain (From a Dissecting Abdominal Aneurysm)

Acute and sudden onset of "tearing" severe low-back/abdominal pain. Presence of abdominal bruit with abdominal pulsation. Patient has signs and symptoms of shock. More common in elderly males, atherosclerosis, White race and smokers.

NORMAL FINDINGS

Joint Anatomy

- *Synovial fluid*: Thick serous clear fluid (sterile) that provides lubrication for the joint
  - Cloudy synovial fluid can be indicative of infection; order C&S
- *Synovial space*: Space between two bones (the joint) filled with synovial fluid
- *Articular cartilage*: The cartilage lining the open surfaces of bones in a joint
- *Meniscus or menisci (plural)*: Crescent-shaped cartilage located in each knee; two menisci in each knee
  - Damage to menisci may cause locking of the knees and knee instability
- *Tendons*: Connects muscles to the bone; ligaments connect bone to bone
- *Bursae*: Saclike structures located on the anterior and posterior areas of a joint that act as padding; filled with synovial fluid when inflamed (bursitis)
  - Cloudy fluid is abnormal and is indicative of infection

Benign Variants

- *Genu recurvatum*: Hyperextension or backward curvature of the knees
- *Genu valgum*: Knock-knees
- *Genu varum*: Bowlegs

EXAM TIP

- **To remember valgum, think of "gum stuck between the knees" (knock-knees). The opposite is varus, or bowlegs.**

EXERCISE AND INJURIES

- Within the first 48 hours, acutely inflamed joints should not:
  - Be exercised in any form (not even isometric exercises)

  - Have applications of heat of any form for 24 to 48 hours (i.e., hot showers or tub baths, hot packs)
  - Engage in any active range-of-motion (ROM) exercises; if done too early, they will cause more inflammation and damage to the affected joints
- Avoid exacerbating activities and protect joint

RICE Mnemonic

Within the first 48 hours after musculoskeletal trauma, follow these rules:

- *Rest*: Avoid using injured joint or limb.
- *Ice*: Apply cold packs on injured area (i.e., 20 minutes on, 10 minutes off) for first 48 hours.
- *Compression*: Use an elastic bandage wrap over joints to decrease swelling and provide support. Joints that are usually compressed are the ankles and the knees.
- *Elevation*: This prevents or decreases swelling. Avoid bearing weight on affected joint.

Isometric Exercise

- Useful during the early phase of recovery before regular active exercise is performed
- Defined as the controlled and sustained contraction and relaxation of a muscle group
- Less stressful on joints than regular exercise
- Usually done first before active exercise postinjury
- Non-weight-bearing exercise:
  - Isometric exercises are non-weight-bearing exercises that are performed in a fixed state in which the muscle is flexed against a stationary object. Examples are pushing one fist against the palm of the other hand, which is stationary, biking, and swimming.
- Weight-bearing exercise:
  - In weight-bearing exercises, the bones/muscles are forced against gravity. Weight-bearing exercise is recommended for treating osteoporosis to help strengthen bone durability. Examples are walking, skiing, yoga, tai chi, lifting weights, etc.

ORTHOPEDIC MANEUVERS

Test both extremities. Use the normal limb as the "baseline" for comparison.

Drawer Sign (Figure 14.2)

Drawer sign is a test for knee stability. It is a diagnostic sign of a torn or ruptured ligament. The positive anterior drawer sign is the test for the anterior cruciate ligament (ACL). The posterior drawer sign is the test for the posterior cruciate ligament (PCL).

Finkelstein's Test (Figure 14.3)

De Quervain's tenosynovitis is caused by an inflammation of the tendon and its sheath, which is located at the base of the thumb. The screening test is Finkelstein's, which is positive if there is pain and tenderness on the wrist (thumb side) upon ulnar deviation (abductor pollicis longus and extensor pollicis brevis tendons).

McMurray's Test (Figure 14.4)

Knee pain and a "click" sound upon manipulation of the knee are positive. A positive McMurray's test suggests injury to the medial meniscus. Gold-standard test for joint damage is the MRI.

Lachman's Sign (Figure 14.5)

Knee joint laxity is positive. Suggestive of ACL damage of the knee. More sensitive than the anterior drawer test for ACL damage.

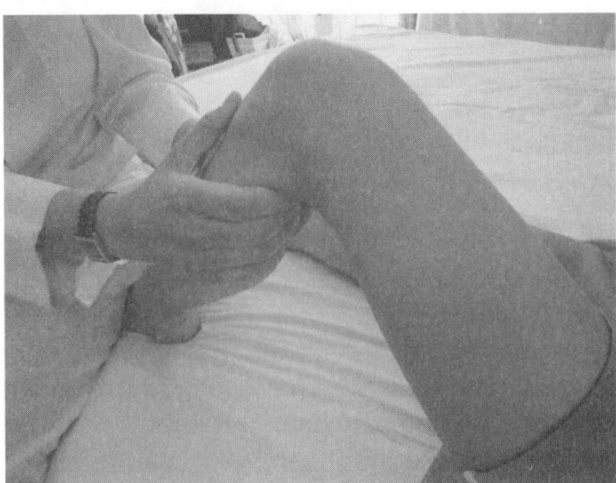

Figure 14.2 Drawer sign.

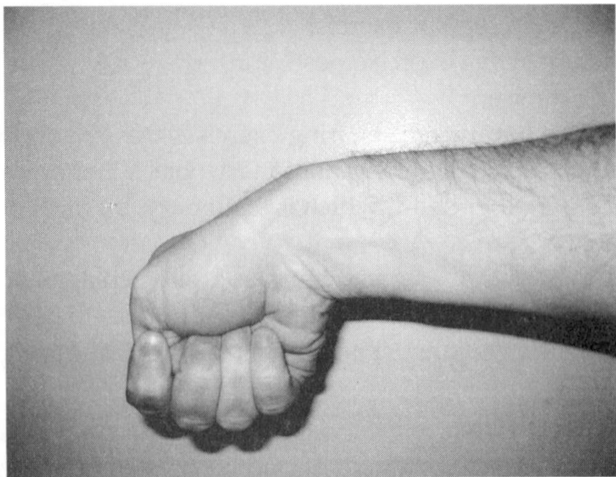

Figure 14.3 Finkelstein's test. This image can be found in color in the app.

Source: Courtesy of InvictaHOG.

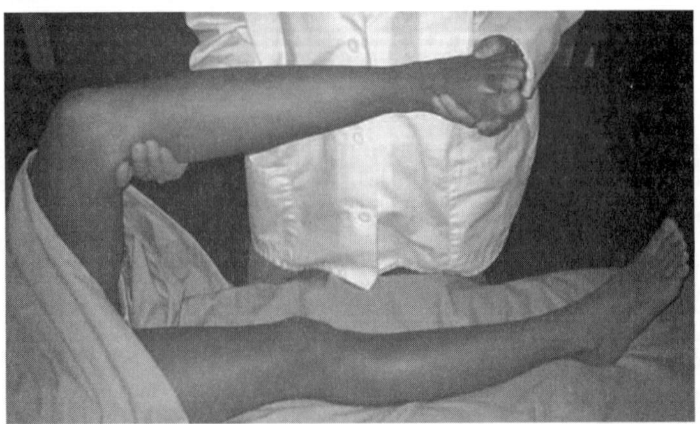

Figure 14.4 McMurray's test.

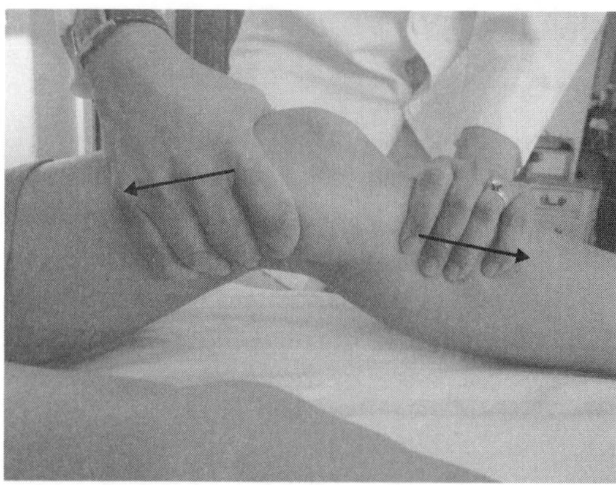

Figure 14.5 Lachman's sign.

Collateral Ligaments (Knees)

Positive finding is an increase in laxity of the damaged knee (ligament tear).

- Valgus stress test of the knee: Test for medial collateral ligament (MCL)
- Varus stress test of the knee: Test for the lateral collateral ligament (LCL)

JOINT INJECTIONS

Administering intra-articular/periarticular joint injections with steroids (e.g., triamcinolone) is a controversial treatment for osteoarthritis (OA). Some expert panels suggest about four injections per joint (such as a knee) in a lifetime. If high resistance is felt when pushing syringe, do not force. Withdraw needle slightly (do not remove from joint) and redirect.

- *Complications*: Tendon rupture, nerve damage, infection, bleeding, hypothalamic–pituitary–adrenal (HPA) suppression, others. Joint injections are contraindicated in patients requiring anticoagulation therapy due to the risk of hemarthrosis.

RADIOGRAPHY, CT SCANS, AND MRI SCANS

- *Plain x-ray films (radiographs):* Show bone fractures, OA (joint space narrowing, osteophyte formation), damaged bone (osteomyelitis, metastases), metal, and other dense objects. Not recommended for soft tissue structures such as the meniscus, tendons, and ligaments.
- *MRI*: Gold standard for injuries of the cartilage, menisci, tendons, ligaments, or any joint of the body. The MRI uses a magnetic field and not radiation (compared with x-rays and CT scans). Can be done with contrast.
  - *Contraindicated:* Metal implants, pacemakers, aneurysm clips, insulin pumps, metallic foreign body in the eye, "triggerfish" contact lens, cochlear implant, electrodes for deep brain stimulation, and metallic joints.
- *CT*: Costs less than MRI. Uses radiation to view structures. Can be done with contrast. Detects bleeding, aneurysms, masses, pelvic and bone trauma, fractures. Uses x-ray images to form three-dimensional picture.

CLINICAL PEARLS

- ***MRI***: **Best for soft tissue injuries such as tendons and cartilage**
- ***X-rays (radiographs)***: **Best for bone injuries such as fractures**

ORTHOPEDIC TERMINOLOGY

Abduction and Adduction

- *Abduction (varus)*: Movement going away from the body
- *Adduction (valgum)*: Movement going toward the body

Hands and Feet

- *Carpal (carpo)*: Refers to the bones of the hands and the wrist
- *Phalanges*: Fingers and the toes; singular form of the term is "phalanx"
- *Tarsal* (tarso): Refers to bones of the feet or the ankle

Proximal and Distal

- *Proximal*: Body part located closer to the body (compared to distal)
- *Distal*: Body part farther away from the center of the body

DISEASE REVIEW

Medial Tibial Stress Syndrome or Fracture

Lower extremity injury caused by overuse resulting in microtears and inflammation of the muscles, tendons, and bone tissue of the tibia. Also known as "shin splints." More common in runners and people with flat feet. If severe, it can progress into a stress fracture. Females are at higher risk of stress fracture, especially those with "female athlete triad" (amenorrhea, eating disorder, and osteoporosis). Onset precipitated or worsened with intensification of activity (increased mileage and/or frequency of training).

Classic Case

Complains of recurrent shin pain in one (or both) leg(s) that becomes more severe over time. The pain is located along the inner border (inside edge) of the tibia and occurs during and after exercise. There may be mild swelling and a focal area of tenderness that is painful on palpation (suggestive of stress fracture of tibia). In contrast, the pain is more vague without localized tenderness with medial tibial stress syndrome.

Treatment Plan

- Follow RICE mnemonic. Several weeks of rest are recommended.
- Use cold packs during acute exacerbation, for 20 minutes at a time, several times a day.
- Compression bandage or sleeve may help decrease swelling. Using cushioned shoes (sneakers) for daily activity helps decrease tibial stress.
- If aerobic exercise is desired, recommend lower impact exercises (e.g., swimming, stationary bike, elliptical trainer). If stress fracture is suspected, advise patient to avoid exercising.
- Imaging test of choice: bone scan and/or MRI. A radiograph (x-ray) does not show stress fractures. Refer to orthopedic specialist.

Plantar Fasciitis

Acute or recurrent pain on the bottom of the feet that is aggravated by walking. Caused by microtears in the plantar fascia due to tightness of the Achilles tendon. Higher risk with obesity (body mass index [BMI] greater than 30), diabetes, aerobic exercise, flat feet, prolonged standing.

Classic Case

Middle-aged adult complains of plantar foot pain (either on one or both feet) that is worsened by walking and weight bearing. Complains that foot pain is worse during the first few steps in the morning, and continues to worsen with prolonged walking.

Treatment Plan

- Nonsteroidal anti-inflammatory drugs (NSAIDs): Naproxen (Aleve) PO BID, ibuprofen (Advil) PO every 4 to 6 hours
- Topical NSAID: Diclofenac gel (Voltaren Gel) applied to soles of feet BID
- Use orthotic foot appliance at night for a few weeks; apply ice pack to affected foot
- Stretching and massaging of the foot: Roll a golf ball with sole of foot several times a day
- Weight loss (if overweight)
- Consider x-ray to rule out fracture, heel spurs, complicated case; refer to podiatrist PRN

Morton's Neuroma

Inflammation of the digital nerve of the foot between the third and fourth metatarsals. Increased risk with high-heeled shoes, tight shoes, obesity, dancers, runners.

Classic Case

Middle-aged woman complains of many weeks of plantar foot pain that is worsened by walking, especially while wearing high heels or tight narrow shoes. The pain is described as burning and/or numbness and is located on the space between the third and fourth toes (metatarsals) on the forefoot. Physical exam of the foot may reveal a small nodule on the space between the third and fourth toes. Some patients palpate the same nodule and report it as "pebble-like."

Mulder Test

This is a test for Morton's neuroma. Done by grasping the first and fifth metatarsals and squeezing the forefoot. Positive test is hearing a click along with a patient report of pain during compression. Pain is relieved when the compression is stopped.

Treatment Plan

- Avoid wearing tight narrow shoes and high heels. Use forefoot pad. Wear well-padded shoes.
- Diagnosed by clinical presentation and history. Refer to podiatrist.

Degenerative Joint Disease (DJD, or OA)

DJD, or OA, occurs when the cartilage covering the articular surface of joints becomes damaged from overuse and with age. Large weight-bearing joints (hips and knees) and the hands are most commonly affected. Risk factors include older age, overuse of joints, and positive family history.

Goal of Treatment

- Relieve pain
- Preserve joint mobility and function
- Minimize disability and protect joint

Classic Case

Gradual onset (over years). Early-morning joint stiffness with inactivity. Shorter duration of joint stiffness (less than 15 minutes) compared to rheumatoid arthritis (RA). Pain aggravated by overuse of joint. During exacerbations, involved joint may be swollen and tender to palpation. May be one sided (e.g., right hip only). Absence of systemic symptoms (not a systemic inflammatory illness like RA).

Heberden's and/or Bouchard's nodes may be noted (Figure 14.6).

- *Heberden's nodes*: Bony nodules on the distal interphalangeal (DIP) joints
- *Bouchard's nodes*: Bony nodules on the proximal interphalangeal (PIP) joints

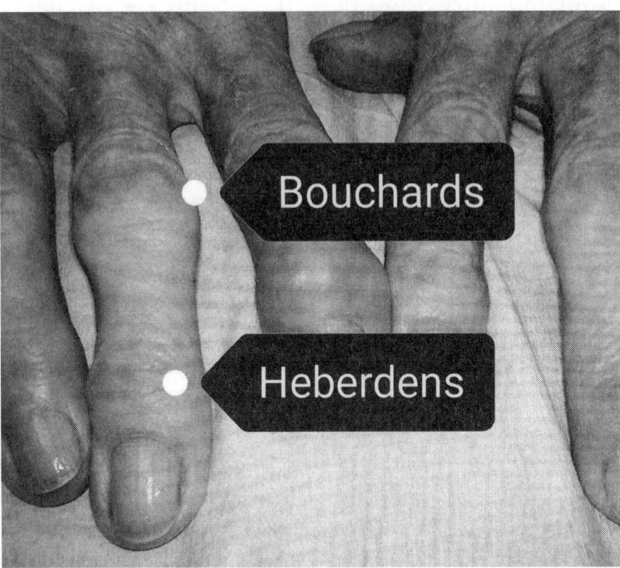

Figure 14.6 Bouchard's and Heberden's nodes. This image can be found in color in the app.

Nonpharmacological Management

- Exercise (with care) at least three times a week. Lose weight. Stop smoking.
- Do isometric exercises to strengthen quadriceps muscles (knee OA).
- Engage in weight-bearing exercise (walking, lifting weights); resistance-band exercises.
- Avoid aggravating activities. Use cold or warm packs and ultrasound treatment.
- Use walking aids. Patellar taping by physical therapist will reduce load on knees.
- Alternative medicine: Use glucosamine supplements, SAM-E, tai chi exercises, acupuncture.

*Treatment Plan**

- First-line medication is acetaminophen 325 to 650 mg every 4 to 6 hours (maximum 4 g/d) PRN.

  or
- Tylenol 325 mg to 1,000 mg every 4 to 6 hours (maximum dose 4 g [4,000 mg] per 24 hours) PRN. Dehydration increases risk of hepatic adverse effects; drink a lot of water.
- If no relief with acetaminophen, switch to a short-acting NSAID.
- Start with NSAIDs, such as ibuprofen (Advil), one to two tablets every 4 to 6 hours or naproxen (Aleve) BID or Anaprox DS one tablet every 12 hours PRN.
- For added GI protection (if long term), add a proton-pump inhibitor (PPI; omeprazole) or misoprostol (Cytotec).

---

*Adapted from the American College of Rheumatology (2012).

- If patient is at high risk for both GI bleeding and cardiovascular side effects, avoid NSAIDs.
  - GI bleed risk factors: History of uncomplicated ulcer, aspirin, warfarin (Coumadin), peptic ulcer disease, platelet disorder
  - Opioid analgesics: Avoid if possible (especially if patient is a recovering addict/ alcoholic)
- Age older than 75 years: Use topical (vs. oral) NSAIDs for treatment
- Rule out osteoporosis and order bone mineral density test

Topical Medicine

- *NSAID*: Diclofenac gel (Voltaren Gel); apply to painful area and massage well into skin QID.
- *Capsaicin cream*: Apply to painful area QID. Avoid contact with eyes/mucous membranes.
- Do not use on wounds/abraded skin. Avoid bathing/showering afterward (so that it is not washed off).
- Capsaicin comes from chili peppers. Also used to treat neuropathic pain (e.g., postshingles).

NSAID Risk

- Highest risk of GI bleeding: Ketorolac (Toradol) and piroxicam (Feldene)
- Lowest risk of GI bleeding: Ibuprofen and celecoxib (Celebrex)
- Highest risk of cardiovascular events: Diclofenac and celecoxib at higher doses
- Lowest cardiovascular risk: Naproxen

EXAM TIPS

- **Heberden's and/or Bouchard's nodes have appeared many times on the exam. Memorize the location of each. The following may help:**
  - **Heberden's: The "-den" ending on the word is the letter "D" for DIP joint. By the process of elimination, Bouchard's is on the PIP joint.**
  - **Another way to distinguish them is by using the alphabet. The letter "B" comes before the letter "H." Therefore, Bouchard's node comes before Heberden's nodes.**
- **Types of treatment methods used for DJD: Analgesics, NSAIDs (PO and topical), steroid injection on inflamed joints (*no* systemic/oral steroids), surgery (i.e., joint replacement).**
- **Do not confuse the treatment options for OA with those for RA.**
- **Recognize signs and symptoms of a medial tibial stress fracture.**

Systemic Lupus Erythematosus (SLE)

A multisystem autoimmune disease that is more common in women (9:1 ratio). Characterized by remissions and exacerbations. More common in African American and Hispanic women. Organ systems affected are the skin, kidneys, heart, and blood vessels. Milder form of lupus is called *cutaneous lupus erythematosus*.

Classic Case

Typical patient is a woman between 20 and 35 years of age. Classic rash is the maculopapular butterfly-shaped rash on the middle of the face (malar rash). May have nonpruritic thick scaly red rashes on sun-exposed areas (discoid rash). UA is positive for proteinuria.

Treatment Plan

Refer to rheumatologist (topical and oral steroids, Plaquenil, methotrexate, biologics).

Patient Education

- Avoid sun between 10 a.m. and 4 p.m. (causes rashes to break out).
- Cover skin with high SPF (UVA and UVB) sunblock.
- Wear sun-protective clothing such as hats with wide brims, long-sleeved shirts.
- Use nonfluorescent light bulbs (more sensitive to indoor fluorescent lighting).

Rheumatoid Arthritis (RA)

Systemic autoimmune disorder that is more common in women (8:1). Mainly manifested through inflammation of multiple joints and possibly joint damage. The goal of treatment is to prevent joint damage. Patients are at higher risk for other autoimmune disorders, such as Graves' disease, pernicious anemia, and others.

Classic Case

Adult, commonly middle-aged, woman complains of gradual onset of symptoms over months with daily fatigue, low-grade fever, generalized body aches, and myalgia. Complains of generalized joint pain, which usually involves the fingers/hands, elbows, wrists, and/or feet. Commonly reports early-morning stiffness/pain and warm, tender, and swollen fingers in the DIP/PIP joints (also called "sausage joints").

Objective Findings

- Joint involvement is symmetrical with more joints involved compared to DJD.
- Most common joints affected: Hands, wrist, elbows, ankles, feet, and shoulders
- "Sausage joints"
- Morning stiffness occurs for at least 1 hour and has been present for more than 6 weeks
- Rheumatoid nodules present (chronic disease)
- Swan neck deformity (50%): Flexion of the DIP joint with hyperextension of the PIP joint
- Boutonniere deformity: Hyperextension of the DIP with flexion of the PIP joint

Labs

- Sedimentation rate: Elevated
- *CBC*: Mild microcytic or normocytic anemia common
- *Rheumatoid factor (RF)*: Positive in 75% to 80% of patients
- *Radiographs*: Bony erosions, joint space narrowing, subluxations (or dislocation)

Treatment Plan

- Refer to rheumatologist for early aggressive management to minimize joint damage
- Surgery: Joint replacement (hip, knees) ameliorates RA
- Careful assessment is necessary: Never prescribe a biologic or anti-TNF medication if signs and symptoms of infection (fever, sore throat, etc.) are present. TB testing should be ordered prior to start of anti-TNF therapy.

Medications

- NSAIDs (i.e., ibuprofen, naproxen sodium) help to relieve inflammation and pain
- Steroids: Systemic oral doses
- Steroid joint injections (synovial space)
- Disease-modifying antirheumatic drugs (DMARDs) such as methotrexate, sulfasalazine, cyclosporine, and hydroxychloroquine (an antimalarial drug)
- If poor response to nonbiologic DMARDs, use other options such as biologic agents, tumor necrosis factor (TNF), and alpha inhibitors
- Anti-TNF biologics: Adalimumab (Humira), etanercept (Enbrel), infliximab (Remicade)
  - *Warnings:* Anti-TNFs increase risk of infections, squamous cell skin cancer, lymphoma.

Complications

- Uveitis (eyes): Inflammation of the uvea (middle layer eyeball). Sudden onset of eye redness, pain, blurred vision. Can cause vision loss. Refer to ophthalmologist *stat*.
- RA increases risk of anterior uveitis, scleritis, vasculitis, pericarditis, etc.
- RA increases risk of certain malignancies, such as lymphoma.
- When prescribing Plaquenil, all patients must have an eye exam prior to starting the medication. Frequent eye-exam monitoring should be performed every 6 months or as recommended by the ophthalmologist to assess and prevent retinal damage, which can lead to blindness.

EXAM TIPS

- **Distinguish between RA and OA in terms of classic presentation. With RA, joint stiffness lasts longer. It involves multiple joints, and has a symmetrical distribution. RA is accompanied by systemic symptoms such as fatigue, fever, normocytic anemia, others.**
- **Treatment of RA includes all DJD treatment methods plus systemic steroids, antimalarials (Plaquenil), antimetabolites (methotrexate), biologics (Humira, Enbrel, etc).**
- **Bouchard's nodes can occur in both OA/DJD and RA (located on PIP). Heberden's nodes are seen only with OA/DJD (located on PIP).**
- **Uveitis: Swelling of the uvea, the middle layer of the eye that supplies blood to the retina (refer to ophthalmologist *stat*). Patient treated with high-dose steroids for several weeks. Higher risk of uveitis with inflammatory disease (ankylosing spondylitis, sarcoidosis, inflammatory bowel disease, others).**
- **Plaquenil is an antimalarial.**
- **Methotrexate is a DMARD. It is contraindicated for use during pregnancy. When prescribing methotrexate to childbearing women, contraception must be prescribed and adhered to while taking methotrexate.**
- **Know the presentation of RA and lab findings. Distinguish between presentation of OA and RA.**
- **NSAIDs injure the GI tract by blocking COX-1 and COX-2, resulting in lower levels of systemic prostaglandins. COX-1 has mucosal protective effect. COX-2 has mucosal lining of stomach versus COX-1 or NSAIDs**
- **Aspirin (acetylsalicylic acid) is a type of NSAID. It affects platelets and clotting.**

Gout

Deposits of uric acid crystals inside joints and tendons due to genetic excess production or low excretion of purine crystals (by-product of protein metabolism). High levels of uric acid crystallize in joints with predisposition for first joint of large toe. More common in middle-aged males older than 30 years of age.

The gold standard for diagnosing gout is performed by joint aspiration of the synovial fluid of the joint. Microscopy exam using a polarized light is used to identify uric acid crystals in the synovial fluid to diagnose gout.

Classic Case

Middle-aged man presents with painful, hot, red, and swollen metatarsophalangeal joint of great toe (podagra). Patient is limping due to severe pain from weight bearing on affected toe. History of previous attacks at same site. Precipitated by ingestion of alcohol, meats, or seafood. Chronic gout has tophi (small white nodules full of urates on ears and joints).

Labs

- *Uric acid level*: Elevated (>7 mg/dL)
  - During the acute phase, uric acid level is normal; uric acid level does not begin to rise until after the acute phase
  - Test uric acid level 2 weeks after acute attack
- *CBC:* WBC level elevated
- *ESR:* Elevated

Treatment Plan

Acute Phase

- *First goal is to provide pain relief.* Two types of NSAIDs are most effective: indomethacin (Indocin) BID and naproxen sodium (Anaprox DS) BID PRN. Do not use narcotics (not effective for gout pain).
- If no relief, combine NSAID with colchicine 1.2 mg (two tablets) at onset of attack and may repeat colchicine 0.6 mg (one tablet) in 1 hour.
- Continue colchicine 0.6 mg one to two times daily until symptoms resolve. May stop therapy when symptom-free for 2 to 3 days.
- After acute phase is over, wait at least 4 to 6 weeks before initiating maintenance treatment.
- Patients taking allopurinol should stop during acute phase and restart 4 to 6 weeks after resolution of symptoms.

Maintenance

- Administer allopurinol (Zyloprim) daily for years to lifetime. Check CBC (affects bone marrow).
- Probenecid (a uricosuric) lowers uric acid.
- Colchicine has anti-inflammatory effects and can be used during acute phase (with NSAIDs) and for maintenance phase. Patients should be instructed to avoid alcohol, high-purine foods, and to remain well hydrated.

Complication

- Joint destruction, kidney failure

Ankylosing Spondylitis

More common in males (two to three times) and those who are HLA-B27 positive. Average age of onset is the 20s to 30s. Chronic inflammatory disorder (seronegative arthritis) that affects mainly the spine (axial skeleton) and the sacroiliac joints. Some other joints affected are the shoulders and hips. Pain improves with exercise and is not relieved by rest.

Classic Case

Young adult man complains of a chronic case of back pain (>3 months) that is worse in the upper back (upper thoracic spine). Joint pain keeps him awake at night. Associated with generalized symptoms such as low-grade fever and fatigue. May have chest pain with respiration (costochondritis). Long-term stiffness improves with activity. Some may have midbuttock pain (sciatica).

Objective Findings

- Causes a marked loss of ROM of the spine such as forward bending, rotation, and lateral bending.
- Decreased respiratory excursion down to less than 2.5 cm (normal 5 cm). Some have lordosis. Hyperkyphosis ("hunchback") occurs after 10 years or more with disease.

- Uveitis (up to 40% patients): Complains of eye irritation, photosensitivity, and eye pain. Scleral injection and blurred vision occur. Refer to ophthalmologist as soon as possible (treated with steroids).

Labs

- Sedimentation rate and C-reactive protein slightly elevated; RF is negative
- *Spinal radiograph*: Classic "bamboo spine"

Treatment Plan

- Refer to rheumatologist.
- Instruct patient in postural training and advise patient to buy a mattress with good support.
- First-line treatment is NSAIDs (dramatic response).
- If high risk of bleeding, prescribe PPI with NSAIDs, or COX-2 inhibitor (celecoxib or Celebrex).
- For severe cases, treatment options are DMARDs, biologics (anti-TNF drugs), spinal fusion.

Complications

- Anterior uveitis
- Aortitis (inflammation of the aorta)
- Fusing of the spine with significant loss of ROM; spinal stenosis

Low-Back Pain

Very common disorder with a lifetime incidence of 85%. Usually due to soft tissue inflammation, sciatica, sprains, muscle spasms, or herniated disks (usually on L5 to S1). Rule out fracture and other etiology (see text that follows).

Further Evaluation (Recommended)

- History of significant trauma
- Suspect cancer metastases
- Suspect infection (osteomyelitis)
- Suspect spinal fracture (elderly with osteoporosis, chronic steroid use)
- Patient age older than 50 with new onset of back pain (rule out cancer) or pain that wakes a patient from sleep
- Suspect spinal stenosis (rule out ankylosing spondylitis)
- Symptoms worsening despite usual treatment
- Herniated disk with symptoms: Common site is at L5 to S1 (buttock/leg pain)

Labs

- *MRI*: Best method for diagnosing a herniated disk. Bone scan may be helpful in identifying occult, lytic lesions.

Treatment Plan

- Treatment depends on etiology. For uncomplicated back pain, use NSAIDs (naproxen sodium); apply warm packs if muscle spasms
- Muscle relaxants if associated with muscle spasms (causes drowsiness; warn patient)
- Abdominal and core-strengthening exercises after acute phase
- Consider chiropractor for uncomplicated low-back pain

> **Note**
>
> Bed rest is not recommended except in severe cases of low-back pain because it will cause deconditioning (loss of muscle tone and endurance) and increased risk of pneumonia.

Complications

Cauda Equina Syndrome

Acute pressure on a sacral nerve root results in inflammatory and ischemic changes to the nerve. Sacral nerves innervate pelvic structures such as the sphincters (anal and bladder). Considered a surgical emergency. Needs decompression. Refer to ED.

Signs

- Bowel incontinence
- Bladder incontinence
- Saddle anesthesia

EXAM TIPS

- **Ankylosing spondylitis: Know signs and symptoms so you are able to diagnose it on the exam. Bamboo spine is pathognomonic for ankylosing spondylitis.**
- **Spinal radiograph will show "bamboo spine."**
- **Name of cast for fractures of the wrist is "thumb spica cast" (also available as a splint).**
- **Learn how to treat gout flare up. If no relief on NSAIDs for gout, combine NSAID with colchicine 1.2 mg (two tablets) at onset of attack and may repeat 0.6 mg (one tablet) in 1 hour. Do not overuse colchicine; will cause GI effects such as abdominal pain and diarrhea.**
- **Learn signs/symptoms of cauda equina. If suspected, refer to ED.**

CLINICAL PEARLS

- **Naproxen is the NSAID with the fewest cardiovascular effects, but it has the same GI adverse effects as other NSAIDs. It can, however, increase BP, so this should be monitored.**
- **The innervation of the bladder and anal sphincter comes from the sacral nerves and, with cauda equina, symptoms include new-onset incontinence of urine (and/or bowel), saddle-pattern paresthesia, sciatica, etc.**

Acute Musculoskeletal Injuries

Treatment

RICE (Rest, Ice, Compression, Elevation)

- Ice is best during first 48 hours postinjury
  - 20 minutes per hour several times/day (frequency varies)
- Rest and elevate affected joint to help decrease swelling
- Compress joints as needed. Use elastic bandage wrap (joints most commonly compressed are knees and ankles); helps with swelling and provides stability
- Administer NSAIDs (naproxen BID, ibuprofen QID) for pain and swelling PRN

Tendinitis (All Cases)

Microtears on a tendon(s) cause inflammation resulting in pain. Usually due to repetitive microtrauma, overuse, or strain. Gradual onset. Follow RICE mnemonic for acute injuries.

Supraspinatus Tendinitis

Common cause of shoulder pain. Also called *cuff tendinitis*. Due to inflammation of the supraspinatus tendon.

Classic Case
Patient complains of shoulder pain with certain movements. Movements that aggravate the pain are arm elevation and abduction (e.g., reaching to the back pocket). There is local point tenderness over the tendon located on the anterior area of the shoulder.

Epicondylitis
Common cause of elbow pain. Lateral epicondyle tendon pain (tennis elbow) or medial epicondyle tendon pain (golfer's elbow).

Lateral Epicondylitis (Tennis Elbow)
Classic Case
Gradual onset of pain on the outside of the elbow that sometimes radiates to the forearms. Pain worse with twisting or grasping movements (opening jars, shaking hands).

Medial Epicondylitis (Golfer's Elbow)
Classic Case
Gradual onset of aching pain on the medial area of the elbow (the side of the elbow that is touching the body). Higher risk in baseball players, bowlers, and golfers. Occurs in the part of the elbow also called the "funny bone."

Complications
Ulnar nerve neuropathy and/or palsy (long-term pressure/damage). Complaint of numbness/tingling on the little finger and the lateral side of the ring finger and weakness of the hand. Worse-case scenario is development of a permanent deformity called "claw hand." Chronic neuropathy is treated with tricyclic antidepressants (TCAs), gabapentin, phenytoin, and pain medications.

SPRAINS

Ottawa Rules (of the Ankle)
- Ottawa rule are used to determine whether a patient needs radiographs of the injured ankle in the ED.
- In mild to moderate sprains during acute phase, use RICE and elastic bandage wrap.

Grade I Sprain
- Mild sprain (slight stretching and some damage to ligament fibers); patient is able to bear weight and ambulate.

Grade II Sprain
- Moderate sprain (partial tearing of ligament); ecchymoses are present, moderate swelling, and pain. Joint tender to palpation. Ambulation and weight bearing are painful. Mild to moderate joint instability occurs. Consider x-ray, referral.

Grade III (Complete Rupture of Ligaments)
- Referral to ED for ankle fracture. Ankle series (done in the ED) needed if:
  - Inability to bear weight immediately after the injury
  - Inability to ambulate at least four steps
  - Tenderness over the posterior edge of the lateral or medial malleolus
  - Other findings (not part of criteria) are resistance to any foot motion, severe bruising, and severe pain

Meniscus Tear (of Knees)

The meniscus is the cartilaginous lining between certain joints that is shaped like a crescent. Tears in the meniscus result from trauma and/or overuse.

Classic Case

Patient may complain of clicking, locking, or buckling of the knee(s). Some patients are unable to fully extend affected knee. Patient may limp. Complains of knee pain and difficulty walking and bending the knee. Some complain of joint line pain. Decreased ROM.

- *Best test*: MRI; refer to orthopedic specialist for repair.

Ruptured Baker's Cyst (Bursitis)

A Baker's cyst is a type of bursitis that is located behind the knee (popliteal fossa). The bursae are protective, fluid-filled synovial sacs located on the joints that act as a cushion and protect the bones, tendons, joints, and muscles. Sometimes when a joint is damaged and/or inflamed, synovial fluid production increases, causing the bursa to enlarge.

Classic Case

Physically active patient (jogs or runs) complains of ball-like mass behind one knee that is soft and smooth. Causes pressure pain or is asymptomatic. If cyst ruptures, will cause an inflammatory reaction resembling cellulitis on the surrounding area (the calf) such as redness, swelling, and tenderness.

Labs

- Diagnosed by clinical presentation and history. MRI if diagnosis is uncertain.
- Rule out plain bursitis from bursitis with infection ("septic joint").

Treatment Plan

- Follow RICE (rest, ice, compression, and elevation) procedures. Gentle compression with elastic bandage wrap.
- Administer NSAIDs as needed.
- Large bursa can be drained with syringe using 18-gauge needle if causing pain. Synovial fluid is a clear, golden color. If cloudy synovial fluid is present and the joint is red, swollen, and hot, order a C&S to rule out a septic joint infection.

Medial Tibia Stress Syndrome (Shin Splints) and Medial Tibial Stress Fracture

More common in runners (higher incidence in females). Overuse results in inflammation of the muscles, tendons, and bone on the tibia.

Classic Case

Female runner reports that she recently increased frequency/distance running and complains of recent onset of pain on the inner edge of the tibia. Pain may be sharp and stabbing or dull and throbbing. Aggravated during and after exercise. Complains of a sore spot on the shin anterior aspect. Focal area of tenderness that is tender when touched. Some may develop a stress fracture on the tibia.

Treatment Plan

- Advise to stop activity and rest (several weeks).
- Apply cold packs for 20 minutes on shin area BID first 24 to 48 hours and then PRN.
- Take NSAIDs (ibuprofen TID or naproxen BID) PRN.
- When pain is gone, wait about 2 weeks after before resuming exercise.

- Stretch before exercise and start at lower intensity. Wear supportive sneakers.
- If suspect stress fracture, imaging tests are bone scan and MRI.

EXAM TIPS

- **Fracture of the wrist: The name of the cast is "thumb spica cast."**
- **Know Baker's cyst presentation.**
- **Plain radiograph of a joint (such as x-ray of knee) will show bony changes or narrowing of joint space (OA), but not soft tissue such as the meniscus. The best imaging test for cartilage, meniscus, or tendon damage is the MRI.**
- **The gold-standard test for assessing any joint damage is the MRI.**

CLINICAL PEARLS

- **Do not forget that NSAIDs increase cardiovascular risk, renal damage, and GI bleeding.**
- **Experts state that dramatic response to NSAIDs is helpful with diagnosing ankylosing spondylitis.**

15

Psychosocial Mental Health Review

DANGER SIGNALS

Suicide Risk Factors

- Older people who have lost a spouse (due to death or divorce)
- Plan involving a gun or other lethal weapon
- History of attempted suicide and/or family history of suicide
- Mental illness such as depression, bipolar disorder
- History of sexual, emotional, and/or physical abuse
- Terminal illness, chronic illness, chronic pain
- Alcohol abuse, substance abuse
- Significant loss (divorce, breakup with boyfriend/girlfriend, job loss, death of someone close to the person)
- Females make more attempts compared to males, but males have a higher success rate
- Bipolar disorder (also known as *manic-depressive disorder*)
  - Two types of bipolar disorder: type 1 (classic manic episodes) and type 2 (hypomanic episodes). Strong genetic component. Peak incidence of onset is in the 20s (ranges from age 14 to age 30 years).
  - Moods cycle between mania and depression. Severe anxiety, rage, and chronic relationship difficulties occur. Classic manic symptoms include labile moods, euphoria, talkativeness, flight of ideas, grandiosity, and less need for sleep.
  - A person with bipolar disorder is at higher risk of suicide during the depression phase of the illness. Look for signs and symptoms of depression and suicide warning signs.

Acute Serotonin Syndrome

Occurs from high levels of serotonin accumulating in the body due to the introduction of a new drug (drug interaction) and an increase in the dose. Has acute onset with rapid progression. Signs and symptoms are sudden onset of high fever, muscular rigidity, mental status changes, hyperreflexia/clonus, and uncontrolled shivering. Look for dilated pupils (mydriasis). Higher risk if combining two drugs that both block serotonin (i.e., selective serotonin reuptake inhibitors [SSRIs], monoamine oxidase inhibitors [MAOIs], tricyclic antidepressants [TCAs], triptans, tryptophan). If switching to another drug affecting serotonin, wait a minimum of 2 weeks. Acute serotonin syndrome is a potentially life-threatening reaction.

Malignant Neuroleptic Syndrome

Rare life-threatening idiopathic reaction from typical and atypical antipsychotics. These drugs affect the dopaminergic system of the brain. Syndrome usually develops following initiation or an increase in dose. Signs and symptoms are sudden onset of high fever, muscular rigidity, mental status changes, fluctuating BP, and urinary incontinence. Look for a history of mental illness and prescription of an antipsychotic(s). This is a potentially life-threatening reaction.

PSYCHIATRIC–MENTAL HEALTH EVALUATION

At-Risk Patients

The Baker Act

The Baker Act allows 72 hours (3 days) of involuntary detention for evaluation and treatment of persons who are considered at very high risk for suicide and/or for hurting others.

Common Mental Health Questionnaires

- Beck Depression Inventory-II
  - A multiple-choice self-report inventory for evaluating depression. Based on the theory that negative cognitions about the self and the world in general can cause depression.
- *Diagnostic and Statistical Manual of Mental Disorders, Fifth Edition* (*DSM-5*; American Psychiatric Association [APA], 2013)
  - The diagnostic manual for mental and emotional disorders used and created by the APA.
- Minnesota Multiphasic Personality Inventory, Second Edition (MMPI-2)
  - A popular questionnaire used to assess for mental illness.
- Mini-Mental State Exam, Second Edition, also known as Folstein Mini-Mental State Exam (MMSE-2; Table 15.1)
  - A questionnaire used to evaluate an individual for confusion and dementia (Alzheimer's, stroke, others).
- Geriatric Depression Scale (GDS)
  - A 30-item (yes/no response) questionnaire. Shorter version contains 15 items. Used to assess depression in the elderly. Self-assessment format.

Table 15.1 Folstein Mini-Mental State Exam (MMSE)

Cognitive Skill	Action Required
Orientation	What is the date today? (current day, month, year)
	Location? (name the city, county, state)
Immediate Recall	
Recall three objects	Instruct that you will be testing his or her memory. Say three unrelated words (pencil, apple, ball). Ask patient to repeat words.
Attention and Calculation	
Counting backward	Say "Starting at 100, count backward and keep subtracting 7."
Backward spelling	Spell the word "WORLD" backward
Writing and Copying	
Writing a sentence	Give person one blank piece of paper and ask him or her to write a sentence.
Copying a figure	Draw intersecting pentagons. Ask patient to copy the pentagons.
Scoring	Maximum score is 30 correctly done. A score of less than 19 indicates impairment.

Source: Adapted from Folstein, Folstein, and McHugh (1975).

PSYCHOTROPIC DRUGS (TABLE 15.2)

Table 15.2 Monitoring Psychiatric Medications

Drug Class	Adverse Effects	Monitor
Atypical Antipsychotics		
Olanzapine (Zyprexa)	Obesity	All can cause weight gain
Risperidone (Risperdal)	Diabetes type 2	Check BMI
Quetiapine (Seroquel)		Check weight every 3 months
Typical Antipsychotics		
Haloperidol (Haldol), chlorpromazine	Elevates lipids/ triglycerides	Labs: Fasting blood glucose and lipid profile
	Malignant neuroleptic syndrome (rare)	*Black Box Warning:* Frail elderly are at higher risk of death from antipsychotics
Anticonvulsants		
Lamotrigine (Lamictal)	Stevens–Johnson syndrome (Lamictal)	Advise patient to report rashes (Stevens–Johnson); some anticonvulsants are also used as a mood stabilizer for bipolar disorder
Carbamazepine (Tegretol)		
Valproate (Depakote)		
SSRIs		
Sertraline (Zoloft)	Anxiety	*Black Box Warning:* May cause suicidal ideation/plans (younger than 24 years of age)
Paroxetine (Paxil)	Insomnia	
Citalopram (Celexa)*	Sexual side effects	Do not discontinue Paxil abruptly Wean gradually
Escitaprolam (Lexapro)*	Serotonin syndrome	
Atypical Antidepressants		
Bupropion (Wellbutrin)	Seizures	Contraindicated with seizures disorder, anorexia, or bulimia
Zyban for smoking cessation		
SNRI		
Venlafaxine (Effexor)	Can precipitate acute narrow-angle glaucoma	Avoid with uncontrolled narrow-angle glaucoma
Duloxetine (Cymbalta**)		
TCAs		
Amitriptyline (Elavil)	Anticholinergic effects	Do not combine with SSRIs or MAOI as it will increase risk of serotonin syndrome
Nortriptyline(Pamelor)	Category X	
Doxepin (Sinequan)		

(continued)

Table 15.2 Monitoring Psychiatric Medications (*continued*)

Drug Class	Adverse Effects	Monitor
Lithium		Used for bipolar disorder; "Ebstein's anomaly" is congenital heart defect caused by lithium
Lithium carbonate (Eskalith)		Check blood levels
		Lithium is a metal

BMI, body mass index; MAOI, monoamine oxidase inhibitor; SNRI, selective norepinephrine reuptake inhibitor; SSRIs, selective serotonin reuptake inhibitors; TCAs, tricyclic antidepressants.
*Lowest number of drug interactions compared to other SSRIs.
**Cymbalta also used for neuropathic pain.

Selective Serotonin Reuptake Inhibitors (SSRIs)

First-line treatment for:

- Major depression, obsessive-compulsive disorder
- Generalized anxiety disorder, panic disorder, social anxiety disorder
- Premenstrual dysphoric disorder

Common SSRIs

- Fluoxetine (Prozac): Longest half-life of all SSRIs and the first SSRI (useful for noncompliant patients)
- Paroxetine (Paxil): Shortest half-life
- Citalopram (Celexa): Has fewer drug interactions compared with other SSRIs
- Escitalopram (Lexapro): Compound derived from citalopram (Celexa)
- Other SSRIs: Sertraline (Zoloft), fluvoxamine (Luvox)

Side Effects

- Causes loss of libido in men and women, erectile dysfunction, anorexia, insomnia
- Avoid with anorexic patients and undernourished elderly (depresses appetite more)
- Paxil: Common side effect is erectile dysfunction

Contraindications

- Avoid SSRIs within 14 days of taking an MAOI (serotonin syndrome)
- Can induce mania with bipolar patients

Tricyclic Antidepressants (TCAs)

- Not considered first-line treatment for depression
- Other uses: Postherpetic neuralgia (chronic pain), stress urinary incontinence
- Avoid if patient at high risk for suicide because may hoard pills and overdose (suicide attempt)
- Overdose will cause fatal cardiac (ventricular arrhythmia) and neurological effects (seizures)
- *Example:* Imipramine (Tofranil), amitriptyline (Elavil), nortriptyline (Norpramin)

Selective Norepinephrine Reuptake Inhibitors

- Increased available serotonin and norepinephrine in the brain
- Duloxetine (Cymbalta): Can treat both depression and neuropathic pain
- Venlafaxine (Effexor)
- Desvenlafaxine (Pristiq)

Monoamine Oxidase Inhibitors (MAOIs)

- Rarely used because of serious food (high tyramine content) and drug interactions
- Phenelzine (Nardil), tranylcypromine (Parnate)

- Do not combine with SSRIs, TCAs, MAO-B (selegiline/Eldepryl), serotonin receptor agonists (sumatriptan/Imitrex, zolmitriptan [Zomig], others)

Contraindications

- Do not combine MAOI with SSRI or TCA
- Wait at least 2 weeks before initiating SSRI or TCA (high risk of serotonin syndrome)

High-Tyramine Foods and MAOIs

- The combination can cause the tyramine pressor response (elevates BP, risk of stroke); avoid combining with fermented foods such as beer, Chianti wine, some aged cheeses, fava beans, and others
- High-tyramine foods can also cause migraine headache in susceptible persons

Benzodiazepines (Tranquilizers)

- Benzodiazepines are indicated for anxiety disorders, panic disorder, and insomnia
- Diazepam (Valium) is also used for severe alcohol withdrawal and seizures
- Do not discontinue abruptly because it increases risk of seizures; wean slowly
- Examples:
  - Ultra-short acting: Midazolam IV only (Versed), triazolam (Halcion)
  - Medium-acting: Alprazolam (Xanax), lorazepam (Ativan)
  - Long-acting: Diazepam (Valium), chlordiazepoxide (Librium), temazepam (Restoril), and clonazepam (Klonopin); avoid with the elderly

DISEASE REVIEW

Major and Minor Depression

Also known as *unipolar depression* (vs. bipolar depression). Minor depression is a milder form. The criteria of signs and symptoms are the same as major depression except that there are fewer symptoms (at least two, but less than five). Attributed to dysfunction of the neurotransmitters serotonin and norepinephrine. Has a strong genetic component.

Symptoms of Depression

- *Mood*: Depressed mood most of the time; may become tearful
- *Anhedonia*: Diminished interest or pleasure in all or most activities
- *Energy*: Fatigued or loss of energy
- *Sleep*: Insomnia or hypersomnia
- *Guilt*: Feelings of worthlessness and inappropriate guilt
- *Concentration*: Diminished concentration and difficulty making decisions
- *Suicide*: Recurrent/obsessive thoughts of death and suicidal ideation
- *Weight*: Weight loss (>5% body weight) or weight gain
- *Agitation*: Psychomotor agitation or retardation

Immediate Goal: Assess for Suicidal and/or Homicidal Ideation or Plan

If patient is considered to be a real and present threat of harm to self or to others:

- Refer to a psychiatric hospital. Patient must be driven by a family member or a friend.
- If none are available, call 911 for police. The police can "Baker Act" the patient. A Baker Act proceeding is a means of providing emergency services for mental health treatment on a voluntary or involuntary basis.

Differential Diagnosis

Rule out organic causes such as hypothyroidism, anemia, autoimmune disorders, vitamin B_{12} deficiency.

Screening Tools for Depression

- Beck Depression Inventory: Contains 21 items
- Beck Depression Inventory for Primary Care (99% specificity): Contains seven items
- Two-item question: Ask these two questions:
  1. During the past month, have you felt down, depressed, or hopeless?
  2. During the past month, have you felt little interest or pleasure doing things?
- If answered yes to either question (or both), positive finding

Labs

- CBC, chemistry profile, thyroid-stimulating hormone (TSH), folate and vitamin B_{12} levels, UA
- Rule out organic causes; toxicology screen to rule out illicit drug use

Treatment Plan

- Rule out diseases such as anemia, diabetes, hypothyroid TSH/thyroid panel), chemistry panel (low potassium for Addison's disease), and vitamin B_{12} anemia
- Refer for psychotherapy. Cognitive behavioral therapy can reduce symptoms (comparable to an antidepressant medication) and is usually effective; if necessary, refer to psychiatrist If psychotic, refer to the ED
- Psychotherapy plus antidepressants work better than either method alone

Medications

- *First-line medication*: SSRIs. Advise patients that antidepressant effect may take from 4 to 8 weeks (up to 12 weeks) to manifest. SSRIs are also first-line therapy for elderly patients because they have fewer side effects.
  - Initiation of medications for elderly patients and patients diagnosed with renal or hepatic disorders should begin at a low dose and increase slowly and gradually as tolerate
  - After initiation, follow up in 2 weeks to check for compliance and side effects
  - Wait for at least 4 to 8 weeks before changing medication
  - Continue SSRI therapy for at least 4 to 9 months after symptoms have resolved (usually on first episode); frequent relapse means patient may need lifetime treatment
- *Other antidepressants*: Administer TCAs (amitriptyline/Elavil, nortriptyline/Pamelor).
  - Prefer bedtime dosing due to sedation. Other uses are postherpetic neuralgia, chronic pain, stress urinary incontinence
  - Avoid TCAs with suicidal patients because the patient may hoard the pills and take an overdose (causes fatal arrhythmia)
- *Food and Drug Administration (FDA) Black Box Warnings*: There is increased risk of death in elderly (with dementia) on antipsychotic drugs such as haloperidol (Haldol) and chlorpromazine (Thorazine)

SSRIs: Special Considerations

- *FDA Black Box Warnings*: Increased risk of suicidal thinking and behavior in children, adolescents, and young adults; the risk of suicidality is increased in young adults ages 18 to 24 years during initial treatment (first 1–2 months)
- *Elderly patients*: Consider using citalopram (Celexa) and escitalopram (Lexapro). These drugs cause fewer drug interactions than other SSRIs; may prolong QT interval
- *Patients with sexual dysfunction caused by an SSRI*: Consider adding bupropion (Wellbutrin) to the SSRI prescription

- *Depressed patient who wants to quit smoking*: Consider bupropion (Zyban). Can be combined with nicotine-avoidance products (patches, gum)
- *Depressed patient with peripheral neuropathy*: Consider duloxetine (Cymbalta), which is also indicated for neuropathic pain
- Depressed patient with postherpetic neuralgia and chronic pain: Consider TCAs
- Depressed patient with stress urinary incontinence: Consider TCAs

Antipsychotics: Adverse Effects

- Pill-rolling, shuffling gait, and bradykinesia caused by chronic use of antipsychotics
- Extrapyramidal symptoms:
  - Akinesia (inability to initiate movement)
  - Akathisia (a strong inner feeling to move, unable to stay still)
  - Bradykinesia (slowness in movement) when initiating activities or actions that require successive steps such as buttoning a shirt
  - Tardive dyskinesia: Involuntary movements of the lips (smacking), tongue, face, trunk, and extremities (more common in schizophrenics)

Anticholinergics: Side Effects

- Many drug classes have strong anticholinergic effects such as antipsychotics, TCAs, decongestants, and antihistamines (e.g., pseudoephedrine)
- Use caution with benign prostatic hyperplasia (BPH; urinary retention), narrow-angle glaucoma, preexisting heart disease
- Use the SAD CUB mnemonic to help remember anticholinergic side effects:
  - *S*edation
  - *A*norexia
  - *D*ry mouth
  - *C*onfusion and constipation
  - *U*rinary retention
  - *B*PH

Complementary/Alternative Treatment

Complementary treatments for depression include various herbs and supplements, guided imagery, and lifestyle measures such as exercise and yoga (Table 15.3). Be aware of herb–drug interactions.

Table 15.3 Alternative Medicine for Depression

Name	Drug Interactions	Adverse Effects
St. John's wort	SSRIs (citalopram/Celexa, paroxetine/Paxil, etc)	Decreases digoxin effectiveness
		Causes breakthrough bleeding that decreases effectiveness of birth control pills
	Tricyclics (amitriptyline/Elavil, imipramine/Tofranil, etc.)	
	MAOIs, Xanax, protease inhibitors (indinavir), and many others	

(*continued*)

Table 15.3 Alternative Medicine for Depression (*continued*)

Name	Drug Interactions	Adverse Effects
Amino acid supplements such as 5-HTP, L-tryptophan	SSRIs and MAOIs	Serotonin syndrome
	Dextromethorphan	Dextromethorphan increases risk of serotonin syndrome
	Triptans (Imitrex, Zomig, others)	
Omega-3 fatty acids (cold-water fish oil such as salmon)	No major drug interactions	High doses of omega-3 fish oil may increase risk of bleeding Supplements are usually stopped about 1 week before surgery
Folate and vitamin B_6 (pyridoxine)		
Exercise, yoga, massage, guided imagery, acupuncture, light therapy		

5-HTP, 5-hydroxytryptophan; MAOIs, monoamine oxidase inhibitors; SSRIs, selective serotonin reuptake inhibitors.

EXAM TIPS

- **Know how to diagnose minor depression and major depression.**
- **Differentiate presentations for bipolar disorder and depression.**
- **Antipsychotics lead to an increased risk of obesity, type 2 diabetes, and hyperlipidemia, metabolic syndrome, and hypothyroidism.**
- **Learn how medication use should be monitored (see Table 15.2).**
- **Know FDA Black Box Warnings of SSRIs and antipsychotics.**
- **Know MAOI and high-tyramine foods to avoid.**
- **Angicholinergics: Use caution with BPH (urinary retention), narrow-angle glaucoma, preexisting heart disease.**
- **In general, there are now more questions on alternative treatments (see Table 15.3).**
  - **St. John's wort is used for depression, menopausal symptoms, and other conditions. Herb–drug interactions of St. John's wort are indinavir (protease inhibitor), cyclosporine, oral contraceptives, SSRIs, TCAs, and others.**
  - **Kava-kava and/or valerian root are both used for anxiety and insomnia. Do not mix with benzodiazepines, hypnotics, or any CNS depressants.**
- **A question on the MMSE (or the MME) will describe an action (such as asking a patient to spell "world" backward). The exam will ask you to indicate the name of the tool that is being used.**

CLINICAL PEARLS

- **Patients starting to recover from depression may commit suicide (from increase in psychic energy). Monitor closely.**
- **If potentially suicidal, be careful when refilling or prescribing certain medications that may be fatal if patient overdoses (i.e., benzodiazepines, hypnotics, narcotics, amphetamines, TCAs). Give the smallest amount and lowest dose possible, with close follow-up.**

Alcoholism

Alcoholism is a compulsive desire to drink alcohol despite personal, financial, and social consequences. Individuals have a strong craving for alcohol and are unable to limit drinking.

With alcohol dependence, a patient experiences cognitive, behavioral, and physiological symptoms that are generated from persistent and chronic use. Abrupt cessation causes withdrawal symptoms. Alcohol abuse occurs when a maladaptive behavior pattern occurs from repeated alcohol use.

Definitions

- Elevated blood alcohol level greater than 0.08% is illegal for driving (blood alcohol or breathalyzer) in all U.S. states
- Standard drink sizes in the United States (considered as "one drink"):
  - Beer: 12-ounce bottle
  - Wine: 5 ounces
  - Liquor/spirits: 1.5 ounces or a "shot" of 80-proof gin, vodka, rum, or whiskey

Dietary Guidelines for Americans (Alcohol Limits)

- *Women*: One drink per day
- *Men*: Two drinks per day
- Binge drinking:
  - A pattern of alcohol consumption that brings the blood alcohol level to 0.08% or higher on one occasion (generally within 2 hours)
  - *Males*: At least five drinks or more in a single occasion
  - *Women*: At least four drinks or more in a single occasion
- Women metabolize alcohol (50%) more slowly than do men

Lab Results

Gamma Glutamyl Transaminase

- Lone elevation (with/without ALT and AST) is a possible sign of occult alcohol abuse

AST/ALT Ratio (Liver Transaminases)

- Both AST and ALT are usually elevated (with or without elevated GGT) in alcoholism
- Ratio of 2:1 with AST/ALT (AST level is double the level of ALT) is associated with alcohol abuse (alcoholic hepatitis)
- ALT is more specific for the liver than AST because AST is also found in the liver, cardiac and skeletal muscle, kidneys, and lungs

Mean Corpuscular Volume (MCV)

- RBCs may be larger size (MCV >100) due to folate deficiency that resembles mild macrocytic anemia.

Quick Screening Tests for Identification of Alcohol Abuse/Alcoholism

CAGE Test

- Positive finding of at least two (out of four) is highly suggestive of alcoholism:
  - **C:** Do you feel the need to *cut down*?
  - **A:** Are you *annoyed* when your spouse/friend comments about your drinking?
  - **G:** Do you feel *guilty* about your drinking?
  - **E:** Do you need to drink *early* in the morning? (an *eye-opener*).
- Examples of some quotes using CAGE:
  - **C:** "I would like to drink less on the weekends." "I only drink a lot on weekends."
  - **A:** "My wife nags me about my drinking." "My best friend thinks I drink too much."
  - **G:** "I feel bad that I don't spend enough time with the kids because of my drinking."
  - **E:** "I need a drink to feel better when I wake up in the morning."

Short Michigan Alcoholism Screening Test (SMAST) Questionnaire

- A 13-item questionnaire that is a shorter version of the original MAST Questionnaire (contains 24 items)

Alcohol Use Disorders Identification Test (AUDIT)

- A 10-question tool that is used with women, minorities, and adolescents

Alcoholic Anonymous (AA)

- One of the most successful methods for recovering alcoholics. Founded by Bill Wilson and Dr. Robert Smith
- Patient is paired with a mentor (a recovered alcoholic); believes in a "higher power"
- Must follow a 12-step program and attend AA meetings (uses "chip" reward)
- Support group for family members and friends is called *Al-Anon (Al-Anon Family Groups)*
- Support group for teen children of alcoholics is called *Alateen*

Acute Delirium Tremens

- This is characterized by a sudden onset of confusion; delusions; transient auditory, tactile, or visual hallucinations; tachycardia; hypertension; hand tremors; disturbed psychomotor behavior (picking at clothes); and grand mal seizures
- Considered a medical emergency so refer to ED

Treatment Plan

- Benzodiazepines (Librium, Valium), antipsychotics if needed (i.e., Haldol)
- Vitamins: Thiamine 100 mg IV, folate 1 mg PO/IV daily, and multivitamins with high-calorie diet
- Refer to AA (12-step program), therapist, and/or a recovery program
- Avoid prescribing a recovering alcoholic/addict drugs with abuse potential such as narcotics or any medication that contains alcohol (cough syrup)

Medications

- *Disulfiram (Antabuse):* Causes severe nausea/vomiting, headache, other unpleasant effects
- *Naltrexone (Vivitrol):* Decreases alcohol cravings

Korsakoff's Syndrome (Wernicke–Korsakoff Syndrome)

This is a complication from chronic alcohol abuse. A neurological disorder with symptoms that include hypotension, visual impairment, and coma. Signs include mental confusion, ataxia, stupor, coma, and hypotension. Treated with high-dose parenteral vitamins, especially thiamine (vitamin B_1).

Korsakoff's Amnesic Syndrome

This is a type of amnesia caused by chronic thiamine deficiency due to chronic alcohol abuse. Problems with acquiring (and learning) new information (antegrade amnesia) and retrieving older information (retrograde amnesia). Symptoms include confabulation, disorientation, attention deficits, and visual impairment. Chronic thiamine deficiency damages the brain permanently.

Smoking Cessation

Tobacco use is the most common cause of preventable death. Discuss smoking cessation at every visit with patients who are smokers.

- Nicotine gum use: Follow "chew and park" pattern. Chew gum slowly until the nicotine taste appears, then "park" next to the cheeks (buccal mucosa) until the taste disappears. Repeat pattern several times and discard nicotine gum after 30 minutes of use.
- Patient cannot smoke while on nicotine patches. Do not use with other nicotine products (e.g., gum, inhaler); patient will overdose on nicotine. Nicotine overdose can cause acute myocardial infarction, hypertension, and agitation in susceptible patients. Nicotine products can be used with bupropion (Zyban).
- Bupropion (Zyban) decreases cravings to smoke. Patients can still smoke while on bupropion; can be combined with nicotine products. Individual eventually loses desire to smoke and finally quits. Contraindications include seizure disorder, history of anorexia/bulimia, abrupt cessation of ethanol, benzodiazepines, antiseizure drugs, severe stroke, and brain tumor. Be careful with depressed patients; may increase risk of suicidal thoughts and behavior.
- Prescribe varenicline (Chantix) therapy for a 12-week course. Advise patient to quit smoking within 1 to 4 weeks after starting varenicline. Take a careful psychiatric history and avoid prescribing to mentally unstable patients or those with a history recent suicidal ideation. Adverse effects include neuropsychiatric symptoms; may impair ability to drive or operate heavy machinery. (The Federal Aviation Administration [FAA] prohibits pilots and air traffic controllers from taking drug.)

Insomnia (Sleep Disorder)

It is thought that 7 to 8 hours of sleep is the ideal amount. About 40 to 70 million Americans (20% of the population) suffer from either transient (<1 week), short-term (1–3 weeks), or chronic (>3 weeks) insomnia. Insomnia in the aged occurs due to changes in sleep pattern, physical activity, health, and increased used of medications. Insomnia can manifest either as difficulty falling asleep (sleep-onset insomnia) or falling asleep but waking up during the night or too early and being unable to go back to sleep. Can cause daytime drowsiness, fatigue, tension headache, irritability, and difficulty concentrating/focusing on tasks.

Patient self-medicating or using alcohol to facilitate sleep may indicate a coexistent alcohol/drug-dependence problem. Abrupt cessation of these agents may cause increased insomnia and/or anxiety.

Risk Factors

Depression, severe anxiety, gastroesophageal reflux disease, female gender, illicit drug use, musculoskeletal illness, pain, chronic health problems, shift work, alcohol, caffeine, and nicotine. Certain medications (SSRIs, cardiac, BP, allergy, steroids) can cause insomnia.

Etiology

Circadian rhythm disorders, psychic issues, mental illness, obstructive sleep apnea, restless leg syndrome, environmental factors, certain medications, idiopathic, and others.

Classification

- *Primary insomnia (25%)*: Not caused by disease, mental illness, or environmental factors
- *Secondary insomnia*: Caused by disease (physical, emotional, mental) or environmental factors
- *Short-term insomnia*: Also known as transient insomnia; duration of less than 3 months; caused by pain, stress, grief, or other factors; expected to resolve when stressor is gone or when patient has adjusted
- *Chronic insomnia*: Presence of symptoms for at least 3 months; occurs at least 3 nights per week; it can be primary or secondary insomnia

Treatment Plan

- Sleep hygiene is first-line treatment
- Improve sleep hygiene (maintain regular sleeping time, nighttime ritual, avoid caffeine/tobacco/heavy meals before bedtime, get out of bed in 30 minutes if not asleep, use bed only for sleep and sex)
- Refer to sleep lab (polysomnography), it is the gold-standard test for sleep apnea; after diagnosis, refer to otolaryngologist

Medications

- Diphenhydramine (Benadryl), an over-the-counter antihistamine, can cause excess sedation and confusion in the elderly. It is the most sedating antihistamine. Avoid with elderly.

Benzodiazepines/Hypnotics (Listed Under Psychotropic Drugs)

Some benzodiazepines are more sedating and are used as hypnotics. This incluces triazolam (Halcion) and temazepam (Restoril).

Hypnotics and "sleeping pills" are ideally used for a short duration. But many insomniacs continue using sleeping pills daily to help them sleep. Physical dependence may develop with long-term use. If a patient has been on a benzodiazepine for a long time, do not discontinue abruptly (will increase risk of seizures). Wean off slowly and gradually.

- *Short acting*: Alprazolam (Xanax), triazolam (Halcion), midazolam (Versed)
- *Intermediate acting:* Lorazepam (Ativan), temazepam (Restoril)
- *Long acting*: Diazepam (Valium), clonazepam (Klonopin), chlordiazepoxide (Librium)

Nonbenzodiazepine Hypnotics

These drugs have quick onset (15–30 minutes). Do not take if unable to get 7 to 8 hours of sleep. Adverse effects include agitation, hallucinations, nightmares, suicidal ideation. There have been cases in which a person wakes up and does his or her normal routine (sleep driving, eating, working) but is unable to recall the incident.

- Zolpidem (Ambien) for sleep-onset or inability to stay asleep
- Eszopiclone (Lunesta) for sleep-onset or inability to stay asleep
- Ramelteon (Rozerem) for sleep-onset insomnia (melatonin agonist)
- Temazepam (Restoril) for sleep-onset insomnia

Complementary/Alternative Treatment for Insomnia

- Kava-kava (avoid mixing with alcohol, tranquilizers, hypnotics; will increase sedation); do not give kava-kava, valerian root, or herbal supplements to children, lactating/pregnant women
- Valerian root (sedating, also used for anxiety)
- Melatonin (also for circadian rhythm disorders such as shift work, jet lag)
- Chamomile tea
- Meditation, yoga, tai chi, acupuncture, regular exercise (avoid 4 hours before bedtime)

EXAM TIPS

- **Lone GGT elevation can be a sign of occult alcohol abuse.**
- **AST/ALT ratio of 2.0 or higher is more likely in alcoholism.**
- **Recognize Korsakoff's syndrome and that it is caused by chronic thiamine deficiency.**
- **Al-Anon is the support group for an alcoholic's family and friends.**
- **A person who drinks one glass of wine or one beer per day is not considered an alcoholic.**

- **Questions may be asked about who is most likely (or least likely) to become an alcoholic.**
- **Do not mix nicotine patches with nicotine gum. Do not smoke while on patches.**
- **Bupropion (Zyban) is for smoking cessation. Patients can smoke while on Zyban.**
- **Women are allowed one drink/day and men are allowed two drinks/day.**
- **Kava-kava and valerian root are natural supplements used for insomnia/anxiety. Do not mix with benzodiazepines or hypnotics.**
- **Discuss smoking cessation with patients (who are smokers) at every visit.**

Bipolar Disorder

Bipolar disorder is characterized by mania and depression. There are two types: bipolar type 1 and bipolar type 2 (has hypomania instead of mania). They are at higher risk of suicide; 10% to 15% die by suicide. Manic symptoms are increased energy/activity, grandiosity, less need for sleep, disinhibition, and euphoric mood. The depressive symptoms are similar to major depression.

- May have psychotic episodes (delusions, hallucinations)
- Bipolar patients have higher rates of substance abuse (40%–60%) and other comorbidities (ADHD, anxiety, OCD, eating disorders)
- Refer to psychiatrist for management

Medications

- Lithium salts (adverse affects kidney and thyroid gland), anticonvulsants (valproate, carbamezapine), and antipsychotics (treats manic episodes)

Schizophrenia

- Psychotic symptoms include delusions and paranoia (disorganized speech and behavior).
- Hallucinations are common (usually auditory) with loss of ego boundaries; flat and restricted affect with poor social skills; executive function is very poor (ability to plan and organize day-to-day activities)
- Onset is usually around the second decade; peak incidence is between 16 and 30 years of age
- Refer patients to a psychiatrist for management

Medications

Safety Issues

- Use of typical antipsychotics increase the risk of sudden death among elderly who are in long-term care
- Antipsychotics can prolong QT intervals (EKG needed) and cause a fatal arrythmia called "torsade de pointes" such as clozapine (Clozaril), thioridazine (Mellaril), ziprasidone (Geodon), haloperidol (Haldol), and others

Anorexia Nervosa

Onset is usually during adolescence. It is an irrational preoccupation with an intense fear of gaining weight along with distorted perception of body shape and weight. Patients tend to be secretive, perfectionistic, and self-absorbed. Characterized by severe restriction of food intake, marked weight loss (BMI <18.5), lanugo (face, back, and shoulders), and amenorrhea for 3 months or longer. If purging, loss of dental enamel may be present. Anorexics engage in severe food restriction or binge eating and purging. Some examples of purging are use of laxatives, vomiting; excessive daily exercise is common.

Complications

- Osteopenia/osteoporosis is due to prolonged estrogen depletion (from amenorrhea) and low calcium intake; higher risk of stress fractures

- Peripheral edema may occur (low albumin from low protein intake)
- Cardiac complications are the most common cause of death (arrhythmias, cardiomyopathy, hypokalemia, etc.)

Posttraumatic Stress Disorder (PTSD)

Characterized by flashbacks, nightmares, intrusive thoughts, avoidance of reminders of trauma, sleep disturbance, and hypervigilance. Causes include being in combat/war, sexual assault (12%), myocardial infarction, stroke, ICU stay (20%). Comorbidity, such as depression, anxiety, antisocial disorder, and substance abuse, is higher in PTSD. Assessment tools include the PTSD checklist (PCL-5), a 20-item self-report measure (screening and for monitoring symptoms over time). The first-line drug treatment of PTSD is SSRIs such as paroxetine (Paxil) and sertraline (Zoloft). A therapeutic trial of SSRIs is needed for at least 6 to 8 weeks to find out whether it is effective. Other treatment includes cognitive behavioral therapy and eye movement desensitization and reprocessing (EMDR).

Munchausen Syndrome

Also known as "factitious disorder imposed on self." Patient falsifies symptoms of factitious disorders (abdominal pain, chest pain, seizures, etc.) and/or injures self and seeks medical treatment, including multiple surgeries. Munchausen by proxy, a related disorder, refers to a parent using a child (and making the child sick) to obtain medical care. These are rare conditions (1%) that are hard to diagnose.

EXAM TIPS

- **Recognize how anorexic patients present (i.e., lanugo, peripheral edema, amenorrhea, BMI <18.5).**
- **Anorexic patients are at higher risk for osteopenia/osteoporosis.**
- **Bupropion (Wellbutrin) is contraindicated for anorexic/bulimic patients. It increases the seizure threshold.**
- **Paroxetine has a short half-life (compared with other SSRIs) and patients need to be weaned. Do not discontinue abruptly; will cause withdrawal symptoms.**
- **A common side effect of paroxetine (Paxil) is erectile dysfunction. Bupropion is used off-label for antidepressant-induced sexual dysfunction caused by SSRIs.**
- **An elderly patient who is depressed (and has multiple medications) can be prescribed citalopram. Citalopram (Celexa) does have drug interactions, but fewer than the other SSRIs.**
- **TCAs: Used for herpetic neuralgia, migraine headache prophylaxis (not acute treatment).**

Abuse: All Types

Abusive behaviors are multifactorial. They may include physical, emotional, and sexual abuse, and/or neglect, as well as economic abuse or material exploitation. Abuse can happen at any age and during pregnancy (higher risk). The state of pregnancy is also associated with a higher incidence of abuse due to jealousy over the pregnancy.

Upon presentation to the ED, for example, the pattern of the injuries is inconsistent with the history given. Elderly who are most likely to be abused are those older than 80 years old and/or who are frail. Children with mental, physical, or other disabilities, and stepchildren are more likely to be abused.

Types of abuse are physical abuse, sexual abuse, emotional/psychological abuse, and neglect. A common finding is a delay in seeking medical treatment for the injury. Intimate partner violence (IPV) is defined as intentional control or victimization performed by a person to another with whom the person has an intimate or spousal relationship. The most significant reason for missing the diagnosis of IPV or other abuse is failure to ask.

Risk Factors That Increase Likelihood of Abuse (All Types)

- Increased stress (partner/parent/caregiver)
- Alcohol/drug abuse
- Personal history of abuse, positive family history of abuse
- Major loss (financial, job loss, others)
- Social isolation
- Pregnancy (domestic abuse)
- Elderly abuse. Frail elderly and those with dementia are more likely to be abused; about two thirds of all elder abuse is perpetrated by family members (usually an adult child or a spouse); most abused elderly also suffer economic abuse.
- Only certain states have mandatory reporting of partner abuse; be mindful of institutional abuse of elderly, children, and the disabled

Physical Exam: Abuse (All Types)

- Another health provider (witness) should be in the same room during the exam.
- Interview victim without abuser in the same room.
- Collect visual evidence of trauma via Polaroid or digital camera to document all injuries. Keep all evidence in a safe place. Use a ruler to identify and document the size of the injuries. Document direct "quotes" in the patient's history.
- Use the abuse assessment screening tool with a body map to document assessment findings.
- Look for spiral fractures (greenstick fracture), multiple healing fractures, especially in rib area, burn marks with pattern, welts, and so forth.
- Look for signs of neglect (dirty clothes, inappropriately dressed for the weather, etc.).
- For partner abuse, focus on developing a plan for safety with the patient when appropriate. Give the patient the phone number of the crisis center and/or a safe place.
- Sexually transmitted disease (STD) testing:
  - Chlamydial and gonorrheal cultures (must use cultures in addition to the Gen Probe)
  - HIV, hepatitis B, syphilis, herpes type 2
  - Genital, throat, and anal area culture and testing must be done
- Abused patient is very fearful and quiet when with the "abuser"

Treatment Plan

- Provide prophylactic treatment against several STDs (with parental consent for minors)
- Teach the patient the cycle of abuse; educate the patient regarding safety issues and having an escape plan ready for use
- Health care professionals must report actual or suspected child abuse
- Be aware of individual state guidelines on reporting suspicion of elder abuse
- Abuse of a disabled person must be reported to the Disabled Person Protective Commission; contact adult protective services or law enforcement agencies with concerns regarding self-neglect

Good Communication Concepts

- State things objectively; do not be judgmental
  - *Example:* Say: "You have bright-red stripes on your back" instead of "It looks as if you have been whipped on your back."

- Open-ended questions are preferred.
  - *Example:* Say: "How can I help you?" instead of "What type of object was used to hurt your back?"
- Do not reassure patients (this stops a patient from talking more about his or her problems).
  - *Example:* Say: "We will make sure you get help" instead of "Don't worry, everything will be fine."
- Let the patient vent his or her feelings. Do not discourage patient from talking.
  - *Example:* Say: "Please tell me why you feel so sad."
- Validate feelings.
  - *Example:* Say: "Yes, I understand your anger when someone hits you."

EXAM TIPS

- **Of all the SSRIs, Paxil is most likely to cause erectile dysfunction.**
- **There will always be a few questions on physical abuse. The questions may address physical abuse, child abuse, sexual abuse, and/or elder abuse.**
- **The abuser is described as a person who does not want the abused person out of sight or interviewed alone.**
- **The abuser typically answers all the questions for the patient and will exhibit "controlling" behaviors toward the abused patient.**
- **Abuse cases: Interview together and then separately.**
- **Any answer choice that reassures patients is always wrong.**
- **Delaying an action (i.e., waiting until the patient feels better, etc.) is always wrong.**
- **Bupropion is used to treat major depression, seasonal affective disorder, and smoking cessation. It increases risk of seizures; avoid if patient at higher risk of seizures (during abrupt discontinuation of ethanol, benzodiazepines).**

Reproductive Review

III

16

Men's Health Review

⚠ DANGER SIGNALS

Priapism

Male complains of a prolonged and painful erection for several hours (at least 2–4 hours). Males with sickle cell disease are at very high risk (6%–45%). Other risk factors are high doses of erectile dysfunction drugs, cocaine, quadriplegia, and others. There are several types of priapism. The ischemic form of priapism is a medical/surgical emergency.

Testicular Cancer

Teenage to young adult male complains of nodule, sensation of heaviness or aching, one larger testicle, and/or tenderness in one testicle. Testicular cancer can present as a new onset of a hydrocele (from tumor pressing on vessels). Usually painless and asymptomatic until metastasis. More common in White males aged 15 to 30 years. Rare in African Americans.

Prostate Cancer

Older to elderly man complains of a new onset of low-back pain, rectal area/perineal pain or discomfort accompanied by obstructive voiding symptoms such as weaker stream and nocturia. May be asymptomatic. More common in older (>50 years), obese, and Black men, and men with a family history of prostate cancer (father, brother).

Torsion of the Appendix Testis (Blue Dot Sign)

School-age boy complains of the abrupt onset of a blue-colored round mass located on the testicular surface. The mass resembles a "blue dot." The appendix testis is a round, small (0.03 cm), pedunculated polyp-like structure that is attached to the testicular surface (on the anterior superior area). The blue dot is caused by infarction and necrosis of the appendix testis due to torsion. More common during childhood. *Not* testicular torsion. Refer to emergency department (ED).

Testicular Torsion

A male (usually adolescent) reports waking up at midnight or in the morning with abrupt onset of an extremely painful and swollen red scrotum. Frequently accompanied by nausea and vomiting. Affected testicle/scrotum is located higher and closer to the body than the unaffected testicle. The cremasteric reflex is missing. Majority of cases (two thirds) occur between the ages of 10 and 20 years.

NORMAL FINDINGS

Spermatogenesis

- Ideal temperature (for sperm production) is from 1° to 2°C (33.8° to 35.6°F) lower than core body temperature
- Sperm production starts at puberty and continues for the entire lifetime of the male
- Sperm are produced in seminiferous tubules of the testes
- Sperm require 64 days (about 3 months) to mature

Testes

- Cryptorchidism (undescended testes) increases risk of testicular cancer
- Production of testosterone/androgens is stimulated by release of luteinizing hormone
- Spermatogenesis is stimulated by both testosterone and follicle-stimulating hormone
- The left testicle usually hangs lower than the right

Prostate Gland

- Heart-shaped gland that grows throughout the life cycle of the male
- Produces prostate-specific antigen (PSA) and prostatic fluid
- Prostatic fluid (alkaline pH) helps the sperm survive in the vagina (acidic pH)
- Up to 50% of 50-year-old men have benign prostatic hypertrophy (BPH)

Epididymis

- Coiled tubular organ that is located at the posterior aspect of the testis. Storage area for immature sperm (sperm takes 3 months to mature). Resembles a "beret" on the upper pole of the testes.

Vas Deferens (Ductus Deferens)

- Tubular structures that transport sperm from the epididymis toward the urethra in preparation for ejaculation. These tubes are cut/clipped during a vasectomy procedure.

Cremasteric Reflex

- The testicle is elevated toward the body in response to stroking or lightly pinching the ipsilateral inner thigh (or the thigh on the same side as the testicle). Reflex is absent with testicular torsion.

Transillumination: Scrotum

- Transillumination is useful for evaluating testicular swelling, mass, bleeding, or cryptorchidism
- Direct a beam of light behind one scrotum (turn off room light)
- Hydrocele will transilluminate (serous fluid inside scrotum)
- Testicular tumor will not transilluminate (solid tumor blocks light)
- Varicocele ("bag of worms") will not transilluminate

DISEASE REVIEW

Testicular Cancer

- Most common tumor in males age 15 to 30 years; more common in White males

Classic Case

Teenage to young adult male complains of nodule, sensation of heaviness or aching, one larger testicle, or tenderness in one testicle. May present as a new onset of a hydrocele (from tumor pressing on vessels). Usually painless and asymptomatic until metastasis.

Objective Findings

- Affected testicle feels "heavier" and more solid
- May palpate a hard, fixed nodule (most common site is the lower pole of the testes)
- Twenty percent of cases will have a concomitant hydrocele

Labs and Treatment Plan

- Ultrasound of the testicle reveals solid mass
- Gold standard of diagnosis: Testicular biopsy
- Refer to urologist for biopsy and management; surgical removal (orchiectomy)

Testicular Torsion

When the spermatic cord becomes twisted, the testis's blood supply is interrupted. Permanent testicular damage results if not corrected within the first few hours (<6 hours). If not corrected within 24 hours, 100% of testicles become gangrenous and must be surgically removed. More common in males with the "bell clapper deformity." Most cases are idiopathic.

Classic Case

A 14-year-old boy reports the sudden onset of severe testicular pain with an extremely swollen red scrotum. Some may have acute hydrocele (severe edema). Complains of severe nausea and vomiting. The affected testicle is higher than the normal testicle. Cremasteric reflex is missing.

Treatment Plan

- Call 911 as soon as possible
- Preferred test in the ED is the Doppler ultrasound with color flow study
- Treatment can be manual reduction or surgery with testicular fixation using sutures

Prostate Cancer

Most common cancer in men (incidence). African American males have a higher risk of prostate cancer. Average age of diagnosis is 71 years. Risk factors are age older than 50 years, African American, obesity, and positive family history (first-degree relative will double the risk). Routine prostate cancer screening (digital rectal exam [DRE] with PSA) is not recommended (USPSTF, 2012). Studies show that absolute risk reduction of prostate cancer deaths with screening is very small. Individualize management, based on patient's risk factors and age.

Objective

Painless and hard fixed nodule (or indurated area) on the prostate gland on an older male that is detected by DRE.

- *Elevated PSA:* Greater than 4.0 ng/mL
- *Diagnostic test:* Biopsy of prostatic tissue (obtained by transurethral ultrasound)
- *Screening test:* PSA level with DRE; if limited life span (<10 years), not recommended

Treatment Plan

- Refer to urologist if PSA greater than 4.0 ng/mL; suspect prostate cancer
- Individualize screening is based on risk factors; discuss risk (bleeding, infection, impotence, procedures, and psychological trauma) versus benefits

- Most cancers are not aggressive and are slowgrowing; watchful waiting/monitoring by urologist is common
- Initiate drug therapy with antiandrogens (Proscar), hormone blockers (i.e., Lupron), others

Benign Prostatic Hyperplasia

- Seen in 50% of men older than age 50 (up to 80% of men >70 years); rarely seen in those younger than age 40; rule out prostate cancer
- Use the American Urological Association (AUA) urinary symptom score/International Prostate Symptom Score (IPSS) questionnaire to assess the severity of the patient's BPH symptoms

Classic Case

Older man complains of gradual development (years) of urinary obstructive symptoms such as weak urinary stream, postvoid dribbling, feelings of incomplete emptying, and occasional urinary retention. Nocturia is very common.

Objective Findings

- PSA is elevated (norm is 0–4 ng/mL)
- Prostate that is symmetrical in texture and size (rubbery texture) is enlarged
- Lifestyle changes may help decrease symptoms and include reduction of caffeine and alcohol intake, avoiding fluids before bedtime, and avoidance of diuretic medications (if possible)

Medications

- *Alpha-adrenergic antagonist:* Terazosin (Hytrin) 5 mg or tamsulosin (Flomax)
- 5-alpha-reductase inhibitors (blocks testosterone): Finasteride (Proscar)
- Duration of treatment ranges from a few months to daily for many years
- *Avoid drugs that worsen symptoms:* Cold medications (antihistamines, decongestants), caffeine
- *Herbal:* Saw palmetto (mild improvement for some); does not work for everyone
- Watch for an adverse effect of alpha blockers, which is orthostatic hypotension
- Advise patients that they may have dizziness due to low BP
- Instruct patients to take medication at bedtime
- Tamsulosin may have less effect on BP than the other alpha blockers (Cunningham & Kadmon, 2017)
- If hypotension is a problem, discontinue and start on a trial of finasteride (Proscar)

EXAM TIPS

- **Finasteride (Proscar) inhibits type 2 5α-reductase (it blocks the androgen receptor) and acts directly on the prostate gland to shrink it (temporarily) while on the medication. If patient stops taking Proscar, the size of the prostate gland returns back to its original size.**
- **The prostate shrinks by 50% while on Proscar (so PSA must be doubled or multiplied by 2).**
- **Proscar is a category X drug (teratogenic). It should not be touched with bare hands by reproductive-aged females (adversely affects male fetus).**
- **Male with BPH and hypertension: Start with alpha-blocker (Hytrin) first. Works by relaxing smooth muscles on prostate gland and bladder neck.**

Chronic Bacterial Prostatitis

Chronic (>6 weeks) infection of the prostate. Some men report a history of acute urinary tract infection (UTI) or of acute bacterial prostatitis. Others are asymptomatic. More common in older men. Caused most commonly by *Escherichia coli* and *Proteus*. Nonbacterial prostatitis has same symptoms but is culture negative.

Classic Case

Elderly man with a history of several weeks of suprapubic or perineal discomfort that is accompanied by irritative voiding symptoms such as dysuria, nocturia, and frequency. Not accompanied by systemic symptoms. Some men are asymptomatic.

Objective Findings

- Prostate may feel normal or slightly "boggy" to palpation; not tender
- *UA:* Normal (unless patient has cystitis)
- Urine mixed with prostatic fluid: Positive for *E. coli*

Labs

- Urine and prostatic fluid cultures
  - Use three tubes: First, urethra; second, bladder; third, urine with prostatic fluid (obtained after prostatic massage)
  - PSA will be elevated (inflammation)

Medications

- Administer trimethoprim–sulfamethoxazole (Bactrim) PO BID for 4 to 6 weeks (if sensitive)
- Some prefer ofloxacin (Floxin) BID or levofloxacin (Levaquin) daily for 4 to 6 weeks

Acute Prostatitis

Acute infection of the prostate. Infection ascends into urinary tract. Most common non–sexually transmitted cause is *Enterobacteriaceae (E. coli, Proteus).* If condition occurs in a male younger than 35 years of age, it is treated like gonococcal or chlamydial urethritis.

Classic Case

Adult to older man complains of sudden onset of high fever and chills with suprapubic and/or perineal pain/discomfort. Pain sometimes radiates to back or rectum. Accompanied by UTI symptoms such as dysuria, frequency, nocturia with cloudy urine. DRE reveals extremely tender prostate that is warm and boggy. The patient may have an accompanying infection of the bladder (cystitis) or epididymitis.

Objective Findings

- Gently examine prostate. Prostate will be extremely tender and warm.
- *Warning:* Vigorous palpation and massage of an infected prostate can cause bacteremia.

Labs

- *CBC:* Leukocytosis with shift to the left (presence of band cells)
- *UA:* Large amount of white blood cells (pyuria), hematuria
- *Urine C&S* (if possible, also obtain urine after gentle prostatic massage)

Medications

- Based on age and presumptive organism:
  - Age younger than 35 years: Ceftriaxone 250 mg IM and doxycycline 100 mg BID × 10 days
  - Age older than 35 or unlikely sexual transmission: Ciprofloxacin or ofloxacin PO BID or levofloxacin (Levaquin) PO daily for 4 to 6 weeks
- *Others:* Levofloxacin (Levaquin) PO daily, Bactrim PO BID
- Antipyretics, stool softener without laxative (Colace), sitz baths, hydration
- Patient should be hospitalized if septic or toxic

EXAM TIPS

- **Learn to distinguish between chronic prostatitis and acute prostatitis.**
- **Chronic is of gradual onset; prostate can feel normal with DRE (older males).**
- **Acute prostatitis presents as sudden onset; prostate is swollen and very tender (younger males).**
- **Selective serotonin reuptake inhibitors (SSRIs) cause erectile dysfunction in men. The SSRI that has the highest risk of erectile dysfunction is paroxetine (Paxil).**

Acute Bacterial Epididymitis

Bacteria ascend the urethra (urethritis) and reach the epididymis, causing an infection. Also known as *bacterial epididymo-orchitis*. Rule out testicular torsion (can mimic condition).

- Sexually active males younger than 35 years of age
  - More likely to be infected with a sexually transmitted disease (chlamydia, gonorrhea)
- Males older than 35 years of age
  - Usually due to gram-negative *E. coli*

Classic Case

Adult to older man complains of acute onset of a swollen red scrotum that hurts. Accompanied by unilateral testicular tenderness with urethral discharge. Scrotum is swollen and erythematous with induration of the posterior epididymis. Sometimes accompanied by a hydrocele, and signs and symptoms of UTI. May have systemic symptoms such as fever.

- *Discharge:* Green-colored purulent or serous clear (chlamydia, viral, chemical, others)
- *Positive Prehn's sign:* Relief of pain with scrotal elevation

Labs

- *CBC:* Leukocytosis
- *UA:* Leukocytes (pyuria), blood (hematuria), nitrites
- Urine C&S and urine for Gram stain
- Testing for gonorrhea and chlamydia (urine or Gen-Probe)

Medications

- Age younger than 35 years (or suspect STD): Doxycycline PO BID × 10 days plus ceftriaxone 250 mg IM × one dose; do not forget to treat sex partner
- Age greater than 35 years: Ofloxacin (Floxin) 300 mg PO × 10 days or levofloxacin (Levaquin) 500 mg PO 7 to 10 days; caution patient regarding risk of tendon injury and discourage vigorous lower extremity exercise while on fluoroquinolone
- Treat pain with NSAIDs (ibuprofen, naproxen) or acetaminophen with codeine (severe pain)
- Employ scrotal elevation and scrotal ice packs; bed rest for few days
- Give stool softeners (i.e., docusate sodium or Colace) if constipated
- Refer to ED if septic, severe intractable pain, abscessed, others

Erectile Dysfunction

Inability to produce an erection firm enough to perform sexual intercourse. Vascular insufficiency, neuropathy (diabetics), medications (selective serotonin reuptake inhibitors, beta-blockers), smoking, alcohol, hypogonadism. May be psychic causation or mixture of both.

- *Organic cause:* Inability to have an erection under any circumstance. Due to neurovascular or vascular damage
- *Psychiatric cause:* Spontaneously has early-morning erections or can achieve a firm erection with masturbation

Medications

- *First line:* Treat with phosphodiesterase type 5 inhibitors drug class
- Take Viagra on an empty stomach for optimal effectiveness; food and fats delay drug action; Levitra can be taken regardless of food intake with one exception—fatty foods have been shown to decrease the onset of effect
- Sildenafil citrate (Viagra) 25/50/100 mg; take one dose 30 to 60 minutes before sex; use only one dose every 24 hours
- Vardenafil (Levitra); take one dose 30 to 60 minutes before sex; duration is 4 hours
- Tadalafil (Cialis) 5 to 20 mg; take 2 hours before sex; duration is up to 36 hours; may also be prescribed as a daily dose for combined BPH and erectile dysfunction (5–10 mg)
- *Adverse effects:* May cause headache, facial flushing, dizziness, hypotension, nasal congestion, priapism.
- *Other forms of treatment:* Vacuum-assisted erection devices, penile self-injection (intracavernosal injection of alprostadil)

Contraindications

- Concomitant nitrates. Use caution with alpha-blockers, recent postmyocardial infarction (MI), postcerebrovascular accident, major surgery, or any condition in which exertion is contraindicated.

Peyronie's Disease

An inflammatory and localized disorder of the penis that results in fibrotic plaques on the tunica albuginea. Results in penile pain that primarily occurs during erection; palpable nodules and penile deformity (crooked penile erections) occur. May resolve spontaneously or worsen over time. Surgical correction if needed.

Labs

- None; clinical diagnosis is used

Treatment Plan

- Refer patient to urologist

Other Conditions

Balanitis

- Candidal infection of the glans penis; more common in uncircumcised men, diabetics, and/or immunocompromised men. Use of sodium-glucose cotransporter 2 (SGLT2) inhibitors for diabetes management, such as canagliflozin (Invokana), dapagliflozin (Farxiga), and empagliflozin (Jardiance) may cause balanitis; this also increases the risk of candidal infections and UTIs. Treated with topical OTC azole creams. If partner has candidiasis, treat at the same time.

Cryptorchidism

- Undescended testicles that remain in the abdominal cavity. Can affect both or only one testicle. Markedly increases the risk of testicular cancer. Usually corrected during infancy.

Phimosis

- Foreskin cannot be pushed back from the glans penis because of edema; usually seen in neonates.

Varicocele (Figure 16.1)

- Varicose veins in scrotal sac (feels like "bag of worms"). New-onset varicocele can signal testicular tumor (20%) or a mass that is impeding venous drainage. Order an ultrasound

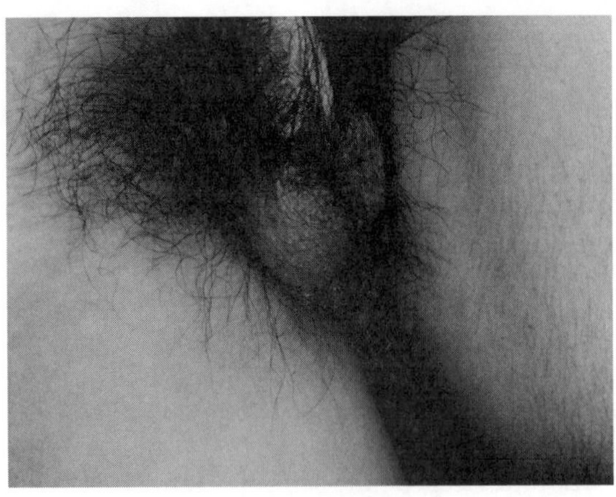

Figure 16.1 Varicocele of left scrotum (adult). This image can be found in color in the app.

Source: Courtesy of Mulief.

of the scrotum. Can contribute to male infertility if large enough (increases temperature of affected testicle). Treatment is surgical removal of varicosities if infertile.

Hydrocele

- More common in infants. Serous fluid collects inside the tunica vaginalis. During scrotal exam, hydroceles are located superiorly and anterior to the testes. Most hydroceles are asymptomatic.
- Will glow with transillumination. If new-onset hydrocele in an adult or enlarging hydrocele, order scrotal ultrasound and refer to urologist.

17

Women's Health Review

DANGER SIGNALS

Dominant Breast Mass/Breast Cancer

Adult to older female with a dominant mass on one breast that feels hard and is irregular in shape. The mass is attached to the skin/surrounding breast tissue (or is immobile). Among the most common locations are the upper outer quadrants of the breast (the tail of Spence). Skin changes may be seen, such as the "peau d'orange" (localized area of skin that resembles an orange peel), dimpling, and retraction. Mass is painless or may be accompanied by serous or bloody nipple discharge. The nipple may be displaced or become fixed. Order a mammogram and refer the patient to breast surgeon.

Paget's Disease of the Breast (Ductal Carcinoma In Situ)

Older female reports a history of a chronic scaly red-colored rash resembling eczema that starts on the nipple and spreads to the areola of one breast. Some women complain of itching, pain, or burning sensation. The skin lesion slowly enlarges and evolves to include crusting, ulceration, and/or bleeding on the nipple.

Inflammatory Breast Cancer

Recent or acute onset of a red, swollen, and warm area in the breast of a younger woman. Can mimic mastitis. Often, there is no distinct lump on the affected breast. Symptoms develop quickly (few weeks to months). The skin may be pitted (peau d'orange) or appear bruised. More common in African Americans. A rare but very aggressive form of breast cancer (1%–5%).

BRCA1- and *BRCA2*-Associated Hereditary Breast and Ovarian Cancer

Patients with a family history of breast cancer (before age 50), male breast cancer, breast cancer that is triple-negative (before age 60), or ovarian and other types of gynecological cancers are at higher risk for *BRCA* (breast cancer susceptibility gene) mutations. In one study of 9,800 female *BRCA* mutation carriers, the "cumulative rate of breast and ovarian cancer until age 80 years were 72% and 44% for *BRCA1* carriers and 69% and 17% for *BRCA2* carriers, respectively" (Peshkin & Isaacs, 2017). Men with *BRCA* mutations are at higher risk of breast cancer and prostate cancer.

A patient who reports being positive for a *BRCA* mutation should be referred to breast specialists. They are screened using both an MRI of the breast and a mammogram. Ask at what age the family member(s) with breast cancer were diagnosed and screen 10 years earlier. For example, if a sister was age 45 when diagnosed with breast cancer, then screening for breast cancer can start at the age of 35 years. *BRCA* mutations are more common among Ashkenazi Jews. Refer high-risk patients for pre- and posttest genetic counseling and *BRCA* mutation testing.

Ovarian Cancer

The typical patient is a middle-aged or older woman with vague symptoms of abdominal bloating and discomfort, low-back pain, pelvic pain, and changes in bowel habits. Look for family history of having two or more first- or second-degree relatives with a history of ovarian cancer or a combination of ovarian cancer, especially women of Ashkenazi Jewish ethnicity with a first-degree relative (or second-degree relatives on the same side of the family) with breast or ovarian cancer (American Cancer Society, U.S. Preventive Services Task Force [USPSTF], 2012). Very-high-risk women with suspected *BRCA 1/BRCA 2* mutations should be referred for genetic counseling pre- and posttest. The screening starts at age 30 years (or 5 to 10 years before the earliest age of first diagnosis of ovarian cancer in a family member).

Ectopic Pregnancy

Sexually active female who has not had a period (or had period with light to scant bleeding) in 6 to 7 weeks complains of lower abdominal/pelvic pain or cramping (intermittent, persistent, or acute). Pain worsens when supine or with jarring. If ruptured, pelvic pain worsens and can be referred to the right shoulder. Medical history of pelvic inflammatory disease (PID), tubal ligation, or previous ectopic pregnancy. Leading cause of death for women in the first trimester of pregnancy in the United States.

☑ NORMAL FINDINGS

Anatomy

Breasts

- Puberty in girls starts with breast buds (Tanner stage II) and ends at stage V.
- During puberty, it is common for both girls and some boys (45%) to have tender and asymmetrical breasts (gynecomastia). One breast may be larger than the other breast.
- The upper outer quadrant of the breasts (called the "tail of Spence") is where the majority of breast cancer is located.
- Very-high-risk factors for breast cancer includes the *BRCA1* or *BRCA2* gene mutation or a history of radiation therapy to the chest between the ages of 10 and 30 years. (Risk factors for breast cancer in men are cryptorchidism, positive family history, others.)
- The diagnostic test for breast cancer (or any type of solid tumor) is the tissue biopsy.

Cervix

- A cervical ectropion looks like bright-red bumpy tissue with an irregular surface on the cervical surface around the os (Figure 17.1). It is a benign finding, made up of glandular cells (same cells that are inside the cervical os). It is more friable (bleeds easily) compared with the squamous epithelial cells on the surface of the cervix (smooth pale pink color cervical surface).
- Some adolescents and adult women taking birth control pills, and pregnant women, may have large ectropions and this is considered a normal finding (due to high estrogen). It can change in size (or shape) and disappear or regress over time.
- If an ectropion is present, it is important to sample the surface of the transformation zone area (or the transitional zone) when performing a Pap test.
- The transformation zone (or the squamocolumnar junction) is an area where abnormal cells are more likely to develop (due to metaplasia). It is the border between the brighter red ectropion and the smoother surface of the cervix.

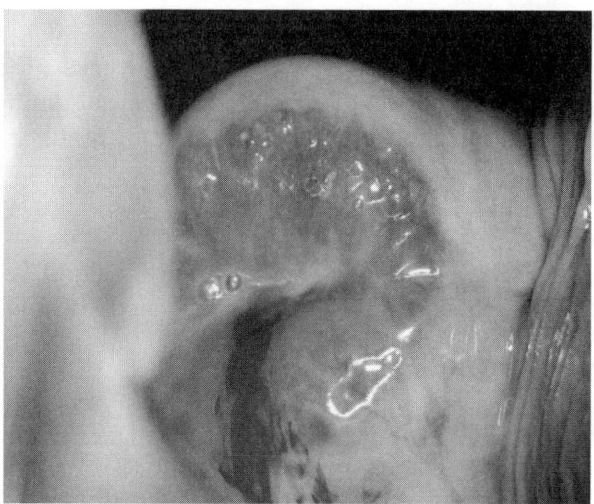

Figure 17.1 Cervical ectropion (6 weeks postpartum). This image can be found in color in the app.

Source: O'Nell Starkey. Beautiful Cervix Project.

Cervical and Vaginal Mucus

- Varies from scant ("dry"), thick white, runny white (white and clear mucus) to clear stringy mucus
- Can be mixed with blood and appear as a red to dark-brownish color during the menstrual cycle

Uterus

- Fibroids (uterine leiomyoma or myoma) can enlarge the uterus. The symptoms are heavy menstrual bleeding (menorrhagia), pelvic pain or cramping, and bleeding between periods.
- Fibroids (uterine leiomyoma/myoma) are usually benign. Can cause heavy menstrual bleeding and cramping, pelvic pain, and urgency (due to fibroid pressing on the bladder).
- On rare occasions, fibroids can be malignant and cause uterine cancer (leiomyosarcoma).

Ovaries

- The ovaries produce estrogen, progesterone, and a small amount of testosterone (androgens).
- Women with polycystic ovary syndrome (PCOS) have multiple cysts on their ovaries and high androgen levels (causes acne, hirsutism, oligomenorrhea, insulin resistance).
- During menopause, the ovaries become atrophied. A palpable ovary in a menopausal woman is always abnormal. Rule out ovarian cancer. Order a pelvic/intravaginal ultrasound and refer to a gynecologist.

Benign Variants

- Supernumerary nipples form a V-shaped line on both sides of the chest down the abdomen and are symmetrically distributed.

MENSTRUAL CYCLE

This example is based on a perfect 28-day menstrual cycle.

Follicular Phase (Days 1 to 14)

Estrogen is the predominant hormone during the first 2 weeks of the menstrual cycle. It stimulates the development and growth of the endometrial lining. Follicle-stimulating hormone (FSH) from the anterior pituitary stimulates the follicles (or the "eggs") into producing estrogen. Also known as the *proliferative phase.*

Midcycle (Day 14): Ovulatory Phase

Luteinizing hormone (LH) is secreted by the anterior pituitary gland, which induces ovulation of the dominant follicle. The follicle migrates to the fimbriae of the fallopian tube.

Luteal Phase (Days 14 to 28)

Progesterone is the predominant hormone during the last 2 weeks of the cycle. It is produced by the corpus luteum and helps to stabilize the endometrial lining.

Menstruation

If not pregnant, both estrogen and progesterone fall drastically, inducing menses. Low hormone levels stimulate the hypothalamus, then the anterior pituitary (FSH), and the cycle starts again.

Fertile Time Period

Sexual intercourse during the 1 to 2 days before ovulation offers the highest chance of pregnancy (Welt, 2017). This time period is characterized by copious amounts of clear mucus that feels thin and elastic in the vagina. This sign is used in the cervical-mucus method of birth control to indicate the fertile period of the cycle. There are now ovulation kits (over the counter) that can detect urinary LH, which appears within 12 hours after it is in the serum (released by the anterior pituitary). False-positive results are possible with women with PCOS, ovarian insufficiency, and menopause.

LABORATORY PROCEDURES

Pap Test and Liquid-Based Cervical Cytology (Table 17.1)

Both the Pap test (also called a Pap smear) and liquid-based cytology are used as cervical screening tests. These tests have a high false-negative rate of 20% to 45%. The liquid-based cervical cytology test (ThinPrep), which is read by a computer, is now more popular in the United States than the conventional Pap smear kit. If the cervix bleeds easily when the brush is inserted to obtain the sample, it may be a sign of inflammation. Rule out cervicitis. Some females may have slight spotting after a Pap test.

- Do not perform a Pap test or liquid-based cytology during the menstrual period.
- The best time to perform a Pap test is between 10 and 20 days after the last menses.
- About 1 to 2 days before the Pap test, tell patient to avoid douching, vaginal foams/ medicines, and intercourse if possible.

Notes

The USPSTF (2012) and the American College of Obstetricians and Gynecologists (ACOG; 2015) provide the following guidelines for cervical cancer screening:

(continued)

- USPSTF: Cervical cancer is rare before age 21 years. Therefore, the USPSTF (2012) does not recommend Pap tests or human papillomavirus (HPV) testing before age 21 years (do not co-test for HPV before age 21). At the age of 30 years, can perform Pap test with co-testing (HPV testing). Can space routine Pap smears to every 5 years if co-testing (except if abnormal Pap).
- ACOG: HIV-positive women are the exception to the recommendation against cervical cancer screening before age 21 years. But ACOG is still against co-testing if younger than age 30 years.

Liquid-Based Cervical Cytology Test (ThinPrep)

Insert the broom-shaped plastic brush into the cervical os and rotate in the same direction for five turns. Place the brush in the liquid medium and swish gently. Remove brush and cover with the plastic cap. The cervical cytology test is read by a computer, and abnormal results are reviewed by a cytologist and/or pathologist.

Conventional Pap Smear

Use wooden spatula to scrape cervical surface (ectocervix). Then insert the brush into the cervical os (endocervix) and twist gently in a circle. Smear the glass slide with both samples. Spray the liquid fixative on the glass slide and label. By sampling the ectocervix first, the chances of bleeding are minimized.

Table 17.1 U.S. Preventive Services Task Force Cervical Cancer Screening Guidelines

Age	Screening Exam	Screening Interval
Age 20 years (or younger)	Do *not* screen (regardless of age of onset of sexual activity)	Do *not* screen
Ages 21–29	Liquid-based cytology or conventional Pap test Against HPV co-testing if younger than 30 years	Every 3 years
Ages 30–65	Liquid-based cytology *or* Conventional Pap smear *or* Liquid-based cytology plus co-testing (for high-risk HPV)	Every 3 years *or* Every 5 years (if co-testing) If *not* co-testing, needs Pap test every 3 years
Age older than 65	Can stop screening	If not otherwise at high risk for cervical cancer*
Hysterectomy (with cervical removal) not due to cancer	Can stop screening*	If not otherwise at high risk for cervical cancer* *No* history of CIN stages 2 to 3, AIS, or cervical cancer

* If no history of CIN stages 2 to 3, AIS, or cervical cancer within previous 20 years.
AIS, adenocarcinoma in situ; CIN, cervical intraepithelial neoplasia; HPV, human papillomavirus.

Source: USPSTF (2012).

The Bethesda System

The Bethesda System (Crum & Huh, 2016; Nayar & Kurtycz, 2014) is a standardized system that is used for reporting cervical cytology results. Cervical cytology (Pap test) combined with HPV testing is used to screen for cervical cancer. A specimen is satisfactory only if both squamous epithelial cells and endocervical cells are present. If lacking either type of cell, specimen is incomplete. Repeat Pap test. If endocervical cells or transformation zone components are missing (unsatisfactory specimen), repeat cytology/Pap test. If cells are obscured by inflammation, treat infection before repeating Pap test.

Atypical Squamous Cells of Undetermined Significance (ASC-US)

- Ages 20 years or younger: Repeat cytology/Pap test in 12 months.
- Ages 21 to 24 years: Preferred is repeat Pap test in 12 months (acceptable is reflex HPV test).
- Ages 25 to 29 years: Preferred is reflex HPV test. Acceptable is repeat Pap test in 12 months.
- Ages 30 years or older: If oncogenic HPV positive (subtypes 16 and 18), refer for colposcopy. If HPV negative, repeat co-testing in 3 years (ACOG, 2016).

Atypical Glandular Cells (AGCs)

- More common in older women (ages 40–69 years). Associated with premalignancy or malignancy in 30% of cases. Risk of cancer goes up with age.
- Presence of endometrial cells: Refer for endometrial biopsy.

Low-Grade Squamous Intraepithelial Lesions (LSIL)

- LSIL means that cervical cells show changes that are mildly abnormal. They are usually caused by an HPV infection.
- Ages 21 to 24 years: Repeat Pap test in 12 months.
- Ages 25 to 29 years: Refer for colposcopy with cervical biopsy.
- Ages 30 years or older: If HPV negative, repeat Pap test in 12 months (or colposcopy). If HPV positive, refer for colposcopy with cervical biopsy. Treatment ranges from cryotherapy or laser therapy (ablative therapy; ACOG, 2016).

High-Grade Squamous Intraepithelial Lesions (HSIL)

- HSIL suggests more serious changes in the cervix than LSIL. They are more likely than LSIL to be associated with precancer and cancer.
- Ages 21 to 24 years: Refer for colposcopy with cervical biopsy.
- Ages 25 years or older: Refer for immediate excisional treatment. It can done by LEEP (loop electrosurgical excision) or cervical conization surgery (ACOG, 2016).

HPV DNA Test (Reflex HPV Testing)

- HPV types 16 and 18 together cause 70% of all cases of cervical cancer in the United States (National Cancer Institute, n.d.). Most cases of cervical cancer are caused by HPV infection.
- Gardasil (males or females) and Cervarix (females only) are Food and Drug Administration (FDA)-approved vaccines given at age 11 or 12 years (or as young as age 9 years through 26 years).

Colposcopy

A colposcope is a specialized "microscope" used to view the cervix. Colposcopy can be performed by a trained physician, nurse practitioner (NP), or physician assistant (PA). The diagnostic test for cervical cancer is a biopsy of the cervix, which is obtained during a colposcopy.

- A vaginal speculum is used to expose the cervix.
- After the cervix is studied, it is washed with acetic acid 3% to 5% (vinegar), which helps remove mucus and causes the abnormal areas of the cervix to turn a bright-white color that resembles leukoplakia (acetowhitening).
- Biopsy samples are obtained from the acetowhitened areas on the cervix, cervical os (glandular cells), and squamocolumnar junction.
- After a colposcopy, a small amount of cramping and bloody spotting is normal (red, brown, black) in the next few days after the procedure.

Loop Electrosurgical Excision Procedure (LEEP)

The loop electrosurgical instrument is a device that is used like a scalpel to cut through the cervix (conization) to treat cervical cancer. Depending on the result of the biopsy (size, depth, and severity), the cancerous cells can be removed by cryotherapy for mild lesions, laser ablation, or surgical conization of cervix.

Potassium Hydroxide Slide

Useful for helping with the diagnosis of fungal infections (hair, nails, skin). Potassium hydroxide (KOH) works by causing lysis of the squamous cells, which makes it easier to see hyphae and spores. Vaginal specimens do not require KOH to visualize *Candida*.

Whiff Test

A test for bacterial vaginosis (BV). A positive result occurs when a strong, fish-like odor is released after one to two drops of KOH are added to the slide (or a cotton swab soaked with discharge).

Tzanck Smear

Used as an adjunct for evaluating herpetic infection (oral, genital, skin). A positive smear will show large abnormal nuclei in squamous epithelial cells. Not commonly used.

EXAM TIPS

- **Recognize menopausal female body changes. If palpable ovary (abnormal), rule out ovarian cancer and order an intravaginal ultrasound.**
- **Be familiar with physical breast exam findings (hard irregular mass that is not mobile) and follow-up of breast cancer.**
- **For patients aged 21 to 24 years with LSIL Pap result, repeat Pap test in 12 months. But if aged 25 to 29 years, follow up with colposcopy with cervical biopsy.**
- **Pap/cytology and HPV testing are not recommended before age 21 years, even if sexually active, has sexually transmitted disease/infection (STD/STI), or multiple sex partners.**
- **If endometrial cells are seen in Pap test, refer for endometrial biopsy. Do not confuse endometrial biopsy with colposcopy, a test used to visualize the cervix and to obtain cervical biopsy.**

CLINICAL PEARLS

- **Using a small amount of K-Y Jelly to lubricate the tips of the speculum (in patients with atrophic vaginitis to reduce pain and vaginal bleeding) will not affect the Pap test results.**
- **In reproductive-age teens or women who present with acute pelvic pain or lower abdominal pain, always perform a pregnancy test (use good-quality urine human chorionic gonadotropin strips).**
- **Girls and teenagers have larger ectropions. Some adult women on birth control pills may develop ectropion.**

CONTRACEPTION

There is up to an 85% chance of becoming pregnant within 1 year of unprotected sexual intercourse. Women seeking to prevent pregnancy can choose from among several options with varying degrees of reported effectiveness (Figure 17.2).

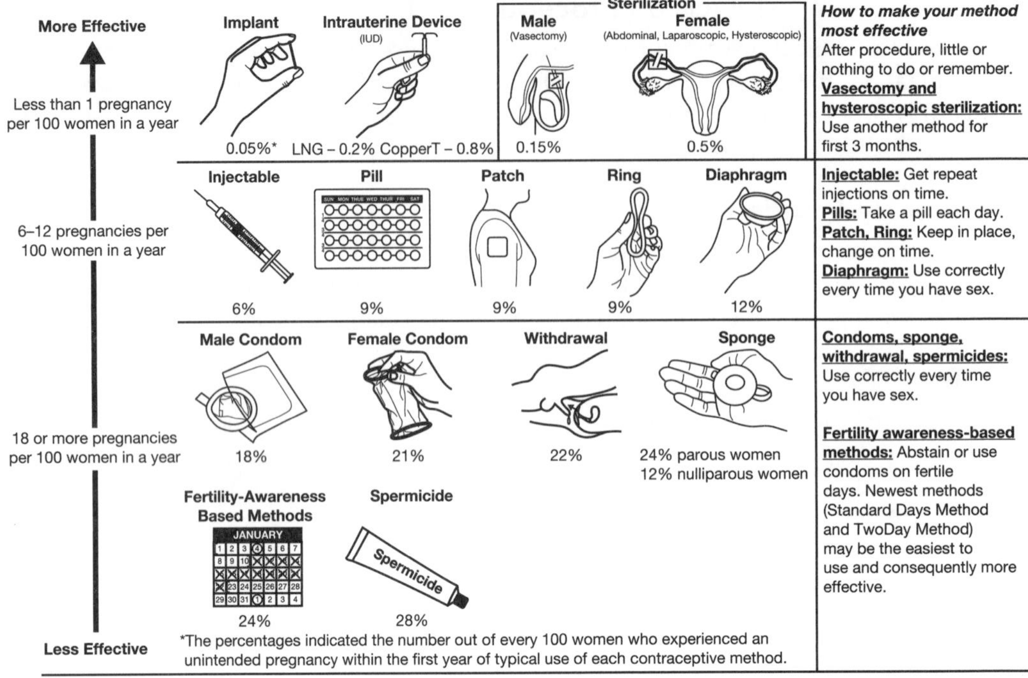

Figure 17.2 Effectiveness of contraceptive methods.

LNG, Levonorgestrel (Mirena).
Source: Association of Reproductive Health Professionals (2014); Centers for Disease Control and Prevention (2016).

ORAL CONTRACEPTIVES

Combined Oral Contraceptives (COCs; 9% Typical Use Failure Rate)

Dosed Monophasic Pills

- *Loestrin FE 1/20:* 21 consecutive days of estrogen/progesterone (same dose daily). For the last 7 days of the cycle, the placebo pills contain iron supplementation (7 days of iron pills).

Biphasic Pills

- *Ortho-Novum 10/11*: Contains two different progesterone doses (two phases). The progesterone dose increases about halfway through the cycle. Other brands are Mircette, Jenest, etc.

Triphasic Pills

- *Ortho Tri-Cyclen:* Contains 21 days of active pills and 7 days of placebo pills. The dose of hormones varies weekly for 3 weeks ("triphasic"). Progestin used is norgestimate. Indicated for acne. Other brands are Cyclessa, Tri-Norinyl, Tri-Levlen, Triphasil, etc.

Extended-Cycle Pills

- *Seasonale:* Contains 84 consecutive days (3 months) of estrogen/progesterone with a 7-day pill-free interval. This method typically results in four periods per year although breakthrough bleeding is not uncommon.

Ethinyl Estradiol and Drospirenone

- *Yaz (24 active pills and four placebo pills)/Yasmin:* Uses drospirenone (a spironolactone analog) as the progestin component. Consider for women with acne, PCOS, hirsutism, or premenstrual dysphoric disorder (PMDD). Higher risk of deep vein thrombosis (DVT) and hyperkalemia.
- *Labs:* Check the potassium level if patient is on an angiotensin-converting enzyme inhibitor (ACEI), angiotensin receptor blocker (ARB), or potassium-sparing diuretic.

Progestin-Only Pills (POPs; 9% Typical Use Failure Rate)

- Safe for breastfeeding women, and most effective if woman is exclusively breastfeeding. Also known as the "minipill."
- It is very important to take the pill at the same time each day. If dose is late (≥3 hours) or a day is missed, the woman should use condoms (backup contraception) or abstain from sexual intercourse for 2 days (Kaunitz, 2017). There is no placebo week with progestin-only pills (Association of Reproductive Health Professionals, 2014).
- *Micronor:* Take one pill daily at about the same time each day (each pack contains 28 pills). Start taking pill on day 1 of menstrual cycle.

Contraindications to Oral Contraceptive Use

Absolute Contraindications

- Any condition (past or present) that increases the risk of blood clotting
  - History of thrombophlebitis or thromboembolic disorders (i.e., DVT)
  - Genetic coagulation defects such as factor V Leiden disease
  - Major surgery with prolonged immobilization
- Smoker older than the age of 35, more than 15 cigarettes per day
  - Also considered a relative contraindication because women younger than 35 years who smoke can take the pill (if no other contraindications exist)
- Any condition that increases the risk of strokes
  - Migraine with aura or focal neurological symptoms or migraine without aura age 35 years or older
  - History of cerebrovascular accidents (CVAs) and transient ischemic attacks (TIAs)
  - Hypertension (if systolic BP >160 mmHg or diastolic BP >100 mmHg)
- Inflammation and/or acute infections of the liver with elevated LFTs
  - In acute infection or inflammation of the liver (i.e., mononucleosis) with elevated LFTs, estrogen is contraindicated
  - When LFTs are back to normal, can go back on birth control pills
  - Hepatocellular adenomas or malignant (hepatoma)
  - Cholestatic jaundice of pregnancy
- Known or suspected cardiovascular disease
  - Moderately to severely impaired cardiac function, complicated valvular heart disease
  - Coronary artery disease (CAD)
  - Diabetes with vascular component
  - Systemic lupus erythematosus
  - Hypertension if SBP is ≥160 or DBP (diastolic blood pressure) 100 mmHg
- Some reproductive system conditions or cancers
  - Known or suspected pregnancy
  - Undiagnosed genital bleeding or breast mass
  - Breast, endometrial, or ovarian cancer (or any estrogen-dependent cancer) less than 21 days postpartum

Absolute Contraindications Mnemonic: "My CUPLETS"

My Migraines with focal neurological aura
C CAD or CVA
U Undiagnosed genital bleeding
P Pregnant or suspect pregnancy
L Liver tumor or active liver disease
E Estrogen-dependent tumor
T Thrombus or emboli
S Smoker age 35 or older

Relative Contraindications

- Migraine headaches
  - Migraine older than age 35 years
  - Migraines with focal neurological findings are an absolute contraindication due to increased risk of stroke
- Smoker younger than age 35 years
- Fracture or cast on lower extremities
- Adequately controlled hypertension

Advantages of the Pill (After 5 or More Years of Use)

- Ovarian cancer and endometrial cancers (decreased by 40%–50%)
- Decreased incidence of:
  - Dysmenorrhea and cramps (decrease in prostaglandins)
  - Decreases symptoms of endometriosis (less pelvic pain)
  - Acne and hirsutism (lower levels of androgenic hormones)
  - Ovarian cysts (due to suppression of ovulation)
  - Heavy and/or irregular periods (due to suppression of ovaries)

New Prescriptions

- Oral contraceptives can be started anytime in the menstrual cycle (rule out pregnancy first).
- All patients should be instructed to use "backup" (condoms) in the first week during the first pill pack.
  - "Quick Start": Start taking the pill on the day prescribed (give samples or prescription). Rule out pregnancy first.
  - "Sunday Start": Take first pill on the first Sunday after the menstrual period starts. Will avoid having a period on a weekend.
  - "Day One Start": Take the first pill during the first day of the menstrual period. Provides the best protection.
- Follow-up: Follow-up visit needed within 2 to 3 months to check BP, any side effects, and to answer patient's questions.

Oral Contraceptive Pill Problems

Unscheduled Bleeding (Spotting)

Term used for menstrual bleeding that occurs outside of usual cycle. The first 3 weeks (21 days) of pills contain active hormones (estrogen/progesterone). During the fourth week (the last 7 days), the pills are hormone free (when the period occurs).

- Educate patient that she may have spotting/light bleeding during the first few weeks after starting birth control pills.
- Discourage patient from switching to another pill brand during the first 3 months because of spotting. Advise patient that most cases resolve spontaneously.

Menstrual Cramps

Menstrual cramps are treated with nonsteroidal anti-inflammatory drugs (NSAIDs), which decrease menstrual cramp pain and bleeding by suppressing prostaglandins. Endometriosis is associated with heavy menstrual periods (menorrhagia) with severe cramping in younger women.

- *Mefenamic acid (Ponstel):* One capsule every 6 hours for pain as needed
- *Naproxen (Aleve):* One enteric-coated tablet every 6 to 8 hours as needed
- *Ibuprofen (Advil)*: One to two tablets every 4 to 5 hours as needed.
- Prescription-strength naproxen sodium (Anaprox, Naprosyn): One tablet BID as needed

Missing Consecutive Days of Oral Contraceptive Pills

Missed 1 Day

- Take two pills now and continue with same pill pack ("doubling up").

Missed 2 Consecutive Days

- Take two pills the next 2 days to catch up and finish the birth control pill pack (use condoms for the current pill cycle).

Drug Interactions With Oral Contraceptives

These drugs can decrease the efficacy of oral contraceptives. Advise patients to use an alternative form of birth control (condoms) when taking these drugs and for one pill cycle afterward.

- *Anticonvulsants:* Phenobarbital, phenytoin
- *Antifungals:* Griseofulvin (Fulvicin), itraconazole (Sporanox), ketoconazole (Nizoral)
- *Certain antibiotics:* Ampicillin, tetracyclines, rifampin
- *St. John's wort:* May cause breakthrough bleeding

Pill Danger Signs (Table 17.2)

Thromboembolic events can happen in any organ of the body. These signs indicate a possible thromboembolic event. Advise patient to report these or to call 911 if symptoms of ACHES:

A Abdominal pain
C Chest pain
H Headaches
E Eye problems; change in vision
S Severe leg pain

Table 17.2 Oral Contraceptive Danger Signs

Complaints	Possible Cause
Chest pain (an acute MI)	Blood clot in a coronary artery
Severe headache	Stroke, TIA
Weakness on one side of the body	Ischemic stroke caused by a blood clot in the brain
Visual changes in one eye	Blood clot in the retinal artery of the affected eye
Abdominal pain	Ischemic pain of the mesenteric area caused by a blood clot
Lower leg pain (DVT)	Blood clot on a deep vein of the leg

DVT, deep vein thrombosis; MI, myocardial infarction; TIA, transient ischemic attack.

Considerations When Choosing an Oral Contraceptive Pill

- Typical use failure rate is 9%.
- Traditional oral contraceptive pills have 21 days of "active" pills and 7 days of placebo pills. The last 7 days are the "hormone-free" days. The menstrual period usually starts within 2 to 3 days after the last active pill was taken (from very low levels of estrogen/progesterone).
- Some brands of birth control pills (e.g., Loestrin FE) contain iron in the pills taken during the last 7 days of the pill cycle (instead of a placebo pill). The last 7 days (hormone-free) of the pill cycle are there to reinforce the habit of daily pill-taking.
- For the *first* pill cycle, advise patient to use "backup" (an alternative form of birth control).
- All the COCs, the patch, and the NuvaRing contain both estrogen (e.g., ethinyl estradiol) and progesterone (e.g., levonorgestrel, norethindrone, desogestrel, others).
- The contraceptive patch (e.g., Ortho Evra) results in higher levels of estrogen exposure compared to COCs (higher risk of blood clots, DVT).
- The estrogen in COCs can elevate blood pressure. Patients' BP should be checked within 4 to 8 weeks.
- Breastfeeding women can use the progestin-only pill ("minipill"; e.g., Micronor, Nor-QD).

OTHER CONTRACEPTIVE METHODS

Intrauterine Device (0.2%–0.8% Typical Use Failure Rate)

The intrauterine device (IUD) is the second most commonly used method of contraception in the world (female sterilization is the first). Paragard is copper-bearing (effective up to 10 years) and Mirena contains the hormone levonorgestrel, which decreases vaginal bleeding. Mirena IUD is effective for up to 5 years and is slightly more effective than copper-bearing IUDs (Cu-IUDs). Typical failure rate of Cu-IUD is 0.5% to 0.8%.

Contraindications

- Active PID or history of PID within the past year
- Suspected or confirmed pregnancy or has STD
- Uterine or cervical abnormality (e.g., bicornate uterus)
- Undiagnosed vaginal bleeding or uterine/cervical cancer
- History of ectopic pregnancy

Increased Risk

- Endometrial and pelvic infections (first few months after insertion only)
- Perforation of the uterus
- Heavy or prolonged menstrual periods

Education

- Educate patient to check for missing or shortened string periodically, especially after each menstrual period. If the patient or clinician does not feel the string, order a pelvic ultrasound.

Depo-Provera (0.05% Typical Failure Rate)

Each dose by injection lasts 3 months. Also known as *depot medroxyprogesterone acetate* (*DMPA*). Highly effective. Check for pregnancy before starting dose. Start within first 5 days of cycle (day 1–5) because females are less likely to ovulate at these times. Women on Depo-Provera for at least 1 year (or longer) have amenorrhea because of severe uterine atrophy from lack of estrogen.

- Do not recommend to women who want to become pregnant in 12 months. Causes delayed return of fertility. It takes up to 1 year for most women to start ovulating.
- *Black Box Warning:*Avoid long-term use (more than 2 years). Increases risk of osteopenia/osteoporosis that may not be fully reversible. Using Depo-Provera for more than 2 years is discouraged.

History of Anorexia Nervosa

Consider testing for osteopenia/osteoporosis (dual-energy x-ray absorptiometry [DXA] scan). Avoid using Depo-Provera in this population because it will further increase their risk of osteopenia/osteoporosis. Recommend calcium with vitamin D and weight-bearing exercises for patients who are on this medicine.

Diaphragm With Contraceptive Gel and Cervical Cap (12% Failure Rate)

- The diaphragm must be used with spermicidal gel. After intercourse, leave diaphragm inside vagina for at least 6 to 8 hours (can remain inside vagina up to 24 hours).
- Need additional spermicide application before every act of intercourse. Apply the spermicidal foam/gel inside the vagina without removing the diaphragm.
- The cervical cap (Prentif cap) can be worn up to 72 hours. Compared with the diaphragm, the Prentif cap may cause abnormal cervical cellular change (abnormal Pap).

Increased Risk

- Urinary tract infections (UTIs) and toxic shock syndrome (rare)

Condoms

Male Condoms (18% Failure Rate)

- More effective than the female condom

Female Condoms (21% Failure Rate)

- Do not use with any oil-based lubricants, creams, etc.

Cervical Ring (9% Failure Rate)

NuvaRing is a plastic cervical ring that contains etonogestrel and ethinyl estradiol and is left inside the vagina for 3 weeks, then removed for 1 week (when woman has her period).

- Educate patient on how to apply and remove (the ring should fit snugly around cervix).
- Absolute and relative contraindications for combined estrogen–progesterone method of contraception are the same as oral contraceptives.
- Do not use NuvaRing if cigarette smoker age 35 years or older.

Ortho Evra Transdermal Contraceptive Patch (9% Failure Rate)

- Higher risk of venous thromboembolism (VTE; releases higher levels of estrogen) compared to oral contraceptive pills. Absolute and relative contraindications for combined estrogen–progesterone method of contraception are the same as oral contraceptives.

Etonogestrel Contraceptive Implant (0.05% Failure Rate)

The contraceptive implant contains a long-acting form of progestin (etonogestrel). Initially, unscheduled bleeding is common, but when the endometrial lining atrophies, amenorrhea results. Ovulation may not occur for a few weeks to 12 months after removal.

- Thin plastic rods are inserted on the inner aspect of the upper arm subdermally (nondominant arm). If keloid scarring occurs, may have problem with removal.
- Norplant II (two rods) is effective up to 5 years. Implanon (now known as *Nexplanon*) (one rod) is effective for up to 3 years.

Emergency Contraception ("Morning-After Pill")

Works best if taken within 72 hours after unprotected sexual intercourse or if 2 consecutive days of birth control pills are skipped. Rule out preexisting pregnancy first.

- Emergency contraception: This is 89% effective.
- Brands include Plan B, My Way, or Next Choice.
- A few birth control pills that contains levonorgestrel (i.e., Triphasil) may be used as morning-after pills but are more likely to cause nausea (because of the estrogen).
- Take first dose taken as soon as possible (up to 72 hours after).
- Take second dose in 12 hours.
- If patient vomits tablet within 1 hour (or less), may need to repeat dose. Over-the-counter (OTC) antiemetics (antihistamine drug class) are dimenhydrinate (Dramamine) and meclizine (Dramamine Less Drowsy).
- Advise patient that if she does not have a period in next 3 weeks, she should return for follow-up to rule out pregnancy.

EXAM TIPS

- Low-dose birth control pills contain 20 to 25 mcg of ethinyl estradiol.
- Desogen, Ortho-TriCyclen, and Yaz/Yasmin are all indicated for treatment of acne.
- Know what to do if 2 consecutive days of the pill are missed (take two pills the next 2 days to finish cycle and use condoms until next cycle starts).
- Avoid using Depo-Provera in anorexic and/or bulimic patients (very high risk of osteoporosis).
- Women taking Seasonale will have only four periods per year.
- Mefenamic acid (Ponstel) is an NSAID that is very effective for menstrual pain.
- Know how to use Plan B (emergency contraception).
- Cu-IUD lasts 10 to 12 years. Mirena (progesterone IUD) lasts 5 years.
- Some questions will ask for the best birth control method for a case scenario. Remember the contraindications or adverse effects of each method (e.g., Depo-Provera).

CLINICAL PEARLS

- Yaz or Yasmin contain estrogen and drospirenone. Has a higher risk of blood clots, stroke, heart attacks, and hyperkalemia.
- Do not recommend Depo-Provera for women who want to become pregnant in 12 to 18 months because it may cause delayed return of fertility. It can take up to 1 year for some women to start ovulating.
- Cu-IUD probably has the broadest indication for use as a contraceptive for women with medical conditions (diabetics, smoker for more than 35 years, on anticonvulsant or antiretroviral therapy, ovarian cancer, ischemic heart disease, liver tumors, etc.).

DISEASE REVIEW

Fibrocystic Breasts

Monthly hormonal cycle induces breast tissue to become engorged and painful. Symptoms occur 2 weeks before the onset of menses (luteal phase) and are at their worst right before the menstrual cycle. Resolves after menses start. Commonly starts in women in their 30s.

Classic Case

Adult to middle-aged woman complains of the cyclic onset of bilateral breast tenderness and breast lumps that start from a few days (up to 2 weeks) before her period for many years. Once menstruation starts, the tenderness disappears and the size of breast lumps decreases. During breast examination, the breast lumps are tender and feel rubbery, and are mobile to touch. Denies dominant mass, skin changes, nipple discharge, or enlarged nodes.

Objective Findings

- Multiple mobile and rubbery cystic masses on both breasts
- Both breasts have symmetrical findings

Treatment Plan

- Stop caffeine intake. Take vitamin E and evening primrose capsules daily
- Wear bras with good support
- Referral needed if dominant mass, skin changes, fixed mass

Polycystic Ovary Syndrome (PCOS)

Hormonal abnormality marked by anovulation, infertility, excessive androgen production, and insulin resistance. These females are at higher risk for type 2 diabetes, dyslipidemia, metabolic syndrome, endometrial hyperplasia, obesity, and obstructive sleep apnea.

Classic Case

Obese teen or young adult complains of excessive facial and body hair (hirsutism 70%), bad acne, and amenorrhea or infrequent periods (oligomenorrhea). Dark thick hair (terminal hair) is seen on the face, cheek, and beard areas.

Treatment Plan

- Transvaginal ultrasound: Enlarged ovaries seen with multiple small follicles (sizes vary).
- Serum testosterone, dehydroepiandrosterone (DHEA), and androstenedione are elevated. FSH levels are normal or low.
- Fasting blood glucose and 2-hour oral glucose tolerance test (OGTT) are abnormal.

Medications

- Use low-dose oral contraceptives to suppress ovaries.
- Spironolactone is used to decrease and control hirsutism.
- If patient does not want oral contraceptives, give medroxyprogesterone tablets (Provera) 5 to 10 mg daily for 10 to 14 days (repeat every 1–2 months to induce menses).
- Metformin (Glucophage) is used to induce ovulation (if desires pregnancy). Warn reproductive-age diabetic females (who do not want to become pregnant) to use birth control.
- Weight loss reduces androgen and insulin levels.

Complications

PCOS patients are at increased risk for:

- Coronary heart disease (CHD)
- Type 2 diabetes mellitus and metabolic syndrome

- Cancer of the breast and endometrium
- Central obesity
- Infertility

Osteoporosis

A gradual loss of bone density secondary to estrogen deficiency and other metabolic disorders. Most common in older women (White or Asian descent) who are thin and with small body frames, especially if positive family history. Treat postmenopausal women (or men aged 50 years or older) who have osteoporosis (T-score −2.5 or less) or history of hip or vertebral fracture.

Other risk groups include:

- Patients on chronic steroids (severe asthma, autoimmune disorders, etc.) are at high risk for glucocorticoid-induced osteoporosis; rule out osteoporosis in older women (or men) on chronic steroids, especially if accompanied by other risk factors (lower testosterone, small frame, thin, White, or Asian)
- Patients who have Anorexia nervosa and bulimia
- Long-term use of proton-pump inhibitors (PPIs) such as omeprazole (Prilosec)
- Gastric bypass, celiac disease, hyperthyroidism, ankylosing spondylitis, rheumatoid arthritis (RA), and others

Lifestyle Risk Factors

- Low calcium intake, vitamin D deficiency, inadequate physical activity
- Alcohol consumption (three or more drinks per day), high caffeine intake
- Smoking (active or passive)

Bone Density Test Scores

- Use DXA to measure the bone mineral density (BMD) of the hip and spine; do baseline and repeat in 1 to 2 years (if on treatment regimen) to assess the efficacy of the medicine; if not on treatment, repeat DXA in 2 to 5 years
- *Osteoporosis:* T-scores of −2.5 or lower standard deviations (SD) at the lumbar spine, femoral neck, or total hip region
- *Osteopenia:* T-scores between −1.5 and −2.4 SD

Treatment Plan

- Weight-bearing exercises most days of the week
  - Swimming and biking are not considered a weight-bearing exercise (but good for severe arthritis)
  - Weight-bearing exercises are walking, jogging, aerobic dance classes, most sports, yoga, tai chi
  - Isometric exercises are not considered a weight-bearing type of exercise
- Calcium with vitamin D 1,200 mg/d, vitamin D_2 (50,000 IU once weekly), and vitamin D_3 (800 mg to 1,000 IU/d)

Medications

Bisphosphonates

- First-line drugs for treating postmenopausal osteoporosis, glucocorticoid-induced osteoporosis (women and men), and osteoporosis in men
- Potent esophageal irritant (advise patients to report sore throat, dysphagia, midsternal pain); may cause esophagitis, esophageal perforation, gastric ulcers, reactivation/bleeding peptic ulcer disease (PUD)
- Increases BMD and inhibits bone resorption
- Fosamax (alendronate) 5 to 10 mg daily or 70 mg weekly

- Actonel (risedronate) 5 mg daily or 35 mg weekly (or 150-mg tablet once a month)
  - Take immediately upon awakening in a.m. with full glass (6–8 ounces) of plain water (do not use mineral water)
  - Take tablets sitting or standing and wait at least 30 minutes before lying down
  - Do not crush, split, or chew tablets; swallow the tablets whole
  - Never take these drugs with other medications, juice, coffee, antacids, vitamins
  - Will cause severe esophagitis or esophageal perforation if lodged in the esophagus
- Alendronate (Fosamax) 10 mg once a day or 70 mg once a week
- Consider prophylaxis for high-risk postmenopausal women with osteopenia
- Repeat dual-energy x-ray absorptiometry (DXA) after 2 years of therapy
- *Contraindications:* Inability to sit upright, esophageal motility disorders, history of PUD or history of GI bleeding
- Osteonecrosis of the jaw (mandible or maxilla) more likely if on intravenous or intramuscular bisphosphonates; complains of jaw heaviness, pain, swelling, and loose teeth

Selective Estrogen Receptor Modulator (SERM) Class

- Evista (raloxifene) blocks estrogen receptors; a category X drug
- Approved for use after menopause. For postmenopausal women with osteoporosis who also need breast cancer (estrogen-receptor positive) prophylaxis
- Do not use to treat menopausal symptoms (aggravates hot flashes)
- Does not stimulate endometrium or breast tissue
- *Black Box Warning*: Increases risk of DVT and pulmonary embolism; increased risk of death from stroke (postmenopausal women with history of heart disease)
- These drugs reduce risk of breast cancer (if taken long term up to 5 years)
- SERMs are an option for patients who cannot tolerate or have contraindications to biphosphanates
- Used as adjunct treatment for estrogen-receptor positive breast cancers

Tamoxifen (Nolvadex)

- Used for breast cancer that is hormone-receptor positive; can be taken up to 5 years
- Increased risk of DVT, endometrial cancer, strokes, and pulmonary emboli
- Common side effects: Causes hot flashes, white or brownish vaginal discharge, weight gain or loss

Parathyroid Hormone (PTH) Analog

- Teriparatide (Forteo) injection is recombinant human parathyroid hormone for treatment of osteoporosis; it comes as a prefilled injector; there is a warning about this drug, as it increased the incidence of osteosarcoma in rats

Other: Miacalcin and Calcitriol

- Calcitonin salmon, derived from salmon; weak antifracture efficacy compared with biphosphonates and PTH
- Calcitriol: Vitamin D analog; must be on a low-calcium diet; monitor patient for hypercalcemia, hypercalciuria, and renal insufficiency; may be effective in preventing glucocorticoid and posttransplant-related bone loss

Women's Health Initiative (WHI)

- Average age of menopause for women in the United States is 51 years.
- The Women's Health Initiative (WHI) showed that combined estrogen-progestin replacement therapy (ERT) increased the risk of stroke, heart disease, venous thromboembolism, breast cancer, and pulmonary embolism.

- The USPSTF does not recommend combined estrogen and progestin or unopposed estrogen for prevention of chronic conditions (heart disease, osteoporosis). But the advice does not apply to women who want hormone therapy for relief of menopausal symptoms. Experts recommend duration of therapy of less than 5 years because of increased risk of breast cancer. Many experts consider it safe for healthy women within 10 years of menopause (younger than 60 years) with no contraindications for estrogen. Women who have a uterus need both estrogen and progesterone (decreases risk of endometrial cancer); use unopposed estrogen for women with hysterectomy.
- Estrogen can alleviate dyspareunia and vaginal/urethral atrophy. Estrogen increases the risk of developing or exacerbating systemic lupus erythematosus (birth control pills are contraindicated in women with lupus).

Ovarian Cancer

Ovarian cancer is the fifth most common cancer in women in the United States. It is seldom diagnosed during the early stages of the disease. Most often, an older woman complains of vague symptoms such as abdominal bloating and discomfort, low-back pain, pelvic pain, urinary frequency, and constipation (frequently blamed on benign conditions) for certain women with *BRCA1* and *BRCA2* mutations. By the time the cancer is diagnosed, it has almost always metastasized. Symptoms in patients with metastatic disease depend on area affected and may include bone pain, abdominal pain, headache, blurred vision, others.

Some experts recommend risk-reducing bilateral salpingo-oophorectomy (BSO) between ages 35 and 40 years (after childbearing complete) for certain women with *BRCA1* and *BRCA2* mutations. BSO has a significant effect in reducing ovarian cancer risk in this population. Although the USPSTF does not recommend routine screening for ovarian cancer in the general population (Grade D), high-risk women with suspected *BRCA 1/BRCA 2* mutations should be referred for genetic counseling. If ovarian cancer screening is done, a transvaginal ultrasound with serum cancer antigen (CA-125) is ordered. The screening starts at age 30 years (or 5 to 10 years before earliest age of first diagnosis of ovarian cancer in a family member).

VULVOVAGINAL INFECTIONS (TABLE 17.3)

Table 17.3 Vaginal Disorders

Type	Signs/Symptoms	Lab Results
Bacterial vaginosis	"Fish-like" vaginal odor; profuse milk-like discharge that coats the vaginal vault	Clue cells no WBCs
	Not itchy/vulva not red; overgrowth of anaerobes	Whiff test: positive pH >4.5 alkaline
Candidal vaginitis	Cheesy or curd-like white discharge	Pseudohyphae, spores, numerous WBCs
	Vulvovagina red/irritated	
Trichomonal vaginitis (trichomoniasis)	"Strawberry cervix"	Mobile protozoa with flagella
	Bubbly discharge	Numerous WBCs
	Vulvovagina red/irritated	
Atrophic vaginitis	Scant to no discharge	Atrophic changes on Pap test
	Fewer rugae, vaginal color pale; dyspareunia (painful intercourse); may bleed slightly during speculum examination (if not on hormones)	Elevated FSH and LH

FSH, follicle-stimulating hormone; LH, luteinizing hormone; WBC, white blood cell.

Bacterial Vaginosis (BV)

Caused by an overgrowth of anaerobic bacteria in the vagina. Risk factors include sexual activity, new or multiple sex partners, and douching. Not an STD; therefore, sexual partner does not need treatment. Pregnant women with BV are at higher risk for intrauterine infections and premature labor.

Classic Case

Sexually active female complains of an unpleasant and fish-like vaginal odor that is worse after intercourse (if no condom is used). Vaginal discharge is copious and has milk-like consistency. Speculum examination reveals off-white to light-gray discharge coating the vaginal walls. There is no vulvar or vaginal redness or irritation (vaginal anaerobic bacteria do not cause inflammation).

Labs

Wet Smear Microscopy

- *Findings:* Clue cells and very few WBCs. May see *Mobiluncus* bacteria (82%), a gram-negative anaerobic rod-shaped bacteria.
- *Clue cells:* Made up of squamous epithelial cells with a large amount of bacteria coating the surface that obliterates the edges of the squamous epithelial cells (Figure 17.3).

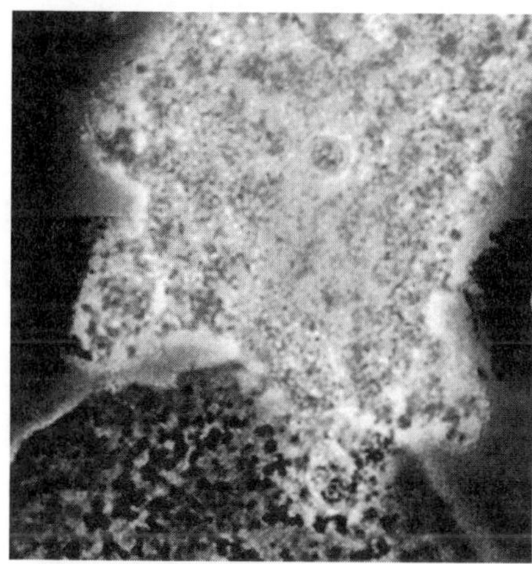

Figure 17.3 Clue cell. This image can be found in color in the app.

Source: Centers for Disease Control and Prevention (2015).

Whiff Test

- Apply one drop of KOH to a cotton swab that is soaked with vaginal discharge.
- *Positive:* A strong "fishy" odor is released.

Vaginal pH

- Alkaline vaginal pH greater than 4.5. Normal vaginal pH is between 4.0 and 4.5 (acidic).

Treatment Plan

- Prescribe metronidazole (Flagyl) BID × 7 days.
- Alternative: Metronidazole vaginal gel one applicator at bedtime for 5 days.
- Watch for disulfiram (Antabuse) effect if combined with alcohol (severe nausea, headache, etc.).
- Prescribe clindamycin (Cleocin) cream at HS × 7 days (oil based).
- Oil-based creams can weaken condoms.
- Sex partners: Treatment is not recommended by the CDC because BV is not an STD.
- Abstain from sexual intercourse until treatment is done.

Candidal Vaginitis

Overgrowth of *Candida albicans* yeast in the vulva/vagina. Considered normal vaginal flora, but can also be pathogenic. Diabetics, those who are HIV-positive, on antibiotics (i.e., amoxicillin), or have any type of immunosuppression are at higher risk. (The male penis can also be infected [balanitis].)

Classic Case

Adult female presents with complaints of white cheese-like ("curd-like") vaginal discharge accompanied by severe vulvovaginal pruritus, swelling, and redness (inflammatory reaction). May complain of external pruritus of the vulva and vagina.

Labs: Wet Smear Microscopy

- Swipe cotton swab with vaginal discharge in the middle of a glass slide.
- Add a few drops of normal saline (to the discharge).
- Cover the sample with a cover slip and examine it under the microscope (set it at high power).
- *Findings:* Pseudohyphae and spores with a large number of WBCs are present.

Treatment Plan

- Miconazole (Monistat), clotrimazole (Gyne-Lotrimin) for 7 days (over the counter)
- *Prescription:* Diflucan 100-mg tablet × 1 dose, terconazole (Terazol-3) vaginal cream/suppository
- If patient is on an antibiotic such as amoxicillin, recommend daily yogurt or lactobacillus pills

Trichomonal Vaginitis (Trichomoniasis)

Trichomonas vaginalis is a unicellular protozoan parasite with flagella that infects genitourinary tissue (both males and females). Infection causes inflammation (pruritus, burning, and irritation) of vagina/urethra.

Classic Case

Adult female complains of very pruritic, reddened vulvovaginal area. May complain of dysuria. Copious grayish-green and bubbly vaginal discharge. Male partners may have dysuria and frequency (urethritis) or may be asymptomatic.

Objective Findings

- "Strawberry cervix" from small points of bleeding on cervical surface (punctate hemorrhages)
- Swollen and reddened vulvar and vaginal area; vaginal pH greater than 5.0
- Dysuria (burning) with urination

Labs

- Microscopy (use low power): Mobile unicellular organisms with flagella (flagellates) and a large amount of WBCs

Treatment Plan

- Metronidazole (Flagyl) 2 g PO × 1 dose (preferred) or 500 mg BID × 7 days
- Treat sexual partner because trichomoniasis is considered an STI; avoid sex until both partners complete treatment

Atrophic Vaginitis

Chronic lack of estrogen in estrogen-dependent tissue of the urogenital tract; results in atrophic changes in the vulva and vagina of menopausal women. Estrogen is the most effective treatment for moderate to severe vaginal atrophy. Low-dosed topical estrogen therapy is preferred because of low systemic absorption.

Classic Case

Menopausal female complains of vaginal dryness, itching, and pain with sexual intercourse (dyspareunia). Complains of a great deal of discomfort with speculum examinations (i.e., Pap tests). Pap test result is "abnormal" secondary to atrophic changes.

Objective Findings

- Atrophic labia with decreased rugae, vulva or vagina may have fissures
- Dry, pale pink color to vagina

Treatment Plan

- If Pap is mildly abnormal (atrophic changes), consider temporary use of topical estrogen vaginal cream for a few weeks and repeat Pap test.
- Topical conjugated estrogen comes in several forms; as a cream, insert, or cervical ring. Apply topical estrogens intravaginally (Premarin, Extrace, Vagifem). Need progesterone supplementation (if intact uterus) if using long term to decrease risk of endometrial hyperplasia.

EXAM TIPS

- Know female body changes in menopause. If palpable ovary (abnormal), order an intravaginal ultrasound.
- Know physical exam findings (hard irregular mass that is not mobile) and follow-up for breast cancer.
- Mefenamic acid (Ponstel) is an NSAID that is very effective for menstrual pain.
- Know how to take bisphosphonates (e.g., Fosamax, Actonel) and their contraindications.
- Know the bone density score for osteoporosis (T-score of >−2.5 SD) and for osteopenia (T-score of −1.5 to −2.4 SD).
- There will be questions on all the types of vaginitis (BV, trichomonal, candidal, atrophic vaginitis). The questions range from diagnosis, workup and lab tests, to treatment.
- Become familiar with BV. "Clue cells" are squamous epithelial cells that have blurred edges due to the large number of bacteria on the cell's surface (see Figure 17.3).

CLINICAL PEARLS

- Become familiar with the vaginal infections, their presentation, and treatment. Wet smear or microscopy is gold-standard diagnosis (bacterial vaginosis, candidal or trichomonal vaginitis).
- Women who have persistent vaginal and urinary tract infections, despite hygiene measures, adequate hydration, and in the absence of sexual exposures from partner(s), should be screened for underlying glucose metabolism disorders and diabetes.

18

Sexually Transmitted Diseases (STDs) or Infections (STIs) Review

⚠ DANGER SIGNALS

HIV/AIDS

The median time between initial HIV infection and AIDS is 10 years (CDC, 2015). AIDS is defined by an absolute CD4 cell count of less than 200 cells/mm^3 along with certain opportunistic infections and malignancies. CD4 levels in healthy people range between 500 and 16,000 cells/mm^3. Signs and symptoms that suggest AIDS are oral candidiasis (thrush), fever, weight loss, diarrhea, cough, shortness of breath, purple to bluish-red bumps on the skin (Kaposi's sarcoma), and certain infections. *Pneumocystis jirovecii*, formerly known as *Pneumocystis carinii*, is the infection that causes the most deaths in patients with HIV.

Acute HIV Infection (Acute Retroviral Syndrome)

Very infectious due to extremely high viral load (>100,000 copies/mL) in blood and genital secretions. The initial immune response may mimic mononucleosis (fever, headache, sore throat, lymphadenopathy, rash, joint ache, and myalgia). These symptoms are seen in 50% to 90% of persons within 2 to 4 few weeks after initial infection with the HIV virus. During this time, the HIV antibody tests may still be negative (window period). Most people (97%) develop antibodies within 3 months after exposure. If you strongly suspect acute HIV infection, order the HIV RNA polymerase chain reaction (PCR) test, which can detect infection 7 to 28 days after exposure.

Disseminated Gonococcal Disease (Disseminated Gonorrhea)

Sexually active adult from high-risk population complains of petechial or pustular skin lesions of hands/soles (acral lesions); swollen, red, and tender joints in one large joint (migratory asymmetrical arthritis) such as the knee. May be accompanied by signs of STD (i.e., cervicitis, urethritis). If pharyngitis, will have severe sore throat with green purulent throat exudate that does not respond to usual antibiotics used for strep throat. Occasionally complicated by perihepatitis (Fitz-Hugh–Curtis syndrome) and rarely endocarditis or meningitis.

NORMAL FINDINGS

- Female normal findings covered in Chapter 17.
- Male normal findings covered in Chapter 16.

STD Screening Recommended by the Centers of Disease Control and Prevention (CDC; 2015)

- Routine annual screening of all sexually active females aged 25 years or younger for *Chlamydia trachomatis* and gonorrhea
  - If infected, retest for chlamydia and gonorrhea 3 months after treatment (to check for reinfection, not for test-of-cure)
- Annual testing for syphilis, chlamydia, and gonorrhea in persons with HIV infection
- Minors do not need parental consent if the clinic visit is related to testing or treating STDs and birth control; no state requires parental consent for STD care

Men Who Have Sex With Men (MSM)

- Annual screening for chlamydia and gonorrhea at sites of contact (urethra, rectum) regardless of condom use. Screen every 3 to 6 months if at increased risk.
- Annual screening recommended for pharyngeal gonorrhea (throat). Screen every 3 to 6 months if at increased risk.
- Annual testing recommended for HIV, syphilis, and for HBsAg. Retest more frequently if at risk.

Pregnant Women

- Screen pregnant women for HIV, chlamydia, gonorrhea, syphilis, and hepatitis B surface antigen (HBsAg) at first prenatal visit.
- Pregnant women treated for chlamydia and/or gonorrhea should have a test-of-cure within 3 to 4 weeks after treatment.
- Retest at 3 months for chlamydia and gonorrhea (check for reinfection, not test of cure).

STD Risk Factors

- Younger ages (females aged 15–24 years); sex initiated at a younger age
- Multiple sexual partners, new sexual partner in past 60 days
- Inconsistent condom use, unmarried status
- History of previous STD infection, illicit drug use
- Genital ulceration (increases risk of HIV transmission)
- Use of alcohol or illicit drugs
- Adolescents

DISEASE REVIEW

Chlamydia Trachomatis

Most chlamydial infections are asymptomatic. The highest prevalence is among persons 25 years of age or younger. *Chlamydia trachomatis* is the most common bacterial STD in the United States. It is an obligate intracellular bacterium (atypical bacterium). Annual screening of all sexually active women younger than 25 years of age is recommended, as is screening of older women at increased risk for infection (e.g., those who have a new sexual partner, more than one sexual partner, a sexual partner with concurrent partners, or a sexual partner with an STI [CDC, 2015]).

Possible Sites of Infection

- *Females*: Cervicitis, endometritis, salpingitis (fallopian tubes), pelvic inflammatory disease (PID)
- *Males*: Epididymitis, prostatitis
- *Both genders*: Urethritis, pharyngitis, proctitis (from receptive anal intercourse)
- *Complications*: PID, tubal scarring, ectopic pregnancy, infertility, Reiter's syndrome (males), Fitz-Hugh–Curtis syndrome

Laboratory Testing (Both Gonorrhea and Chlamydia)

- Nucleic acid amplification tests (NAATs) are highly sensitive tests for both gonorrhea and chlamydia. Swab samples (vagina, cervix, urethra, rectum, pharynx) or urine specimen can be collected for both males and females.
- Vaginal swab specimens can be collected by a provider or self-collected in a clinical setting. Self-collected vaginal swab specimens are equivalent in sensitivity and specificity to those collected by a clinician using NAATs.
- Preferred diagnostic test for men is urine specimen for NAAT. Collect the first part of the urinary stream (15–20 mL) from the first void of the day.
- For samples from pharynx or rectum, swab using a NAAT test. Another option for gonorrhea is to order gonorrheal culture (Thayer–Martin or chocolate agar).
- Chlamydial cultures are not used in primary care (use NAAT test).
- Gram stain: Polymorphonuclear leukocytes with gram-negative intracellular diplococci are used for males with gonorrheal urethritis. Not commonly used in primary care.

Treatment Plan

Uncomplicated Infections

Chlamydia (Cervicitis, Urethritis, Sexual Partners)

- No test-of-cure is necessary for azithromycin or doxycycline regimen
- Azithromycin 1 g PO in a single dose (directly observed treatment [DOT] preferred) *or* doxycycline 100 mg BID × 7 days
  - Swallow with large amount of water; may cause esophagitis if tablet gets stuck in throat (difficulty and/or pain with swallowing, acute-onset heartburn, nausea/vomiting)
  - Nausea, GI upset, photosensitivity (avoid sun or use sunscreen)
  - Category D drug (stains growing tooth enamel)

Sexual Partners

- Administer azithromycin 1 g PO in a single dose. Patient and partner abstain from sex for 7 days.
- Expedited Partner Therapy (EPT) is the practice of treating the sexual partner(s) of a patient diagnosed with an STD without the sexual partner being seen or evaluated by the health care provider.
  - EPT is permissible (CDC, 2017) in 41 states, potentially allowable in seven states, and prohibited in two states (Kentucky, South Carolina). Use the following CDC website to check if EPT is legal in your state (www.cdc.gov/std/ept/legal/default.htm)

Pregnant Women

- Test-of-cure 3 weeks after completion of treatment (to detect therapeutic failure)
- Azithromycin 1 g PO in a single dose *or* amoxicillin 500 mg PO TID × 7 days
- Test-of-cure recommended 3 to 4 weeks after treatment and retest again within 3 months

Complicated Infections

Pelvic Inflammatory Disease

- Ceftriaxone (Rocephin) 250 mg IM × one dose *plus* doxycycline PO BID × 14 days *with or without* metronidazole (Flagyl) PO BID × 14 days

Neisseria gonorrhoeae

A gram-negative bacterium that infects the urinary and genital tracts, rectum, and pharynx. Unlike chlamydia, gonorrhea can become systemic or disseminated if left untreated. If positive for *N. gonorrhoeae*, cotreat for both (even if negative chlamydial tests) because of the high rate of coinfection. Do not use quinolones to treat gonorrhea due to high-level resistance.

Laboratory Tests

Discussed in chlamydia section in this chapter.

Classic Case

Sexually active female complains of purulent green-colored vaginal discharge. May walk using shuffling gait to avoid pelvic pain. Speculum examination reveals purulent discharge on the cervix, which may be friable (bleeds easily). Males will have penile discharge and dysuria and may report staining of underwear with green purulent discharge. History of new partner (<3 months) or multiple sexual partners. Inconsistent condom use. Signs and symptoms depend on the organ/site that becomes infected.

Signs and Symptoms (by Site)

- Cervicitis (mucopurulent cervix, pain, mild bleeding after intercourse, dyspareunia)
- Urethritis (scant to copious purulent discharge, dysuria, frequency, urgency)
- Proctitis (pruritus, rectal pain, tenesmus, or feeling urge to defecate even if rectum is empty, avoidance of defecation due to pain)
- Pharyngitis (severe sore throat unresponsive to typical antibiotics, purulent green-colored discharge on the posterior pharynx)
- Bartholin's gland abscess (cystic lump that is red and warm [or has purulent discharge] that is located on each side of the introitus or vestibule)
- Endometritis (menometrorrhagia, or heavy prolonged menstrual bleeding)
- Salpingitis (fallopian tubes) and PID (one-sided pelvic or lower abdominal pain, adnexal pain, dyspareunia or painful intercourse and/or cervical motion tenderness)
- Epididymitis and prostatitis (discussed in Chapter 16)

Syphilis

Screen for syphilis if HIV infection, MSM, presence of any genital ulcer (especially if painless chancre), previous STD, pregnancy, intravenous drug use, or high risk.

Treponema pallidum (spirochete) infection becomes systemic if untreated.

Classic Case

Signs and symptoms are dependent on stage of infection.

Primary

- Painless chancre (heals in 6–9 weeks if not treated)
- Chancre has clean base, well demarcated with indurated margins

Secondary (More Than 2 Years)

- Condyloma lata (infectious white papules in moist areas that look like white warts)
- Maculopapular rash on palms and soles that is not pruritic (may be generalized)

Latent Stage

- Asymptomatic but will have positive titers

Tertiary (3–10 Years)

- Neurosyphilis, gumma (soft tissue tumors), aneurysms, valvular damage, and so on

Labs

Two types of syphilis serologic tests (treponemal and nontreponemal tests) are needed to diagnose syphilis.

- *Step 1*—Order screening test (nontreponemal tests): Rapid plasma reagin (RPR) or Venereal Disease Research Laboratory (VDRL). If reactive, order confirmatory test.
- *Step 2*—Order confirmatory test (treponemal tests): Fluorescent treponemal antibody absorption (FTA-ABS), microhemagglutination test for antibodies to *T. pallidum* (MHA-TP), *T. pallidum* particle agglutination assay (TPPA), others; darkfield microscopy (not commonly used anymore).
- If both RPR (or VDRL) and FTA-ABS (or other treponemal test) are reactive: This is diagnostic for syphilis.
- During treatment, if initial test used is RPR, order sequential RPR to document treatment response. If initial test is VDRL, order sequential VDRL. Use the same laboratory to monitor.
- If RPR or VDRL shows a fourfold or higher (>1:4) decrease in titers, patient is responding to treatment.

Treatment Plan

Primary Syphilis (Chancre), Secondary Syphilis, or Early Latent Syphilis (<1 Year)

- Benzathine penicillin G (Bicillin L-A) 2.4 million units IM × one dose

Latent Syphilis (>1 Year), Latent Unknown Duration Syphilis

- Benzathine penicillin G 2.4 million units IM once per week × 3 weeks
- Penicillin allergy: Doxycycline, tetracycline, and for neurosyphilis, ceftriaxone; use these therapies with close clinical and laboratory follow-up; refer to specialist

Follow-Up

- Recheck RPR or VDRL at 6 and 12 months after treatment (look for at least a fourfold decrease in the pretreatment and posttreatment titers).
- Treat sexual partner(s) from previous 90 days before patient's diagnosis even if their RPR or VDRL is negative. Test patient and partner(s) for HIV and other STDs.
- Refer to infectious disease specialist for suspected neurosyphilis, poor response to treatment, penicillin allergy, or if primary clinician not familiar with syphilis management.

EXAM TIPS

- **RPR or VDRL are the screening tests for syphilis.**
- **If positive RPR or VDRL (nontreponemal test), confirm with FTA–ABS (treponemal test). If reactive RPR and reactive FTA–ABS, this is diagnostic for syphilis.**
- **If gonorrheal infection, always co-treat for chlamydia.**
- **Gonorrhea treated with ceftriaxone IM 250 mg x one dose (for both uncomplicated/complicated cases) plus co-treat for chlamydia.**
- **Learn treatment of PID and proctitis.**
- **Do not confuse condyloma acuminata (genital warts) with condyloma lata (secondary syphilis).**

- **Know tertiary syphilis treatment.**
- **Acute retroviral syndrome or primary HIV infection flu-like or mono-like infection is very infectious at this stage of HIV infection. Best if HIV is treated as early as possible.**

CLINICAL PEARLS

- **False-positive RPR can be caused by pregnancy, Lyme disease, autoimmune diseases, chronic or acute disease.**
- **Recheck syphilitic chancre in 3 to 7 days after injection (should start healing).**
- **Nontreponemal titers (RPR or VDRL) usually decline after treatment, but in some persons, nontreponemal antibodies can persist for a long time (serofast reaction). Most patients with reactive nontreponemal tests will be reactive for the rest of their lives (low titers), but 15% to 25% revert to being serologically nonreactive in 2 to 3 years.**

CDC-RECOMMENDED STD TREATMENT REGIMENS (TABLE 18.1)

Uncomplicated Infections of the Cervix, Urethra, Rectum, and Pharynx

First-Line Therapy

- Ceftriaxone (Rocephin) 250 mg IM × one dose *plus* cotreat for chlamydia
- Azithromycin 1 g orally × one dose *or* doxycycline 100 mg orally × 7 days
- Test-of-cure (i.e., repeat testing 3 to 4 weeks after treatment) is not needed (except pregnant women). If symptoms persist, obtain specimen for gonococcal culture and sensitivity.

Management of Sexual Partners

- Treat male partners of women with PID if sexual contact during the 60 days preceding the patient's symptoms.
- Avoid sex until both partners finish treatment and no longer have symptoms.

Complicated Gonococcal Infections

PID, Acute Epididymitis, Acute Prostatitis, Acute Proctitis

- Ceftriaxone (Rocephin) 250 mg IM × one dose *plus* cotreat for chlamydia
- Doxycycline 100 mg PO BID × 14 days *with or without* metronidazole (Flagyl) 500 mg PO BID × 14 days

Disseminated Gonococcal Infection

Refer to emergency department or infectious disease specialist. Administer ceftriaxone (Rocephin) 1 g IM or IV every 24 hours.

Table 18.1 Sexually Transmitted Diseases: Treatment Guidelines

Diseases and Organism	Uncomplicated Infections	Complicated Infections
Chlamydia		
Chlamydia trachomatis	Azithromycin 1 g × one dose	Doxycycline 100 mg
Pregnancy*	*or*	BID × 14 days
Azithromycin 1 g × one dose	Doxycycline 100 mg	PID, salpingitis
	BID × 7 days	Tubo-ovarian abscess

(continued)

Table 18.1 Sexually Transmitted Diseases: Treatment Guidelines (*continued*)

Diseases and Organism	Uncomplicated Infections	Complicated Infections
	Mucopurulent cervicitis Urethritis	Males
	Sexual partner treatment	Epididymitis, prostatitis
Gonorrhea		
Neisseria gonorrhoeae Pregnancy*	Ceftriaxone 250 mg IM ×one dose *plus*	Ceftriaxone 250 mg IM × one dose *plus*
Ceftriaxone 250 mg IM × one dose *plus* Azithromycin 1 g × once	Azithromycin 1 g × one dose or Doxycycline 100 mg BID × 7 days	Doxycycline 100 mg BID × 14 days
	Mucopurulent cervicitis	PID, salpingitis
	Urethritis	Tubo-ovarian abscess
	Proctitis	Males
	Sexual partner treatment	Epididymitis, orchitis, prostatitis
		Disseminated gonorrhea
		Asymmetric arthritis and maculopapular rash
Syphilis		
Treponema pallidum	Benzathine penicillin G 2.4 mU IM × one dose	Benzathine penicillin G 2.4 mU IM weekly × 3 weeks
	Primary or secondary syphilis or early latent <1 year	More than 1 year's duration or latent syphilis; refer
	Treat sexual partners	Follow-up of cases is mandatory (any stage of disease)
	Retreat if clinical signs recur or sustained fourfold titers	

*Doxycycline is contraindicated in lactation/pregnancy (category D).
BID, two times a day; IM, intramuscular; PID, pelvic inflammatory disease.

Source: Adapted from the Centers for Disease Control (2017).

Risk Factors for PID

- History of PID: 25% recurrence
- Multiple partners
- Age 25 years or younger

Labs

- Reproductive-aged females: Rule out pregnancy first
  - Women can insert a swab inside the vagina for NAAT test (vaginal fluid)
  - Both men and women can obtain urine specimen for NAAT by using initial urinary stream (first urine of the day)
  - Gonorrhea (anaerobic cultures), such as the Thayer–Martin or chocolate agar, is an alternative to test rectum or pharynx infection

Gram Stain

- Useful for gonorrhea only; look for gram-negative diplococci in clusters

Other STD Testing

- HIV, syphilis, hepatitis B (HBsAg), herpes simplex type 2 (HSV-2)
- Partners should be tested and treated; no sex until both complete treatment

UNUSUAL COMPLICATIONS

Fitz-Hugh–Curtis Syndrome (Perihepatitis)

Chlamydial and/or gonococcal infection of the liver capsule (not the liver itself). There is extensive scarring between the liver capsule and abdominal contents (e.g., colon). Scars look like "violin strings" (seen on laparoscopy). A complication of PID (10%) due to chlamydia and/or gonococcal infection.

Classic Case

Sexually active female with symptoms of PID complains of right upper quadrant (RUQ) abdominal pain and tenderness on palpation. The liver function tests are normal. Treated as a complicated gonorrheal/chlamydial infection (ceftriaxone [Rocephin] 250 mg IM plus doxycycline PO BID × 14 days).

Jarisch–Herxheimer Reaction

Acute febrile reaction that can occur during the first 24 hours after treatment of syphilis and other spirochete infections (e.g., Lyme disease). Look for acute-onset fever, chills, headache, myalgias. An immune-mediated reaction that usually resolves spontaneously within 12 to 24 hours. Treatment is supportive.

Reiter's Syndrome

More common in males. An immune-mediated reaction secondary to infection with certain bacteria (e.g., chlamydia) that spontaneously resolves. Treatment is supportive (e.g., NSAIDs).

Classic Case

A male with current history of chlamydia genital infection (i.e., urethritis) complains of red and swollen joints that come and go (migratory arthritis in large joints such as knee) and ulcers on the skin of the glans penis.

Mnemonic: "I can't see (conjunctivitis), pee (urethritis), or climb up a tree (migratory arthritis in large joint such as the knee)."

EXAM TIPS

- **Use ceftriaxone (Rocephin) 250 mg IM × one dose for both uncomplicated and complicated gonorrheal infection.**
- **Recognize proctitis symptoms and treatment. Become familiar with the treatment regimens for chlamydia and gonorrhea.**
- **If gonorrheal test is positive, always cotreat for chlamydia even if the chlamydial test result is negative.**
- **Inverse is not true. If chlamydia, do not give prophylaxis against gonorrhea unless indicated.**
- **Azithromycin used for pregnant patients who have chlamydia. Test-of-cure needed 3 to 4 weeks after treatment.**
- **HSV-1 infection more common on oral mucosa and HSV-2 more common on the genitals.**

- **Learn presentation of Fitz-Hugh–Curtis or Jarisch–Herxheimer syndrome.**
- **If STD symptoms with new onset of swollen red knee on side (or another joint), may be caused by disseminated gonorrheal infection (DGI).**

CLINICAL PEARLS

- **PID is a clinical diagnosis. Even if both gonorrheal and chlamydial tests are negative, treat a sexually active patient who has signs and symptoms of PID combined with a sexual history.**
- **Probably better to "overtreat" than to miss treating possible PID infections.**
  - **A large study found that adnexal tenderness is the most sensitive physical exam finding for PID (compared with cervical motion tenderness, which may be negative).**
- **After treating a patient for PID, follow up within 72 hours and perform vaginal bimanual examination to check for improvement of adnexal tenderness and/or cervical motion tenderness.**
- **For STDs treated with azithromycin 1 g × one dose (chlamydia), instruct patient and partner not to have sex for at least 7 days.**

HIV INFECTION

HIV attacks the CD4 T-lymphocytes. In the United States and worldwide, HIV-1 is the most common strain. In West Africa, HIV-2 is more common. Currently, 36.7 million people worldwide are living with HIV/AIDS. Almost 15% of HIV-infected persons in the United States are unaware of their HIV infection.

Risk Factors

- Sexual intercourse with an HIV-infected person, or with gay or bisexual men
- Received blood products between 1975 to March 1985, history of illicit drug use
- History of other STDs, multiple partners, homeless status, prisoners in jails, and so on

Diagnostic Tests: CDC Fourth-Generation Testing (Table 18.2)

- *Step 1*: Order HIV-1/HIV-2 antibodies and P24 antigen (combination assay) with reflexes. "Reflex" means that if positive, the lab will automatically perform the follow-up test to confirm the results.
- *Step 2*: If positive, the lab will perform the HIV-1/HIV-2 antibody differentiation immunoassay (to confirm the result of the initial combination assay).
  - Detects if infection is from HIV-1, HIV-2, or both viruses
  - If test result is indeterminate, order an HIV RNA test.
- HIV RNA PCR
  - Detects HIV-1 RNA (actual viral presence). Order to test infant if HIV(+) mother, or if the HIV-1/HIV-2 antibody differentiation test is indeterminate. Can detect HIV infection as early as 7 to 28 days after exposure.
  - *Opt-out HIV screening*: Notify patient that HIV testing will be performed. If patient declines HIV testing, known as "opt-out HIV testing."

Viral Load

- Number of HIV RNA copies in 1 mL of plasma. Test measures actively replicating HIV virus; progression of disease and response to antiretroviral treatment.
- The best sign of treatment success is an undetectable viral load (<50 copies/µL).
- If suspect acute or early HIV infection, order combination antigen/antibody immunoassay with viral load test.

CD4 T-Cell Counts (norm 500–1,500 cells/mL)

- Used to stage HIV infection and to determine response to ART.
- If CD4 count goes up (with decrease in viral load), it means that patient is responding to ART (immune system improved).
- Values vary throughout the day. Check at the same time of the day using the same laboratory each time you remeasure CD4.

Prophylaxis for Opportunistic Infections (Primary Prevention)

- *Pneumocystis jirovecii* pneumonia (previously known as *Pneumocystis carinii* pneumonia or PCP).
- CD4 lymphocyte count is less than 200 cells/mm^3.
- *First line*: Trimethoprim–sulfamethoxazole (Bactrim DS) one tablet daily. If develops a severe reaction to sulfas, the next step is dapsone 100 mg daily or atovaquone suspension.
- *Alternatives*: Use dapsone, atovaquone, or aerosolized pentamidine.

> **Note**
>
> With dapsone, first check patient for glucose-6-phosphate dehydrogenase (G6PD) anemia due to risk of hemolysis (10% of African American males have G6PD).

Toxoplasma gondii Infections (Protozoa)

- CD4 count is less than 100 cells/mm^3.
- *First line*: Administer trimethoprim–sulfamethoxazole (Bactrim DS) one tablet daily.
- Infection causes brain abscesses (headaches, blurred vision, confusion, imbalance, others).
- Avoid cleaning cat litter boxes and eating undercooked meats.

Monitoring Viral Load: Antiretroviral Therapy (ART) or Highly Active Antiretroviral Therapy (HAART)

- Best response if HIV infection is treated with ART in early stage. ART will suppress HIV virus level and increase CD4 counts.
- Check every 1 to 2 months until viral load is undetectable, then every 3 to 4 months.

Lab Monitoring With Medications

- Tenofovir disoproxil fumarate: Check urinalysis every 6 months (nephrotoxic).
- Zidovudine (ZDV): Check CBC with differential (bone marrow suppression).

Recommended Vaccines

HIV and AIDS patients can receive inactivated vaccines such as hepatitis A, hepatitis B, annual influenza vaccine, pneumococcal vaccine, Td/Tdap every 10 years, HPV (up until age 26 years), others as needed. Vaccines work best if CD4 counts exceed 200 copies/mm^3.

HIV Education

- Do not handle cat litter or eat uncooked or undercooked meat (risk of toxoplasmosis).
- Avoid bird stool since it contains histoplasmosis spores.
- Turtles, snakes, and other amphibians may be infected with salmonella.
- Use gloves when cleaning animal cages or when handling stool.

Preventing HIV Transmission

- Use condom every single time you have sex. Genital ulcers increase risk for HIV.
- Do not share needles or syringes if you inject drugs.
- Do not share any toothbrushes, razors, or other items that may have blood on them.

Table 18.2 HIV Tests

Types of HIV Tests	Rationale
HIV-1/HIV-2 antibody with p24 antigen with reflexes	Also known as the *combination assay* (fourth generation). Screening test to diagnose HIV infection. If positive, lab will perform HIV-1/HIV-2 antibody differentiation immunoassay to confirm initial test.
ELISA	Older screening test (antibody test). If positive, next step is Western blot test (done automatically by lab if positive for ELISA).
Western blot	Older confirmatory test. If positive, next step is HIV RNA PCR test.
Rapid HIV testing kits or point-of-care tests	Also used for screening. Result available in <30 minutes (antibody test). Can be done at home. If positive, follow-up with blood testing.
HIV PCR	Tests for HIV virus directly. Used for infants of HIV-positive mothers. Diagnoses acute HIV infection (window stage). Use if indeterminate result on antibody-antigen testing.
CD4 T-cell counts (normally >500 cells/mm^3)	Check before starting ART, staging HIV infection, disease progression, and treatment response. If on ART, check at same time as viral load.
Viral load (antigen)	Monitor treatment response. If on ART, monitor every 1–2 months until nondetectable, then every 3–4 months.

ART, antiretroviral therapy; ELISA, enzyme-linked immunosorbent assay; PCR, polymerase chain reaction.

- For mothers with HIV infection, do not breastfeed your baby.
- Limit your number of sexual partners.

Occupationally Acquired HIV Infection

- Of all health care occupations, nurses have the highest rate of occupationally acquired HIV/AIDS.
- At highest risk if trauma with large-bore hollow needles that contain contaminated material from patients with high viral loads such as retroviral syndrome, symptomatic patients, or AIDS.

Preexposure Prophylaxis (PrEP)

- PrEP has been shown to reduce HIV transmission by more than 90%.
- Daily oral PrEP is recommended as a prevention option for sexually active individuals at substantial risk of HIV such as:
  - Anyone with ongoing sexual relationship with an HIV-infected partner.
  - Gay, heterosexual, bisexual, or transgender men who do not use condoms and engage in high-risk sexual behaviors.
- Do not confuse with postexposure prophylaxis (PEP). Check for HIV infection before starting medications and check for HIV every 3 months thereafter.

Postexposure Prophylaxis: Health Care Workers

- Exposure to infectious fluid with portal of entry (percutaneous, mucous membrane, nonintact skin).

- Infectious fluids are blood; semen; vaginal fluid; amniotic fluid; breast milk; CSF; pericardial, peritoneal, pleural, or synovial fluid and can transmit HIV, HBV, and HCV. Note that saliva, vomitus, urine, feces, sweat, tears, and respiratory secretions do not transmit HIV (unless visibly bloody).
- Baseline labs: HIV (rapid HIV test and HIV antibody/antigen immunoassay), HCV RNA, HBsAg, HBV surface antibody, etc.
- The best time to start PEP is as soon as possible. If you think you have been exposed to HIV at work, during sex, sharing needles, or through sexual assault, go to your health provider or ED right away.
- About 72 hours postexposure is the outer limit of effective PEP. Do not wait for lab results before starting PEP unless it is available within 1 to 2 hours.
- A minimum of three antiretroviral drugs are used.

EXAM TIPS

- **PCP prophylaxis when CD4 is less than 200 copies/mL.**
- **If a patient on ART has a CD4 count that increases (from CD4 200 to 400 copies/mL), it means that their immune system is getting better.**
- **Bactrim DS PO is first line, used first; if allergic to sulfa, use dapsone 100 mg PO daily.**
- **Bactrim DS is used for both prophylaxis or treatment of PCP.**
- **HIV-infected pregnant women: Start AZT as soon as possible.**
- **Hairy leukoplakia of tongue, recurrent candidiasis, thrush: Rule out HIV infection.**
- **Acute retroviral syndrome or primary HIV infection: Influenza-like or similar to mononucleosis infection, very infectious at this stage of HIV infection. Best if HIV treated as early as possible.**

CLINICAL PEARLS

- **It can take from 3 to 12 weeks for HIV antibody tests to detect HIV infection.**
  - **The HIV antibody/antigen test can detect infection in 2 to 6 weeks (may be positive within 2 weeks after infection).**
  - **NAAT can detect HIV infection in 7 to 28 days.**
- **For job-related exposures, contact National Clinician's Postexposure Prophylaxis Hotline (Pipeline) toll free at (888) 448-4911 for advice (open 24/7).**

HIV Infection: Pregnant Women

- The HIV drug that is considered the "safest" to use during pregnancy is zidovudine (Retrovir, ZDV, AZT). Avoid breastfeeding.
- *Newborns*: Start treatment with zidovudine (AZT) within first 6 to 12 hours of delivery.

Zidovudine

- Drug of choice for treating pregnant women and infants
  - Check CBC with differential baseline and monitor for bone marrow suppression.
- Reduces rate of perinatal transmission by 70%
- Start ZDV as soon as HIV is diagnosed or, if established HIV diagnosis, start as soon as pregnancy is diagnosed

OTHER STDs

Condyloma Acuminata (Genital Warts)

External genital warts appear as soft flesh-colored pedunculated, flat, or papular growths.

- Human papillomavirus (HPV) high-risk oncogenic types are 16 and 18. Can occur at any age.
- Cervical HPV infection is usually asymptomatic. Infected cervix can appear "normal."
- HPV vaccine (e.g., Gardasil): Give at age 11 to 12 years (both girls and boys). Only two doses are needed (6–12 months apart) for adolescents aged 9 to 14 years. Another HPV vaccine, Cervarix (girls only) has pulled out of the U.S. market since late 2016. HPV vaccine is also recommended for gay men.
- *Genital sites:* Warts may appear on the vagina, external genitals, urethra, anus.
- Other sites are the anus, penis, nasal mucosa, oropharynx, conjunctiva.

Medications

Self-Administered Topical Medications (Patient-Applied Methods)

- Podofilox (Condylox) 0.5% gel or cream (antimitotic drug). Contraindicated in pregnancy.
  - Apply to external genital warts twice a day for 3 consecutive days (max 0.5 mL/d).
  - Hold treatment for 4 days, then repeat this cycle up to four times.
- Imiquimod (Aldara) 5% or Zyclara (3.75% imiquimod) immune-modulating (or immune response modifier) drug that stimulates the local production of interferon and other cytokines. Contraindicated in pregnancy.
  - Apply a thin layer three times/wk at bedtime for up to 16 weeks. Do not cover with dressing.
  - Leave cream on skin for 6 to 10 hours. Wash off skin with soap and water after.
  - *Side effects*: May cause irritation, ulceration/erosions, hypopigmentation.
- Sinecatechins 10% ointment (Veregne). Sinecatechins is a botanical, derived from green tea polyphenols, used for external anogenital warts (not for vagina or anus).
  - Apply 0.5-cm-size strand of ointment on each wart with a finger (use gloves), up to three times/d for up to 16 weeks.
  - Wash off skin before sexual contact or before inserting tampon in vagina.
  - Can weaken condoms and diaphragms.
- Provider-applied methods: Other treatment methods include Corry laser, electrocautery, bichloracetic or trichloroacetic acid (caustic acids) surgical excision is done in the clinic.

Herpes Simplex: HSV-1 and HSV-2

Asymptomatic shedding (intact skin) also occurs intermittently and patient is still contagious.

- *HSV-1*: Usually oral infection, sometimes genital
- *HSV-2*: Causes most cases of recurrent genital herpes, can be oral

Classic Case

May have prodrome (i.e., itching, burning, and tingling) on site. Sudden onset of groups of small vesicles sitting on an erythematous base. Easily ruptures and is painful. Vesicle fluid and crust are contagious. Primary episode is more severe and can last from 2 to 4 weeks. Recurrent breakouts.

Treatment Plan

- *Diagnostic test*: Herpes viral culture or RPR assay for HSV-1 and HSV-2 DNA (more sensitive)

Tzanck Smear

An "old test." If herpes virus infection (herpes simplex or varicella), shows multinucleated giant cells.

First Episode (Primary Genital Herpes)

- Acyclovir (Zovirax) 400 mg three times/d for 7 to 10 days (or 200 mg five times/d for 7–10 days)
- Famciclovir (Favier) 1 g BID for 7 to 10 days
- Valacyclovir (Valtrex) TID for 7 to 10 days

Episodic Treatment (Flare-Up)

- Best if treatment started within 1 day of lesion onset
- Famciclovir (favor) 125 mg BID for 5 days
- Zovirax BID or TID × 5 days or Valtrex BID × 5 days

Suppressive Treatment

- Acyclovir (Zovirax) 400 mg PO BID *or* famciclovir (Favier) 250 mg PO BID

Evaluation

- For all cases of genital ulcers: Always rule out syphilis and HSV (genital herpes) infection

EXAM TIPS

- **Know first-episode treatment for herpes (Zovirax five times/d or Valtrex three times/d or favor BID for 7 to 10 days).**
- **Know flare-up treatment (Zovirax or Valtrex or Favier BID × 5 days).**
- **Imiquimod is an immune-modulator treatment for genital warts and patient can use at home.**
- **Treatments contraindicated in pregnancy are podofilox, podophylla, imiquimod.**
- **For pregnant women, mechanical methods are used to destroy genital warts (curio, laser, excision, etc.).**
- **HPV strains 16 and 18 are oncogenic/carcinogenic (memorize).**
- **Tzanck smear shows multinucleated giant cells with herpesvirus infection (varicella, herpes simplex).**
- **Genital herpes treatment duration for 7 to 10 days for treating primary genital herpes infection. For breakouts, duration is 5 days.**

19

Women's Health: Pregnancy and Childbirth Review

⚠ DANGER SIGNALS

Placental Abruption (Abruptio Placentae)

Pregnant woman who is in the late third trimester of pregnancy complains of sudden onset of vaginal bleeding accompanied by a contracted uterus that feels hard (hypertonic) and is very painful. Associated with a sudden onset of dark-red-colored vaginal bleeding. Up to 20% of women do not have vaginal bleeding (blood is trapped between placenta and uterine wall). If mild, blood is reabsorbed and affected area reimplants. Severe cases cause hemorrhage; fetus must be delivered to save mother's life. Higher risk in females with history of hypertension, preeclampsia/eclampsia, cocaine use, or history of abruptio placentae.

Placenta Previa

A multipara who is in the late second to third trimester complains of new onset of painless vaginal bleeding that is worsened by intercourse. Blood is bright red in color. Uterus is soft and nontender. If cervix is not dilated, treatment is strict bed rest. Administer intravenous magnesium sulfate if there is uterine cramping. Uterus will usually reimplant itself if mild. Any vaginal or rectal insertion or stimulation is an absolute contraindication (can precipitate hemorrhage). If cervix is dilated or if hemorrhaging, fetus is delivered by cesarean section (C-section). Severe cases cause hemorrhage; fetus must be delivered to save mother's life.

Severe Preeclampsia

A primigravida who is in the late third trimester of pregnancy (>34 weeks) complains of a sudden onset of severe recurrent headaches, visual abnormalities (blurred vision, scotomas), and pitting edema. Edema easily seen on the face/eyes and fingers. Sudden rapid weight gain within 1 to 2 days (>2 to 4 1b/wk). New onset of right upper quadrant abdominal pain. BP more than 140/90 mmHg. Urine protein 1+ or higher. Sudden decrease in urine output (oliguria). Nausea and vomiting are worrisome signs (encephalopathy). If seizures occur, condition is reclassified as eclampsia. Earliest time period that preeclampsia/eclampsia can occur is at 20 weeks gestation (and up to 4 weeks postpartum). Only known "cure" is delivery of fetus or baby.

HELLP (Hemolysis, Elevated Liver Enzymes, and Low Platelets) Syndrome

Serious but rare complication of preeclampsia/eclampsia. Classic patient is a multipara older than 25 years of age who is in the third trimester of pregnancy. Presents with the signs and symptoms of preeclampsia accompanied by right upper quadrant (or midepigastric) abdominal pain with nausea/vomiting and malaise (may be mistaken for viral illness). Symptoms can present suddenly. Lab abnormalities are elevation of AST, ALT, total bilirubin (>1.2 mg/dL), and lactate dehydrogenase (LDH) with decreased number of platelets (<100,000 cells/mcL) and hemoglobin and hematocrit.

LABORATORY TESTING (TABLE 19.1)

Table 19.1 Laboratory Results During Pregnancy

Test	Elevated	No Changes
Liver function	Alkaline phosphatase	AST, ALT, GGT
Lipid profile	Total cholesterol, triglycerides	Wait 4–6 weeks after pregnancy to check lipids
Thyroid function	Total T3	Free T3, free T4, TSH
CBC	WBC Sedimentation rate	Platelet count
Renal function	GFR	Lower serum creatinine

Normal reference ranges for laboratory values in pregnancy.
ALT, aspartate aminotransferase; AST, alanine aminotransferase; CBC, complete blood count; GFR, glomerular filtration rate; GGT, gamma glutamyl transpeptidase; TSH, thyroid-stimulating hormone; WBC, white blood cell.

Source: Bastian and Brown (2017).

Urinalysis (UA; Dipstick)

Obtain midstream urine before gynecologic exam (minimizes contamination from vaginal discharge). Check protein, leukocytes, nitrite, blood, glucose.

- Protein: Negative (trace, 1+ to 4+)
- If 20 weeks gestation or more, rule out preeclampsia.
- If proteinuria present, order 24-hour urine for protein and creatinine.

Liver Function Tests

- ALT, AST, bilirubin, and gamma glutamyl transpeptidase (GGT) remain the same except for alkaline phosphatase.

Alkaline Phosphatase

- Expected to increase during pregnancy due to the growth of the fetal bones. Values higher in multiple gestation pregnancies.

White Blood Cells (WBCs)

- WBC count is elevated throughout pregnancy, especially during the third trimester. May climb as high as 16,000 cells/mm^3 in the third trimester. (WBC in nonpregnant adults: range is 4,500–10,500 cells/mm^3.)
- Leukocytosis with neutrophilia is "normal" during pregnancy (if it is not accompanied by signs of infection).

Hemoglobin and Hematocrit

- Both values go down during pregnancy due to hemodilution. The hemoglobin value may be as low as 10.5 g/dL, and the hematocrit value may go down to about 30% (by the third trimester).
- To rule out iron-deficiency anemia, check the MCV. It is not affected by pregnancy.

Erythrocyte Sedimentation Rate

- Increases during pregnancy: By the third trimester, the sedimentation rate ranges from 13 to 70 mm/hr.
- Erythrocyte sedimentation rate (nonpregnant): 0 to 20 mm/hr.

Thyroid Function Tests

- Total triiodothyronine (T3) is higher during pregnancy because of increased levels of thyroid-binding globulin (TBG).
- Thyroid-stimulating hormone (TSH), free T3, and free T4 results remain unchanged.

Serum Alpha-Fetoprotein (AFP)

- AFP is manufactured by the liver of the fetus and mother.
- Majority of maternal AFP comes from the fetus (liver, fetal yolk sac, GI tract).

Low AFP

- Mature maternal age is the most common risk factor for Down syndrome (35-year-old or older woman has a 1:200 chance).
- If AFP is low, order the triple screen test (AFP, human chorionic gonadotropin [hCG], and estriol) or the quadruple screen test (AFP, hCG, estriol, inhibin-A) to evaluate for Down syndrome (trisomy 21).

High AFP

- Rule out neural tube defects or multiple gestation. Most common reason for a high AFP is pregnancy dating error.
- If AFP is high, order the triple screen or the quad screen test and sonogram to rule out neural tube abnormalities (higher sensitivity than AFP alone).
- To prevent neural tube defects: Ingest folic acid 400 mcg (0.4 mg) per day (found in leafy green vegetables, fortified cereals). To reduce risk, advise patients to take prenatal vitamins when planning to become pregnant.

Triple Screen Test

- The triple screen test combines the AFP, beta hCG, and estriol serum level values. The hormone level results are used in a formula to figure out the risk for a Down syndrome infant.
- Diagnostic test for genetic anomalies is chromosome testing.

Quadruple Screen Test

- Combination of the triple screen hormones plus inhibin-A (hormone release by the placenta). The triple or quadruple screen tests are more sensitive than the AFP alone (but have a higher rate of false positives).
- Gold-standard test for genetic disorders is testing of fetal chromosomes/DNA.

Screening for Genetic Disorders

- Jewish descent (Tay–Sachs disease); this fatal neurological disease, with no known cure, is more common among Eastern Europeans of Jewish descent (Ashkenazi Jews)
- Whites screen (cystic fibrosis)
- African Americans (sickle cell anemia)

Amniocentesis and Chorionic Villus Sampling (CVS)

- Can be done earlier (10–12 weeks) than the amniocentesis (15–18 weeks). Specimens contain fetal cells.
- Fetal chromosomes/DNA are tested for abnormalities.

Beta Human Chorionic Gonadotropin (hCG)

- This is manufactured by the chorion (early placenta) by day 8.
- High-quality urine home pregnancy tests (e.g., "First Response," EPT) can detect pregnancy as early as the first missed period (2 weeks after conception).
- There are higher levels of hCG with twins/multiple fetuses.

Doubling Time

Doubling time is an important indicator of the viability of a pregnancy. Useful only in the first trimester; thereafter, it loses its predictive value (do not use after week 12).

- Normal finding: Human chorionic gonadotropin doubles every 48 hours during the first 12 weeks (first trimester) in a normal pregnancy.
- Ectopic pregnancy: The hCG has lower values than normal. Values increase slowly and do not double as expected.
- Inevitable abortion: Values of hCG start decreasing rapidly; there is no doubling. Cervix is dilated.

Vaginal Cultures

- Group B *Streptococcus* (GBS) is tested for at 35 to 37 weeks. Swab vaginal introitus and rectum (insert up to anal sphincter) for C&S. If positive, administer intrapartum antibiotic prophylaxis with penicillin G 5 million units IV, followed by 2.5 to 3 million units IV every 4 hours until delivery.
- If allergic to penicillin: Use clindamycin or erythromycin instead.

Sexually Transmitted Diseases (STDs)

- Screen for HBsAg, HIV, gonorrhea, chlamydia, syphilis, herpesvirus types 1 and 2.

Titers

- Check rubella titer.
- Check varicella titers (if no proof of infection).

DRUGS AND VACCINES DURING PREGNANCY

The new Federal Drug Administration (FDA) Pregnancy and Lactation Labeling Rule (PLLR) will eventually replace the pregnancy letter categories (A, B, C, D, and X) with new labeling. The new rule is discussed in Chapter 3. Since most of the drugs on the exam were released before the PLLR, the FDA letter categories will still be covered in this edition. Most of the drugs used in pregnancy are FDA category B drugs. Because it is unethical to experiment on pregnant women, a number of drugs used during pregnancy are found to be safe only through many years of use by pregnant women (e.g., penicillins, macrolides).

Category A Drugs

Animal and human data show no risk to pregnant women. Examples are:

- Prenatal vitamins (high-dose multivitamins are not used during pregnancy)
- Insulin
- Thyroid hormone

Category B Drugs

Animal studies show no risk. No human data available. Examples:

- Antacids (Tums, Maalox) are safe for pregnant women.
- Docusate sodium (Colace). Colace is a stool softener and is approved for pregnant women. It is not a laxative.
  - Avoid laxatives (e.g., ex-lax, Bisacodyl), especially in the third trimester (may induce labor).
- Analgesics (acetaminophen preferred to nonsteroidal anti-inflammatory drugs [NSAIDs] especially in the third trimester; see "Category C Drugs," which follows.

Antibiotics for Pregnant Women

The following antibiotics are category B.

- Penicillins
  - Amoxicillin (Amoxil), penicillin, dicloxacillin
- Cephalosporins
  - *First generation*: Cephalexin (Keflex), cefadroxil (Duricef)
  - *Second generation*: Cefuroxime axetil (Ceftin), cefaclor (Ceclor), cefprozil (Cefzil)
  - *Third generation*: Ceftriaxone (Rocephin) injections, cefdinir (Omnicef), cefixime (Suprax)
  - *Fourth generation*: Cefepime (Maxipime) injection/IV (used mainly in hospitals)
- Macrolides
  - Erythromycins
  - Erythromycin ethylsuccinate (E-mycin)
    - Erythromycin estolate (EES) can cause hepatotoxicity in pregnant women and its use in pregnancy is not recommended.
  - Azithromycin (Zithromax)
    - Clarithromycin (Biaxin) is the only macrolide that is a category C. Avoid use during pregnancy. Consult with physician before use and discuss risk versus benefits.
- Nitrofurantoin
  - Nitrofurantoin (Furadantin, Macrobid)
  - Do not use with glucose-6-phospate dehydrogenase deficiency (G6PD anemia) because it will cause hemolysis (anemia, jaundice, dark urine)

Antihypertensives for Pregnant Women

Used for women with preexisting hypertension or for moderate to severe preeclampsia or eclampsia. Use of antihypertensive drugs to control mild hypertension does not alter the course of the disease or diminish perinatal morbidity or mortality of preeclampsia.

- Methyldopa (Aldomet)
- Calcium channel blockers (Procardia)
- Labetalol (Normodyne)

Category C Drugs

Adverse effects seen in animal studies. No human data available.

- Sulfa drugs
  - Considered category C in third trimester because they can cause hyperbilirubinemia. Sulfa drugs displace bilirubin from albumin. High blood levels of unconjugated bilirubin can cross the blood–brain barrier and cause brain damage (mental retardation, seizures, deafness, etc.).
- Trimethoprim-sulfamethoxazole (e.g., Bactrim DS, Septra)
  - Clarithromycin (Biaxin) is the only category C macrolide antibiotic. Avoid use in pregnant women. Consult with physician before using category C drugs during pregnancy.

- NSAIDs
  - Avoid using in the third trimester (especially the last 2 weeks) because it blocks prostaglandins. Classified as either category B or C (depends on type of NSAID).
  - Ibuprofen (Advil) is category B (first and second trimesters) and category D (third trimester).

Category D Drugs

Evidence of fetal risk. Benefits should outweigh the risk of using the drug.

- Angiotensin-converting enzyme (ACE) inhibitors and angiotensin receptor blockers (ARBs)
  - Causes fetal renal abnormalities, renal failure, and hypotension
  - Captopril (Capoten) and losartan (Hyzaar)
  - Category C in first trimester
  - Category D in second and third trimester
- Fluoroquinolones
  - Affects fetal cartilage development; a rare side effect is Achilles tendon rupture in athlete; contraindicated in pregnant or lactating women and children younger than 18 years
  - Ciprofloxacin (Cipro)
  - Ofloxacin (Floxin)
  - Levofloxacin (Levaquin)
- Tetracyclines
  - Stains growing tooth enamel
  - Tetracycline, minocycline (Minocin)
  - Avoid in the third trimester
- NSAIDs
  - Block prostaglandins and may cause premature labor; avoid using, especially in the last 2 weeks of pregnancy
- Sulfa drugs
  - Risk of hyperbilirubinemia (neonatal jaundice or kernicterus); sulfa drugs displace bilirubin from albumin; high levels of unconjugated bilirubin will cross the blood–brain barrier and cause brain damage (mental retardation, seizures, deafness, etc.)

Category X Drugs

Proven fetal risks outweigh the benefits.

- Accutane (isotretinoin, a vitamin A derivative)
  - Used for severe cystic and nodular acne recalcitrant to treatment; it is highly teratogenic.
- Methotrexate (antimetabolite)
  - Used for some types of autoimmune diseases (psoriasis, rheumatoid arthritis) and certain cancers.
- Proscar (antiandrogen)
  - Used for benign prostatic hyperplasia (BPH) and prostate cancer.
- Misoprostol (prostaglandin analog)
  - Used as one of the drugs in medical abortions (a component of the "abortion pill").
- Evista and tamoxifen (selective estrogen receptor modulator [SERM])
  - Use reduces risk of reoccurrence of estrogen receptor-positive breast cancer.
- All hormonal drugs (natural or synthetic) are category X in pregnancy—all forms of estrogens, progesterone, testosterone, finasteride (Proscar), mifepristone (RU-86).
- Any drug that blocks hormone synthesis or binding
- Depo Lupron is used for infertility, hormone-dependent cancers, and endometriosis

Drugs to Avoid (Third Trimester of Pregnancy)

- NSAIDs (blocks prostaglandin)
- Aspirin and salicylates (affects platelets)
- Sulfa-containing drugs (trimethoprim–sulfamethoxazole, nitrofurantoin): Higher risk of hyperbilirubinemia, jaundice, kernicterus

Live Vaccines

- Mumps, measles, and rubella (MMR), oral polio, varicella, FluMist are contraindicated in pregnancy.
- Influenza vaccine is an inactivated virus and is safe to use in pregnant women.
  - Recommend for pregnant women especially if they are pregnant during the fall and winter seasons. Only use the injectable flu vaccine (no FluMist).
  - Live attenuated influenza virus vaccine (LAIV) flu vaccine via nasal spray (FluMist) is contraindicated.
  - For the 2017 to 2018 flu season, the CDC recommends against using FluMist because of poor immune response.

Note

After a live virus vaccine, advise reproductive-age women not to get pregnant (and use reliable birth control) in the next 4 weeks (MMR) or 3 months (varicella and shingles vaccine).

Teratogens

Agents that can cause structural abnormalities during pregnancy:

- Alcohol: Fetal alcohol syndrome
- Aminoglycosides: Deafness
- Cigarettes: Intrauterine growth retardation (IUGR), prematurity
- Cocaine: Cerebrovascular accidents (CVAs), mental retardation, abruptio placentae
- Isotretinoin (Accutane): CNS/craniofacial/ear/cardiovascular defects
- Lithium: Cardiac defects (Ebstein's anomalies)

Chronic hyperglycemia during pregnancy (poorly controlled diabetes or gestational diabetes mellitus [GDM]) is a teratogenic state. It increases the risk of neural tube defects and craniofacial defects.

HEALTH EDUCATION

- Take prenatal vitamins with 400 mcg of folic acid daily (start 3 months before conception).
- Always wear seatbelt (lap-style seatbelt below uterine fundus).
- Avoid soft cheeses (blue cheese, brie), uncooked meats, raw milk (listeria bacteria).
- Sex is safe except during vaginal bleeding, incompetent cervix, placenta previa, or preterm labor.
- Cat litter or raw/undercooked meat can cause toxoplasmosis (congenital infection).
- Do not eat raw shellfish or raw oysters (*Vibrio vulnificus* infection).
- Be careful with cold cuts, uncooked hot dogs, and "deli" meat (listeria bacteria). Pregnant women are 20 times more likely to become infected with *Listeria monocytogenes*.
- Smoking (IUGR) and alcohol (fetal alcohol syndrome) are contraindicated.
- Regular coffee (8 oz/d) is okay. Do not consume an excessive amount of caffeine (premature labor).
- Do not use hot tubs, saunas, or expose oneself to excessive heat.

Weight Gain

- Most weight is gained in third trimester (about 1–2 lbs per week).
- Best weight gain: A total gain of 25 to 35 lbs (11.3–15.9 kg) if healthy weight before pregnancy (body mass index [BMI] of 18.5–24.9) is ideal.
- Underweight patients (BMI <18.5): Gain a total of 28 to 40 lbs (12.7–18.1 kg).
- Obese patients (BMI >30): Gain a total of up to 11 to 20 lbs (4.98–9.07 kg).
- After delivery: Loss of up to 15 to 20 lbs (6.8–9.1 kg) in first few weeks is appropriate.
- Twins: Increased weight gain (37–54 lbs [16.8–24.5 kg]) is appropriate but weight gain should not be double that for a single fetus.

SIGNS OF PREGNANCY

Positive Signs

- Palpation of fetus by health provider
- Ultrasound and visualization of fetus
- Fetal heart tones (FHTs) auscultated by health provider
  - 10 to 12 weeks by Doppler/Doptone
  - 20 weeks by fetoscope/stethoscope

Probable Signs

- Goodell's sign (4 weeks): Cervical softening
- Chadwick's sign (6–8 weeks): Blue coloration of the cervix and vagina
- Hegar's sign (6–8 weeks): Softening uterine isthmus
- Enlarged uterus
- Ballottement (seen in midpregnancy). When the fetus is pushed, it can be felt to bounce back by tapping the palpating fingers inside the vagina
- Urine or blood pregnancy tests (beta hCG)

Presumptive Signs

The following are the "softest" and least objective signs. Can be caused by many other conditions besides pregnancy.

- Amenorrhea
- Nausea/vomiting (most common in first trimester in the morning, usually disappears by the second trimester)
- Breast changes (swollen and tender)
- Fatigue
- Urinary frequency
- Slight increase in body temperature
- "Quickening": Mother feels the baby's movements for the first time; starts at 16 weeks

EXAM TIPS

- **Palpation of fetal movements by the mother is not considered a positive sign of pregnancy (quickening). It is classified as a "presumptive sign."**
- **Urine/serum pregnancy tests are considered probable signs (do not confuse them as "positive signs"). Beta hCG presents also in molar pregnancy and ovarian cancer.**
- **Questions asking for one of the signs will mix them up (mix a positive sign with a probable sign) on the exam. Make sure the answer option contains the two signs from the same category.**

- **Memorize the three positive signs of pregnancy. This is the shortest list to memorize. By the process of elimination, you can rule out (or in) the correct answer choice.**

CLINICAL METHODS FOR DATING PREGNANCY

Fundal Heights

12 Weeks (Third Month)

- Uterine fundus first rises above symphysis pubis.
- FHTs are heard by Doppler by 10 to 12 weeks.

16 Weeks (Fourth Month)

- Uterine fundus between symphysis pubis and the umbilicus

20 Weeks (Fifth Month)

- Uterine fundus at level of the umbilicus
- FHTs are heard with fetoscope or stethoscope by 20 weeks

From 20 to 35 Weeks Gestation

- Measure the distance between upper edge of pubic symphysis and the top of the uterine fundus using a tape measure. Fundal height in centimeters equals number of weeks gestation (±2 cm). For example, a 32-week-gestation fetus should have a fundal height of between 30 and 34 cm.

Size and Date Discrepancy

Defined as a difference of 2 cm (or more) in uterine size from the number of weeks gestation. If present, order an ultrasound for further evaluation.

For example, if a 30-week gestation with a 26-cm uterus, the uterus is smaller than expected (small for gestational age), and the fetus may not be growing normally. Fetus may have IUGR or other problem.

PHYSIOLOGICAL CHANGES DURING PREGNANCY

CARDIAC SYSTEM

Position of the Heart

- Heart is shifted anteriorly and toward the left.
- It rotates toward a transverse position as the uterus enlarges.

Heart Rate

- Increases during pregnancy by 15 to 20 beats/min.

Heart Sounds

- Heart sounds are louder in pregnancy.
- The S3 heart sound is common in pregnant women (but not S4).
- There is wide splitting of S1.
- In the third trimester, splitting of S2 may be heard.

Murmurs

- A systolic ejection murmur (grade II/IV) over the pulmonary and tricuspid areas is common.

- A mammary soufflé (systole or continuous) is heard over the breasts later in pregnancy and during lactation (breastfeeding).

Cardiac Output

- Increases by 30% to 50% and peaks at about 28 to 34 weeks gestation
- Reduction of systemic vascular resistance and systolic BP

Plasma Volume

- Plasma volume increases by almost 50% by the end of the second trimester.
- Hemodilution results in physiological anemia of pregnancy (hematocrit decreased).

Physiological Anemia of Pregnancy

- Physiological anemia of pregnancy is most obvious during the second and third trimesters.
- Hemoglobin and hematocrit are decreased because of the hemodilution from increased plasma volume. The hemoglobin can decrease to as low as 10.5 g/dL.

Preload and Afterload

- Preload increases because of higher blood volume.
- Afterload goes down because of the decrease in peripheral vascular resistance that occurs during pregnancy.

Blood Pressure (BP)

- Systolic and diastolic BP starts to decrease in the first trimester and continues in the second trimester. Many mothers who are hypertensive before pregnancy can be off prescription antihypertensives at this time.
- By the third trimester, BP gradually returns back to prepregnancy levels. Antihypertensives used for pregnant women are methyldopa (Aldomet) or labetalol (Normodyne; beta-blocker).

Vena Cava

- Compression by enlarged uterus decreases blood return to the brain, resulting in orthostatic hypotension. Advise women to lie on the left side and to change positions slowly.

Coagulation Factors

- Pregnancy is a hypercoagulable state (clotting factors go up), especially after labor (puerperium or postpartum period).

OTHER CHANGES

Lungs

- Presence of basal rales that disappear with coughing or deep breathing
- Feeling of breathlessness (innocent hyperpnea) and decreased exercise tolerance
- The gravid uterus pushes up the diaphragm as it gets larger; the diameter of the thorax is increased
- No change in forced expiratory volume in one second (FEV1), but total lung capacity drops slightly from 4.2 to 4 L

Thyroid

- Diffusely enlarged (size up to 15% larger), with higher metabolic activity.

Gastrointestinal (GI) System

- Decreased peristalsis from progesterone effects (constipation, heartburn).

Integumentary System (Skin and Hair)

Pigmentary Changes

- Pigmentary changes from increase in melanocyte-stimulating hormone from higher levels of estrogen. Causes the linea nigra (dark pigmented "line" that extends from mons pubis to the umbilicus located midline).
- The nipples and areola darken.

Chloasma (Melasma)

- Blotchy hyperpigmentation on forehead, cheeks, nose, and upper lip seen in pregnant women and in some birth control pill users. Usually gets lighter and regresses within 1 year, but in some women, hyperpigmentation may be permanent.
- Condition is more common in darker skins (olive skins and darker).

Striae Gravidarum (Stretch Marks)

- Most common locations are abdomen, breasts, and thighs. Other less common areas are upper arms, lower back, and buttocks.

Telogen Effluvium (Hair Loss)

- During the postpartum period, hair loss may accelerate, but it is temporary.

Renal System

- Kidney size increases during pregnancy. The ureters and renal pelvis become dilated (physiologic hydronephrosis).
- GFR is much higher in pregnancy due to higher cardiac output and renal blood flow.

Ear, Nose, Throat Changes

- Some women develop nasal congestion and/or epistaxis due to increased blood flow to the nasopharynx during pregnancy.
- Rule out acute sinusitis if purulent mucus seen in posterior pharynx.

Varicose Veins

- Varicose veins become more severe during pregnancy.

Edema

- Peripheral edema is considered normal in pregnancy. Mild edema of the lower extremities and the feet is most noticeable in the third trimester.

NAEGELE'S RULE

- This is used to estimate date of delivery (EDD) during the first trimester.
- Assumes regular 28- to 30-day menstrual cycle. Not as useful for irregular menstrual cycles. A full-term pregnancy is 40 weeks (280 days).

- There are two different ways to use Naegele's rule. They are equivalent; pick the one with which you feel most comfortable (LMP = last menstrual period).
  - Method 1: LMP + 9 months + 7 days
  - Method 2: LMP – 3 months + 7 days

Example

A 28-year-old woman who is at 8 weeks gestation reports that her LMP was on February 20, 2017. Using Naegele's rule, which of the following dates is correct for her expected EDD?

A) November 10, 2017
B) November 27, 2017
C) December 10, 2017
D) December 27, 2017

Solution

Method 1: LMP: 2/20/2017

1. Add 9 months to February: 2 + 9 = 11 (November)
2. Add 7 days to date of the LMP: 20 + 7 = 27
3. EDD = November 27, 2017

Method 2: LMP: 2/20/2017

1. Subtract 3 months from February = November
2. Add 7 days to date of the LMP: 20 + 7 = 27
3. EDD = November 27, 2017

EXAM TIPS

- **There is usually one question about the EDD (use Naegele's rule).**
- **The LMP month on the exam will either be January (01), February (02), or March (03).**

If LMP is:	Expected EDD:
January	October
February	November
March	December

- **S3 heart murmur is normal finding in pregnancy.**
- **Chloasma/melasma is due to high estrogen level.**
- **Placenta previa is vaginal bleeding (bright red) without a hypertonic tender uterus.**
- **Placenta abruptio is vaginal bleeding that is intermittent with hypertonic, hard, and tender uterus.**
- **Fundus at 12 weeks is above symphysis pubis.**
- **Fundus at 16 weeks is between the symphysis pubis and the umbilicus.**
- **Fundus at 20 weeks is at the umbilicus.**
- **Ashkenazi Jews (European Jews) should be screened for Tay–Sachs disease.**
- **If hypertensive, reproductive-age sexually active females do not use birth control. ACE inhibitors and ARBs are not the best choice.**
- **Preferred medications for hypertension in pregnancy are methyldopa (Aldomet) or labetalol (beta-blocker).**
- **For methyldopa, check LFTs at baseline and periodically (contraindicated if active hepatic disease). Discontinue if jaundice, abnormal LFTs, or unexplained fever occur.**

Obstetric History (Table 19.2)

Table 19.2 Obstetric History (G-T-P-A-L)

Term	Definition
Gravida or G	Number of pregnancies (twins or multiples counted as one pregnancy)
Term or T	Number of deliveries after 37 weeks
Preterm or P	Number of deliveries after 20 weeks (up to 38 weeks)
Abortion or A	Number of deliveries before 20 weeks (induced or spontaneous)
Living or L	Number of living children

Example

G: 5 (five pregnancies total)
T: 3 (three pregnancies full term)
P: 1 (one pregnancy preterm born at 30 weeks)
A: 1 (one abortion)
L: 5 (five living children because she had one set of twins)

Postpartum (or Puerperium)

- Occurs immediately after delivery and generally lasts about 6 weeks

Uterine Involution

- It is normal for postpartum women to have uterine contractions (spontaneous or with breastfeeding) during the first 2 to 3 days after giving birth. After delivery, the uterus is the size of a 20-week pregnancy (fundi at the umbilicus).
- A soft boggy uterus accompanied by heavy vaginal bleeding is a sign of atony (inadequate contraction).
- Uterine involution takes about 6 weeks.

DISEASE REVIEW

Rh-Incompatibility Disease

In Rh-negative mothers with Rh-positive fetuses, the maternal immune system develops antibodies against Rh-positive blood if not given RhoGAM (gamma globulin against Rh factor). Give RhoGAM for all pregnancies of Rh-negative mothers—even if they terminate in miscarriages, abortions, or tubal or ectopic pregnancies.

RhoGAM

Also known as *anti-D immune globulin*. It is made from pooled IgG antibodies against Rh (rhesus) factor. It is an immunoglobulin that helps prevent maternal isoimmunization (self-immunization) or alloimmunization (immunity against another individual of the same species). If RhoGAM is not given to Rh-negative pregnant women, this will result in fetal hemolysis and fetal anemia in her future pregnancies.

- Coombs test: Detects presence of Rh antibodies in the mother (indirect Coombs test) and the infant (direct Coombs test). This test is done as part of the labs performed early in pregnancy.
- RhoGAM 300 mcg IM first dose is at 28 weeks.
- Give second dose within 72 hours (or sooner) after delivery.
- RhoGAM decreases the risk of isoimmunization of the maternal immune system by destroying fetal Rh-positive RBCs that have crossed the placenta.

Gestational Diabetes Mellitus (GDM)

GDM is diabetes that occurs during pregnancy. GDM mothers are at high risk for type 2 diabetes. GDM has high rates of reoccurrence (33%–50% chance) in future pregnancies. GDM has concomitant higher rates of neural tube defects (anencephaly, microcephaly), congenital heart disease, birth trauma (shoulder dystocia), preeclampsia, and neonatal hypoglycemia. Risk factors are history of GDM in a previous pregnancy, obesity, ethnicity (Asian, Native American, Pacific Islander, African American, Hispanic), macrosomic infant (>9 1bs), and age (older than 35 years).

Evaluation

Screen at the first visit if history of GDM and/or presence of risk factors.

- If not high risk for GDM, screen at 24 to 28 weeks gestation.
- There are two methods of testing for GDM (one-step or two-step strategy).

CLINICAL PEARLS

- **GDM is diagnosed in the second to third trimester.**
- **A woman with diabetes in the first trimester has type 2 diabetes.**
- **An A1C <6% (second to third trimesters) has the lowest risk for large-for-gestational-age infants.**

One-Step Method

- Administer 75-g oral glucose tolerance test (OGTT; check fasting, 1 hour, and 2 hours). Overnight fast of at least 8 hours. Perform test in the morning.
- Diagnostic criteria (American Diabetes Association, 2017)
  - Fasting: equal or >92 mg/dL
  - 1 hour: equal or >180 mg/dL
  - 2 hours: equal or >153 mg/dL
- If one value is elevated in this test, it is diagnostic of GDM.
- The 75-gram OGTT is the preferred test.

Two-Step Method

- Screening: 50-g glucose load (nonfasting), check plasma glucose at 1 hour
- If 140 mg/dL or higher: rule out GDM. Order 100-g OGTT (fasting, 1 hour, 2 hours, and 3 hours).
- Diagnostic criteria (American Diabetes Association, 2017)
  - Fasting: equal or >95 mg/dL
  - 1 hour: equal or >180 mg/dL
  - 2 hour: equal or >155 mg/dL
  - 3 hour: equal or >140 mg/dL

Treatment Plan

- Glycemic targets in pregnancy are:
  - Preprandial: 95 mg/dL or less
  - 1-hour postmeal: 140 mg/dL or less
  - 2-hour postmeal: 120 mg/dL or less
  - A1C goal: 6% to 6.5%
- First-line treatment is lifestyle (follow a meal plan and scheduled physical activity).
  - Eat three meals per day plus two to three snacks. Limit carbohydrates.
  - Exercise 30 minutes per day at least 5 days a week (total of 2 hours per week).
- Low-impact exercises such as walking and swimming are preferred.
  - Perform frequent home glucose monitoring (four to six times per day).
  - If medication needed, human insulin is the preferred agent. Insulin injections needed if unable to control blood glucose with diet and exercise.

- May need to self inject insulin from three to six times per day.
- American Diabetes Association (ADA) and American Congress of Obstetricians and Gynecologists (ACOG) have endorsed use of oral antihyperglycemic drugs glyburide or metformin.

- Glucose monitoring: Check blood glucose at least four times per day (fasting, 1 or 2 hours after the first bite of each meal).

Follow-Up

- Test for GDM 6 to 12 weeks postpartum and at least every 3 years afterward (future).

Note

The FDA does not endorse the use of any oral antidiabetic drugs for pregnant women, but the ADA and ACOG have endorsed their use for GDM (ADA, 2017).

EXAM TIPS

- **There are two methods of screening for GDM.**
- **One-step method uses the 75-g OGTT (both for screening and diagnosis).**
- **Two-step method uses 50-g OGTT test (nonfasting) as the screening test.**
- **If 50-g OGTT is abnormal (postprandial >140 mg/dL or fasting >95 g/dL), follow-up test is 100-g OGTT (must fast for at least 8 hours).**
- **First-line treatment for GDM is lifestyle change (correct diet and scheduled exercises).**
- **Learn the risk factors for GDM.**
- **Learn action of RhoGAM (Rh antibodies that hemolyze fetal Rh-positive fetal RBCs).**

Urinary Tract Infections (UTIs)

Acute cystitis can occur alone or it may be complicated by acute pyelonephritis. The most common organism is *Escherichia coli* (75%–95%). The signs and symptoms include dysuria, frequency, urgency, and nocturia. Higher risk of preterm birth and low birth weight.

Asymptomatic Bacteriuria

Pregnant women with asymptomatic bacteriuria are always treated because they are at high risk for acute pyelonephritis (25%). Diagnosis is based on midstream urine C&S results. Obtain specimen before antibiotic treatment and after (to check for eradication of infection). UTIs increase the risk of preterm birth, low birth weight, and perinatal mortality.

Treatment Plan

- Urine dipstick: WBCs (leukocyte esterase): positive; nitrite: may be positive or negative
- Send midstream urine for UA and urine C&S
- Document resolution of infection by ordering posttreatment urine C&S 1 week after completing antibiotic therapy
- If suspect pyelonephritis, refer to ED or a physician

Medications

- Nitrofurantoin (Macrobid) BID × 5 to 7 days (avoid using during the last trimester)
  - Do not use sulfa drugs (e.g., Bactrim) or nitrofurantoin near term because of the risk of hyperbilirubinemia. Causes hemolysis if the mother (or both mother and baby) has G6PD anemia.

- Amoxicillin–clavulanate (Augmentin) BID for 3 to 7 days
- Amoxicillin BID for 3 to 7 days
- Cephalexin BID for 3 to 7 days
- Fosfomycin 3-g single dose

Nitrofurantoin and Sulfa Drugs

- Nitrofurantoin and sulfa drugs should be avoided near term (38–42 weeks), during labor, and during delivery. They are also contraindicated in neonates younger than 4 weeks of age.
- These drugs increase the risk of hyperbilirubinemia (bilirubin is toxic to nerves and CNS).
- Complication of hyperbilirubinemia is called "kernicterus" (serious nerve/brain damage).
- Do not use if G6PD anemia is suspected (causes hemolysis).
- Nitrofurantoin causes serious adverse effects, such as pulmonary reactions (interstitial pneumonitis, pulmonary fibrosis), liver damage, neuropathy, and others.

EXAM TIPS

- **Always treat asymptomatic bacteriuria and UTIs in pregnant women.**
- **UTIs in pregnant women are classified as "complicated UTIs."**
- **A count of 10^3 cfu/mL or higher in a symptomatic pregnant woman is considered a UTI.**
- **In a nonpregnant healthy adult, a UTI is defined as 100,000 CFU or 10^5 CFU of one organism.**
- **Signs and symptoms of UTI in pregnant women are the same as in nonpregnant state.**
- **Amoxicillin is not the first-line drug for empiric UTI treatment (high resistance rates).**
- **There are usually only a few questions that address pregnancy. Do not overstudy this subject area for the exam because the number of questions has decreased over the past few years.**

Spontaneous Abortion

Also known as a *miscarriage*. Spontaneous loss of the fetus before it is viable (<20 weeks).

Threatened Abortion

Vaginal bleeding occurs but cervical os remains closed. Most of these cases will result in an ongoing pregnancy.

Inevitable Abortion

Cervix is dilated and unable to stop process. Fetus will be aborted.

Complete Abortion

Vaginal bleeding with cramping occurs. Placenta and fetus are expelled completely. Cervical os will close and bleeding stops.

Incomplete Abortion (Abortion With Retained Products of Conception)

Vaginal bleeding with cramping occurs. Placental products remain in the uterus. Cervical os remains dilated and bleeding persists; pieces of tissue may be seen at the cervical os. Vaginal discharge is foul smelling (bacterial vaginosis). Treatment is dilation and curettage (D&C) and antibiotics.

OBSTETRIC COMPLICATIONS

Preeclampsia (Pregnancy-Induced Hypertension)

Most cases of preeclampsia occur in the late third trimester (34 weeks gestation or later). It can occur up to 4 weeks after childbirth (postpartum period). Mild cases of preeclampsia may not have symptoms such as headaches, blurred vision, or right upper quadrant abdominal pain.

Will cause multiorgan damage to the brain (stroke), kidneys (acute renal failure), lungs (pulmonary edema), liver (hepatic rupture), as well as disseminated intravascular coagulation (DIC), and fetal and/or maternal death. Older name is "toxemia." The exact etiology of preeclampsia is unknown. If seizures develop, the woman will be diagnosed with eclampsia.

Risk factors include primigravida, multipara, older than 35 years of age, obesity, prior history of preeclampsia, hypertension, or kidney disease.

Diagnostic Criteria

Classic triad: Hypertension, proteinuria, and edema that occur after 20 weeks gestation and up to 4 weeks postpartum. Take at least two separate readings (at least 6 hours apart).

- *Systolic* BP: 140 mmHg or greater *or*
- *Diastolic* BP: 90 mmHg or greater
- *Proteinuria*: More than 0.3 g protein in a 24-hour urine specimen. Proteinuria ranges from trace to 1+ to 4+ (severe cases).
- Rapid weight gain of from 2 to 5 lbs per week. The edema is most obvious in the face, around the eyes, and on the hands.

Treatment Plan

Refer to obstetrician for management. The only definitive "cure" for preeclampsia and eclampsia is delivery of the placenta/fetus.

Preexisting/Chronic Hypertension

Defined as the presence of an elevated BP (>140/90 mmHg) before the 20th week of gestation. Do not confuse this condition with preeclampsia. May be on a prescription. If on an ACE inhibitor or ARB, discontinue ASAP and monitor BP closely. Most pregnant women with preexisting hypertension can usually get off their BP medications (temporarily) during the first to second trimester because of the lowering of BP during pregnancy (less peripheral vascular resistance).

Placenta Abruptio (Placental Abruption)

Premature partial to complete separation of a normally implanted placenta from the uterine bed. Rupture of the maternal blood vessels from the decidua basalis. Bleeding ranges from mild to hemorrhage. Controllable risk factors are smoking, cocaine use, hypertension, and encouraged seatbelt use.

Classic Case

Sudden onset of vaginal bleeding (mild to hemorrhage) with abdominal and/or back pain. Painful uterine contractions. Uterus is rigid (hypertonic) and very tender.

Treatment Plan

- Refer to the ED.
- Initial ED labs are CBC, PT/PTT, blood type, cross-match, Rh factor, and so on.
- Abdominal ultrasound and blood transfusion needed.

- If mild contractions, give magnesium sulfate ($MgSO_4$) IV. Strict bed rest is needed.
- Deliver fetus by C-section if mother's life is threatened. Give steroids if fetus is viable.

Placenta Previa

This is an abnormally implanted placenta. The placenta implants too low either on top of cervix or on the cervical isthmus/neck. Most cases get better spontaneously (will reimplant). Some cases are asymptomatic. Higher risk if previous history of placenta previa or C-section, multipara, older age, smoking, fibroids, or cocaine use.

Classic Case

A woman who is a multipara who is at the late second to third trimester of pregnancy complains of the sudden onset of bright-red vaginal bleeding (light to heavy) accompanied by mild contractions. The uterus feels soft and is not tender.

Treatment Plan

- Refer to ED.
- Avoid bimanual examination because palpation of the uterus may cause severe hemorrhage.
- Use abdominal ultrasound only. No intravaginal ultrasound. No rectal exams.
- Avoid any vaginal/rectal sexual intercourse.
- Bed rest required. Close fetal and maternal monitoring.
- If contractions, give magnesium sulfate ($MgSO_4$) IV. If mild cases, pregnancy can be salvaged and the placenta will reimplant. Perform C-section if mother's life is in danger.

BREASTFEEDING

Colostrum and Breast Milk

During the first few days (day 1–2) of breastfeeding, colostrum is produced (thick yellow-color), which contains maternal antibodies (passive immunity). By the third to the fourth day, mature breast milk is produced (contains fat, sugar/lactose, water, protein, and antibodies). The full-term healthy infant can be exclusively breastfed for the first 6 months of life, with no supplemental fluids unless ill or dehydrated.

Vitamin D

- All breastfed infants need vitamin D supplementation started within first few days.
- Formula-fed infants should only be given iron-fortified formula (has vitamin D).

Breastfeeding Technique

- Breastfeed within the first hour of birth. It provides the baby with colostrum and helps the uterus contract.
- A new mother should be taught proper breastfeeding technique. Refer to specialist if having problems; follow up at home.
- If noisy, assess for improper latch on (check positioning, sucking, clicking noises). Swallowing noises are normal, but not clicking noises.
- For clicking, advise the mother to use her index finger to pull down the baby's chin so that the baby's lower lip will be outside. The baby should have the entire nipple and most of the areola inside his mouth.
- Newborns will nurse about eight to 12 times per 24 hours.

Sore Nipples

- Advise the mother not to stop breastfeeding. This causes breast engorgement (painful).
- If poor latch, the infant may have to suck harder which causes pain.

- This results from babies having difficulty "latching on" to an engorged breast.
- Nipple pain is worse during the first week and usually disappears by the second week.
- If nipple pain persists, assess nipples for fissures and infection.
- Start nursing on the less painful breast first.
- Initiate "letdown reflex" of milk by massage/warm shower.
- Apply lanolin or breast milk to nipple after nursing to protect from skin breakdown.
- Avoid using plastic nipple shields, alcohol, and soap. Wear nursing bras with good support.
- May need referral to a lactation specialist (e.g., La Leche League)

Maternal Benefits

- Stimulates uterine contractions (speeds up uterine involution after delivery).
- Increases maternal bonding with infant (oxytocin effect).
- Speeds up weight loss after pregnancy.
- Lowers risk of breast/ovarian cancer.
- Can delay ovulation if mother breastfeeds exclusively.

Fetal Health Benefits

- Lowers risk of infections (necrotizing enterocolitis, acute otitis media).
- Lowers risk of bacterial and viral infections such as otitis media and diarrhea.
- Lower incidence of asthma and allergies in breastfed babies.
- Young infants who are exclusively breastfed get enough fluids and do not need extra water. Juices should be avoided because they increase the risk of dental caries.
- Lowers risk of sudden infant death syndrome (SIDS) and future obesity.

EXAM TIPS

- **Swallowing noises may be heard in breastfeeding, especially in younger babies.**
- **If clicking noises are heard during breastfeeding, it is abnormal. Advise the mother to use her index finger to pull down the baby's chin so that the baby's lower lip will latch better onto the areola.**
- **If a question describes a mother who complains of sore nipples, do not advise her to stop breastfeeding, to supplement with formula, or to use formula at nighttime feedings. The best answer is to advise the mother that it is a common problem during the first 2 weeks and will resolve.**

Breastfeeding Mastitis (Lactational Mastitis)

Most common in the first 2 months of breastfeeding. Skin fissures on the nipple(s) allow bacterial entry. Most common organism is *Staphylococcus aureus* (gram positive). Consider methicillin-resistant *S. aureus* (MRSA) bacterial infection (becoming more common). If severe or toxic, refer to ED or admit to the hospital.

Prevention

Frequent and complete emptying of breast and proper breastfeeding technique. Breast engorgement and poor technique increases risk of mastitis.

Classic Case

Patient who is breastfeeding complains of the sudden onset of a red, firm, and tender area (induration) on one breast. May also have fever/chills and malaise (flu-like symptoms). May have adenopathy on the axilla by the affected breast.

Labs

- Usually not needed; this is a clinical diagnosis.
- CBC shows leukocytosis. Order C&S of milk if hospital acquired, severe, or not responding to antibiotic treatment.

Medications

If Low Risk of MRSA

- Dicloxacillin 500 mg PO QID or cephalexin (Keflex) 500 mg PO QID for 10 to 14 days.
- Do not use sulfas during the newborn period, due to increased risk of kernicterus.

If High Risk of MRSA

- Trimethoprim–sulfamethoxazole (Bactrim) one to two tablets PO BID for 10 to 14 days *or* clindamycin 300 mg PO QID for 10 to 14 days
- Continue to breastfeed on affected breast during antibiotic treatment. If unable to breastfeed, pump milk from infected breast (and discard) to prevent engorgement.
- If breast abscess is suspected, order an ultrasound and refer for incision and drainage.
- Administer ibuprofen for pain as needed. Apply cold compresses on indurated breast area.
- Refer to lactation consultant if suspect poor breastfeeding technique.

Uncomplicated Chlamydia Infection (Cervicitis, Urethritis)

- Treating *Chlamydia trachomatis* infection in the mother will help to prevent the transmission (vertical transmission) of the infection to the newborn through the birth canal.
  - *Example*: trachoma (or inclusion conjunctivitis of the newborn) and pneumonia

Labs

- Obtain nucleic acid amplification tests (NAATs) such as the Gen-Probe, Amplicor, or ProbeTec.
- Gen-Probe can only be used on the cervix and urethra. Do not use to collect specimens from the eyes.
- Test-of-cure needed in 3 weeks after completing treatment.

Treatment Plan

- *First line*: Azithromycin 1 g orally (single dose)
- Alternative: Amoxicillin 500 mg PO TID × 7 days (lower cure rate than azithromycin)

Sexual Partners

- *First line*: Azithromycin 1 g orally (single dose)
- Doxycycline 100 mg PO BID × 7 days
- Avoid sexual activity for 7 days; avoid unprotected intercourse until both partners are treated; test for other STDs (gonorrhea, syphilis, HIV)

Postpartum Contraception

- Women who exclusively breastfeed (at least every 4 hours daily) with amenorrhea and who are less than 6 months postpartum are much less likely to ovulate than a woman who does not breastfeed exclusively (lactational amenorrhea method).
- In women who do not breastfeed, ovulation resumes (average) at 39 days postpartum. During the postpartum period and with breastfeeding, birth control pills or any contraceptive method containing estrogen (pregnancy category X) is contraindicated.

- Postpartum women or women who cannot take estrogens can use methods such as intrauterine devices (IUDs; copper or levonorgestrel) or progesterone-only contraception such as etonogestrel (Nexplanon), depot medroxyprogesterone (Depo-Provera), progestin-only pills, or barrier methods (condoms, diaphragm, cervical cap).
  - The progestin-only contraceptive pill norethindrone (Micronor) contains 28 active pills that are taken daily (no pill-free week).
  - For maximum effectiveness, pill must be taken at the same time each day (very important). If more than 3 hours late, take dose as soon as possible and use backup (condom) for the next 2 days. Will probably have vaginal spotting for the next few days.

Pediatrics and Adolescents Review

IV

20

Pediatrics Review: Newborns

⚠ DANGER SIGNALS

Failure to Thrive (FTT)

Defined as weight for age that falls below third to fifth percentile for gestation-corrected age and gender when plotted on appropriate growth chart (on more than one occasion). Also, infants whose rate of weight change decreases over two or more major percentile lines (90th, 75th, 50th, 25th, and 5th) exhibit FTT (e.g., a child at the 50th percentile goes down to 5th percentile over a few months). Use World Health Organization (WHO) growth charts until the age of 2 years, then Centers for Disease Control and Prevention (CDC) growth charts. In most cases seen in primary care, causes are usually inadequate dietary intake, diarrhea, malabsorption (celiac disease, cystic fibrosis, food allergy), poor maternal bonding, frequent infections, and others.

Down Syndrome

A genetic defect caused by trisomy of chromosome 21 (three copies instead of two). The most common chromosomal disorder; the average life span is 60 years in the United States.

Affected persons have a round face that appears "flat" (decreased anterior–posterior diameter), accompanied by upward-slanting eyes (palpebral fissures) and low-set ears. Chronic open mouth caused by enlarged tongue (macroglossia). Shorter neck with short broad hands with transverse palmar crease (simian crease). Newborns have hypotonia and poor Moro reflex. Higher risk of congenital heart defects (50%), congenital hearing loss, visual problems, cataracts, sleep apnea, and early onset of Alzheimer's disease (average age 54 years).

Educate parents about high-risk sports (risk of spinal cord injury): contact sports (football, soccer), trampoline, or gymnastics. Avoid trampoline use, especially before age 6 years.

Fetal Alcohol Syndrome (FAS)

Classic FAS facies is a small head (microcephaly) with shortened palpebral fissures (narrow eyes) with epicanthal folds and a flat nasal bridge. There is a thin upper lip with no vertical groove above the upper lip (smooth philtrum). Ears are underdeveloped. Also known as *fetal alcohol spectrum disorder* and can range from severe disease with mental retardation to mild developmental defects that may not be obvious until adolescence (i.e., attention deficit disorder [ADD]). There is no safe dose or time for alcohol during pregnancy. Alcohol adversely affects the CNS, somatic growth, and facial structure development.

Cryptorchidism (Undescended Testicle)

Empty scrotal sac(s). Most cases involve undescended testicles. One or two testicles may be missing. Testis does not descend with massage of the inguinal area. Majority of cases (90%)

of cryptorchidism are associated with patent processus vaginalis. Infant should be sitting and the exam room should be warm to relax muscles when massaging the inguinal canal. Another option is to examine child after a warm bath.

Increased risk of testicular cancer if testicles are not removed from the abdomen. Surgical correction necessary within the first year of life if testicles does not spontaneously descend (orchiopexy).

Gonococcal Ophthalmia Neonatorum

Symptoms usually show within 2 to 5 days after birth. Infection can rapidly spread, causing blindness. Do not delay treatment by waiting for culture results. Symptoms include injected (red) conjunctiva with profuse purulent discharge and swollen eyelids. Majority of cases of congenital gonorrhea infection are acquired during delivery (intrapartum). Coinfection with chlamydia is common with gonococcal infection. Any neonates with acute conjunctivitis presenting within 30 days or less from birth should be tested for chlamydia, gonorrhea, herpes simplex, and bacterial infection.

Order gonococcal culture (Thayer-Martin), herpes simplex culture, and chlamydial polymerase chain reaction (PCR) with Gram stain of eye exudate. Hospitalize and treat with high-dose intravenous or intramuscular ceftriaxone. Preferred prophylaxis is with topical 0.5% erythromycin ointment (1-cm ribbon per eye) immediately after birth. Test (and treat) mother and sexual partner for sexually transmitted diseases (STDs).

Chlamydial Ophthalmia Neonatorum (Trachoma)

Symptoms will show 4 to 10 days after birth. Eyelids become edematous and red with profuse watery discharge initially that later becomes purulent. When obtaining a sample, collect not only the exudate, but also conjunctival cells as well. Rule out concomitant chlamydial pneumonia. Treated with systemic antibiotics such as azithromycin IM or oral erythromycin base or erythromycin ethylsuccinate syrup QID × 14 days. Treatment only 80% effective. May need second course. Use only systemic antibiotics. Prophylaxis is with topical 0.5% erythromycin or tetracycline ointment (1-cm ribbon per eye). Reportable disease. Test (and treat) mother and sexual partner for STDs.

Chlamydial Pneumonia

In infants with ophthalmia neonatorum, also rule out concomitant chlamydial pneumonia. Obtain nasopharyngeal culture for chlamydia. Infant will have frequent cough with bibasilar rales, tachypnea, hyperinflation, and diffused infiltrates on chest x-ray. Treated with erythromycin QID × 2 weeks. Daily follow-up. Reportable disease.

Sudden Infant Death Syndrome (SIDS)

Unexplained and sudden death in apparently healthy infants younger than 12 months. Higher risk with prematurity, low birth weight, maternal smoking and/or drug use, and poverty. Cause unknown; theories range from CNS abnormalities; cardiac arrhythmias; suffocation from soft, thick bedding; and so on. To decrease risk, position infants on their backs (supine) only. Avoid side-lying and prone positions. Avoid "overheating" infant and use of thick quilts, soft beds, pillows, and so on.

Weight Loss (More Than 7%)

Newborns are expected to lose a little weight during the first 5 to 7 days of life. Formula-fed infants may lose up to 5% and breast-fed infants may lose 7% to 10% of their birth weight.

Weight loss (up to 7%) of birth weight should be regained within 10 to 14 days. Weight loss beyond 7% in neonates is considered abnormal. Assess the infant for dehydration and the mother and infant for lactation difficulties.

Dehydration

Signs of severe dehydration (>10% weight loss) in an infant are weak and rapid pulse, tachypnea or deep breathing, parched mucous membranes, anterior fontanelle that is markedly sunken, skin turgor shows tenting, cool skin, acrocyanosis, anuria, and change in LOC (lethargy to coma). Refer severely dehydrated infants to the ED for IV hydration. Severe dehydration due to acute gastroenteritis is one of the leading causes of death of infants in the developing world.

SKIN LESIONS

Mongolian Spots

Most common type of pigmented skin lesions in newborns. Present in almost all Asians (85%–100%) and in more than half of Native American, Hispanic, and Black neonates. Blue- to black-colored patches or stains. A common location is the lumbosacral area (but can be located anywhere on the body). May be mistaken for bruising or child abuse. Usually fade by age 2 to 3 years.

Milia, Miliaria, or "Prickly Heat"

Most common in neonates. Multiple white 1- to 2-mm papules located mainly on the forehead, cheeks, and nose. Common locations are the nose and the cheeks. Due to retention of sebaceous material and keratin. Resolves spontaneously.

Erythema Toxicum Neonatorum

Small pustules (whitish yellow color) that are 1- to 3-mm in size and surrounded by a red base. Erupts during the second to the third day of life. Located on the face, chest, back, and extremities. Lasts from 1 to 2 weeks and resolves spontaneously.

Seborrheic Dermatitis ("Cradle Cap")

Excessive thick scaling on the scalp of younger infants. Treated by softening and removal of the thick scales on the scalp after soaking scalp a few hours (to overnight) with vegetable oil or mineral oil. Shampoo scalp and gently scrub scales with soft comb. Prevention is by frequent shampooing with mild baby shampoo and removing scales with soft brush or comb. Self-limited condition that resolves spontaneously within a few months.

Faun Tail Nevus

Tufts of hair overlying spinal column usually at lumbosacral area. May be a sign of neural tube defects (spina bifida, spina bifida occulta). Perform neurological exam focusing on lumbosacral nerves (fecal/urinary incontinence, problems with gait). Order ultrasound of lesion to rule out occult spina bifida.

Café au Lait Spots

Flat, light-brown to dark-brown spots greater than 5 mm (0.5 cm). If six or more spots larger than 5 mm (0.5 cm) in diameter are seen, rule out neurofibromatosis or von Recklinghausen's disease (neurological disorder marked by seizures, learning disorders, etc.). Refer to pediatric neurologist if the spots meet the same criteria to rule out neurofibromatosis.

VASCULAR LESIONS

Port Wine Stain (Nevus Flammeus)

Neonates with pink to red, flat, stain-like skin lesions located on the upper and lower eyelids or on the V_1 and V_2 branches of the trigeminal nerve (CN V) should be referred to a pediatric ophthalmologist to rule out congenital glaucoma. Blanches to pressure. Irregular in size and shape. Large lesions located on half the facial area may be a sign of trigeminal nerve involvement and Sturge–Weber syndrome (rare neurological disorder). The lesions do not regress and grow with the child. These lesions can be treated with pulse-dye laser (PDL) therapy.

Hemangioma (Strawberry Hemangioma)

Raised vascular lesions ranging in size from 0.5 to 4.0 cm that are bright red in color and feel soft to palpation. Usually located on the head or the neck. The lesions grow during the first 12 months of life, but the majority will involute spontaneously over time. Watchful waiting is the usual strategy. Can be treated with PDL therapy.

SCREENING TESTS

VISION SCREENING

Newborn Vision

- Newborns are nearsighted (myopia) and have a vision of 20/400.
- They can focus best at a distance of 8 to 10 inches.
- During the first 2 months, the infant's eyes may appear crossed (or wander) at times (normal finding). If one eye is consistently turned in or turned out, refer to pediatric opthalmologist.
- Human face is preferred by newborns.
- Newborns do not shed tears because the lacrimal ducts are not fully mature at birth.
- Caucasian neonates are born with blue–gray eyes. It is normal for their eye color to change as they mature.
- Retinas (CN II) are immature at birth and reach maturity at age 6 years; at which time vision is 20/20.

Infant Screening

- *1 month*: Infant can fixate briefly on the mother's face. Prefers the human face.
- *3 months*: Infant will hold the hands close to the face to observe them. Hold a bright object or a toy in front of the infant. Watch behavior as the infant fixates on the toy for a few seconds. Avoid using objects/toys that make noises when testing vision.
- *6 months*: Makes good eye contact. Scans surroundings with 180-degree visual field.
- *12 months*: Makes prolonged eye contact when spoken to. Will actively turn head around 180 degrees to observe people and surroundings for long periods. Recognizes parents and favorite people from a longer distance.
- *Retina and optic disc*: Set funduscope lens at 0 to –2 diopters. Fundus appears dark orange to red (red reflex). The red reflex of both eyes should be symmetrical in shape and color.

Abnormal Findings

Strabismus

- Misalignment of the eye. Horizontal strabismus may be esotropia (inward turning of the eyes) or exotropia (outward turning of the eyes). Vertical strabismus may be hypertropia (one eye higher than the other) or hypotropia (one eye lower than the other).

- Uncorrected strabismus can result in permanent visual loss and abnormal vision such as diplopia (double vision). Treatment can range from eyeglasses, eye exercises, prism, and/or eye muscle surgery.

Amblyopia ("Lazy Eye")

- If corrected early, affected eye can have normal vision.

Esotropia

- Misalignment of one or both eyes ("cross-eyed"). Infants (younger than 20 weeks) may have intermittent esotropia, which usually resolves spontaneously.
- Some infants with obvious epicanthal folds appear "cross-eyed" (pseudostrabismus). Refer to pediatric opthalmologist if in doubt.

Indications for Referral

- Abnormal red reflex (rule out retinoblastoma, cataract, glaucoma)
- Presence of white reflex (rule out retinoblastoma)
- Strabismus (rule out CN III, IV, and VI abnormalities, retinoblastoma)
- Greater than two-line difference between each eye
- Esodeviation present after 3 to 4 months of age
- Corneal light reflex test with abnormal result
- Shape/appearance of pupils not equal
- New onset of strabismus (retinoblastoma, brain mass, bleeding, lead poisoning, etc.)

Red Reflex

Screening test for cataracts and retinoblastoma. Abnormal if there are white-colored opacities (cataracts) or white spots (leukocoria). Determine presence of white reflex, rule out retinoblastoma, and refer infant to pediatric ophthalmologist as soon as possible. Even if the test is normal during the visit, but a parent reports that one eye appears white on a digital photograph, refer. If absence or decreased intensity of red reflex, rule out cataract and refer to pediatic opthalmologist.

- *Procedure*: Perform test in a darkened room. Use a direct ophthalmoscope and shine light about 12 to 18 inches away from the infant. Normal finding is symmetrical and round orange-red glow from each eye.

Congenital Cataracts

- Red reflex exam on neonate shows a round, white-colored pupil.

Light Reflex Test or Corneal Light Reflex (Hirschberg Test)

Screening test for strabismus. Abnormal if corneal light reflex is not clear or if it is "off-center."

- *Procedure*: Shine light directly in eyes (24 inches away) using a fixation target. Infant or child must look directly forward with both eyes aligned. Observe for the symmetry and brightness of light reflecting from both eyes.

HEARING SCREENING

Universal screening for hearing loss is done while in nursery before discharge.

Newborns

- Each state has its own rules about neonatal hearing exams.

Auditory Brainstem Response (ABR)

- Measures the CN VIII by the use of "click" stimuli

Otoacoustic Emissions (OAEs)

- Gross hearing test: As a response to loud noise, look for startle response (neonates), blinking, turning toward sound.
- Measures the middle ear mobility only. Less sensitive than the ABR.

Mnemonic Device (HEARS) for High-Risk Factors for Hearing Loss:

H (hyperbilirubinemia)
E (ear infections that are frequent)
A (Apgar scores low at birth)
R (rubella, cytomegalovirus [CMV], toxoplasmosis infections)
S (seizures)

Premature infants and infants admitted to NICUs have a higher incidence of hearing loss compared with full-term infants.

LABORATORY TESTS

Testing varies from state to state. Blood is obtained by heel stick or from cord blood. A spot of blood is blotted into filter paper for stable transport.

Thyroid-Stimulating Hormone (TSH)

TSH testing is federally mandated. Lack of thyroid hormone results in mental and somatic growth retardation. Treated by thyroid hormone supplementation.

Phenylketonuria (PKU)

PKU testing is federally mandated. Severe mental retardation results if not treated early. Disorder is an inability to metabolize phenylalanine to tyrosine because of a defect in the production of the enzyme phenylalanine hydroxylase. Perform test only after infant has protein feeding (breast milk or formula) for at least 48 hours. Higher risk of false negatives if done too early (<48 hours). Treated by following special diet (phenylalanine-free diet).

Sickle Cell Disease

The required test can detect four types of hemoglobin (hemoglobin F, S, A, and C).

Hemoglobin and Hematocrit

Normal newborns have hemoglobin F (fetal hemoglobin) and hemoglobin A. Healthy infants have enough iron stores to last up to 6 months. Screening for anemia is done in late infancy (9–12 months) for full-term, healthy infants. Not screened at birth because hemoglobin is elevated from maternal RBCs mixed in fetal RBCs.

Lead Screening

High-risk children should be screened at age 1 to 2 years (12 and 24 months).

PHYSIOLOGICAL CONCERNS IN INFANCY

Nutritional Intake

Breastfeeding is preferred over formula. If formula chosen, start with one fortified with iron. (See Chapter 19 for breastfeeding concerns in newborns.)

Breastfeeding

Give vitamin D drops (400 IU of vitamin D) starting in the first few days of life if breastfeeding because breast milk alone does not provide adequate levels of vitamin D (CDC, 2009). Infant formula is supplemented with vitamin D, iron, other vitamins, and essential fatty acids.

- Breast milk or formula contains 20 calories per ounce
- Decreases risk of infections (i.e., otitis media) during the first few weeks of life

Colostrum

Sticky and thick yellowish fluid that comes before breast milk. Secreted first few days after the birth and contains large amounts of maternal antibodies and nutrients.

Cow's Milk

- Avoid cow's milk the first year of life (causes GI bleeding)
- Common cause of iron-deficiency anemia in babies younger than 12 months

Meconium

Thick dark-green to black-colored stool that is odorless. Most full-term neonates pass meconium stool within a few hours of birth. Failure to pass meconium within 24 hours of birth is worrisome and may be a sign of intestinal obstruction or cystic fibrosis.

Solid Foods

- Can start at 4 to 6 months. Start with rice cereal (fortified with iron) before other types of cereal or food.
- Introduce one food at a time for 4 to 5 days (if allergic, easier to identify offending food).

Head Findings

Caput succedaneum is diffused edema of the scalp that crosses the midline. Caused by intrauterine and vaginal pressure from prolonged or difficult vaginal labor. The scalp becomes molded and "cone-shaped." Self-limited and resolves spontaneously.

Head Circumference

Also known as the *occipitofrontal circumference (OFC)*. Use paper tape (cloth tapes stretches) and place above the ear.

- Average head circumference at birth is 13.7 inches (35 cm).
- Head circumference is measured at each wellness visit until the age of 36 months (3 years).
- In newborns, chest is about 1 to 2 cm smaller in size than the head circumference.
- Head circumference will increase by 12 cm during the first 12 months.
- Fastest rate of head growth is during the first 3 months of life (2 cm per month).

Abnormal Finding: Cephalohematoma

Traumatic subperiosteal hemorrhage. Rule out skull fracture (order radiographs of the skull). Swelling does not cross the midline or suture lines.

Weight Gain and Length

Birth Weight

Neonates lose up to 7% of body weight but should regain it by 2 weeks of age. They double their birth weight by 6 months and triple their birth weight by 12 months.

Infant Weight

- *0 to 6 months*: 6 to 8 ounces per week and 1 inch per month
- *6 to 12 months*: 3 to 4 ounces per week and 1/2 inch per month

If the child's weight and/or length decelerates across two or more major percentiles, rule out FTT (see "Danger Signals," earlier). In addition, any child who is at the third to fifth percentile is considered to have FTT. Of the many causes of FTT, the most common in primary care are undernutrition and malnutrition. Evaluate the child, including maternal bonding and depression.

Length and Height

Length (linear growth) of infants is measured from birth to about 24 months. Starting at age of 2 years, measure height (child is standing up) and body mass index (BMI). Plot the measurements on the infant's or child's percentile growth chart.

Dentition

First Tooth (Primary Teeth)

Both the left and right teeth erupt bilaterally at the same time (symmetrical). Symptoms are drooling, chewing on objects, irritability, crying, and fever.

- *6 to 10 months of age*: Lower central incisors (lower front teeth)
- *2½ years of age*: Has complete set of primary teeth (20 teeth)

First Permanent Teeth (Deciduous Teeth)

- *6 years of age*: Central incisors and the first molars

Genitourinary Anomalies

- *Hypospadias*: Urethral meatus located on the ventral aspect of the penis. Location may be at the glans or on the shaft. Some have two urethral openings; one opening is normal and the other opening is lower on the glans or shaft. Refer to pediatric urologist.
- *Epispadias*: Urethral meatus is located on the dorsal aspect (upper side) of the penis.
- *Hydrocele*: Presence of fluid inside the scrotum (tunica vaginalis/processus vaginalis) that results in swelling of the affected scrotum. Skin is normal color and temperature. Fairly common in newborn males. Incidence rate is 10 to 20 cases out of every 1,000 live births.
- *Transillumination*: Affected testicle(s) will show increased size in the "glow" of light compared with the normal scrotum. Darken the room and place the light source on the scrotal skin. Compare each scrotum.
- *Newborn female vagina swollen with small amount of blood*: Caused by maternal hormones and will disappear within a few days.
- *Cryptorchidism*: Retention of one or both testicles in the abdominal cavity or the inguinal canal. Markedly increases risk of testicular cancer. Order inguinal and abdominal ultrasound. Corrected surgically after 4 months of age.

EXAM TIPS

- **Weight loss of 5% to 7% starts after birth, but neonates should regain birth weight in 2 weeks.**
- **Birth weight doubles at 6 months and triples at 12 months.**
- **Head circumference: Grows by up to 12 cm (first 12 months).**
- **Caput succedaneum crosses midline and cephalohematoma does not (blood blocked by scalp sutures).**
- **Colostrum (IgG antibodies) looks like thick yellow fluid and is secreted the first few days of breastfeeding before milk release.**
- **Avoid cow's milk during first 12 months of life (causes GI bleeding, iron-deficiency anemia).**
- **Breastfeeding: Supplement with vitamin D the first few days of life.**
- **Epstein's pearls: White papules found on gum line resembles an erupting tooth.**

- **Do not confuse questions asking for the "first tooth" with the "first permanent tooth."**
- **Hypospadias: Urethral opening under glans/shaft (refer to pediatric urologist)**
- **Epispadias: Urethral opening on top of glans/shaft (refer to pediatric urologist)**
- **Cryptorchidism increases risk of testicular cancer. Refer to pediatric urologist for evaluation between 4 to 12 months of age.**
- **Transillumination is used to assess for hydrocele, empty scrotal sac, and scrotal masses.**
- **Hydrocele is fluid collection inside the scrotum (tunica vaginalis/processus vaginalis).**
- **Infant with hydrocele and transillumination: Scrotal sac with hydrocele will appear "brighter" or will have more light glow compared with scrotum with a testicle (solid objects block light, so less glow of light).**

REFLEX TESTING

Anal Wink

Gently stroke the anal region. Look for contraction of the perianal muscle. Absence is abnormal and suggestive of a lesion on the spinal cord (i.e., spina bifida).

Plantar Reflex (Babinski Reflex)

Upward extension of the big toe with fanning of the other toes. Starting on the heel, stroke firmly the outer side of the sole toward the front of the foot.

Palmar Reflex (Grasp Reflex)

Place a finger on the infant's open palm. The infant closes his or her hand around the finger. Pulling away the examiner's finger causes the infant's grip to tighten.

Moro Reflex (Startle Reflex)

Sudden loud noise will cause symmetric abduction and extension of the arms followed by adduction and flexion of the arms over the body. Disappears by 3 to 4 months.

- *Absence on one side*: Rule out brachial plexus injury, fracture, or shoulder dystocia.
- *Absence on both sides*: Rule out spinal cord or brain lesion.
- *Older infant*: Persistence of Moro reflex is abnormal. Rule out brain pathology.

Step Reflex

Hold baby upright and allow the dorsal surface of one foot to touch the edge of a table. Baby will flex the hip and knee and place the stimulated foot on the tabletop (stepping motion). Absent with paresis and breech births. Disappears by 6 weeks.

Blink Reflex

Eyelids will close in response to bright light or touch.

Tonic Neck Reflex (Fencing Reflex)

Turning head to one side with jaw over shoulder causes the arm and leg on the same side to extend. The arm and leg on the opposite side will flex.

Rooting Reflex

Stroking the corner of the mouth causes baby to turn toward stimulus and suck. Disappears by 3 to 4 months.

EXAM TIP

- **A strong Moro reflex in an older infant (age 6 months or older) is abnormal and indicative of brain damage.**

IMMUNIZATIONS (TABLE 20.1)

Table 20.1 Immunization Schedule (Birth to 6 Years)

Vaccine	Birth	2 Months	4 Months	6 Months	12 Months	4–6 Years
Hepatitis B	#1 (#2 at 1 to 2 mo)			#3 at 6 to 18 mo		
Rotavirus		#1	#2	#3*		
Diphtheria, tetanus, acellular pertussis (DTaP)		#1	#2	#3	#4 at 16 to 18 mo	#5
Haemophilus influenzae type b conjugate vaccine (Hib)		#1	#2	#3**	#4**	
Pneumococcal conjugate form of vaccine (PCV4)		#1	#2	#3	#4 at 12 to 15 mo	
Inactivated polio (IPV)		#1	#2	#3 at 6 to 18 mo		#4
Measles, mumps, rubella (MMR)					#1	#2
Varicella					#1	#2

*Rotarix (RV) is two doses and RotaTeq (RV5) needs three doses.
**There are five forms of Hib vaccine that require from two to four doses.

Source: Adapted from the Centers for Disease Control and Prevention (2017). Most vaccines have a range (from 3 to 6 months) when they can be given. For a complete list of all vaccine schedules, visit the CDC website at www.cdc.gov/vaccines.

Mumps, Measles, and Rubella (MMR) and Varicella Vaccine

Live attenuated virus vaccine. Not recommended before the age of 12 months (not effective due to immaturity of immune system). If dose given before 12 months of age, must be repeated.

- Avoid salicylates for 6 weeks (theoretical risk of Reye's syndrome). Children (ages birth to 12 years) should not be given any aspirin or any aspirin products (Pepto-Bismol, Pamprin, Alka Seltzer, Kaopectate, etc.).
- *First dose (MMR and varicella)*: 12 months
- *Second dose (MMR and varicella)*: Age 4 to 6 years (preschool age)
- *Proof of varicella*: Documentation of chickenpox or herpes zoster on the chart by a health care provider, record of two doses, or a positive varicella titer

Influenza Vaccine

Beginning with the 2016–2017 influenza season, the CDC recommended use of injectable flu vaccines. The nasal spray form (live attenuated influenza vaccine) is not to be used.

- Do not give influenza vaccines before age of 6 months because they are not effective (immature immune system). It takes 2 weeks to produce antibodies after vaccination.
- Recommended for everyone age 6 months or older (with rare exceptions), but especially for children 6 months to 4 years of age; people with congenital heart disease, asthma, cystic fibrosis, sickle cell anemia, heart disease, and chronic obstructive pulmonary disease (COPD); women who will be pregnant during the influenza season; Native Americans/Alaska Natives; health care personnel; elderly; and others.

- Trivalent inactivated influenza vaccines (protects against three types of influenza virus)
  - Minimum age is 6 months. Administer fall to winter as injection.
  - FLUAD trivalent contains an adjuvant (makes it more immunogenic) for people aged 65 years or older.
- Quadrivalent influenza vaccines (protects against four types of influenza virus)
  - Intradermal formulation of quadrivalent influenza shot is approved for people aged 18 to 64 years.

Contraindications

Influenza Injection (Trivalent Inactivated Vaccine)

- Age younger than 6 months
- Severe egg allergy
  - If history of egg allergy (hives *only*), can receive the flu vaccine injection. *But*, if severe reaction to eggs (hypotension, wheezing, nausea and vomiting) requiring medical treatment or epinephrine, the patient can only receive the flu vaccine in an outpatient or inpatient clinic that has a health provider who can treat anaphylaxis (epinephrine, intubation, O_2, etc.)
- Moderate to severe illness with fever (wait until patient is better)
- History of Guillain–Barré syndrome

Live Influenza Nasal Spray (FluMist)

As of 2017–2018 flu season, live influenza nasal spray is not recommended by the CDC. See CDC website for updates (www.cdc.gov). Avoid giving the FluMist vaccine to the following groups of children. Use the inactivated injection form of the influenza vaccine.

- Children younger than age 2 years
- Children aged 2 to 4 years who had wheezing within the past 12 months
- Children who have any other underlying condition that predispose them to influenza complications; use inactivated form of the influenza vaccine (injection form) for these children

Diphtheria, Tetanus, Pertussis (DTaP) Vaccines

Diphtheria, tetanus, acellular pertussis (DTaP) is the form of vaccine used in the United States. Has fewer side effects compared to older DTP form.

- *Diphtheria–tetanus (DT)*: This form is used for infants and children younger than age 7 years unable to tolerate pertussis component.
- *Tdap vaccine*: For age 7 years and older. At age 11- to 12-year visit, give the Tdap. Or if due for tetanus booster, give Tdap once in a lifetime. Then gets Td every 10 years for lifetime.

If incomplete DTaP series and child age 7 years or older, give Tdap instead (Immunization Action Coalition, 2017). Can be given to breastfeeding mothers. Tdap given to child younger than age 7 years is *not* valid (use DTaP).

Side Effects: DTaP/DT

- Fever (defined as 100.4°F) in up to 50% of patients
- Swelling, pain, and/or redness at injection site in up to 50% of patients
- Irritability in up to 50% of patients
- Acute encephalopathy one in 110,000

Contraindications

- Severe allergic reaction
- Encephalopathy (i.e., prolonged seizures, change in level of consciousness [LOC]) not attributable to another cause within 7 days of administration of the vaccine

Precautions

- Fever equal to or greater than 105°F (within 48 hours of dose)
- Seizures (within 3 days or less of dose)
- Collapse or shock-like state within 48 hours after dose

Not Considered Contraindications to DTP/DTaP Vaccination

- Family history of seizures
- Family history of SIDS
- Fever less than 105° F from prior DTaP vaccination

Vaccine Adverse Event Reporting System (VAERS)

A national postmarketing vaccine safety surveillance program in the United States managed by both the CDC and the Food and Drug Administration (FDA). Report vaccine adverse events at www.vaers.hhs.gov.

Immunizations Tips

By age 15 to 18 months, the following vaccines are usually completed (for most infants):

- Hepatitis B vaccine (three doses)
- *Haemophilus influenzae* type b (Hib) vaccine (several types of Hib vaccines, may require from two, three, or four doses)
- Pneumococcal vaccine (PCV 13; four doses)
- Rotavirus vaccine (two to three doses)

EXAM TIPS

- **Do not give varicella and MMR vaccine before age of 12 months.**
- **Youngest age for influenza vaccine is 6 months.**
- **Only vaccine given at birth is hepatitis B.**
- **If HBsAg-positive mother, give the neonate hepatitis B immunoglobulin (HBIG) and the hepatitis B vaccine.**
- **Do not use DTaP if age 7 years or older. Use Td or Tdap form of vaccine.**
- **Give Tdap vaccine at age of 11 to 12 years as a booster. If older, then replace one dose of Td with a Tdap (once in a lifetime).**
- **Any vaccine that has a time range (e.g., third dose of IPV can be given from 6 to 18 months; third dose of hepatitis B can be given between 6 and 18 months) does not appear on the exam.**
- **The vaccines listed in Table 20.1 in this chapter contains only the childhood vaccines that must be given by a definite age (no "wiggle room"). For example, the first dose of the hepatitis B vaccine must be given at birth.**

GROWTH AND DEVELOPMENT

Newborns

- Strong primitive reflexes (e.g., Moro, rooting, fencing, etc.)
- Head lag
- Grasp finger tightly if placed on the baby's hand (grasp reflex)
- Pasty yellow stool after each feeding (especially if breastfed)
- Eats every 2 to 3 hours or nurses from eight to 10 times a day

- Newborns do not produce tears when crying; tear ducts are not yet mature at birth
- Sleeps 16 hours per day
- *Report*: High-pitched cry, "cat-like" cry, hypotonic microcephaly

2 Months Old

- Follows objects past midline
- Coos vowels (e.g., "aa") and makes gurgling sounds
- Lifts head up 45 degrees when prone
- Smiles in response to another

4 Months Old

- Smiles spontaneously (social smile)
- Begins to babble

Fine Motor

- Brings hands to mouth
- Can swing at dangling toys

Gross Motor

- Holds head steady and unsupported
- Rolls from front to back (supine to prone)

6 Months Old

Fine Motor

- Has palmar grasp of objects
- Reaches for toys using palmar grasp
- Brings things to mouth
- Starts to pass things from one hand to the other

Gross Motor

- Begins to sit up independently without support
- Rolls over in both directions (back/supine to stomach and stomach to the back/supine)

Language

- Starts to say consonants (e.g., "da-da, ba-ba")
- Is very curious and will look around environment

Other

- Report failure to follow objects past midline (180 degrees), poor eye contact

9 Months Old

Fine Motor

- Pincer grasp starts and can pick up things (e.g., food) between thumb and forefinger
- Waves "bye-bye"
- May clap hands and play clapping games such as pat-a-cake

Gross Motor

- Pulls self up to stand
- Crawls and "cruises"
- Bears weight well

Language

- Plays peek-a-boo
- "Stranger anxiety" very obvious
- Report absence of babble, inability to sit alone, strong primitive reflexes such as the Moro (startle reflex) or fencing (tonic neck reflex)

12 Months Old

Fine Motor

- Can use "sippy" cup

Gross Motor

- Stands independently
- May walk independently
- Starts to cruise (moves from one piece of furniture to the next for support)

Language

- Knows at least two to four words
- Can say exclamations, such as "uh-oh!"
- Knows first name

Other

- Growth rate slows down
- Follows simple directions, such as "pick up toy"
- Report absence of weight bearing, inability to transfer objects hand to hand

15 Months Old

Fine Motor

- Feeds self with spoon
- Can drink from a cup

Gross Motor

- Walks independently for longer distances

Language

- Follows commands with gestures
- Knows four to six words

18 Months Old

Fine Motor

- Turns pages of book

Gross Motor

- Can walk up steps

Language

- Can point to four body parts
- Knows 10 to 20 words

Safety Education

- Advise parent to learn infant cardiopulmonary resuscitation (CPR; basic life support [BLS] course)
- Avoid heating formula in the microwave
- Do not leave a baby on the changing table (e.g., to answer phone)

- Do not position cribs next to strings or cords. When the child is crawling, hide electrical cords
  - Close toilet seats (safety lock); lock bathroom doors; lock all cleaning products
- Turn pot handles away from the edge of stove; use rear burners on the stove
- Use safety locks for stove handles, low cabinets, and doors

Choking

- Remove objects smaller than 2 inches
- Cut up food into small pieces (e.g., hot dogs, carrots, grapes)
- Examples of choking sources are: grapes, raw carrots, hot dogs, latex balloons, coins, buttons
- Avoid giving hard candy to children younger than 6 years of age
- Encourage at least one parent to attend infant BLS course

Car Safety (Table 20.2)

- Infants and toddlers up to the age of 2 years should be in a rear-facing car seat.
- Safest place in the car for infant or child younger than 13 years of age is in the back seat.
- Avoid used infant safety seat if its parts are missing or if it is damaged.
- Air bags in cars can cause serious brain injury if they hit the child's head or neck area.
- Turn off the air bag on the front seat if the person who is using the seat is under the weight limit, which is usually set at 100 lbs (check car manual).

Table 20.2 Car Safety Seats

Age Group	Type of Seat	Notes
Infants and toddlers	Rear-facing car seat with three-point seatbelt until age of 2 years. Convertible car seats can be used as rear-facing and front-facing car seats	Children under age 2 years are 75% less likely to be killed or injured in a car crash if they are in a rear-facing seat
Toddler to preschool	Safest if rear-facing seat up to age of 2 years. Forward-facing car seat with three-point safety harness Weight limit ranges from 80 to 100 lbs (depends on brand)	Children aged 2 years or older (or if over the weight or height limit for rear-facing car seat) until they have reached the weight limit
School age	Booster seats (belt-positioning booster seats)	Use until child has reached 4 feet, 9 inches or is 8 to 12 years of age Shoulder belt should cross the middle of the child's chest and shoulders
Older child to teenager	Seat belt with lap belt	All children aged 13 years or younger should sit in the back seat and use a seat belt with the lap belt

Other

- Chronic exposure to second-hand smoke increases rates of SIDS, otitis media, bronchitis, pneumonia, and wheezing and coughing. It also affects lung development and exacerbates asthma.

DISEASE REVIEW

Jaundice

- Jaundice at birth or within first day of life (usually due to hemolysis or bleeding in utero)
  - Infant's color is bright yellow or the soles of the feet are yellow

- Jaundice of full-term infant after 2 weeks of age
  - Bilirubin level increases too rapidly (>0.2 mg/dL per hour) or is too high; total bilirubin levels greater than 13 to 15 mg/dL

Physiological Jaundice

Also known as *neonatal unconjugated hyperbilirubinemia* and *neonatal icterus*. Jaundice first appears on the head/face (sclera is yellow) and progresses downward to the chest, abdomen, legs, and soles of the feet. Jaundice appears when bilirubin level is 5 mg/dL or higher.

Physiological jaundice starts after 24 hours and will usually clear up within 2 to 3 weeks. The total bilirubin levels in Caucasians and African American infants can peak at 7 to 9 mg/dL, but Asian infants have higher peak values (10–14 mg/dL).

Breast Milk Jaundice

Onset is later than physiological jaundice. Breast jaundice usually starts to show after 7 days of life. It peaks in 2 to 3 weeks and can take more than 1 month to clear. It is thought to be caused by insufficient breast milk intake and/or breast milk from some mothers who have a substance that slows down hepatic conjugation of bilirubin.

Bilirubin

Bilirubin (breakdown product from old RBCs) binds to the brain and the nerves (neurotoxic). Elevation is due to increased breakdown of fetal RBCs combined with exceeding the infant liver's capacity to conjugate bilirubin.

Treatment Plan

- Check bilirubin level. Use noninvasive methods first (bilirubinometers).
- If suspect pathological jaundice, order serum fractionated bilirubin level, Coombs test, CBC, reticulocyte count, and peripheral smear.
- Treatment is usually not needed. Keep baby well hydrated with breast milk or formula.
- Feed infant every 2 to 3 hours (10–12 times per day).
- First-line treatment is phototherapy. Light used in the blue spectrum is the most effective wavelength. The skin converts bilirubin into a nontoxic water-soluble form so that it is excreted in the urine.
- All newborns should be seen for follow-up within the first 5 days of life to check for jaundice.

Complications

- *Kernicterus*: Neurological disorder caused by high levels of unbound bilirubin in circulation that damaged the infant's CNS. Associated with severe mental retardation and seizures.

Physiological Anemia of Infancy

Hemoglobin drops at the lowest level in life (nadir) at 6 to 8 weeks of age. Full-term infants' hemoglobin decreases from 9 to 11 g/dL. Caused by the temporary decrease in erythropoietin production by the kidneys. When the hemoglobin level is at its lowest, it stimulates erythropoietin production, which prompts the bone marrow to produce more RBCs.

Congenital Lacrimal Duct Obstruction (Dacryostenosis)

Also known as *congenital nasolacrimal duct obstruction*. Occurs in up to 20% of newborns. Usually spontaneously resolves within 6 months in the majority (95%) of infants.

Classic Case

An infant's mother reports persistent tearing and crusting in the morning on one or both of the baby's eyes. When the lacrimal duct is palpated, reflux of mucoid discharge or tears may be seen. Yellow- to green-colored purulent eye discharge is abnormal and is due to secondary bacterial infection.

Acute Dacryocystitis

Look for redness, warmth, tenderness, and swelling on one of the lacrimal ducts. Culture discharge and treat with systemic antibiotics for 7 to 10 days. Usually caused by streptococcal or staphylococcal organisms. Severe cases may spread and cause orbital cellulitis.

Treatment Plan

- *Lacrimal sac massage*: Place finger on lacrimal sac and massage downward toward mouth. Perform maneuver two to three times per day.

Infant Colic (Rule of 3s)

The goal when evaluating an infant with colic is to rule out conditions causing pain and/or discomfort, infections, environment, and formula "allergy."

- Crying and irritability lasting a total of 3 hours a day in an infant younger than 3 months. Crying usually occurs at the same time each day.
- Crying occurs more than 3 days in a week.
- Colic usually resolves by 3 to 4 months.

Coarctation of the Aorta

Congenital narrowing of a portion of the aorta. Usual location is the aortic area that is distal to the subclavian artery. Newborn may be asymptomatic if mild case or patent ductus arteriosus (PDA). Severe cases will have heart failure or shock when PDA closes. Up to 30% of infants with this condition have Turner's syndrome. Female infants should get tested with karyotype analysis.

Screening

Compare the femoral and brachial pulses simultaneously. Absence or delay of the femoral pulse when it is compared to the brachial pulse is diagnostic. Neonate is pale, irritable, dyspneic, and diaphoretic. If abnormal, order cardiac echocardiogram, EKG, and chest x-ray.

Older Infants

May be asymptomatic. Take BP measurements of both arms and thighs.

- *Normal finding*: Systolic BP is higher in legs than in arms.
- *Abnormal*: Systolic BP higher in arms than in thighs. Palpate pulse in all four extremities. There is a delay or change in amplitude of pulses. Bounding radial pulses compared with femoral pulse.

Developmental Dysplasia of the Hip (DDH)

There is higher risk with breech births, female gender, family history, oligohydramnios.

Screening

Birth to 3 Months

- Look for asymmetry in the creases of the legs. Examine infant front and back without diapers. Check that gluteal, thigh, and popliteal folds match.

Ortolani Maneuver/Test

Hold each knee and place your middle finger over the greater trochanter (outer thigh over the hips). Rotate the hips in the frog leg position (abduction, then adduction). During abduction, resistance may be felt at 30 to 40 degrees.

- *Positive*: "Click" or "clunk" sound and/or if examiner palpates the trochanter becoming displaced (temporarily) from the hip socket

Barlow Maneuver/Test

Place your index and middle finger over the greater trochanter. Gently push both knees together at midline downward, then pull upward. Will hear "clunk" sound when the trochanter slips back into the acetabulum (reducible dislocated hip).

- *Positive*: "Clunk" sound or palpating trochanter being displaced by the index/middle finger

Abnormal

- If either screening exam is positive, refer to a pediatric orthopedist. Order an ultrasound of the hips.

Older Infants

- Look for leg that is turned outward.
- One femur appears shorter when infant is supine (Galeazzi sign).
- Hip has limited range of motion.
- *Abnormal*: If preceding findings are present, order a hip ultrasound and refer to orthopedic specialist.

Note

Avoid performing both tests too many times per visit because the ligaments on the hips can become damaged.

EXAM TIPS

- **Ortolani and Barlow are screening tests for DDH. Positive sign is if "click" or "clunk" sound is heard and/or if examiner palpates the trochanter becoming displaced (temporarily) from the hip socket. Refer to pediatric orthopedic specialist.**
- **Asymmetry of thigh/gluteal folds: Rule out congenital hip dysplasia or hip fracture.**
- **Rolls from front to back and back to front at 6 months.**
- **Plays pat-a-cake and peek-a-boo at 9 months.**

21

Pediatrics Review: Toddlers (Ages 2 to 3 Years)

DANGER SIGNALS

Neuroblastoma

Most common presentation is a painful abdominal (retroperitoneal or hepatic) mass that is fixed, firm, irregular, and frequently crosses the midline. The most common site is the adrenal medulla (sits on top of the kidneys). About half of patients present with metastatic disease. May be accompanied by weight loss, fever, Horner's syndrome (miosis, ptosis, anhidrosis), periorbital ecchymoses ("racoon eyes"), bone pain, hypertension, others. Most are diagnosed in children between the ages of 1 and 4 years. Elevated urinary catecholamines and anemia. Initial imaging test is the ultrasound. Refer to nephrologist.

Wilms' Tumor (Nephroblastoma)

Asymptomatic abdominal mass that extends from the flank toward the midline. The non-tender and smooth mass rarely crosses the midline (of the abdomen). Some patients have abdominal pain and hematuria. One fourth of patients have hypertension. Higher incidence in Black, female children. Peak age is 2 to 3 years. The most common renal malignancy in children. While performing the abdominal exam, palpate gently to avoid rupturing the renal capsule (causes bleeding and seeding of abdomen with cancer cells). Initial imaging test is an abdominal ultrasound.

Epiglottitis

Acute and rapid onset of high fever, chills, and toxicity. Child complains of severe sore throat and drooling saliva. Will not eat or drink, muffled (hot potato) voice, and anxiety. Characteristic tripod sitting posture with hyperextended neck with open-mouth breathing. Stridor, tachycardia, and tachypnea. Usually occurs between ages 2 and 6 years. Before the Hib vaccine was used, most cases were due to *Haemophilus influenzae* type b (Hib; 75%). Other pathogens are *Staphylococcus aureus, Streptococcus pyogenes*, fungi, others. Now rare due to the Hib conjugate vaccine. Prophylaxis with rifampin (duration is 4 days) for close contacts. Reportable disease to the public health department. A medical emergency. Call 911.

Osteomyelitis

More common in infants and children. Infected bone or joint is red, swollen, warm, and tender to touch. Patient is febrile and irritable. If patient walks with a limp, may have infection on the hip, knee, or leg. If infection involves the upper extremities, will favor infected limb (avoids

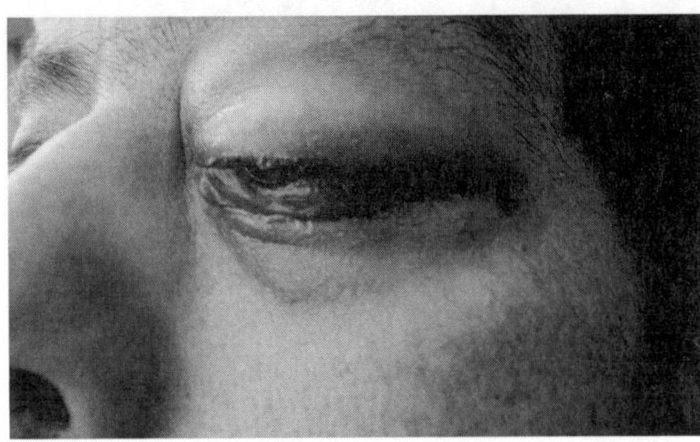

Figure 21.1 Periorbital cellulitis. This image can be found in color in the app.
Source: Courtesy of Bobjgalindo.

using the limb). Growth plate infection results in growth stunting of the affected limb. Refer for hospitalization and high-dose antibiotics.

Orbital Cellulitis

Young child complains of abrupt onset of deep eye pain that is aggravated by eye movements and is accompanied by a high fever and chills. Affected eye will appear to be bulging (proptosis or exophthalmos). Extraocular eye movements (EOMs) exam will be abnormal due to ophthalmoplegia (limited movement of eyeball) form infection of the ocular fat pads and muscles. More common in younger children. Ethmoid sinusitis is more likely to cause orbital cellulitis compared with frontal/maxillary sinusitis. Can be life-threatening. A serious complication of rhinosinusitis, acute otitis media, or dental infections. Refer to emergency department (ED). CT scan or MRI is done in the ED.

Pretectal Cellulitis (Periorbital Cellulitis; Figure 21.1)

More common than orbital cellulitis. An infection of the anterior portion of the eyelid that does not involve the orbit/globe or the eyes. Rarely causes serious complications (compared with orbital cellulitis). Younger children are most likely to be affected. Young child complains of the new onset of red swollen eyelids and eye pain (sometimes none). Eye movements do not cause pain and EOM exam is normal (both are abnormal with orbital cellulitis). No visual impairment. May be hard to distinguish from orbital cellulitis. Refer to ED.

Child Abuse

The majority of perpetrators are parents (82%), with other relatives accounting for 6%. About 16% of the perpetrators are persons whom the child is exposed to such as day care staff and unmarried partners. Multiple healed skull and/or rib fractures. Greenstick fractures. Bruises in the trunk area.

Delay in seeking medical care. Explanations for injuries inconsistent with presentation. Infants and children who are developmentally or physically disabled are at higher risk. Nurses, nurse practitioners, and several other professionals are required to report suspected or actual child abuse to authorities.

U.S. Health Statistics: Toddlers

Top Three Causes of Death

Ages 1 to 4 Years

- Accidents or unintentional injuries
- Congenital and genetic anomalies
- Assault (homicide) (Heron, 2016)

Cancer in Children

Top Three Cancers in Children

- Leukemia (34%)
- Brain and nervous system tumors (27%)
- Neuroblastoma (7%)

The most common cancer in children is leukemia. The most common type of leukemia in children is acute lymphocytic leukemia (ALL). The remaining cases are due to acute myelogenous leukemia (AML). Medulloblastomas are the most common type of childhood brain cancer (most occur before age 10 years). The most common renal malignancy in children is Wilms' tumor.

GROWTH AND DEVELOPMENT

Table 21.1 summarizes normal and abnormal childhood development from birth through 5 years of age. See Chapter 20 for corresponding discussions of newborn through 1 year, and Chapter 22 for preschool and school-age child, ages 4 and older.

2 Years Old

Language

- Speaks in two- to three-word sentences (intelligible mostly by family)
- Understands simple commands
- Knows first name

Fine Motor

- Stacks six cubes
- Can copy straight line

Gross Motor

- Goes up stairs using same foot
- Runs, jumps, and climbs
- Is very active and energetic

Behaviors

- Temper tantrums are common at this age
- Easily frustrated and says "no" often; oppositional behaviors
- May have a favorite stuffed toy (transitional object)
- Toilet training is now in progress
- Report loss of speech, social skills, or previously learned skills; flapping hands; avoids social interaction (rule out autism)

3 Years Old

Language

- Speaks in complete sentences using three to five words
- Speech is understood by most strangers
- Knows full name, age, sexual identity
- Magical thinking is prominent at this age (ages 3–5 years); may have an imaginary friend; a girl may think that she is a fairy with special powers

Fine Motor

- Copies a circle (but not a cross)
- Can throw a ball overhead
- Can stack nine cubes

Gross Motor

- Pedals a tricycle
- Knows three numbers and three colors
- Walks up (ascends) stairs with alternating feet

Behaviors

- Freud classified this age as the "Oedipal stage" (phallic stage): The child expresses the desire to marry the parent of the opposite sex; occurs between the ages of 3 and 5 years (preschool)
- Plays with other children, (group play) but does not like to share toys or to take turns
- Imagination is becoming more active (pretends that a broom is a "horse")

Table 21.1 Growth and Development Milestones: Infancy Through Preschool

Age	Characteristics	Abnormal
Neonate	Strong reflexes. Minimum of six to eight bowel movements per day. Urinates eight times a day.	Jaundice at birth (hemolysis). High-pitched cry. Irritable. "Floppy" (hypotonic). Poor reflexes.
3rd month	Smiles. Able to coo. Makes gurgling sounds. Can hold head up. Starts to recognize parents.	Inability to hold head up. Avoids eye contact. Floppy.
6th month	Sits up without support. Rolls in both directions (front to back, back to front). Says single-syllable sounds "ba, da, ma." Tries to get things out of reach by "raking" (uses palms to reach).	Lack of babbling. Does not laugh. Inability to turn head past midline (180 degrees).
9th month	Pincer grasp (fine motor). Plays "pat a cake" and "peek-a-boo." Says "good-bye." May be afraid of strangers (can be clingy). Can stand holding on. Crawls.	Infantile reflexes strong. Persistence of primitive reflexes (startle, fencing, etc.). Does not babble. Does not bear weight on legs with support. Unable to sit with help.
1 year (12 months)	Supports own weight. Walks with hands held. Parallel play. Separation anxiety. Can "climb" stairs by crawling up or down. Starts to cruise (moves from one piece of furniture to the other for support).	Unable to support own weight. Lack of babbling. No response to smiles, poor eye contact, loss of previously learned skills (autism).
2 years	Walks. Runs. Climbs stairs up and down on own by holding onto handrails. Speech mostly understood by family. Follows two- or three-step instructions. Copies a line.	Unable to speak meaningful two-word "sentences." Does not understand simple commands. Loss of speech, social skills, previously learned behaviors and/or does not say words by 16 months (autism).
3 years	Speaks three- to four-word sentences; understood by strangers. Copies a circle with crayon or pencil. Rides tricycle. Builds towers of more than six blocks. Runs and climbs easily.	Speech hard to understand or unclear speech. Unable to understand simple commands. Falls down often. Does not speak in sentences. No eye contact. Loses skills he or she once had.
4 years	Draw a cross. Draws person with three body parts. Plays "Mom" and "Dad." Hops and stands on one foot up to 2 seconds. Cooperates with other children. Names some colors and some numbers.	Unable to speak in full sentences. Inability to skip, run, hop. Cannot put on clothes without help. Unable to play with other kids. Unable to follow three-part commands.
5 years	Can draw a person with six body parts. Counts 10 or more things. Is aware of gender. Speaks clearly.	Unusually withdrawn. Not active. Trouble focusing on one activity for more than 5 minutes.

Source: Centers for Disease Control and Prevention (2016).

HEALTH EDUCATION, SAFETY, AND SCREENING

Nutrition

Limit fruit juice intake. Do not serve whole raw carrots or whole hot dogs. Cut solid food into bite-size pieces. Avoid hard foods, such as nuts, gum drops, jelly beans, grapes (cut in quarters), and hard candies, because they can cause choking. Have regular mealtimes and snacks.

Toilet Training

Clues that a child is ready: Child is walking, can reach potty chair, indicates when diaper is dirty, child can pull down his own pants, can stay dry for up to 2 hours at a time, interested about the toilet or potty seat. Make sure that child can understand basic instructions.

Most children are ready for "potty" training at 18 to 24 months. Some children may not be ready until 36 months of age. During toilet training, signs that a child is ready to use the potty are squirming, holding genital area, or squatting.

Most children master daytime bladder and bowel control by age 3 to 4 years. Nighttime control of urine is usually the last toileting skill that is mastered. Complete nighttime control may not happen until child is 4 to 5 years of age. If a child who is 5 years of age or older is not dry at night, the child needs to be evaluated.

Car Safety

- Infants from birth to age 2 years: As stated by the American Academy of Pediatrics (AAP), all infants and toddlers should ride in rear-facing car safety seats until the age of 2 years.
  - Air-bag safety: Never place an infant younger than age 1 (or less than 20 lbs or 9 kg) on the front seat of a car.
- Toddlers and preschooler (up to 40 lbs or about 18 kg): Place car safety seat on the back seat facing forward. Make sure anchors and tethers are used correctly.
- Children younger than age 12 should be restrained in the back seat.

Safety Education

- Use rear burners on stove. Turn pot handles away from reach.
- Child should be supervised at all times.
- Hold child's hand when crossing the street or when shopping.
- Keep tools and sharp objects out of reach. Inspect toys for loose parts or breakage.
- Water safety education needed. Put fences around pools. Never leave child alone in the pool.

Autism

Signs of autism spectrum disorder may appear as early as 18 months. Screening starts at age 18 to 24 months. Usually, autism becomes more apparent in early childhood (ages 2 to 6 years).

Five behaviors to look for:

- Does not point/wave/grasp by 12 months
- No babbling or cooing (by 12 months). Does not say single words (by 16 months)
- Does not say two-word phrases on his own (by 24 months)
- Any loss of language or social skills (by 24 months)
- Does not gesture (waving, grasping, pointing) at 24 months

Classic Case

An autistic 3-year-old boy is enrolled in a preschool program. The mother goes inside the school to drop the child off at the classroom. After she gives him a hug, she leaves the room. How would the child react after his mother leaves?

- At this age, a 3-year-old boy (who is not autistic) would most likely cry, protest, and cling to his mother's legs when she tries to leave.
- An autistic child will not protest, cling, or cry when his mother leaves (as would be expected in a child who does not have autism). If the mother hugs him, an autistic 3-year-old child will probably hold his body stiffly and not return the hug. Some may push the mother away because they do not like to be touched.

EXAM TIPS

- **Wilms' tumor (crosses midline) is a congenital tumor of the kidneys. More common in African American girls.**
- **Epiglottitis presentation: Sitting posture with hyperextended neck with open-mouth breathing.**
- **Speech of a 2-year-old is understood mostly by family members.**
- **Speech of a 3-year-old can be understood by strangers.**
- **Three-year-old can ride a tricycle. Can ride a bicycle at the age of 6 to 7 years.**
- **Three-year-old can copy a circle. (An easy way to memorize this fact is that when you take the "3" and join the two halves, it forms a circle.)**
- **Four-year-old can copy a cross (the number "4" resembles a cross at the center).**
- **Oedipal stage is when the child (age 3–6 years) expresses the desire to marry the parent of the opposite sex.**
- **Can draw a "stick person" with three body parts by age 4 years.**
- **Can draw a person with at least six body parts at age of 5 years.**
- **Recognize autistic child behavior (see "Classic Case").**

22

Pediatrics Review: School-Age Children (Including Preschool)

⚠ DANGER SIGNALS

Kawasaki Disease/Syndrome

Onset of high fever (up to 104°F) and enlarged lymph nodes in the neck. Bright-red rash (more obvious on groin area). Conjunctivitis (dry, no discharge), dry cracked lips, "strawberry tongue." Swollen hands and feet. After fever subsides, skin peels off hands and feet. Treated with high-dose aspirin and gamma globulin.

Most cases (75%) occur in children younger the age of 5 years. Resolves within 4 to 8 weeks but may have serious sequelae, such as aortic dissection, aneurysms of the coronary arteries, and blood clots. Close follow-up with pediatric cardiologist done for several years because effects may not be apparent until child is older (or an adult).

Leukemia

Complains of extreme fatigue and weakness. Pale skin and easy bruising. May have petechial bleeding (pinpoint to small red spots). May have bleeding gums and nosebleeds. Some have bone or joint pain, lymphadenopathy, or swelling in the abdomen. The most common type in children is acute lymphocytic leukemia. Leukemias are the most common type of cancer in children and adolescents.

Acute Lymphocytic Leukemia (ALL)

Fast-growing cancer of the lymphoblasts, which are immature lymphocytes. CBC will show very high WBC count (>50,000 cells/mm^3). Girls have slightly higher chance of cure compared with boys. African American and Hispanic children tend to have a lower cure rate compared with children from other races.

Acute Myelogenous Leukemia (AML)

Fast-growing cancer of the bone morrow that affects immature or precursor blood cells, such as myeloblasts (WBCs), monoblasts (macrophages, monocytes), erythroblasts (RBCs), and megakaryoblasts (platelets). Children with Down syndrome who have AML tend to have better cure rates, especially if the child is younger than age 4 years.

Reye's Syndrome

History of febrile viral illness (chickenpox, influenza) and aspirin or salicylate intake (Pepto-Bismol, etc.) in a child. Abrupt onset with quick progression. Death can occur within a few hours to a few days. Mortality rate of up to 52%. Although most cases are in children, disease has been seen in teenagers and adults. This disease is now rare.

Five Stages of Progression

- *Stage 1*: Severe vomiting, diarrhea, lethargy, stupor, elevated ALT and AST
- *Stage 2*: Personality changes, irritability, aggressive behavior, hyperactive reflexes
- *Stages 3 to 5*: Confusion, delirium, cerebral edema, coma, liver damage, seizures, death

Theoretical risk of Reye's syndrome after varicella immunization; avoid using aspirin before, during, and after immunization.

Down Syndrome: Atlantoaxial Instability

Up to 17% of Down syndrome patients have atlantoaxial instability (increased distance between the C1 and C2 joints). Medical clearance is necessary for sports participation. All children/ adolescents (or older) with Down syndrome who want to participate in sports need cervical spine x-rays (including lateral view). Patients with atlantoaxial instability are restricted from playing contact sports (i.e., basketball, tackle football, soccer, etc.) and other high-risk activities (i.e., trampoline jumping). Persons with Down syndrome without evidence of atlantoaxial instability may participate in low-impact sports and sports not requiring extreme balance. For more information about medical conditions and athletic participation, see Table 22.1.

Absence Seizures

Brief episodes during which child stares and suddenly stops whatever he or she is doing. If in school, teacher may tell parent that child is daydreaming and inattentive. A common type of pediatric seizure. Also called *petit mal seizure*. Refer to pediatric neurologist.

Still's Murmur

A benign systolic murmur that is described as having a vibratory or musical quality. Becomes louder in supine position or with fever. Minimal radiation. Grade I or II intensity. Most common in school-age children. Usually resolves by adolescence.

U.S. Health Statistics: School-Age Children

Top Causes of Death

Age 1 to 24 Years (Toddlers to Young Adults)

- Accidents or unintentional injuries

Table 22.1 Medical Conditions and Sports Participation

Condition	Rationale
Hypertrophic cardiomyopathy	Sudden cardiac death
Atlantoaxial instability (Down syndrome, juvenile rheumatoid arthritis)	Instability between C1 and C2
Marfan syndrome with aortic aneurysm	Aortic aneurysm risk: Lens eyes displacement, joint hypermobility
Ehlers–Danlos syndrome (vascular form)	Cerebral or cervical artery aneurysm, spondylolisthesis, joint hypermobility
Acute rheumatic fever with carditis	Worsens condition, heart inflamed
Mitral valve prolapse, especially if significant mitral valve pathology	Sudden cardiac death
Fever	Heat stroke
Infectious diarrhea	Contagious
Pink eye	Contagious

Note: Some are approved to play low-contact or noncontact sports. List is not all inclusive.

Source: American Academy of Pediatrics (2008).

Age 5 to 14 Years

- Accidents or unintentional injuries
- Cancers
- Developmental and genetic conditions

IMMUNIZATIONS

Preschool (Ages 4 to 6 Years)

- Administer vaccines: Measles, mumps, rubella (MMR); varicella, inactivated poliovirus vaccine (IPV); and diphtheria, tetanus, acellular pertussis (DTaP)
- If history of chickenpox and documented on chart by health provider, does not need varicella.
- If child is 7 years or older, give Tdap instead of DTaP.

Middle School (Ages 11 to 12 years; Table 22.2)

- Tdap booster
- Meningococcal conjugate vaccine/Menactra (MCV4)
- Human papillomavirus (HPV) vaccine/Gardasil

Notes

- HPV vaccine is now indicated for both girls and boys. Need a total of three doses of vaccine. Gardasil used for both genders.
- Age 13 to 14 years (or older): Give Tdap if did not receive it at age 11 to 12 years.
- If no history of varicella immunization (or the disease), then give the varicella vaccine.
- If child did not complete hepatitis B series (fewer than three doses), administer hepatitis B booster. Do not restart hepatitis B series.

Meningococcal Vaccines

- There are six types of meningococcal vaccines, only two of which are discussed here.
  - MenACWY-D (Menactra): Youngest age is 9 months or older
  - MenACWY-CRM (Menveo): Youngest age is 2 months or older
- Administer Menactra or Menveo vaccine first dose age 11 to 12 years. If missing, catch-up age is 13 to 15 years. Booster (second dose) at age 16 years.
- Also used for first-year college students (living in dorms) and people with asplenia, functional asplenia (sickle cell), splenectomy, HIV infection, complement deficiencies, and others at higher risk.

Primary Series of Vaccination: Missing or Not Done

After Seventh Birthday (Never Been Vaccinated)

- Td (three doses primary, then every 10 years); substitute Tdap for one dose of Td (once in a lifetime)
- IPV (three doses)
- Hepatitis B (three doses)
- MMR (two doses)
- Varicella (two doses) if no history of chickenpox
- HPV (three doses; give if younger than age 26 years)

Table 22.2 Immunizations: Age 10 and Older*

Vaccine	Immunizations
Hepatitis B	Total of three doses over 6 months. If missing a booster, give until total of three doses. Do not repeat series.
Measles, mumps, rubella (MMR)	Give second dose (if needs to catch up). Live virus precautions.
Varicella	Give second dose (if needs to catch up) if no proof of varicella. Live virus precautions.
Tetanus	Give Tdap at age 11 to 12 years (or older if missed this dose). Replace one Td booster with Tdap.
Hepatitis A	Needed for high-risk groups (homosexuals) and endemic areas (certain areas of southwestern United States).
Influenza	Needed annually after age of 6 months.
Human papillomavirus	Indicated for boys and girls. Give first dose at age 11 to 12 years. Catch-up dose at age 13 years if missed. Gardasil: Need three doses. Give second dose 1 to 2 months after first dose. Give third dose 6 months after the first dose.
Meningococcal	First does at age 11 to 12 years. Give booster at age 16 years. Meningococcal conjugate vaccine (MCV4) needed for all college freshmen living in dormitories.

*This table is a simplified version and is designed for studying for the certification exams only. Do not use this table as a guideline for clinical practice.

Source: Adapted from Centers for Disease Control and Prevention (2017).

GROWTH AND DEVELOPMENT

4 Years Old (Preschool)

Fine Motor

- Can copy a cross
- Draws a person with two parts

Gross Motor

- Rides a bicycle; hops on one foot
- Dresses with little assistance

Other

- According to Piaget, children between 1 and 4 years are at the preoperational stage
- Child is ready to learn the alphabet, spell or read short words, and learn basic math concepts

5 Years Old (Preschool)

Fine Motor

- Copies square
- Can draw a person with four body parts

Gross Motor

- Can ride a bicycle (use bike helmet)
- Likes to help parent with certain household chores; child at this age likes to help adults; can dress and undress self

6 Years Old (Kindergarten)

Gross Motor

- Copies a triangle (copies a diamond at age 7)
- Ties shoes
- Rides a bicycle

Age 7 to 11 Years (Middle Childhood)

Freud classified this age group under the "latency stage." The major task for this age group is to succeed in school and to interact with their peer group. May have a "best" friend(s). Starts to think of the future. Some girls may start puberty at age 8 years. According to Piaget, this age group is in concrete operations stage (early abstract thinking starts at about age of 11 years).

TV and Electronics Use

Limit to 2 hours a day or less. Use parental-control software.

DISEASE REVIEW

Autism

This is a developmental disorder that affects the normal development of communication and social skills. The exact cause is unknown. Autism affects more boys than girls. There are several theories about the cause, but they are unproven (thimerosal, mercury, vaccines, etc.). Autism is hard to diagnose before the age of 18 months.

Classic Case

Child who is extremely sensitive to noises, touch, smells, and/or textures. Will refuse to wear tight or rough-textured clothes because they feel "itchy." Prefers to be alone. Has poor eye contact. Does not interact with others. Slow to poor language development. Has repeated body movements such as flapping arms. Some may appear to be progressing normally but suddenly regress. Language, physical, and social skills disintegrate.

Treatment Plan

- Refer to psychiatrist or psychologist for testing and evaluation
- Intensive rehabilitation needed at younger ages (i.e., occupational therapy [OT], physical therapy [PT], speech therapy)
- Medications: Risperidone (Risperdal) is an antipsychotic that is prescribed for some patients

Fragile X Syndrome

Classic Case

Child has large head circumference and mental retardation. Delayed physical developmental milestones, such as crawling and walking. Autism is common. Hyperactive behavior exhibited. Tends to avoid eye contact. Patient has a long face with prominent forehead, jaw, and large ears. Large body with flat feet.

Treatment Plan

- Refer for genetic testing
- Refer patient to developmental pediatrician or psychiatrist/psychologist for psychosocial, behavioral, and mental evaluation

Hand–Foot–Mouth Disease

A common acute viral illness that mainly affects children younger than 10 years of age. Most common cause is the coxsackievirus A16. Spread through direct contact with nasal discharge, saliva, blister fluid, or stool. Patient is most contagious during the first week of the illness.

Classic Case

Acute onset of fever, severe sore throat, headache, and anorexia. Multiple small blisters appear on the hands, feet, and diaper area. Ulcers are present inside the mouth, throat, tonsils, and the tongue. Child will complain of sore throat and mouth pain with acidic foods.

Treatment Plan

- Treatment is symptomatic; self-limited illness; complete recovery usually occurs within 5 to 7 days.
- Ibuprofen or acetaminophen for pain and fever every 4 to 6 hours; do not use aspirin
- Use salt-water gargle (1/2 teaspoon salt in one glass of warm water)
- Drink cold fluids (avoid soda, orange or lemon juice, tomato juice)

Childhood Rashes

See Table 22.3. Be familiar with the appearance of these for the exam.

Table 22.3 Childhood Rashes

Condition	Appearance of Rash
Hand–foot–mouth disease	Multiple small blisters appear on the hands and the feet. Small ulcers are inside the mouth, throat, tonsils, and the tongue.
Impetigo	"Honey-colored" crusted lesions. Fragile bullae (bullous type). Pruritic.
Measles (rubeola)	Koplik's spots are small white papules inside the cheeks (buccal mucosa) by the rear molars.
Varicella	Generalized rash in different stages; new lesions appear daily. Papules → vesicles → pustules → crusts. Pruritic. Very contagious.
Scarlet fever	"Sandpaper" rash with sore throat. Strawberry tongue is not specific (but also seen in Kawasaki disease).
Pediculosis capitis or head lice	Ovoid white nits on hair hard to dislodge. Red papules that are very itchy and nits are initially located in the hairline area behind the neck and the ears.
Molluscum contagiosum	Smooth wax-like round (dome-shaped) papules 5 mm in size. Central umbilication with white plug.
Scabies	Located in interdigital webs of hands, waist, axillae, penis, etc. Very pruritic, especially at night.

Functional Constipation (Encopresis)

Rome IV criteria diagnosis of functional constipation in children (age 4 years or older; criteria are slightly different for infants and toddlers up to 4 years of age). Must meet two (or more) of the criteria at least once per week (for at least 1 month).

- History of withholding of stool
- History of painful or hard bowel movements
- History of large-diameter stools that may obstruct the toilet
- Presence of large fecal mass in rectum
- Two or fewer defecations in toilet per week
- At least one episode of fecal incontinence per week (thin fluid with feces that bypasses a large stool mass and leaks around it); ask patient whether fecal soiling of underwear

- Up to 80% of children with functional fecal incontinence may also have constipation (Sood, 2017).
- Order a plain film (x-ray) of the abdomen to check for retained stool.

EXAM TIPS

- All 11- to 12-year-old children should be vaccinated with single dose of quadrivalent meningococcal vaccine (MenACWY); brand names are Menactra or Menveo.
- Recognize hand–foot–mouth disease, scabies, impetigo, and varicella.
- Recognize how fragile X syndrome looks.
- Immunizations are needed at age 11 to 12 years (Tdap, HPV, MCV4).
- Child at age of 11 years is at "early abstract" thinking stage (Piaget).
- Recognize molluscum photos. Molluscum is caused by the poxvirus.
- HPV vaccine (Gardasil): Know that youngest age group for vaccination is 9 years.
- Rubeola is measles. Koplik's spot appearance is described in Table 22.3.

23

Adolescents Review

⚠ DANGER SIGNALS

Acetaminophen Poisoning (Intentional Ingestion)

Acetaminophen damages the liver, resulting in mild to severe fulminant liver failure. Acetaminophen also known as *paracetamol* and sold as Tylenol and others.

- Stage 1 (up to 24 hours after overdose): Patients are usually asymptomatic but may have nausea and vomiting and, with very large doses, lethargy, and malaise.
- Stage II (24–72 hours after overdose): Patients complain of right upper quadrant pain and have high LFTs, PT, and INR, with possible nephrotoxicity (elevated BUN, creatinine) and/or pancreatitis (serum amylase and lipase elevated). Most deaths from liver failure occur within 72 to 96 hours.

With acute overdose, serum acetaminophen concentration should be measured as soon as possible but at least 4 hours must have passed since ingestion to obtain accurate blood level (if less than 4 hours, blood level is not accurate). Antidote is N-acetylcysteine given intravenously.

Testicular Torsion (Acute Scrotum)

Pubertal male awakens with abrupt onset of unilateral testicular pain that increases in severity. Pain may radiate to the lower abdomen and/or groin. Almost all patients (90%) also have nausea and vomiting. Ischemic changes result in severe scrotal edema, redness, induration, and testicular pain. Ipsilateral (same-side) cremasteric reflex is absent. Highest incidence is during puberty. UA is negative for WBCs. Doppler ultrasound is the initial diagnostic test. Testicle is not functional after 24 hours if not repaired. Refer to ED. This is a surgical emergency.

Testicular Cancer

Teenage to adult male complains of a testicular or scrotal mass that may be tender to touch or asymptomatic. Some patients may have testicular discomfort, but not pain. The patient reports a sensation of heaviness in the affected testicle. The affected testicle has a firm texture. More common in males from the age of 15 to 35 years. Cryptorchidism is a strong risk factor.

Hodgkin's Lymphoma

Patient presents with enlarged and painless cervical, axillary, and supraclavicular lymphadenopathy associated with fever (Pel-Ebstein sign) and night sweats. May report having severe pain on or over malignant areas a few minutes after drinking alcohol. The most common cancers in teens aged 15 to 19 years are Hodgkin's lymphoma (16%) and germ cell tumors (16%) such as testicular and ovarian cancer.

NORMAL FINDINGS

Adolescence

Defined as the onset of puberty until sexual maturity.

Most Common Cause of Death

- Accidents (i.e., motor vehicle crashes)

Puberty

The period in life when secondary sexual characteristics start to develop because of hormonal stimulation. Girls' ovaries start producing estrogen and progesterone. Boys' testes start producing testosterone. All of these changes result in reproductive capability.

Girls

- Precocious puberty if puberty starts before age 8 years
- Delayed puberty if no breast development (Tanner stage II) by age 12 years

Growth Spurt

Majority of somatic changes occur between the ages of 10 and 13 years.

- Majority of skeletal growth occurs before menses. Afterward, growth slows down.
- Girls start their growth spurts 1 year earlier than boys.

Growth Timeline

Breast development → peak growth acceleration → menarche. Most of a girl's height is gained before menarche. Skeletal growth in girls is considered complete within 2 years after menarche.

Mittelschmerz

Unilateral midcycle pelvic pain that is caused by an enlarged ovarian follicle (or ruptured follicle). Pain may last a few hours to a few days. May occur intermittently.

Menarche

- Average age is about 12 years (12.34 years) in the United States (range age 8–15 years)
- The first few months after the onset of menarche, it is common to have irregular periods because of irregular ovulation (may skip a month or longer intervals, lighter bleeding)
- After Tanner stage II starts (breast bud stage), girls start menses within 1 to 2 years
- Delayed puberty if no secondary sexual characteristics appear by age 12 to 13 years

Menstrual Cycle

- Average duration is 28 days; in younger teens, cycles range from 21 to 45 days; in adults, they can range from 21 to 35 days
- Average duration of menstrual bleeding is about 3 to 5 days (range 2–7 days)
- Day 1 of the menstrual cycle starts as spotting, then blood flow becomes heavier for 2 to 3 days, and then bleeding lightens until it stops
- The most fertile period in the cycle is about 3 days before and during ovulation (days 11–14)

Dysmenorrhea

- Painful periods due to severe menstrual cramps caused by high levels of prostaglandins
- Treatment is use of heating pads and nonsteroidal anti-inflammatory drugs (NSAIDs) such as ibuprofen (Advil, Motrin) and naproxen (Aleve)

Boys

- Precocious puberty if starts before age 9 years
- Delayed puberty if no testicular/scrotal growth by age 14 years

Growth Spurt

- Boys' growth spurts are 1 year later than girls' (ages 11–15 years)

Spermarche

- Average age is 13.3 years

TANNER STAGES (TABLE 23.1)

Boys

- Stage I: Prepuberty
- Stage II: Testes begin to enlarge, with increased rugation of scrotum
- Stage III: Penis elongates; testicular/scrotal growth continues; scrotal color starts to darken.
- Stage IV: Penis thickens and increases in size; testes are larger and scrotal skin darker
- Stage V: Adult pattern

Girls

- Stage I: Prepuberty
- Stage II: Breast bud (onset of thelarche, or breast development)
- Stage III: Breast tissue and areola are in one mound
- Stage IV: Areola/nipples separate and form a secondary mound
- Stage V: Adult pattern

Pubic Hair (Both Genders)

- Stage I: Prepuberty
- Stage II: Sparse growth of straight hair that is easily counted
- Stage III: Hair is darker and starts to curl
- Stage IV: Hair is curly but not on medial thigh yet as in adult; hair is coarser
- Stage V: Adult pattern; hair spreads to medial thigh and lower abdomen

Table 23.1 Tanner Stages

Stage	Girls	Boys	Pubic Hair
I	Prepuberty	Prepuberty	None
II	Breast bud	Testes enlarges Scrotal rugae	Few straight, fine hairs
III	Breast and areola One mound	Penis lengthens	Darker, coarse Starts to curl
VI	Breast and areola Secondary mound	Penis widens	Thicker, curly Darker, coarse
V	Adult pattern	Adult pattern	Adult pattern Spreads to inner thigh

IMMUNIZATION SCHEDULE FOR ADOLESCENTS

The schedule in Table 23.2 is for patients who did not complete immunization or were not immunized as infants.

Table 23.2 Immunization Schedule (Age 7–18 Years)

Vaccine	Immunizations
Tdap (Boostrix, Adacel)	All 11- or 12-year-olds: Give Tdap as booster, then Td every 10 years for lifetime.
HPV (Gardasil)	All 11- or 12-year-olds: Give to girls and boys.
	Minimum age (HPV vaccines): 9 years old
	All 11- or 12-year-olds: Give first shot. Needs two doses, from 6 to 12 months apart.
	From age 15 to 26 years needs three doses.
Meningococcal (ACWY-D [Menactra], MenACWY-CRM [Menveo], MenB-4C [Bexsero], MenB-FHbp [Trumenba])	All at age 11–12 years, give single dose of Menactra or Menveo vaccine at age 11–12 years with booster at age 16 years. Catch-up: age 13–18 years, give Menactra or Menveo. If first dose at age 13–15 years, needs booster at age 16–18 years. But if first dose at age 16 years, no booster dose is needed. Clinical discretion: Young adults 16–23 years may be vaccinated with either Bexsero or Trumenba.*
Influenza inactivated	Vaccinate everyone from age 6 months and older.
Hepatitis B (Recombivax HB)	Catch-up: Give the third dose if not completed.
Hepatitis A (HAVRIX, VAQTA)	Recommended for children with certain health or lifestyle conditions placing them at risk.
MMR	Catch-up: Give the second dose if not completed.
Varicella	If no reliable history of chickenpox (verbal OK). Live virus is contraindicated.

*Recommendations as per Centers for Disease Control and Prevention (2017). Centers for Disease Control and Prevention (CDC) Recommended Immunization Schedule for Children and Adolescents Aged 18 Years or Younger, United States, 2017

HPV, human papillomavirus; Tdap, tetanus, diphtheria, and pertussis.

Source: Adapted from CDC (2017). This table is a simplified version and is designed for studying for the certification exams only. Do not use this table as a guideline for clinical practice.

EXAM TIPS

- *Meningococcal vaccine is now required for all*, starting at age 11 to 12 years (not only for college freshmen living in dormitories).
- Antidote of acetaminophen poisoning is IV N-acetylcysteine.
- Recognize presentation of testicular torsion and testicular cancer.
- Hodgkin's lymphoma presents as enlarged lymph nodes with fever, night sweats, and pain (lymph nodes) after drinking alcohol.
- *Vaccine Adverse Event Reporting System (VAERS):* Government program to report clinically adverse events.
- Centers for Disease Control and Prevention recommends HPV vaccine for females until age 26 years; for males until age 21 years (except males who have sex with males); and for gay, bisexual, or males who have sex with males until age 26 years.

LABORATORY TESTS

Elevated Alkaline Phosphatase

Children and adolescents normally have higher blood levels compared to adults due to growing bone. It is produced by the osteoblasts.

LEGAL ISSUES

Right to Consent and Confidentiality

No parental (or guardian) consent is necessary for the following:

- Contraception
- Treatment for sexually transmitted diseases (STDs)
- Diagnosis and management of pregnancy

Emancipated Minor Criteria

These minors may give full consent as an adult without parental involvement:

- Legally married
- Active duty in the armed forces

Confidentiality

Confidentiality can be broken in the following situations:

- Gunshot wounds and stab wounds, which must be reported to the police (regardless of victim's age)
- Child abuse (actual or suspected abuse), which must be reported to the authorities
- Suicidal ideation and/or attempt (discharge to parents/guardians or hospital)
- Homicidal ideation or intent (especially mental health providers)

"Mature Minor Rule"

A mature minor is an unemancipated minor (from 15 to 17 years of age) with the mental capacity (and intelligence) to understand the consequences of a decision (such as refusing a surgical procedure or medical treatment). The mature minor has the right to refuse or to request treatment (even if the parents disagree with this decision). There are statutory and/or common laws at the state level. Each state has its own laws and statutes.

Example

A 17-year-old male who is scheduled for a procedure calls the nurse practitioner (NP) and tells her that he does not want to have the procedure. After the NP speaks with the patient and listens to his rationale (the patient understands the consequences), she decides to call the hospital's patient liaison/advocate (or ombudsman) to speak with the patient first (instead of calling the parents first).

HEALTH PROMOTION

During a physical examination or wellness visit, assess teenager for high-risk behaviors. Intensive behavior counseling is recommended. The following are high-risk behaviors to screen for:

- *Sexual activity:* Use of condoms, birth control, intimate partner violence (i.e., rape), signs/symptoms of STDs
- *Safety:* Driver safety, seatbelt/helmet use, smoking, alcohol and drug use
- *Social history:* Family, peers, school performance, work
- Signs/symptoms of depression and antisocial behaviors (i.e., gangs)

EXAM TIPS

- **Puberty starts at Tanner stage II in girls (breast bud) or boys (testicular enlargement and scrotal rugation/color starts to become darker). Puberty ends at Tanner stage V (adult stage).**
- **Tanner stage III in boys is elongation of the penis (testes continues to grow). Only Tanner stages II to IV need to be memorized for the exam.**
- **There is no need to memorize pubic hair changes for either gender. Memorize only the breast changes (girls) and the genital changes (boys).**
- **There will be one question about Tanner staging (girl or boy).**
- **Adolescent health history is obtained from both parent and child initially, then the adolescent is interviewed alone without the parent.**
- **Memorize the criteria for an emancipated minor. Do not confuse the right to confidentiality with emancipated minor status.**
- **Recognize presentation of testicular torsion.**

DISEASE REVIEW

Primary and Secondary Amenorrhea

- *Primary amenorrhea:* No menarche by the age of 15 years (with or without development of secondary sexual characteristics). Half of cases are caused by chromosomal disorders (50%) such as Turner syndrome.
  - Puberty is delayed if there is no breast development by age 13 years, absence of pubic hair at age 14 years, and no menarche by age 15 years.
- *Secondary amenorrhea:* No menses for three cycles, or 6 months if previously had menses. Most common cause is pregnancy. Others are ovarian disorders, stress, anorexia, polycystic ovary syndrome (PCOS).

Secondary Amenorrhea Associated With Exercise and Underweight

- Excessive exercise and/or sports participation have a higher incidence of amenorrhea (and infertility) due to relative caloric deficiency
- "Female athlete triad"; anorexia nervosa/restrictive eating, amenorrhea, and osteoporosis

Labs

- Pregnancy test (serum human chorionic gonadotropin [hCG])
- Serum prolactin level (rule out prolactinoma-induced amenorrhea)
- Serum TSH; also follicle-stimulating hormone (FSH) and luteinizing hormone (LH; rule out premature ovarian failure)
- If amenorrhea for more than 6 months, measure bone density

Treatment Plan

- Educate about increasing caloric intake and decreasing exercise
- Prescribe calcium with vitamin D 1,200 to 1,500 mg daily and vitamin E 400 IU daily

Complications

- Osteopenia/osteoporosis (stress fractures)
- Myocardial atrophy, arrhythmia (sudden death), bradycardia, hypotension
- Hypoglycemia, dehydration, electrolytes
- Lanugo (fine downy hair), telogen effluvium (hair loss), xerosis (dry skin), infertility
- Low body mass index (BMI), cachexia, anemia, respiratory failure

Anorexia Nervosa

- Usual onset is during adolescence. Involves an irrational preoccupation with and intense fear of gaining weight.
- *Two types:* Patient engages in restriction (dieting, excessive exercise) or binge eating and purging. Some examples of purging are excessive use of laxatives, enemas, diuretics, vomiting.

Clinical Findings

- Marked weight loss (BMI ≤18.5), low pulse (≤40 beats/min), vital signs unstable, hypotension
- Lanugo (increased lanugo especially in the face, back, and shoulders)
- Stress fractures (osteopenia or osteoporosis from estrogen depletion and low calcium intake)
- Swollen feet (low albumin), dizziness, abdominal bloating

EXAM TIPS

- **Recognize how anorexic patients present (i.e., lanugo, peripheral edema, amenorrhea, significant weight loss >10% of body weight).**
- **Increased risk of osteoporosis or osteopenia. For birth control, avoid Depo Provera and other progesterone-only contraceptives because they can cause bone loss.**
- **Low albumin level results in peripheral edema.**

Gynecomastia (Figure 23.1)

Excessive growth of breast tissue in males. Can involve one or both breasts. Physiological gynecomastia is benign and is more common during infancy and adolescence. Normal in up to 40% of pubertal boys (peaks at age 14). Most cases resolve spontaneously within 6 months to 2 years.

Classic Case

Pubertal to adolescent male is brought in by a parent who is concerned about gradual onset of enlarged breasts or asymmetrical breast tissue (one may be larger). Child is embarrassed and scared about breast changes. Affected breast may be tender to palpation.

Objective Findings

Round, rubbery, and mobile mound (disk-like) under the areola of both breasts. Skin has no dimpling, redness, or changes. If mass is irregular, fixed, or hard or rapid growth in breast size, or suspect secondary cause, refer to specialist.

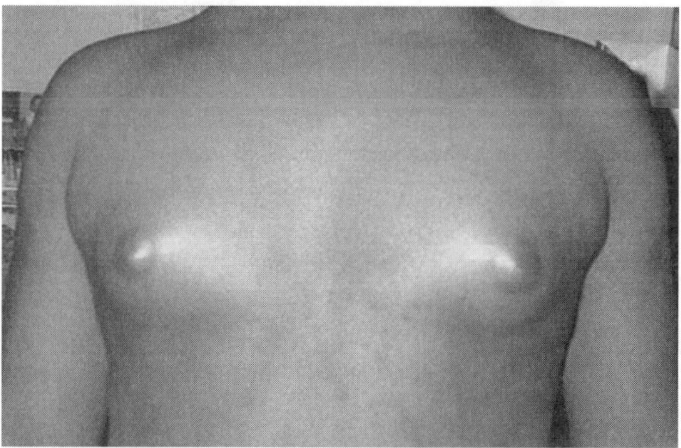

Figure 23.1 Gynecomastia (male aged 14 years).

Treatment Plan

- Evaluate for Tanner stage (check testicular size, pubic hair, axillary hair, body odor).
- Check for drug use: both illicit and prescription (i.e., steroids, cimetidine, antipsychotics).
- Rule out serious etiology (testicular or adrenal tumors, brain tumor, hypogonadism, etc.).
- Recheck patient in 6 months to monitor for changes.

Pseudogynecomastia

Bilateral enlarged breast is due to fatty tissue (adipose tissue). Common in obese boys and men. Both breasts feel soft to touch and are not tender. No breast bud or disk-like breast tissue is palpable.

Labs

None. Diagnosed by clinical presentation.

Adolescent Idiopathic Scoliosis (Figure 23.2)

Screening Test: Adam's Forward Bend Test

Lateral curvature of the spine that may be accompanied by spinal rotation. More common in girls (80% of patients). Painless and asymptomatic. Scoliosis will most likely worsen (66% of cases) if it starts in the beginning of the growth spurt. Rapid worsening of curvature is indicative of secondary cause (Marfan or Ehlers–Danlos syndrome, cerebral palsy, myelomeningocele, etc.)

Classic Case

Pubertal to young teen complains that one hip, shoulder, breast, or scapula is higher than the other. No complaints of pain.

Adam's Forward Bend Test (or Forward Bend Test)

Bend forward with both arms hanging free. Look for asymmetry of spine, scapula, thoracic, and lumbar curvature. Check height. Measure the Cobb angle (degree of spinal curvature). Full-spine x-rays are used to measure degree of curvature.

Scoliosis Treatment Parameters

- Curves less than 20 degrees: Observe and monitor for changes in spinal curvature

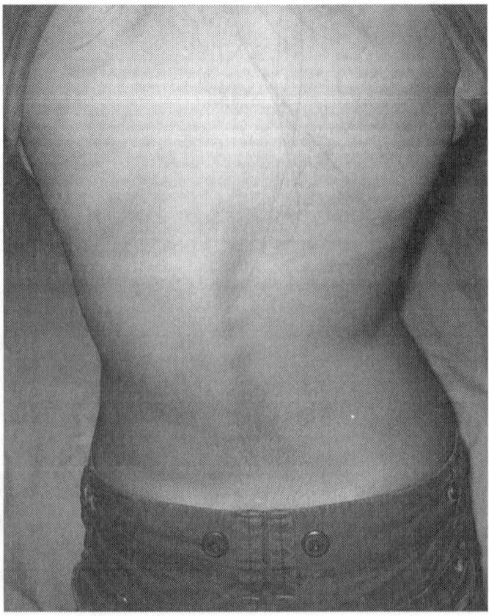

Figure 23.2 Scoliosis (female aged 18 years).

- Curves of 20 to 40 degrees: Bracing (i.e., Milwaukee brace)
- Curves greater than 40 degrees: Surgical correction with Harrington rod used on spine and other options

Management

- Check Tanner stage (Tanner stages II–V).
- Order spinal x-ray (PA view) to measure Cobb angle.

CLINICAL PEARL

Refer all patients with scoliosis to a pediatric orthopedic specialist.

Osgood–Schlatter Disease

A common cause of knee pain in young athletes. Caused by overuse of the knee. Repetitive stress on the patellar tendon by the quadriceps muscle causes pain, tenderness, and swelling at the tendon's insertion site (the tibial tuberosity). Usually affects one knee, but can be bilateral. Most common during rapid growth spurts in teenage males who are physically active and/or play sports that stress the patellar tendon (i.e., basketball, soccer, running). Condition abates when growth stops.

Classic Case

A 14-year-old male athlete undergoing a rapid growth spurt complains of a tender bony mass over the anterior tubercle of one knee. The pain is worsened by some activities (squatting, kneeling, jumping, and climbing up stairs). The knee pain improves with rest and avoidance of aggravating activity. Reports the presence of bony mass on the anterior tibial tubercle that is slightly tender. Almost all cases resolve spontaneously within a few weeks to months. Rule out avulsion fracture (tibial tubercle) if acute onset of pain posttrauma (order lateral x-ray of knee).

Treatment Plan

Follow RICE: Rest affected knee. Use ice pack three times/day for 10 to 15 minutes. Avoiding aggravating activities or sport will typically reduce or resolve pain. Adolescent may continue to play based on degree of pain after sports participation. Play does not necessarily worsen the condition. Use acetaminophen (Tylenol) or NSAIDs for pain as needed. Quadriceps strengthening and quadriceps/hamstring stretching exercises aimed at stabilizing the knee joint may also be beneficial.

Klinefelter Syndrome

A condition in which males are born with an extra X chromosome (i.e., 47, XXY). Condition occurs approximately in one in 1,000 live births. It is one of the causes of primary hypogonadism (deficiency in testosterone). Testicles are small and firm with small penis. Tall stature, wider hips, reduced facial and body hair, and higher risk of osteoporosis (compared with normal males). Treatment includes testosterone replacement and fertility treatment.

Turner's Syndrome (Figure 23.3)

Females with complete or partial absence of the second sex chromosome (45, X). Occurs in approximately one in 2,500 live-born females. Congenital lymphedema of hands and feet, webbed neck, high-arched palate, and short fourth metacarpal. Short stature (height usually below 50% percentile). Ovarian failure, cardiovascular and renal issues, ear malformations, and other health problems, as well as amenorrhea due to premature ovarian failure (infertility).

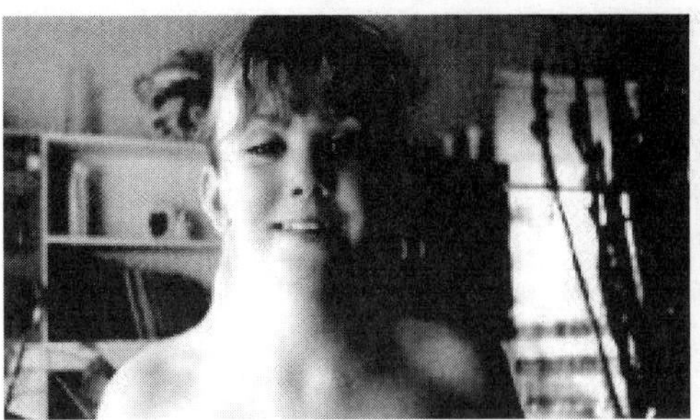 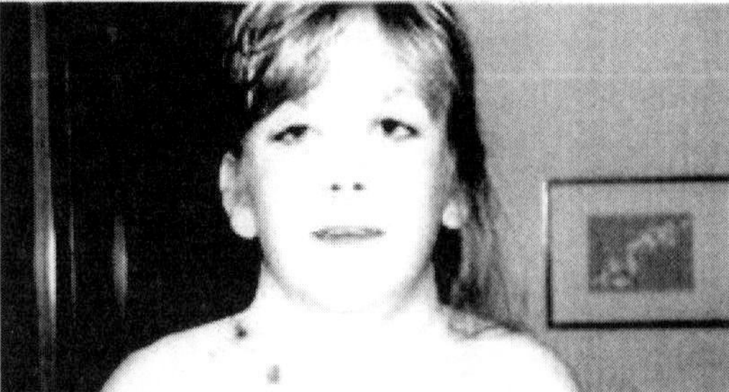

Figure 23.3 Turner syndrome (before and after surgery to correct neck webbing). This image can be found in color in the app.

Source: Courtesy of Johannes Nielsen.

EXAM TIPS

- **Scoliosis treatment needed for a 10-degree curve (observe for worsening).**
- **Screening test for scoliosis is the Adam's forward bend test.**
- **For Klinefelter syndrome, understand how patient looks.**

Delayed Puberty

- Absence of secondary sexual characteristics by the age of 13 years for girls (such as a breast bud) or at the age of 14 years for boys. The child remains in Tanner stage I (prepubertal).
- *Primary amenorrhea*: Menarche has not occurred by age 15 years.

Labs

- Serum pregnancy test
- Check prolactin level. If prolactin level is elevated, next step is to order a CT scan of the sella turcica (location of pituitary gland inside the skull).
- For primary amenorrhea (no menses by age 15 years), rule out hypogonadism by checking hormone levels (i.e., estrogen, progesterone, dehydroepiandrosterone [DHEA], FSH, TSH). Rule out chromosomal disorders, absence of uterus/vagina, imperforate hymen. X-ray of the hand is used for estimating "bone age":
  - When the long-bone epiphyses (growth plates) are fused, skeletal growth is finished.
  - Refer to pediatric endocrinologist if no growth spurt, delayed puberty, others.

EXAM TIPS

- **Know the Osgood–Schlatter presentation.**
- **Understand gynecomastia versus pseudogynecomastia (know the difference).**
- **No parental consent is needed for health services related to sexual activity (STD testing, pregnancy tests, birth control prescriptions).**
- **If not related to sexual activity, then need parental consent (dysmenorrhea, headache, upper respiratory infection [URI]).**
- **Know the emancipated minor definition.**
- **Know the presentation of anorexia nervosa (lanugo, low albumin causes pedal edema, etc.).**

Gerontology Review

V

24

Body and Metabolic Changes in the Older Adult

Skin and Hair

With aging, the skin atrophies; the epidermis and dermis thin and there is less subdermal fat and less collagen (less elasticity). Skin is fragile and slower to heal. Oil production is lower and skin drier (xerosis) due to decreased sebaceous and sweat gland activity. There is a decrease in the skin's sensory ability and reduction in vitamin D synthesis. Fewer melanocytes lead to graying of hair.

Seborrheic Keratoses

Soft wart-like skin lesions that appear "pasted on." Mostly seen on the back and trunk. Benign.

Senile Purpura

Bright purple-colored patches with well-demarcated edges. Located on the dorsum of the forearms and hands. Lesions eventually resolve over several weeks. Benign.

Lentigines

Also known as "liver spots." Tan- to brown-colored macules on the dorsum of the hands and forearms caused by sun damage. More common in light-skinned individuals. Benign.

Stasis Dermatitis

Statis dermatitis affects primarily the lower legs and ankles secondary to chronic edema (from peripheral vascular disease [PVD])

Senile Actinic Keratosis (Solar Keratosis)

Condition is secondary to sun exposure and has the potential for malignancy. It has the potential to be a precancerous lesion of squamous cell carcinoma.

Nails

Growth slows and nails become brittle, yellow, and thicker. Longitudinal ridges develop.

Eyes

Presbyopia is caused by loss of elasticity of the lenses, which makes it difficult to focus on close objects. Close vision is markedly affected. Onset is during early to mid-40s. Can be remedied with "reading glasses" or bifocal lenses. Cornea is less sensitive to touch. Arcus senilis, cataracts, and glaucoma are more common.

Arcus Senilis (Corneal Arcus)

Opaque grayish-to-white ring at the periphery of the cornea. Develops gradually and is not associated with visual changes. Caused by deposition of cholesterol and fat. In patients younger than 40 years, can be a sign of elevated cholesterol. Check fasting lipid profile.

Cataracts

Cloudiness and opacity of the lens of the eye(s) or its envelope (posterior capsular cataract). There are three types (nuclear, cortical, and posterior capsular). Color of the lens is white to gray. Cataracts cause gradual onset of decreased night vision, sensitivity to glare of car lights (driving at night), and hazy vision. The red reflex disappears.

Test: Red reflex (reflection is opaque gray versus orange-red glow)

Macular Degeneration

Loss of central visual fields results in loss of visual acuity and contrast sensitivity. May find drusen bodies. Use Amsler grid to evaluate central-vision changes.

Ears

Presbycusis (Sensorineural Hearing Loss)

High-frequency hearing is lost first (e.g., a speaking voice is an example of high-frequency). Presbycusis starts at about age 50 years. There are degenerative changes of the ossicles, fewer auditory neurons, and atrophy of the hair cells resulting in sensorineural hearing loss.

Heart

Elongation and tortuosity (twisting) of the arteries occurs. Thickened intimal layer of arteries and arteriosclerosis result in increased systolic BP due to increased vascular resistance (isolated systolic hypertension). The mitral and aortic valves and may contain calcium deposits.

Baroreceptors are less sensitive to changes in position. There is decreased sensitivity of the autonomic nervous system. BP response is blunted. Maximum heart rate decreases. There is higher risk of orthostatic hypotension. S4 heart sound is a normal finding in the elderly if not associated with heart disease. The left ventricle hypertrophies with aging (up to 10% increase in thickness).

Lungs

Total lung capacity remains relatively the same as we age. Forced vital capacity (FVC) decreases with age. Forced expiratory volume in 1 second (FEV1) decreases with age. Residual volume (air left in the lungs at the end of expiration) increases with age due to decrease in lung and chest wall compliance. The chest wall becomes stiffer and the diaphragm is flatter and less efficient.

Mucociliary clearance (fewer cilia) and coughing are less efficient. The airways collapse sooner during expiration. Responses to hypoxia and hypercapnia decreases. Decreased breath sounds and crackles are commonly found in the lung bases of elderly patients without presence of disease. Instruct the patient to "cough" several times to inflate the lung bases (the benign crackles will disappear). There is increased anterior–posterior (AP) diameter related to normal body changes.

Liver

Liver size and mass decreases due to atrophy (20%–40%). Liver blood flow and perfusion decrease (up to 50% in some elders). Fat (lipofuscin) deposition in the liver is more common.

The liver function test result (ALT, AST, alkaline phosphatase) is not significantly changed. Metabolic clearance of drugs is slowed by 20% to 40% because the cytochrome P450 (CYP450) enzyme system is less efficient. The LDL and cholesterol levels increase with aging.

Renal System

Renal size and mass decrease by 25% to 30%. The steepest decline in renal mass occurs after the age of 50. Starting at the age of 40 years, the glomerular filtration rate (GFR) starts to decrease. By age 70, up to 30% of renal function is lost. Renal clearance of drugs is less efficient. The serum creatinine is a less reliable indicator of renal function in the elderly due to the decrease in muscle mass, creatine production, and creatinine clearance. Serum creatinine can be in the normal range, even if renal function is markedly reduced. The risk of kidney damage from nonsteroidal anti-inflammatory drugs (NSAIDs) is much higher. The renin–angiotensin levels are lower in the elderly.

Genitourinary System

The amount of urine that remains in the bladder after urination is completed (residual urine) increases with age. Normally, the bladder holds approximately 300 to 400 mL. In postmenopausal women, the urethra becomes thinner and shortens and the ability of the urinary sphincter to close tightly decreases (due to declining estrogen). Urinary incontinence is two to three times more common in women. According to the Cleveland Clinic, erectile dysfunction affects 40% of men aged 40 years and 70% of men aged 70 years.

Musculoskeletal System

Older adults can lose a total of 1 to 3 inches (2.5–2.7 cm) in height; this loss becomes more rapid after age 70. Compression fractures of vertebrae are a sign of osteoporosis (kyphosis) and contribute to loss of height.

Deterioration of articular cartilage is common after age of 40. Stiffness in the morning that improves with activity is a common symptom of osteoarthritis (degenerative joint disease [DJD]). Fat mass increases but muscle mass and muscle strength markedly decrease, with more muscle loss in the legs compared with the arms. Bone resorption is more rapid than bone deposition in women compared with men (4:1). Fractures heal more slowly because of decrease in the number of osteoblasts.

Gastrointestinal System

Receding gums and dry mouth are common. Decreased sensitivity of the taste buds results in decrease in appetite. There is decreased efficiency in absorbing some vitamins (i.e., folic acid, vitamin B_{12}) and minerals (e.g., calcium) by the small intestines. Delayed gastric emptying occurs. Higher risk of gastritis and GI damage from decreased production of prostaglandins. Diverticuli are common. Large bowel (colon) transit time is slower. Constipation is more common. Increased risk of colon cancer (age >50 years is strongest risk factor). Fecal incontinence common due to drug side effects, underlying disease, neurogenic disorders, or a combination of these factors. Fecal impaction may lead to a small amount of runny soft stool. Laxative abuse is more common.

Endocrine System

Minor atrophy of the pancreas occurs. Increased levels of insulin are seen along with mild peripheral insulin resistance. Changes or disorders of the circadian rhythm hormonal secretion (growth hormone, melatonin, and other hormones) can cause changes in sleep patterns.

Sex Hormones

Testes are active for the entire life cycle. Less dehydroepiandrosterone (DHEA) and testosterone are produced.

Estrogen and progesterone production decrease significantly in women due to ovarian failure (menopause). Higher serum testosterone concentration in some postmenopausal women may cause frontal balding on the head and excess hair growth on the mustache area and/or on the chin.

Adipose tissue is able to synthesize very small amounts of estrogen. In the United States, up to 53% of those aged 65 to 74 years are sexually active (Stewart & Graham, 2013).

Immune System

Older adults are less likely to present with fever during infections. Typical body temperature is slightly lower. There is a decreased antibody response to vaccines. Immune system is less active and there is higher risk of infection.

Cellular immunity is affected more by aging than humoral immunity. Cellular or cell-mediated immunity involves the activity of T-lymphocytes, macrophages, and the cytokines. Humoral immunity is associated with B-lymphocytes and antibody (immunoglobulins or IgG) production.

Hematological System

There are no changes in the RBC life span, the blood volume, or the total number of circulating leukocytes. There is a higher risk of thrombi and emboli due to increased platelet responsiveness. Increased risk of iron and folate-deficiency anemia due to decreased efficiency of the GI tract to absorb vitamin B_{12} and folate.

Neurological System

Cranial nerve testing may show differences in ability to differentiate color, papillary response, and decreased corneal reflex. Gag reflex decreases. Deep tendon reflexes may be brisk or absent. Neurological testing may be impaired by medications, causing slower reaction times. Benign essential tremor is more common.

Pharmacological Issues

Drug clearance is affected by renal impairment, less efficient liver CYP450 enzyme system, slow gastric emptying, increased gastric pH, decreased serum albumin, and relatively higher ratio of fat:muscle tissue (extends fat-soluble drugs). Older adults have an increased sensitivity to benzodiazepines and anticholinergic drugs such as hypnotics, tricyclic antidepressants (TCAs), antihistamines, and antipsychotics. The American Geriatrics Society has made a list of inappropriate medications for the elderly (Beers criteria; Agency for Healthcare Research and Quality, National Guideline Clearinghouse, & American Geriatrics Society, 2015).

EXAM TIPS

- **Seborrheic keratosis (benign) appears as a wart-like growth that look pasted on; found mostly on the back, color can range from tan, brown, to black.**
- **Presbycusis is a sensorineural type of hearing loss (inner ear). Hearing loss initially occurs in the high frequency range.**
- **Arcus senilis (corneal arcus) is a white or grey ring in the margin of the cornea or on the periphery of the iris (cholesterol deposits).**

- S4 in elderly is not associated with heart disease symptoms and is considered normal.
- FEV1 and FVC decrease with age, but residual volume increases.
- Actinic keratosis is a precursor of squamous cell cancer. Memory tip: the letter "C" in *actinic* is a reminder for cancer.
  - Do not confuse this with seborrheic keratosis, which is benign (common mistake).
- Most common cause of blindness in the United States is macular degeneration. In developing countries, cataracts are the most common cause of blindness.
  - Cataracts increase sensitivity to glare of car lights (driving at night). Red reflex test on cataracts appear as grayish-to-white reflection (mature cataracts appear white).
- Cellular immunity is affected more by age than humoral immunity.
- Anticholinergic drugs cause constipation, urinary retention (especially men with BPH), blurred vision, dry mouth, and orthostatic hypotension.

25

Common Disorders in Geriatrics

⚠ DANGER SIGNALS

Retinal Detachment

New onset or sudden increase in number of floaters or specks on the visual field, flashes of light, and the sensation that a curtain is covering part of the visual field. Considered a medical emergency that can lead to blindness if it is not treated. Risk factors are extreme nearsightedness, history of cataract surgery, and family or personal history of retinal detachment. Treated with laser surgery or cryopexy (freezing).

Temporal Arteritis (Giant Cell Arteritis)

Temporal headache (one sided) with tenderness or induration over temporal artery; may be accompanied by sudden visual loss in one eye (amaurosis fugax). Scalp tenderness on affected side. Screening test is the sedimentation rate, which will be elevated. Considered a medical emergency (can cause blindness).

Acute Angle-Closure Glaucoma

Older adult with acute onset of severe eye pain, severe headache, and nausea and vomiting. The eye(s) is(are) reddened with profuse tearing. Complains of blurred vision and halos around lights. Call 911. Do not delay treatment. Tonometry is done in the ED to quickly measure the intra-ocular pressure.

Cerebrovascular Accident (CVA)

Sudden onset of neurological dysfunction that worsens within hours. Also called a "brain attack." Deficits can include changes such as blurred vision, slurred speech, one-sided upper and/or lower extremity weakness, hemianopsia, confusion. Signs and symptoms are dependent on location of infarct. In comparison, a transient ischemic attack (TIA) is a temporary episode that generally lasts less than 24 hours.

Actinic Keratosis (Precursor of Squamous Cell Carcinoma)

Small rough pink to reddish lesions that do not heal. Located in sun-exposed areas such as the cheeks, nose, back of neck, arms, chest, and so on. More common in light-skinned individuals. Squamous cell precancerous skin lesions. Diagnostic method of choice is biopsy. Small number of lesions can be treated with cryotherapy. Larger numbers with wider distribution are treated with 5-fluorouracil cream.

Fractures of the Hip

Acute onset of limping, guarding, and/or inability or difficulty with bearing weight on the affected side. New onset of hip pain; may be referred to the knee or groin. Unequal leg length. Affected leg is abducted (turned away from the body). History of osteoporosis or osteopenia. Fractures of the hip are a major cause of morbidity and mortality in the elderly. Up to 20% of elderly with hip fractures die from complications (e.g., pneumonia).

Colorectal Cancer

Unexplained iron-deficiency anemia (23%), blood on rectum (37%), hematochezia, melena, abdominal pain (34%), and/or change in bowel habits. No symptoms during early stages, diagnosed due to screening. Presentation depends on location. Rectal cancer can present with tenesmus, rectal pain, and diminished-caliber stools (ribbon-like stools). About 20% of cases have distant metastases at time of presentation. Refer to a gastroenterologist.

Severe Bacterial Infections

Atypical presentation is common. Older adults/elderly with bacteremia or sepsis may be afebrile. About one third to one half of people with severe bacterial infections do not develop fever and/or chills. Some present with slightly lower than normal body temperature (<37°C [98.6°F]). The WBC can be normal. Atypical presentations also include a sudden decline in mental status (confusion, dementia), the new onset of urine/bowel incontinence, falling, worsening inability to perform activities of daily living (ADL), and/or loss of appetite. Serious infections include pneumonia, pyelonephritis, bacterial endocarditis, sepsis, and others. The most common infection in older adults (>65 years) is urinary tract infection (UTI).

Elder Abuse

- Presence of bruising, skin tears, lacerations, and fractures that are poorly explained
- Presence of sexually transmitted disease, vaginal, and/or rectal bleeding, bruises on breasts are indicators of possible sexual abuse
- Malnutrition, poor hygiene, and pressure injuries
- Screen for abuse and financial exploitation

Interview Elder Alone With These Three Questions

- Do you feel safe where you live?
- Who handles your checkbook and finances?
- Who prepares your meals?

Top Three Leading Causes of Death (Older Than Age 65 Years)

- Heart disease (myocardial infarction [MI], heart failure, arrhythmias)
- Cancers (lung and colorectal)
- Chronic lower respiratory diseases (chronic obstructive pulmonary disease [COPD])

CANCER IN OLDER ADULTS

Aging and advancing age are the most common risk factors for cancer. Up to 60% of newly diagnosed malignancies occur in older adults (age 65 years or older). Cancers among older adults may be caused by gene-related DNA damage, familial genetics, decrease in immunity, decreased healing rates, environment, and hormonal influences.

- Cancer with highest mortality: Lung and bronchial cancer (both genders)
- Cancer with second highest mortality: Colorectal cancer

Median Age of Diagnosis of Certain Cancers

- Breast cancer: 61 years old
- Prostate cancer: 68 years old
- Lung cancer: 70 years old

Lung Cancer

The cancer with the highest mortality (both genders). About one out of four cancer deaths are caused by lung cancer. Most patients with lung cancer are older adults. Fewer than 2% of people diagnosed with lung cancer are younger the age 45 years (American Cancer Society, 2016).

- *Most common risk factor:* Smoking (causes 90% of cases); other risk factors include radon exposure (10%), occupational exposures to carcinogens (9%–15%), and outdoor pollution (1%–2%)
- *Most common type of lung cancer:* Non–small cell lung (90%) carcinoma
- *Screening:* The U.S. Preventive Services Task Force (USPSTF) recommends annual screening for lung cancer in adults (aged 55–80 years) who have a 30-pack-year smoking history and currently smoke (or have quit within past 15 years); screening test is low-dose computed tomography (LDCT)
  - Discontinue screening: Patient stops smoking for 15 years or longer or develops a health problem that substantially limits life expectancy (or the ability or willingness for curative lung surgery)

Classic Case

An older male smoker (or ex-smoker) presents with a new onset of cough that is productive of large amounts of thin mucoid phlegm (bronchorrhea). Some patients have blood-tinged phlegm. The patient complains of worsening shortness of breath or dyspnea. Some will report persistent and dull achy chest pain that does not go away. If the tumor is obstructing a bronchus, it can result in recurrent pneumonia of the same lobe. Some may have weight loss.

Treatment Plan

- Order chest radiograph (nodules, lesions with irregular borders).
- The next imaging exam needed is a CT scan. Gold standard is a positive lung biopsy.
- Baseline labs include CBC, fecal occult blood test (FOBT), chemistry panel, and UA.
- Refer patient to a pulmonologist for bronchoscopy and tumor biopsy.

Colorectal Cancer

The second most common cause of cancer deaths in the United States. About 20% of cases have distant metastases at time of presentation. It is staged using the tumor-node-metastasis (TNM) staging system (stages I to IV).

- *Risk factors:* Advancing age (most common), inflammatory bowel disease, or a family history of colorectal cancer, colonic polyps
- *Lifestyle risk factors:* Lack of regular physical activity, high-fat diet, low-fiber diet, obesity, etc.
- *Screening:* Start at age 50 years with baseline colonoscopy (repeat every 7 to 10 years; abnormal findings dictate more frequent rescreening), sigmoidoscopy (every 5 years), or a high-sensitivity FOBT (annually). A DNA-based screening fecal occult test (Cologuard) is now available in place of the screening colonoscopy, but it is only for average risk individuals with no prior history of abnormal colonoscopy findings and/or no family history of colon cancer.

Classic Case

An older adult who presents with a change in bowel habits with hematochezia or melena and/or abdominal pain, but may be asymptomatic, and presents with unexplained iron-deficiency anemia (23%). The patient may report anorexia and unintentional weight loss. Asymptomatic during early stages; diagnosed by screening. Presentation depends on location. Patients with rectal cancer can present with tenesmus, rectal pain, and diminished-caliber stools (ribbon-like stools).

Treatment Plan

- Baseline labs include CBC, FOBT, chemistry panel, and UA.
- Check occult blood in stool (guaiac-based, stool DNA, others).
- Refer to gastroenterologist for colonoscopy and management.

Multiple Myeloma

Myeloma is a cancer of the bone marrow that affects the plasma cells of the immune system (production of monoclonal immunoglobulins). The racial background with the highest incidence are people of African descent (doubled or tripled compared with Whites). Multiple myeloma is a cancer found mostly in older adults.

Classic Case

Typical patient is an older to elderly adult who complains of bone pain with generalized weakness. The bone pain is usually located on the chest and/or the back and usually does not occur at night. The majority have anemia (73%).

Treatment Plan

- Baseline labs include CBC, FOBT, chemistry panel, and UA
- Refer patient to a hematologist

Pancreatic Cancer

The most lethal cancer. The 5-year survival rate is 8.2%. More than 95% of cases arise from the exocrine portion of the pancreas. Most patients already have metastases by time of diagnosis. The most common presentation is weight loss (85%), anorexia, jaundice, weakness (asthenia), and abdominal pain.

Treatment Plan

- Initial labs: AST, ALT, alkaline phosphatase, bilirubin, lipase, amylase
- Refer to a GI surgeon for Whipple procedure or other interventions, as determined

EXAM TIPS

- **Ribbon-like stool (low-caliber stool) in older adult with iron-deficiency anemia; rule out colon cancer**
- **Know signs and symptoms of retinal detachment**
- **Know signs and symptoms of acute angle-closure glaucoma**
- **Hip fracture signs and symptoms**
- **Actinic keratosis is precancer of squamous cell skin cancer**
- **Temporal arteritis: Check sedimentation rate with/without C-reactive protein (CRP; both elevated)**
- **Top cause of death is heart disease**

CLINICAL PEARLS

- **Any patient with unexplained iron-deficiency anemia who is older, male, or postmenopausal should be referred for a colonoscopy (GI bleed, colon cancer).**
- **If the chemistry profile shows marked elevations in the serum calcium and/or alkaline phosphatase, it is usually indicative of cancerous metastasis of the bone.**

DISEASE REVIEW

Atypical Presentations in the Elderly

Atypical disease presentations are more common in this age group. The immune system becomes less robust as people age and is less likely to become stimulated by bacterial and viral infections. Vaccines may not be as effective in the elderly as in the young because of decreased immune response in the former (result is lower antibody production).

Older adults and the elderly are more likely to be asymptomatic or to present with subtle symptoms. The elderly are less likely to have a high fever during an infection. Instead, they are more likely to suffer acute cognitive dysfunction such as confusion, agitation, and delirium. Cognitive dysfunction in the elderly may also result from use of multiple prescriptions to manage multiple comorbid conditions. Polypharmacy increases the chances of adverse drugs reactions and drug–drug interactions.

For management of diseases not included in this chapter, see the other system review chapters in this book. For example, the management and treatment of pneumonia is covered in Chapter 8.

Bacterial Pneumonia

Fever and chills may be missing or mild (oral temp >100 F or rectal >99.5 F). Coughing may not be a prominent symptom. The cough may be mild and produce little to no sputum (especially if the patient is dehydrated). May stop eating and drinking water and start losing weight. More likely to become confused and weak with loss of appetite. May become incontinent of bladder and bowel. Tachycardia usually present. Increases the risk of falls. The WBC count may be normal or mildly elevated. Streptococcal pneumonia causes the most deaths from pneumonia in the elderly.

Urinary Tract Infections (UTIs)

The most common infection in elderly nursing home residents and in adults age 65 and older. Patients usually have no fever or can be asymptomatic. May become acutely confused or agitated. May become septic with mild symptoms. New onset of urinary incontinence. At higher risk of falls.

Acute Abdomen

Elderly patients may have more subtle symptoms such as the absence of abdominal guarding and other signs of acute abdomen. The abdominal pain may be milder. The WBC count may be only slightly elevated or it may be normal. Patient may have low-grade fever with anorexia and weakness.

Acute Myocardial Infarction (MI)

May be asymptomatic. Symptoms may consist of new-onset fatigue, back pain and/or mild chest pain.

Hypothyroidism

Subtle and insidious symptoms such as sleepiness, severe constipation, weight gain, and dry skin. Hypothyroidism is very common in patients aged 60 years or older. Problems with memory. If severe, may mimic dementia. Slower movements. Appears apathetic.

Urinary Incontinence

Should not be considered a "normal" aspect of aging. Evaluate all cases. May be short term and temporary (e.g., UTI, high intake of tea or coffee) or chronic. Two to three times more common in women. Risk factors are obesity, pregnancy, vaginal delivery, menopause, age, and diabetes. Some foods and drinks worsen urinary incontinence because of their diuretic effect (tea, caffeine, alcohol, carbonated drinks, citrus fruits, spicy foods), and medications (diuretics, sedatives) may have a similar effect. Table 25.1 describes the types of urinary incontinence.

Table 25.1 Types of Urinary Incontinence

Type	Description
Stress incontinence	Increased intra-abdominal pressure (laughing, sneezing, bending, lifting) causes involuntary leakage of small to medium volume of urine Highest incidence in middle-age women (peak at 45 to 49 years) **Plan**: Kegel exercises; decongestant (pseudoephedrine) if no contraindications
Urge incontinence	Sudden and strong urge to void immediately. Involuntary loss of urine can range from moderate to large volumes. Condition also known as "overactive bladder" Highest incidence in older women **Plan**: Trial of anticholinergics (oxybutynin/Ditropan) or tricyclic antidepressant (imipramine)
Overflow incontinence	Frequent dribbling of small amounts of urine from overly full bladder; due to blockage of flow (e.g., benign prostatic hyperplasia [BPH]) or underactive detrusor muscle (e.g. spinal cord injury, multiple sclerosis) Highest incidence in older men **Plan**: BPH treatment (discussed in Chapter 16)
Functional incontinence	Problems with mobility (walking to the toilet) or inability to pull down pants in a timely manner **Plan**: Bedside commode, raised toilet seats with handles, physical therapy for strengthening and gait
Mixed incontinence	Symptoms that are a mixture of stress and urge incontinence

Treatment Plan

- First-line treatment: Lifestyle modifications for all types (stress, urge, mixed). If obese, advise weight loss. Smoking cessation if smoker.
- Dietary: Avoid certain beverages (alcohol, coffee, tea, carbonated drinks). Avoid excessive fluid intake (>64 ounces) and decrease fluid intake before bedtime.
- Kegel exercises (pelvic floor exercises): All types of urinary incontinence, especially stress incontinence. Kegel exercises have been found to help with fecal incontinence.
- Use absorbent pads and absorbent underwear made for urinary incontinence.
- For moderate to advanced pelvic organ prolapse (cystocele, rectocele, enterocele, uterine prolapse, vaginal eversion), refer to urologist or gynecologist specializing in urinary incontinence and pelvic organ prolapse repair.

Kegel Exercises

Tell the patient to:

- Identify the muscles used to stop urinating (stop urinating midstream to confirm this). Do not tighten muscles of the abdomen, buttocks, thighs, and legs at the same time.

- Squeeze and hold these muscles and slowly count to five.
- Relax and release these same muscles to a slow count of five.
- Repeat this 10 times. Aim for at least three sets of 10 repetitions each day.

Behavioral Bladder Training

- Bladder training to delay urination after feeling the urge to urinate. At first, have the patient try holding off urinating for 10 minutes each time. The goal is to lengthen the time between trips to the bathroom to every 2 to 4 hours.
- Double voiding helps to empty the bladder more completely to avoid overflow. Double voiding means urinating, then waiting a few minutes and voiding again.

Medications for Urinary Incontinence

Anticholinergics

- Oxybutynin (Ditropan) 2.5 to 5 mg PO TID (immediate release); other formulations: Extended release, transdermal patch (twice/week), transdermal gel
- Contraindications: Urinary retention, gastric retention, severe decreased motility of GI tract, uncontrolled narrow-angle glaucoma, benign prostatic hyperplasia (BPH)

Tricyclic Antidepressants (TCAs)

- Imipramine (Tofranil) PO 25 mg at HS
- TCAs have anticholinergic and antimuscarinic effects, which helps to decrease bladder spasms and increases urethral resistance. Adverse effects: urinary retention, dry mouth, drowsiness, constipation; contraindicated in glaucoma.
- Pseudephedrine helps stress incontinence by increasing the muscle tone of the bladder neck. It is an alpha receptor agonist and the bladder neck has numerous alpha receptors.

Oral Decongestant

- Pseudoephedrine (Sudafed) PO 30 to 60 mg BID
- Adverse effects: Hypertension, arrhythmias, insomnia, headache, tremor. Be careful with the elderly.

Pelvic Organ Prolapse in Women

Herniation of the bladder (cystocele), rectum (rectocele), uterus (uterine prolapse), enterocele, or vagina (vaginal vault prolapse; Table 25.2). Caused by weakening of pelvic muscles and supporting ligaments. During early stage, pelvic organ prolapse is usually asymptomatic. Advise the patient to avoid heavy lifting or excessive straining, which can worsen condition, and to avoid chronic constipation because straining worsens pelvic organ prolapse.

Evaluation

During the gynecological exam (bimanual exam, speculum exam), instruct the patient to cough (cover mouth to increase intra-abdominal pressure) so that herniation becomes more visible and palpable.

Table 25.2 Pelvic Organ Prolapse

Organ	Description
Cystocele (bladder)	Bulging of the anterior vaginal wall; early stage is usually asymptomatic in all types of pelvic organ prolapse. Symptoms: Stress urinary incontinence (60%), frequency and urgency (35%), difficulty voiding (23%) **Plan**: Refer for pessary placement (Figure 25.1), surgical repair

(continued)

Table 25.2 Pelvic Organ Prolapse *(continued)*

Organ	Description
Rectocele (rectum)	Bulging on the posterior vaginal wall; herniation ranges from mild to rectal prolapse Symptoms: Feeling of rectal fullness or pressure, sensation that rectum does not completely empty; rectal prolapse can cause fecal incontinence **Plan**: Kegel exercises; avoid straining during bowel movement; treat constipation; refer for pessary placement (Figure 25.1), surgical repair
Uterine prolapse	Cervix descends midline (apical) into vagina; cervix feels firm with pale pink color and os visible; with third-degree full prolapse, a tubular sac-like protrusion is seen outside of the vagina Symptoms: Sensation of vaginal fullness, feeling that something is falling in the vagina, low-back pain **Plan**: Avoid heavy lifting and straining; refer for pessary placement (Figure 25.1) or surgical repair by urologist specializing in pelvic organ prolapse
Enterocele (small intestines)	Small bowel slips into the area between the uterus and posterior wall of the vagina, bulging external vagina Symptoms: Pulling sensation inside pelvis, pelvic pressure or pain, low-back pain, dyspareunia

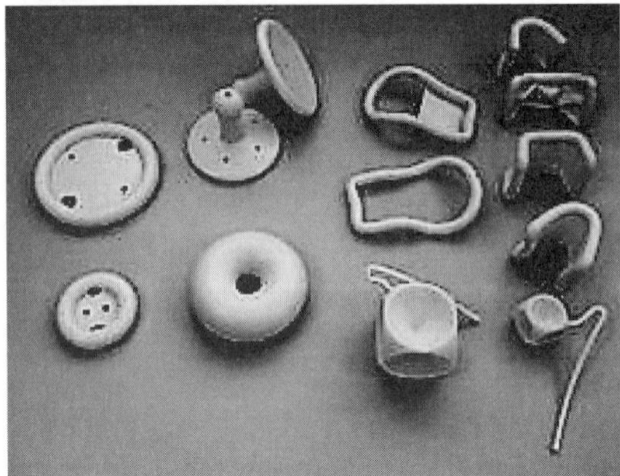

Figure 25.1 Pessaries.

Chronic Constipation

There are two types of constipation: idiopathic and functional constipation. Constipation is the most common GI complaint. Self-treatment is common with over-the-counter (OTC) fiber and laxatives. Constipation has many secondary causes such as prescription and OTC drugs, neurological disease (Parkinson's disease, dementia), irritable bowel syndrome (IBS), diabetes, hypothyroidism, and others. Lifestyle factors that contribute to constipation are immobility, low-fiber diet, dehydration, milk intake, and ignoring the urge to have bowel movement.

Drugs that cause constipation are iron supplements, beta-blockers, calcium channel blockers, antihistamines, anticholinergics, antipsychotics, opiates, and calcium-containing antacids.

Classic Case

Older adult complains of history of long-term constipation (years). Describes stool as dry and hard "ball-like" pieces or as large-volume stools that are difficult to pass. Reports of straining often to pass the stool. Accompanied by feelings of fullness and bloating. Some patients take laxatives daily (laxative abuse). Usually accompanied by hemorrhoids, which may become exacerbated (reports bright-red blood on toilet paper and blood streaks on stool surface).

Treatment Plan

- Education and behavior modification (bowel retraining). Teach "toilet" hygiene such as going to the bathroom at the same time each day; advise not to ignore the urge to defecate.
- Dietary changes such as eating dried prunes and/or drinking prune juice. Increase intake of fruit and vegetables.
- Ingest bulk-forming fibers (25–35 g/d) once to twice a day. Do not take with medication (will absorb drugs). Take with full glass of water (can cause intestinal obstruction).
- Increase physical activity, especially walking.
- Increase fluid intake to eight to 10 glasses/day (if no contraindication).
- Consider laxative treatment (Table 25.3). Avoid using laxatives daily (except for fiber supplements) and chronic treatment with laxatives.

Table 25.3 List of Laxatives

Type of Laxative	Name	Notes
Bulk forming	Psyllium (Metamucil) Wheat dextrin (Benefiber) Methylcellulose (Citrucel) Polycarbophil (FiberCon)	Two types: Soluble or insoluble fiber (bran, psyllium); absorbs water, adding bulk to stool; constipation, IBS, diverticulitis
Stimulants (irritants)	Bisacodyl (Dulcolax), oral and suppository Senna extract (Senokot), oral Aloe vera juice	Stimulates colon directly causing contractions; drug class: Anthraquinone
Osmotics (hyperosmotic agents)	Sorbitol Lactulose (Cephulac) Polyethylene glycol or PEG 3350 (MiraLAX) Glycerin suppositories	Draws fluid by osmosis to increase fluid retention in the colon Rectal use only
Saline laxatives	Magnesium citrate Magnesium hydroxide (Milk of Magnesia) Magnesium sulfate (Epsom salts)	Saline attracts water into the intestinal lumen (small and large intestines) Side effects: Fluid and electrolyte imbalance
Guanylate cyclase-C receptor agonist	Linaclotide Linzess	Stimulates intestinal fluid secretion and transit; for IBS, chronic idiopathic constipation
Chloride channel activators	Lubiprostone (Amitiza)	Idiopathic chronic constipation, IBS Contraindications: History of mechanical obstruction
Lubricants	Mineral oil	Lubricants are not absorbed
Stool softeners	Docusate sodium (Colace)	Softens stool (does not stimulate colon) Stool becomes soft and slippery

IBS, irritable bowel syndrome; PEG, polyethylene glycol.

Bowel Retraining Program

- Choose time of the day patient prefers for bowel movements. Usually in mornings about 20 to 40 minutes after eating breakfast.
- Spend about 10 to 15 minutes on the toilet each day at the same time. Avoid straining.

SCREENING FOR DEMENTIA AND COGNITIVE IMPAIRMENT

- The most common cause of dementia in elderly is Alzheimer disease (60%–80%).
- The second most common cause is vascular dementia (CVA).
- One of the most helpful methods of diagnosing dementia is by eliciting a thorough history of the changes in the patient's memory, behavior, function, and personality from family members and close contacts of the patient.
- Cognitive testing of the patient is important (cognitive performance scales).
- Ruling out secondary causes is done by ordering laboratory tests for syphilis, vitamin B_{12} deficiency, thyroid-stimulating hormone (TSH), CBC, heavy metals, others.
- Best brain imaging test is the MRI scan of the brain.

Cognitive Performance Scales

- Folstein Mini-Mental State Exam
- Mini-Cog Test
- Addenbrookers Cognitive Examination Revised (ACE-R)
- Beck Depression Inventory-II
- ADL Self-Performance Hierarchy Scale
- Index of Social Engagement Scale

Folstein Mini-Mental State Exam (MMSE)

A brief screening exam to assess for cognitive impairment. High sensitivity and specificity.

- Orientation
  - Ask about year/season/date/day/month
  - Where are we now? Name state (county, town/city, hospital, floor)
- Short-term memory
  - Name three unrelated objects and instruct the patient to recite all three words
- Attention and calculation
  - Serial 7s (ask the patient to count backward from 100 by sevens)
  - Alternative: Instruct the patient to spell "world" backward
- Recall
  - Say to the patient, "Earlier I told you the names of three things. Can you tell me what they were?"
  - Show the patient two simple objects (i.e., pencil, coin). Instruct patient to name them.
  - Instruct the patient to repeat the phrase "No ifs, ands, or buts."
  - Give the patient one blank piece of paper. Instruct patient to "take the paper in your right hand, fold it in half, and put it on the floor."
  - Write on the paper "Close your eyes." Instruct the patient to read and do what it says.
- Writing a sentence
  - Instruct the patient to make up and write a sentence about anything.
- Copying a design
  - Use a questionnaire with a picture of two pentagons that intersect.
- The maximum score is 30 points: Score of 0 to 10 (severe), 10 to 20 (moderate), 20 to 25 (mild), 25 to 30 (questionable significance–mild deficits).

"Mini-Cog" Test

A 3-minute tool to screen for cognitive impairment in older adults in the primary care setting (Borson, Scanlan, Brush, Vitaliano, & Dokmak, 2000). High sensitivity and specificity.

- Step 1: Three-word recognition (one point for each word)
  - Instruct the patient to repeat three words. There are six versions of words that can be used (two examples listed here):
    - Banana, sunrise, chair (version 1)
    - Leader, season, table (version 2)
- Step 2: Clock drawing (score as normal or abnormal)
  - Instruct the patient to draw a clock by putting in the numbers first and then ask him or her to indicate a specific time by saying "set the hands to 10 past 11" or "set the hands at 20 minutes after 8."
- Step 3: Three-word recall
  - Ask the patient to recall the three words you stated in Step 1.
- Score range: 0 to 3; dementia if score 0 to 2 points; no dementia if score of 3 to 5

Delirium (Acute Confusional State)

A reversible, temporary process. Duration is usually brief (hours to days). Acute and dramatic onset. Patient may be excitable, irritable, and combative, with short attention span, memory loss, and disorientation. Secondary to medical condition, drug, intoxication, adverse reaction to medicine.

Etiology

- Prescription medications (opioids, sedatives, hypnotics, antipsychotics, polypharmacy)
- Substance abuse (alcohol, heroin, hallucinogens), plants (jimson weed, Salvia)
- Drug–drug interactions, adverse reactions, psychiatric illness
- Abrupt drug withdrawal (alcohol, benzodiazepines, drugs)
- Preexisting medical conditions, ICU patients with sensory overload
- Infections, sepsis (UTIs and pneumonia most common infections)
- Electrolyte imbalance, heart failure, renal failure

Treatment Plan

- Remove and/or treat illness, infection, or metabolic derangement, and delirium will resolve

"Sundowning" Phenomenon

- This condition occurs in both delirium and dementia
- Starting at dusk/sundown, the patient becomes very agitated, confused, and combative; symptoms resolve in the morning; seen more with dementia; recurs commonly

Treatment Plan

- Avoid quiet and dark rooms
- Have well-lit room with a radio, TV, or clock
- Familiar surroundings are important. Do not move furniture or change decor
- Avoid drugs that affect cognition (antihistamines, sedatives, hypnotics, narcotics)

Dementia

An irreversible brain disorder that involves loss of learned cognitive and physical/motor skills. The presentation and the signs and symptoms are determined by the etiology and location of the brain damage (Table 25.4). Gradual and insidious onset except if caused by stroke or acute brain damage).

Dementia affects executive skills adversely. *Executive function* is defined as self-regulation skills, attention, planning, multitasking, self-control, motivation, and decision-making skills. These higher level cognitive skills are regulated in the frontal lobes of the brain.

Table 25.4 Types of Dementia

Disease	Brain Pathology	Presentation
Alzheimer's disease (#1 cause of dementia)	Deposits of beta amyloid protein and neurofibrillary tangles on the frontal and temporal lobes	Early signs are short-term memory loss such as difficulty remembering names and recent events, plus wandering, apathy, apraxia, aphasia, and agnosia Progression to impaired judgment, executive skills, confusion, and behavioral changes. Terminal stage is characterized by difficulty speaking, swallowing, and walking
Vascular dementia (#2 cause of dementia)	Ischemic damage due to atherosclerotic plaques, bleeding, and/or blood clots	Symptoms of stroke with cognitive symptoms such as memory loss, impaired executive function, impaired judgment, and apathy; location of infarct determines symptoms
Dementia with Lewy bodies (DLB)	Alpha-synuclein protein (Lewy bodies)	Causes sleep disturbance, visual hallucinations, executive function is impaired plus parkinsonism (muscle rigidity, tremors), with fluctuations in alertness and cognition
Parkinson's disease	Loss of dopamine receptors in the basal ganglia of the substantia nigra	Causes rigidity, bradykinesia, difficulty initiating voluntary movements, pill-rolling tremor, masked facies, depression, plus features of DLB (sleep disturbance, visual hallucinations)
Frontotemporal dementia (Pick's disease)	Orbital and frontal areas of brain (orbitofrontal)	Causes personality change, social withdrawal, loss of spontaneity, loss of motivation/desire to do task (abulia), impulsive, disinhibition; utilization behavior (i.e., uses and reuses same object as in using a spoon to eat, comb hair, waving it, etc.) occurs
Mixed dementia	Mixture of two or more types (e.g., Alzheimer's and vascular dementia)	If Alzheimer's and vascular dementia, symptoms of both conditions are present
Wernicke–Korsakoff dementia (or Wernicke's encephalopathy)	Chronic thiamine (vitamin B_1) deficiency due to chronic alcohol abuse causes brain damage	Causes confusion, disorientation, indifference, horizontal movement nystagmus (both eyes); thiamine IV in high doses can help, but if late diagnosis, permanent brain damage. If caught early, treatment with high-dose thiamine may reverse some symptoms. Most have permanent brain damage.
Normal pressure hydrocephalus	Increased amount of cerebrospinal fluid (but normal intracranial pressure)	Causes difficulty walking (body bent forward, legs wide apart, slow). Impaired thinking, executive function impaired, reduced concentration, apathy, changes in personality

Etiology

- Alzheimer's disease: Most common cause of dementia in the United States.
- Vascular (multi-infarct) dementia is the second most common type of dementia.

- DLB: Symptoms are sleep disorder/insomnia, visual hallucinations, cognitive fluctuations, and parkinsonism (rigidity, bradykinesia, resting tremor, postural instability). Very sensitive to adverse effects of neuroleptics.
  - Deficiency in executive functioning is usually seen earlier with DLB compared with Alzheimer's disease. Memory loss shows up earlier with Alzheimer's disease.
- Dementia patients are very sensitive to adverse effects of neuroleptics.
- Parkinson's disease: Up to 40% of Parkinson's patients develop dementia.
- Normal pressure hydrocephalus is caused by excess cerebrospinal fluid. Symptoms may resemble Alzheimer's disease. Brain shunt surgery to decrease intracranial pressure (ICP) may help.

Differential Diagnosis

- Rule out correctable causes such as vitamin B_{12} deficiency, hypothyroidism, major depression, infection, adverse/drug interactions, heavy metal poisoning, neurosyphilis, and others.
- Parkinson's dementia and DLB may resemble each other.
- Remember that normal pressure hydrocephalus can cause dementia-like symptoms.

Treatment Plan

- It is important to obtain a thorough health/medical/drug history.
- The patient should be accompanied by family during the interview. Family members (and friends) will report patient's signs and symptoms. Refer to neurologist for further assessment.
- The preferred imaging test for dementia signs/symptoms is an MRI of the brain.

Alzheimer's Disease

Rare before age 60 years. Accumulation of neurofibrillary plaques/tangles causes permanent damage to brain. Decrease in acetylcholine production. Average life expectancy of person age 65 years or older (when diagnosed) is 4 to 8 years. Seizures occur in 10% to 20% of patients with Alzheimer's disease.

- Three As: Aphasia, apraxia, agnosia
  - Aphasia (difficulty verbalizing)
  - Apraxia (difficulty with gross motor movements such as walking)
  - Agnosia (inability to recognize familiar people or objects)

Classic Case

- *Mild (from 2 to 4 years):* Problems coming up with the right word when talking. Getting lost on familiar routes. Problems managing personal finances and money. Forgets important dates. Repeats same questions. Poor judgment. Becomes withdrawn, anxious, and/or depressed. Easily upset. Personality changes.
- *Moderate (from 2 to 10 years):* Wanders and gets lost. Problems with speech and following instructions. Stops paying bills. May start a conversation and forget to complete sentences. Loses ability to read and write. Has problems recognizing familiar people (agnosia).
- *Severe/Stage 3 (from 1 to 3 years):* Needs total care. Unable to feed self. Incontinent of bowel and bladder. Stops walking. Uses wheelchair or bedridden. Incoherent or mute. Apathetic.

Treatment Plan

Most patients with Alzheimer's disease are taken care of at home by a family member or care-giver during the early stages of the disease. As disease progresses, many patients are placed in skilled nursing facilities, or assisted-living dementia units. In later stages of the disease, families may consider hospice care.

Medications

- Mild to moderate (MMSE 10–26): Begin trial of a cholinesterase inhibitor (increases acetylcholine synthesis): Donepezil (Aricept), rivastigmine (Exelon), galantamine, Memantine (Namenda) PO daily to BID.
- Moderate to advanced dementia (MMSE <17): Add memantine (10 mg BID) to cholinesterase inhibitor or use memantine alone.
- Severe dementia (MMSE <10): Continue memantine or discontinue drug.
  - Vitamin E 2,000 IU daily (not recommended for other forms of dementia)
- Improvement within 3 to 6 months. Stop if no longer effective.

Adjunct Treatment

- Physical activity and exercise have been shown to decrease the risk of dementia.
- *Ginkgo biloba:* May help with memory (do not mix with aspirin or warfarin).
- Use omega-3 fatty acids, vitamin B supplementation.
- Axona (caprylidene): Prescription triglyceride-rich medical food (consumed as a shake) that addresses diminished cerebral glucose metabolism by assisting the body in metabolizing ketone bodies as an alternative fuel source for the brain.

Rehabilitation

- Cognitive rehabilitation: May help during early stages of dementia.
- Exercise programs: May slow functional decline.
- Occupational therapy: May improve performance of ADL.

Driving and Early-Stage or Mild Dementia

- Evaluate for safety and monitor regularly.
- Ask family or close contacts about patient's driving ability, traffic accidents, getting lost, difficulty making decisions, etc.

Complications

- Death is usually due to an overwhelming infection such as pneumonia and sepsis.
- Hip fractures are also a common cause of death (from complications).

Parkinson's Disease

Progressive neurodegenerative disease marked decrease of dopamine receptors. More common after 60 years of age. Depression is common (up to two thirds of all patients). The classic three symptoms are tremor (worse at rest), muscular rigidity, and bradykinesia. Parkinson's dementia is common (up to 40%).

Classic Signs

An elderly patient complains of a gradual onset of motor symptoms such as pill-rolling tremors of the hands, cogwheel rigidity with difficulty initiating voluntary movement. Walks with slow shuffling gait. Has poor balance and falls often (postural instability). Generalized muscular rigidity with masked facies. Mood disorders such as anxiety and depression. Excessive daytime sleepiness. Difficulty with executive function (making plans, decisions, tasks). May have signs and symptoms of dementia. Worsening of seborrheic dermatitis (white scales, erythema).

Treatment Plan

Consider treatment for significant bradykinesia or gait disturbance, moderate to severe hand tremors (dominant hand), depending on patient preference, and the degree that the tremors interfere with ADL, work, and social function.

Medications

- First-line drug: Carbidopa-levodopa (Sinemet) TID (dopamine precursor)
  - Start at low doses Sinemet 25/100 mg (half tab) PO BID to TID with meal or snack to avoid nausea. Titrate up slowly to control symptoms.
  - Sudden withdrawal or dose reductions of levodopa or dopamine agonists (bromocriptine, ropinirole, etc.) may be associated (rarely) with akinetic crisis or parkinsonism-hyperpyrexia syndrome (fever, autonomic dysfunction, muscular rigidity, altered mental status).
  - Adverse effects: Motor fluctuations (wearing-off phenomenon), dyskinesia, dystonia, dizziness, somnolence, nausea, headache. Eventually will develop tardive dyskinesia (treat with benztropine, amantadine, others).
- Dopamine agonists: Ergot type, such as bromocriptine (Parlodel) used in Parkinson's; newer dopamine agonists are non-ergot type, such as pramipexole (Mirapex)
  - Do not abruptly discontinue dopamine agonists. Dopamine withdrawal syndrome (8%–19%) causes panic attacks, anxiety, craving drug.
  - Adverseeffects:Cancauseimpulsecontroldisorders(compulsivegambling,sex,orshopping).
- MAO-B inhibitors: Selegiline (Eldepryl) or rasagiline (Azilect)
  - Does not have dietary restrictions like monoamine oxidase inhibitors (MAOIs).
  - Adverse effects: May cause insomnia, jitteriness, hallucinations. Do not combine with MAOIs or serotonin antagonist (selective serotonin reuptake inhibitors [SSRIs], triptans). Does not have dietary restrictions like MAOIs.
- Treatment for tardive dyskinesia (extrapyramidal symptoms)
  - Administer anticholinergics: Benztropine (Cogentin).
  - Administer amantadine (Symmetrel): Antiviral (treats type A influenza) and antiparkinson agent.
- Nonpharmacological: Exercise, physical therapy, speech therapy
- Surgery: Consider deep brain stimulation

Complications

- *Acute akinesia:* Loss of voluntary movement; sudden exacerbation of Parkinson's disease
- Dementia (40%)
- Frequent falls may result in fractures of the face, hips, and so on
- Drug-related adverse effects such as tardive dyskinesia, dystonia, motor fluctuations

Essential Tremor

The most common type of action or postural tremor. Usually seen in the arms or the hands and may be progress to include the head. Exact etiology is unknown. Essential tremor can occur in children and adults. It is not curable, but the symptoms can be controlled by medication. In some patients with essential tremor, the tremors can worsen with anxiety. Medications can be taken PRN (anxiety) or daily.

Treatment Plan

- Propranolol 60 to 320 mg per day. Long-acting propranolol (Inderal LA) is also effective but it provides the same response as "regular" propranolol
  - Contraindications (beta-blockers): Asthma, COPD, second- to third-degree heart block, bradycardia
- Primidone (Mysoline) 25 to 750 mg per day at bedtime
- Refer to neurologist for evaluation and treatment

NEUROCOGNITIVE FINDINGS

- *Abulia*: Loss of motivation or desire to do tasks, indifference to social norms (e.g., urinates in public)
- *Akathisia*: Intense need to move due to severe feelings of restlessness
- *Akinesia*: Reduced voluntary muscle movement (e.g., Parkinson's disease)
- *Amnesia*: Memory loss; anterograde amnesia is memory loss of recent events (occurs during disease) and retrograde amnesia is memory loss of events in the past (before the onset of disease)
- *Anomia*: Problems recalling words or names
- *Aphasia*: Difficulty using (speech) and/or understanding language; can include difficulty with speaking, comprehension, and written language
- *Apraxia*: Difficulty with or inability to remember learned motor skill
- *Astereognosis*: Inability to recognize familiar objects placed in the palm (place a coin on palm with eyes closed and ask patient to identify object)
- *Ataxia*: Difficulty coordinating voluntary movement
- *Broca's aphasia*: Ability to speak is intact but ability to comprehend language is lost
- *Confabulation*: "Lying" or fabrication of events due to inability to remember the event
- *Dyskinesia*: Abnormal involuntary muscle rigidity
- *Dystonia*: Involuntary repetitive muscle movements resulting in abnormal movements and postures (continuous muscle spasms)

EXAM TIPS

- **A question will ask you to identify the MMSE "activity" that is being performed.**
- **When a person is asked to interpret a proverb (given by the nurse practitioner [NP]), it is a test of abstract thinking.**
- **Korsakoff–Wernicke dementia brain damage is caused by vitamin B_1 (thiamine).**
- **The MMSE is the most popular screening test for dementia, and the most commonly used test for Alzheimer's disease.**
- **Alzheimer's disease is the most common cause of dementia in the United States.**
- **Vascular dementia is second most common cause of dementia.**
- **Recognize classic presentation of Parkinson's and Alzheimer's diseases.**
- **Recognize the "sundowning" phenomenon.**
- **First-line treatment for Parkinson's disease is levodopa (Sinemet) immediate-release.**
- **Selegiline (Eldepryl) is an MAO-B drug without food interactions. It affects the serotonin system; any drug that alters serotonin will increase risk of serotonin syndrome. Drugs that alter serotonin are the SSRIs, SNRIs, TCAs, MAOIs, and triptans. Allow at least 14 days (or longer) to pass before starting another drug that affects serotonin.**
- **Essential tremor is an "action," or postural tremor (not a resting tremor).**
- **First-line treatment for essential tremor is beta-blockers (propranolol).**

Sample Question

A nurse practitioner instructs a patient to copy a square (or spell "world" backward, subtract 7 from 100, etc.). Which of the following tests is being performed?

A) MMPI (or Minnesota Multiphasic Personality Inventory; for personality testing)
B) CAGE (for alcohol abuse screening in primary care)
C) MMSE
D) Beck's Inventory (a depression screening tool)

The correct answer is option C, the MMSE

CLINICAL PEARLS

- **Refer patients with suspected Alzheimer's disease and Parkinson's disease to a neurologist for diagnostic evaluation and management.**
- **UTI is one of the most common causes of acute mental status changes in the elderly. Order a UA in all elderly patients with acute mental status changes or delirium.**
- **Idiopathic Parkinson's disease is associated with low serum vitamin B_{12} levels due to levodopa. Check the vitamin B_{12} level.**
- **Some clinicians postpone levodopa use in early-onset Parkinson's disease (younger than 60 years) because of higher incidence of levodopa-related dyskinesia.**
- **Cholinergic drugs can exacerbate or worsen Parkinson's disease symptoms.**

OTHER COMMON GERIATRIC CONDITIONS

These diseases are covered under their respective organ systems.

- Acute diverticulitis (Chapter 10)
- Anemia (Chapter 13)
- Bacterial pneumonia (Chapter 8)
- COPD (Chapter 8)
- Congestive heart failure (Chapter 7)
- Diabetes type 2 (Chapter 9)
- Glaucoma (Chapter 5)
- Heart disease/murmurs (Chapter 7)
- Hyperlipidemia (Chapter 7)
- Hypertension (Chapter 7)
- Macular degeneration (Chapter 5)
- Menopause/atrophic vaginitis (Chapter 17)
- Temporal arteritis (Chapter 12)

PHARMACOLOGICAL ISSUES: OLDER ADULTS

Drug clearance is affected by renal impairment, a less efficient liver cytochrome P450 system, malabsorption, and relatively higher fat:muscle tissue (extends half-life, fat-soluble drugs). Older adults have an increased sensitivity to benzodiazepines, hypnotics, TCAs, and antipsychotics. The American Geriatrics Society has made a list of inappropriate medications for the elderly (Agency for Healthcare Research and Quality, National Guideline Clearinghouse, & American Geriatrics Society, 2015; Table 25.5).

Table 25.5 Potentially Inappropriate Medications for Older Adults (Beers List Criteria)*

Drug Class	Drugs to Avoid
Antihistamines	Diphenhydramine/Benadryl and others; newer generation has lower incidence (Claritin)
Benzodiazepines	Risk confusion, delirium, falls, fractures
Short–intermediate acting	Alprazolam (Xanax), lorazepam (Ativan), triazolam (Halcion)
Long acting	Diazepam (Valium), clonazepam (Klonopin)

(continued)

Table 25.5 Potentially Inappropriate Medications for Older Adults (Beers List Criteria) *(continued)*

Drug Class	**Drugs to Avoid**
Antipsychotics	Thioridazine (Mellaril), mesoridazine (Serentil)
Atypical antipsychotics	Quetiapine (Seroquel), olanzapine (Zyprexa)
Tricyclic antidepressants	Amitriptyline (Elavil), imipramine (Tofranil), doxepin
Cardiac drugs	Orthostatic hypotension
Alpha-blockers	Terazosin (Hytrin), clonidine (Catapres), higher risk hypotension
Atypical antipsychotics	Black box warning: Higher risk mortality in elderly from nursing homes
Sulfonylureas (avoid long-acting first-generation)	Glyburide (DiaBeta), chlorpropamide (Diabinese)
NSAIDs (indomethacin, ketorolac, others)	High risk of GI bleeding and PUD, especially aged >75 years or taking corticosteroids or anticoagulants
Mineral oil (oral) Proton-pump inhibitors	Aspiration pneumonia with mineral oil; long-term PPIs may increase risk of aspiration pneumonia
Zolpidem (Ambien), eszopiclone (Lunesta)	Adverse effects similar to benzodiazepines; minimal improvement in sleep latency
Antispasmodics	Dicyclomine (Bentyl), scopolamine, belladonna
Other	Metoclopramide (Reglan except for gastroparesis)
	Sliding-scale insulin dosing

* List is not all inclusive.

GI, gastrointestinal; NSAID, nonsteroidal anti-inflammatory drug; PPI, proton-pump inhibitor; PUD, peptic ulcer disease.

Source: Adapted from the American Geriatrics Society (2015). Updated Beers Criteria.

Professional Issues Review

VI

26

Ethical Guidelines and Advanced Practice Law

ETHICAL CONCEPTS

Beneficence

The obligation to help the patient—to remove harm, prevent harm, and promote good ("do no harm"). Acting in the patient's best interest. Compassionate patient care. The core principle in patient advocacy.

Examples:

- Educating patient with a new prescription about how to take the medication
- Encouraging a patient to stop smoking and enroll in smoking cessation program
- Calling the surgeon to get a prescription for stronger pain medications (a narcotic) for a postsurgical patient who complains of severe pain

Nonmaleficence

The obligation to avoid harm. Protecting a patient from harm.

Example: A middle-aged woman with osteoporosis wants to be treated with bisphosphonates. The nurse practitioner (NP) advises that the patient is not a good candidate for these drugs because of her past medical history of GI bleeding and peptic ulcer disease (PUD). The NP decides not to prescribe bisphosphonates.

Utilitarianism

The obligation to act in a way that is useful to or benefits the majority. The outcome of the action is what matters with utilitarianism. It also means to use a resource (e.g., tax money) for the benefit of most. It may resemble justice (see next definition), but it is not the same concept.

Example: The Special Supplemental Nutrition Program for Women, Infants, and Children food (WIC) are only for pregnant women and children, not other adults and elderly men. The reason may be that it would cost society more if women (and their fetuses), infants, and children are harmed by inadequate food intake (affects the brain growth, etc.).

Justice

The quality of being fair and acting with a lack of bias. The fair and equitable distribution of societal resources.

Example: A homeless alcoholic man without health insurance presents to the ED with abdominal pain. The patient is triaged and treated in the same manner as the other patients who have health insurance.

Dignity

The quality or state of being worthy of ethical and respectful treatment. Respect for human dignity is an important aspect of medical ethics. A person's religious, personal, and cultural beliefs can influence greatly what a person considers "dignified" treatment.

Examples:

- Hospital gowns should be secured correctly so that when patients get up to walk, their backs are not visible.
- Foley catheter urine bags should not be visible to visitors so patients are not embarrassed. NPs should move urine bags to the opposite bed rail so that they are not visible to outsiders.

Fidelity

The obligation to maintain trust in relationships. Dedication and loyalty to one's patients. Keeping one's promise.

Example: The relationship between a patient and her health care team is important. The primary care NP should try his or her best to develop a trusting relationship with a patient.

Confidentiality

The obligation to protect the patient's identity, personal information, test results, medical records, conversations, and other health information. This "right" is also protected by the Health Insurance Portability and Accountability Act (HIPAA; which restricts release of patient information). Psychiatric and mental health medical records are protected information and require separate consent.

Example: The HIPAA Privacy Rule protects most "individually identifiable health information" in any format (oral, paper, electronic). It is known as "protected health information" (PHI). The PHI includes demographic information (name, address, date of birth, Social Security number) as well as the individual's past, present, or future physical/mental health and provision of care.

Autonomy

The obligation to ensure that mentally competent adult patients have the right to make their own health decisions and express treatment preferences. If the patient is mentally incapacitated (dementia, coma), the designated surrogate's choices are respected. See later discussion on advance health care directives A mentally competent patient can decline or refuse treatment even if his or her adult children disagree.

Example: An alert elderly woman who has breast cancer decides to have a lumpectomy after discussing the treatment options with her oncologist. The woman's daughter tells the NP that she does not want her mother to have the surgery because she thinks her mother is too old. The NP has a duty to respect the patient's decision. This case is also a good example of the NP acting as the patient advocate.

Accountability

Health care providers are responsible for their own choices and actions and do not blame others for their mistakes.

Example: An NP has an adult male patient with acute bronchitis who complains of acute onset of chest pain. He is diagnosed with pleurisy. The patient goes to the ED and is diagnosed with an acute MI. The NP made an error in diagnosis; she is held accountable for her decision and actions in a court of law.

Notes

Paternalism describes situations in which one person interferes with or overrules the autonomy of another. In health care, it occurs when a provider makes decisions for a patient because he or she "believes" that it is in the patient's best interest. The opinion (or desire) of the patient is minimized or ignored. The patient is "powerless."

Example: A 92-year-old man does not want to be on a ventilator if he "codes." The son disagrees and quietly tells the NP and physician that he wants his father to be aggressively treated with life support, if necessary.

Veracity

The obligation to present information honestly and truthfully. In order for patients to make an informed and rational decision about their health care, pertinent information (including "bad" news) should not be withheld or omitted.

Example: The mammogram result of a 64-year-old female patient is highly indicative of breast cancer. The patient's son does not want his mother to know about the results. The NP has a duty to discuss the mammogram results with the patient and to refer her to a breast surgeon.

EXAM TIP

- **Become familiar with some of the ethical concepts (e.g., beneficence, veracity, nonmaleficence, justice) and how they are applied (look at the examples provided here).**

The American Nurses Association (ANA) *Code of Ethics for Nurses*

The new ANA *Code of Ethics for Nurses with Interpretive Statements* (2015) contains "the goals, values and ethical precepts that direct the profession of nursing." According to the ANA, the Code "is nonnegotiable." Each nurse "has an obligation to uphold and adhere to the code of ethics."

For example, under Provision 4.4, "Nurses may not delegate responsibilities such as assessment and evaluation; they may delegate selected interventions according to state nurse practice acts" (ANA, 2015).

LEGAL TERMS

Ombudsman

A person who acts as an intermediary (or as a liaison) between the patient and an organization (long-term care facilities or nursing homes, hospitals, governmental agencies, courts). The ombudsman investigates and mediates the complaint from both sides and attempts to reach a fair conclusion.

Guardian Ad Litem

An individual who is assigned by a court (and has the legal authority) to act in the best interest of the ward. The ward is usually a person who is a child, or someone who is frail or vulnerable.

Advance Health Care Directives

Living Will

A document that contains the patient's instructions and preferences regarding health care if the patient becomes seriously ill or is dying. It contains the patient's preferences (or not) for aggressive life-support measures. Health care providers should ensure that there is a copy of the document in the patient's chart.

Health Care Power of Attorney

A document that indicates that if a patient becomes incapacitated (physical and/or mental) in the future, his or her preferences for medical care (including life-prolonging procedures) are listed. Also known as an "advance directive for medical decisions," "health care proxy," "durable medical power of attorney," or "health care surrogate." The patient designates a person (family member or a close friend) who has the legal authority to make future health care decisions for the patient in the event that the patient becomes mentally incompetent or incapacitated (i.e., comatose).

It goes into effect when the patient's doctor has determined that he or she is physically or mentally unable to communicate in a willful manner. The patient designates a person (family, close friend) to be his or her health care surrogate (or health care proxy). To be legal, the advance directive must be signed in the presence of two adult witnesses who must also sign the document (the designated surrogate cannot act as a witness). Power is only for health care decisions (not financial assets).

Power of Attorney

A document whereby the patient designates a person (the "agent") who has the legal authority to make all decisions for the incapacitated patient. The document should be signed and notarized. Also known as the "durable power of attorney." This role is broader and encompasses not only health care decisions but also other areas of the patient's life, such as those relating to financial affairs.

Health Insurance Portability and Accountability Act (HIPAA)

Also known as the "HIPAA Privacy Rule" (or Public Law 104–191). The law was passed by the U.S. Congress and enacted in August, 1996. The law provides protections for "the use and disclosure of individuals' health information"—called "protected health information" by organizations subject to the Privacy Rule, which are called "covered entities."

Covered Entities

All health care providers, health insurance companies, health care plans, laboratories, hospitals, skilled nursing facilities (SNFs), and third-party administrators (TPAs) who electronically transmit health information must follow the HIPAA regulations.

What Is a TPA?

A TPA is the organization that does the processing of claims and administrative work for another company (health insurer, health plan, retirement plan).

HIPAA Requirements (Not Inclusive)

- Health providers are required to provide each patient with a copy of their office's HIPAA policy (patient to sign the form).
- The HIPAA form must be reviewed and signed annually by the patient.
- Patients have the right to review their medical files.
- A mental health provider has the right to refuse patients' requests to view their psychiatric and mental health records.
- When patients request to review their medical records, the health provider has up to 30 days to comply.
- Patients are allowed (under HIPAA) to correct errors in their medical records.
- Providers must keep identifying information (name, date of birth, address, Social Security number) and any diagnosis/disease or health concerns private except under certain conditions (see list that follows).

When Patient Consent Is Not Required

- To contact the health plan/insurance company that is paying for the medical care
- To contact a third party or business associate (e.g., accounting, legal, administrative) that the insurance company or doctor's office hires to assist in payment of their services (e.g., medical billing services)
- To perform certain health care operations (medical services review, sale of health care plan, audits)
- To contact collection agency for unpaid bills
- To report abuse/neglect or domestic violence
- To consult with other health care providers

HIPAA Case Scenarios (Table 26.1)

Examples

- If a staff member (who is not involved in the patient's care) calls the attending NP and wants to discuss a patient's progress, the NP cannot release information to the staff member.
- How to communicate results of lab tests or procedures? Ask the patient how he or she would like this to be handled. If the patient advises the health care provider to "leave it on my voice mail" and gives a phone number, then it is not a HIPAA violation to do so rather than relaying this information directly to the patient. Unless the patient has directed the clinician to leave the results on the voicemail, the clinician cannot assume that the voicemail is private and restricted to that individual (Buppert, 2012).

HIPAA, Psychotherapy, and Mental Health Records

Psychotherapy records made by a mental health professional are treated differently under HIPAA. They should be separated from the patient's other medical records. A separate consent form is needed to release psychotherapy records. The exceptions are mandatory reporting of abuse and "duty to warn" when the patient threatens serious and imminent harm to others. "In situations where the patient is given an opportunity and does not object, HIPAA allows the provider to share or discuss the patient's mental health information with family members or other persons involved in the patient's care or payment for care" (HHS, 2017).

Table 26.1 HIPAA and Patient Care

Situation	Description	Notes
Putting patient charts on door box	Place the chart so that the front of the chart is facing the door (so that patient name is hidden).	Nonstaff members are in the hallways.
Having sign-in sheets on front desk	This is allowed if it does not list patient's diagnosis.	Attendance list can show names, dates, and time.
Calling a patient in the waiting room to go inside the clinic exam room	Use only first name. If more than one person with same first name, use the first letter of last name.	If you have two patients named "Ann" (e.g., Ann Lee and Ann Smith), use Ann L. and Ann S.
Leaving messages on voicemail	When calling, first provide your name and contact information. Be concise. Limit to 60 seconds. Maximum of three calls per week.	When a patient lists a phone number as a contact, it constitutes express consent for telephone calls to be made, subject to certain HIPAA restrictions.

(*continued*)

Table 26.1 HIPAA and Patient Care *(continued)*

Situation	Description	Notes
	Information that can be given may includes appointment reminders, notifications about prescriptions, and preoperative and postoperative instructions.	Text messages should be restricted to 160 characters. There should be a limit of one text message per day.
Having a colleague who works in same clinic or hospital call, wanting information about a patient's progress	If staff member is not part of the health care team, no patient information can be released to that person.	HIPAA also does not allow such a person to access a friend's or family member's records without permission.
Having a family member call, wanting information about a patient's progress	Put on hold, and tell patient about the call. If patient gives permission, you can speak with the family member.	If patient does not consent, then advise the family member about the patient's decision. Do not release patient information.
Having inappropriate access of health information on the computer	Viewing the records of your relatives, friends, or coworkers information is a HIPAA violation.	Do not allow someone to use your computer password, or leave a computer terminal with the patient's information displayed on the screen (log out first).
Using personal devices (smart phones, laptops, tablets)	Ideally, it is best to avoid using personal devices at work. Requirements: secure WiFi with passwords, regular encrypted backups, antivirus software, policies, etc.	If you want to use a personal device, discuss it with your manager and/or consult information technology. Best practice is to use the facility's or clinic's devices.
Discussing a patient's drugs and other instructions with a health aide who is with the patient	Discussing information is allowable.	If patient has the capacity to make health care decisions, discussing information is allowable.
Discussing patient's treatment in front of a patient's friend who is visiting	Discussing treatment with the patients' friend if the patient gives consent or requests that the friend come inside the treatment room.	Discussing patient information with others is allowable if patient agrees to it.

HIPAA, Health Insurance Portability and Accountability Act.

Source: HIPAA Journal (2015).

Minors

The health records of a minor (by law, an individual younger than 18 years of age) can be released to parents or legal guardians without the minor's consent. If authorization is needed to release a minor's medical record, the parent or legal guardian must sign for it (except for emancipated minors). Emancipated minors can sign their own legal documents.

EXAM TIPS

- **Become familiar with how HIPAA is applied in real life. Study the HIPAA case scenarios in the table.**
- **Regarding leaving any laboratory results on voicemail, it is a HIPAA violation unless the patient has given specific consent such as "you can leave the lab results in my voicemail at this phone number." If not, then call and leave your name and contact information.**

- **Understand the role of an ombudsman, guardian ad litem, and others who act on behalf of a patient.**
- **A TPA is the organization that does the processing of claims and administrative work for another company (health insurer, health plan, retirement plan).**

HEALTH INSURANCE

The Affordable Care Act (ACA; 2010)

This national health insurance legislation, officially known as the Patient Protection and Affordable Care Act and unofficially nicknamed Obamacare, was enacted in March 2010 with the goal of expanding health insurance for the millions of Americans who were then uninsured. Signed by President Obama in March 2010 (and upheld by the U.S. Supreme Court in 2012), the ACA expanded health coverage through various provisions (e.g., allowing adult children younger than age 26 to be insured under their parents' health care insurance). This comprehensive reform of U.S. health insurance law prohibits an insurance company from rejecting people with preexisting health conditions. There is also a penalty for employers (and individuals) who choose not to participate in the national health plan. Although increased numbers of American gained insurance as a result of the law's passage, many millions more still lack coverage.

Consolidated Omnibus Budget Reconciliation Act of 1985 (COBRA)

Also known as "COBRA coverage." Provides for the continuation of coverage of preexisting group health insurance (from the employer) for workers and their families who lose their coverage (between jobs, quit job, or are fired) for a fixed period of time. COBRA coverage is generally offered for 18 months (up to 36 months in some cases).

Managed Care

Both HMOs and PPOs are classified as "managed health care plans."

Health Maintenance Organizations (HMOs)

Patients are assigned a primary care provider (PCP), who is the "gatekeeper." The patient has a set "copay" per visit, and the participating physician/health provider is paid a set fee (per patient) monthly. The physician receives a monthly check from the HMO.

- Specialist/consultant: The PCP must first approve the referral. The patient is limited to seeing the physicians/specialists who are enrolled in the HMO's network.
- "Out-of-network physicians" or not referred by the PCP: The visit may not be covered or it will be reimbursed at a lower rate.

Preferred Provider Organization (PPO)

The patient can visit any provider in the network without a referral. Not assigned a PCP (as in HMOs). The patient can choose his or her own PCP. No referral is needed to see a specialist who is part of the PPO panel. PPOs are usually more expensive than HMOs.

MEDICARE AND MEDICAID

Both the Medicare and Medicaid programs are under the aegis of the Centers for Medicare & Medicaid Services (CMS). The CMS is one of the agencies under the U.S. Department of Health and Human Services (DHHS).

Medicare Part A (Inpatient Hospitalization)

"Automatic" at age 65 if the person paid the premiums (automatically deducted from paycheck by the employer). If the person never paid the premiums (e.g., full-time housewife), the person is not eligible for Medicare coverage. Also covers persons with end-stage renal diseases at any age.

Certain religious groups (e.g., Amish, Mennonites) do not participate in Medicare.

- Medicare Part A will pay for the following "medically necessary" services:
  - Inpatient hospitalization (including inpatient psychiatric hospitalization
  - Hospice care
  - Home health care
  - Skilled nursing facility care
- Medicare Part A will not pay for custodial care (nursing homes, retirement homes).

Medicare Part B (Outpatient Insurance)

Medicare Part B is a voluntary program with monthly premiums. One must enroll during the "general enrollment period."

- Medicare Part B will pay for the following "medically necessary" services:
  - Outpatient visits (including walk-in clinics, urgent care clinics, ED visits)
  - Laboratory and other types of tests (EKG, x-rays, CT scans)
  - Durable medical equipment
  - "Second opinions" with another physician (surgery)
  - Kidney dialysis (outpatient), self-dialysis equipment/supplies, organ transplants, and many others
- Medicare Part B does not pay for:
  - Most eyeglasses and eye exams (except following cataract surgery that implants an intraocular lens)
  - Hearing aids
  - Most dentures and dental care
  - Cosmetic plastic surgery (unless it is medically necessary)
  - Over-the-counter drugs and most prescription drugs
- Medicare Part B does pay for some health prevention services:
  - Abdominal aortic aneurysm screening
  - Influenza shots once a year and Pneumovax and Prevnar 13 (each once in a lifetime)
  - Screening mammogram (once every 12 months for women age 40+)
  - Hepatitis B vaccine series for individuals at medium or high risk
  - Hepatitis C screening if high risk
  - Screening colonoscopy or flexible sigmoidoscopy (aged 50 years or older) every 10 years if low risk
  - Routine Pap smears (once every 2 years, or once every 12 months for women at high risk)
  - Prostate cancer screening (digital rectal exam [DRE] and prostate specific antigen [PSA] once a year after age 50)
  - Bone density testing allowed once every 24 months if at risk for osteoporosis, taking prednisone, bisphosphonate therapy to monitor progress
  - HIV screening; sexually transmitted disease/infection screenings covered once every 12 months.
  - Physical exams (once a year)
  - Smoking-cessation counseling and treatment

- Alcohol misuse screening and counseling
- Diabetes screening (twice yearly if at risk)
- Cardiovascular disease screening

Medicare Advantage (Medicare Part C)

Medicare Advantage Plans cover both inpatient care (Part A) and outpatient care (Part B), and some plans cover some prescription drugs. They are administered by private health insurance companies approved by Medicare.

Medicare Part D

- Also known as the Medicare prescription drug benefit. Only individuals who are enrolled (or eligible) for Medicare Part A and/or Part B are eligible. One type of Part D coverage is called the Medicare Advantage (MA) plan.
- All prescription drug plans have a list of preferred drugs (the formulary). If a non-formulary drug is used, it may not be covered and the patient has to pay for it "out-of-pocket."

Medicaid

Authorized by Title XIX of the Social Security Act. A federal and state matching program. Provides health insurance coverage for low-income individuals and their families who meet the federal poverty-level criteria. Covers children, pregnant women, adults, seniors, and individuals with disabilities (i.e., blindness). Pays for health care and prescription drugs.

Currently, Medicaid is the single largest payer for mental health services in the United States. It covers care offered by substance use disorder and family planning services (including contraception) as well as by maternal and infant health programs.

Children's Health Insurance Programs

The Children's Health Insurance Program (CHIP) and the Children's Health Insurance Program Reauthorization Act of 2009 (CHIPRA) cover uninsured children (infancy to adolescents) and pregnant women.

CASE MANAGEMENT

Case Managers

Health care case managers are usually experienced RNs who act as coordinators for the outpatient management of patients with certain diagnoses (usually chronic, resource-intensive diseases). The process is called "case management." Case management is mainly done by telephone.

Examples: Asthma (children), chronic obstructive pulmonary disease (COPD), chronic heart failure, diabetes

Patient-Centered Medical Home (PCMH)

PCMH is a health care delivery model that is also known as the "primary care medical home." It is another way to deliver patient-centered primary care. In PCMH, the patient and family are considered important members of the health care team. Most of the patient's health care needs are taken care of in the home setting. Other team members may include physicians, advanced practice nurses, physician assistants (PAs), nurses, pharmacists, nutritionists, social workers, educators, and care coordinators (Agency for Healthcare Research and Quality, n.d.).

Delivery of health care is coordinated to ensure smooth transition between home and the hospital, home health agency, and community services. The patient and/or family has 24/7 access to a member of the team by phone, video chat, or email.

Quality-Improvement Programs

Quality improvement involves monitoring, identifying problems, measuring outcomes, and establishing new parameters for improved performance. The goal of these programs is to improve the quality of care, decrease complications, decrease hospitalizations, lower patient mortality, decrease system errors, and increase patient satisfaction. Patient outcomes are important indicators of a health system's quality.

Example: A "problem" is identified (diabetic complications such as peripheral neuropathy, retinopathy, etc.). Then outcome measures are identified (e.g., hemoglobin A1C <6.5%, etc.). Be familiar about what a good outcome is for a disease (for diabetics, a good outcome is A1C <6.5%) and what a poor outcome is (A1C >8%).

Risk Management in Health Care

Risk management is an important aspect of quality-improvement/quality-assurance programs in the health care setting. It is the systematic organizational process used to identify risky practices to minimize adverse patient outcomes and corporate liability. For example, high-risk areas that are usually checked by risk managers are medication errors, hospital-acquired infections, patient identification problems, and falls. Risk management promotes safe and effective patient care practices.

Accreditation

Accreditation is a voluntary process through which a nongovernmental association evaluates and certifies that an organization (e.g., hospital, clinic, nursing program) has met the requirements and excels in its class. For example, the American Nurses Credentialing Center and the National League for Nursing Accrediting Commission are accreditation organizations.

The Joint Commission (TJC)

An independent, not-for-profit organization that accredits health care organizations (hospitals, nursing homes, home care, laboratories) via inspection and evaluation of their facilities (charged a fee). Achieving TJC certification means that a facility has met or surpassed the organization's strict requirements. "The ultimate purpose of The Joint Commission's accreditation process is to enhance quality of care and patient safety" (The Joint Commission, 2017).

Sentinel Event (SE) Reporting

An SE is a patient safety event (not primarily related to the natural course of the patient's illness or condition) that results in any of the following: death, permanent harm, and/or severe temporary harm with "intervention required to sustain life" (The Joint Commission, 2017). When an SE occurs, the health care organization is expected to conduct a root cause analysis, make improvements to reduce risk, and monitor effectiveness of the improvements. Accredited organizations are strongly encouraged but are not required to report SEs to the TJC.

Examples of SEs

- Suicide that occurs while receiving care in a staffed around-the-clock facility or within 72 hours discharge
- Unanticipated death of an infant or discharge of infant to the wrong family
- Rape or assault of a staff member, visitor, or vendor
- Invasive procedure on the wrong patient, or the wrong procedure is done on a patient or is done to the wrong limb
- Unintended retention of a foreign object
- Fire, flame, or unanticipated smoke or heat during an episode of patient care

Root Cause Analysis (RCA)

A process used in health care to identify the contributing factors that result in an error. "RCA is a structured facilitated team process to identify root causes of an event that resulted in an undesired outcome and develop corrective actions" (The Joint Commission, 2017). The TJC has mandated the use of RCA to analyze SEs.

The gathered data are analyzed for the root causes (usually a combination of human, environmental, and system factors). The goal is to identify the system breakdowns that resulted in an inadvertent mistake and to propose at least one corrective action to reduce or eliminate each root cause. When an SE occurs, an RCA is recommended. The focus is on the system and not on blaming individuals. A small team usually does the investigations.

Outcomes Analysis

Outcomes analysis refers to analysis and tracking of patient outcomes by using outcome measures (i.e., surveys, questionnaires).

HOSPICE

The majority of hospice care in the United States takes place in patient's homes (59% die in their own homes). The goal is palliative care, not curative care. Ensuring the patient's quality of life and comfort are the ultimate goals of hospice care. Hospice care is available for both pediatric and adult patients.

An interdisciplinary team provides hospice care. This team usually consists of the patient's primary physician, hospice physician, registered nurse, nursing assistants, therapists, social workers/grief counselor, and clergy. Hospice staff are on call 24 hours a day. They provide grief-and-loss counseling for patients and family members.

Hospice is covered under Medicare Part A, Medicaid, and most health insurance plans. Hospice patients are allowed to have physical therapy (PT), occupational therapy (OT), and speech therapy if prescribed (see www.medicare.gov/coverage/hospice-and-respitecare.html).*

Eligibility Criteria for Hospice

- The hospice physician and the patient's physician certify that the patient is terminal and has 6 months (or less) to live. The hospice physician approves of admission.
- Patient is rapidly declining or exhibits worsening symptoms.
- Patient needs assistance with two or more activities of daily living (ADL).
- Patient accepts palliative care, not curative care. If he or she does not want to be in hospice (even if all criteria are met), then patient is not eligible.

*Your Medicare Coverage. Hospice & respite care.

Examples of Terminal Conditions

- Metastatic cancers (e.g., lung cancer, colon cancer)
- End-stage lung disease (e.g., COPD)
- End-stage heart disease (e.g., congestive heart failure [CHF] class III or IV)
- End-stage liver disease
- HIV/AIDS with comorbidities and refusal/discontinuation of antiretrovirals
- End-stage renal disease with plan to discontinue dialysis
- Amyotrophic lateral sclerosis, Parkinson's disease, stroke, coma
- End-stage dementia (e.g., Alzheimer's disease)

Respite Care

This refers to short-term respite care for the primary caregiver is reimbursed by Medicare. This gives the primary caregiver a break, even if it is only a few hours. For example, resite care gives the caregiver a chance to go see a movie and to "relax" and rest.

HUMAN GENETIC SYMBOLS

New to the exam are questions about genetic symbols. The symbol for a healthy male is an empty square and for a diseased/affected male, it is a filled square. The symbol for a healthy female is an empty circle and for a diseased/affected female, it is a filled circle. A diagonal dash across a symbol means that the person is dead.

Gender	Symbol	Description
Healthy male	□	Empty square
Diseased male	■	Filled square
Healthy female	○	Empty circle
Diseased female	●	Filled circle
Death	⍁	Diagonal dash across a symbol

EXAM TIPS

- **A patient may meet the criteria for hospice admission, but if the patient refuses hospice care, then the patient is not eligible.**
- **If the patient meets the criteria for hospice care, Medicare Part A will reimburse hospice.**
- **Medicare Part B will pay for an ambulance for emergency care only. If the ambulance is used for transportation purposes, Medicare will not reimburse this type of service.**
- **Medicare Part B does not reimburse for dentures, eyeglasses, or hearing aids.**
- **COBRA is a law that allows a person to continue group health insurance coverage from a job even if he or she has quit (the individual has to pay the insurance premiums).**
- **No separate consent is required for entities that pay or process the patient's health bills, such as health insurance companies, HMOs, medical billers, or collection agencies (or third-party contractors hired by the company to pay or to process claims).**
- **The "medical home" is a method of primary health care delivery. Health care providers and therapists (physical, occupational, speech) deliver care in the patient's home, with**

the family. These patients have chronic long-term illness. To communicate, technology is used such as phone, video chat, or email.

- Use common sense in answering questions on quality improvement and risk management. Keep in mind the goals of these processes: to improve the quality of care, decrease complications, decrease hospitalizations, lower patient mortality, decrease system errors, and increase patient satisfaction. Look for the answer that fits these goals.
- Learn the human genetic symbol for a diseased (or affected) male and female.

27

Professional Roles and Reimbursement

THE NURSE PRACTITIONER ROLE

History

Loretta C. Ford, PhD, RN, FAAN, and Henry K. Silver, MD, started the first nurse practitioner (NP) program at the University of Colorado in 1965. Initially, it was a certificate program and later became a master's program in the 1970s. The first NPs were pediatric NPs who practiced in poor rural areas where there were no physicians (because of a severe shortage of primary care physicians).

Regulation of Nurse Practitioners

Educational Requirements

An NP must meet the minimal educational requirements that are mandated by the nurse practice act of the state (where he or she plans to practice).

State Nurse Practice Act

The nurse practice act is enacted into law by the state legislature. Therefore the NP's legal right to practice is derived from the state legislature. Each state has its own nurse practice act that contains regulations that dictate the educational requirements, responsibilities, and the scope of practice for NPs and for other nurses (e.g., RNs, licensed practical nurses, midwives, etc.) who practice in the state. NP practice is not regulated by the federal government, the AMA, or the DHHS..

State Board of Nursing

The state board of nursing (SBON) is responsible for enforcing the state's nurse practice act. The SBON is a formal governmental agency that has the statutory authority to regulate nursing practice. The SBON has the legal authority to license, monitor, and to discipline nurses. The SBON is also authorized to revoke a nurse's license (after formal hearings).

Title Protection

Professional designations, such as RN, or NP, advanced registered nurse practitioner [ARNP], or advanced practice registered nurse [APRN]), are protected by law. It is illegal for any person to use these titles without a valid license. Title protection is under mandate by a state's nurse practice act. Title protection protects the public from unlicensed "nurses."

Licensure and Certification

Licensure is a legal requirement to practice as an NP. It is obtained through a governmental entity, the SBON. The NP must meet the minimal educational and clinical requirements in order to become licensed.

Certification is generally a "voluntary" process and is done through a nongovernmental entity such as a professional nursing association or specialty organization. The majority of states in the United States now mandate board certification (or certification) as a condition to obtain licensure.

Standards of Professional Nursing Practice

Standards are authoritative statements of the duties that all registered nurses, regardless of role, population, or specialty are expected to perform (Bickford, Marion, & Gazaway, 2015). According to the American Nurses Association (ANA), these include both the Standards of Practice and the Standards of Professional Performance (Bickford, Marion, & Gazaway, 2015). They are developed by professional societies (e.g., ANA) as well as specialty organizations. For example, the American Association of Nurse Practitioners (AANP) publishes *Standards of Practice for Nurse Practitioners* (AANP, 2013).

Collaborative Practice Agreements

A written agreement between a physician and NP outlining the NP's role and responsibility to the clinical practice. A copy of the collaborative practice agreement must be kept at the NP's practice setting and mailed to the state board of nursing. Most states require an annual review of the agreement that contains signatures of the individuals involved and dates.

The state practice environment differs for each specific state. Some states allow full practice under the exclusive authority of the SBON. Some states allow reduced practice, and some have restricted practice. In these states, the NP must be under the supervision or delegation of an outside health discipline such as the Board of Medicine.

Agreements With Physicians and Dentists

NPs can sign collaborative practice agreements with physicians (MDs), osteopaths (doctors of osteopathy [DOs]), and dentists/dental surgeons (doctors of medicine in dentistry [DMDs]/ doctors of dental surgery [DDSs]). Chiropractors (DCs) and naturopaths (NDs) are not considered physicians under nurse practice acts. In most states, physicians are the only practitioners who can legally sign a death certificate.

Prescription Privileges

The majority of states require NPs to have a written practice protocol with a supervising physician in order to prescribe drugs. The protocol usually contains the list of drugs (by name, by class, or by condition) that an NP is allowed to prescribe. As of January 1, 2017, all states now allow NPs to prescribe certain controlled drugs, but with limitations.

Prescription Pads

The NP's prescription pad should contain the following:

- NP's name, designation, and license number
- Clinic's name, address, and phone number; if the practice has several clinics, the other clinics where the NP practices should also be listed on the pad
- To reduce fraud, it is best if the drug enforcement agent (DEA) number is not list (only for controlled substance prescriptions)

Food and Drug Administration (FDA) Controlled Substances

- Tamper-resistant prescription pads are required by Medicare and Medicaid, as well as when prescribing FDA controlled substances.
- A controlled substance prescription can be typed, but it must be signed by the prescribing practitioner the day it is issued.

FDA Schedule II Drug Prescriptions

- Substances in this schedule have a high potential for abuse with severe psychological or physical dependence.
- These cannot be called in. They must be written on tamper-resistant pads and signed by the prescriber (not stamped).
- There is some variation among the different state laws regarding prescriptions of Schedule II drugs.

Examples:

Codeine, morphine, hydrocodone, oxycodone, opium, fentanyl, methadone, amphetamines, etc.

E-Prescribing (Electronic Prescriptions)

- A method of sending prescriptions electronically directly to the pharmacy
- Preferred method of prescribing by Medicare and Medicaid

The Four Generations of Nurses

This may be the first time that four generations of nurses are working side by side. Each generation behaves differently. Table 27.1 describes each generation.

Table 27.1 Generation Types

Generation	Description
"Silent Generation"	Born from 1925 to 1945. Disciplined and loyal. Traditional work ethic. More action oriented. The youngest nurses from this generation are now in their 70s and most have retired.
Baby boomers	Born from 1946 to 1964. Hard workers. Like to achieve. More susceptible to burnout and stress-related illness.
Generation X (Gen Xers)	Born from 1965 to 1980. Question authority, expect immediate results. They are loyal to peers over the company.
Generation Y (Millennials)	Born from 1981 to 2000. Multitaskers who seek learning and career development, but also value free time to socialize.

Source: Frandsen (2014).

NURSING LEADERSHIP STYLES

Situational Leadership

Leader is flexible and can adjust his or her leadership style to fit the changing needs of an organization. Can establish rapport easily and bring out the best in people. The result is that staff members are engaged with the goals of the organization and are more productive. Situational leadership theory was developed by Ken Blanchard and Paul Hersey.

Transformational Leadership

Leader has the ability to communicate vision to staff members. May have charismatic personality. Good communication skills. Staff members usually have higher job satisfaction with this type of leader.

Laissez-Faire Leadership

Leader engages in minimal supervision and direction of staff members. Prefers "hands off" approach. May not like to make decisions. This style of leadership works well if workers are experienced, like autonomy, and are self-directed. New or unexperienced staff may feel anxious with this type of authority due to minimal supervision and feedback.

Authoritarian Leadership (Autocratic)

Leader likes control and structure and prefers to give directions. May have many rules. Makes decisions without (or minimal) staff input. Motivated, independent, and self-directed staff may be unhappy in this type of environment.

Democratic Leadership

Leader may like to have more frequent staff meetings because he or she values staff members' input and feedback. Team shares in decision-making process, which may be slow due to desire to include all of staff in process. Leader values relationships and staff opinions.

Servant Leadership

Leader likes to work along with staff on the unit. May assume many roles. Develops relationships with staff members and treats staff as individuals, which results in high job satisfaction for staff. But this type of leader may not like to make decisions that can "anger" staff members.

MALPRACTICE INSURANCE

The two types of malpractice insurance are claims-based and occurrence-based.

Claims-Based Policy

This type of malpractice insurance will cover claims only if the incident occurred when the NP paid the premium *and* only if the NP is still enrolled with the same insurance company at the time the claim is filed in court. The claim will not be covered (in the future) if he or she does not have the same insurance company as when the lawsuit was filed. Buying "tail coverage" can help address this issue.

Tail coverage insurance will cover the NP for malpractice claims that may be filed against him or her in the future. When an NP with claims-based malpractice insurance retires or changes jobs, it is advisable to buy tail coverage insurance.

Example: An NP who has been retired for 2 years has a claim filed against her for an incident that occurred while she was employed and insured. The NP discontinued her claims-based malpractice insurance when she retired. In this case, the claim will not be covered. But if she bought tail coverage, then it would be covered.

Occurrence-Based Policy

This type of malpractice policy is not affected by job changes or retirement. If a claim is filed against the NP in the future, it is covered if he or she had an occurrence-based policy at the time the incident occurred.

Example: An NP who has been retired for 2 years has a claim filed against her for an incident that occurred while she was employed and insured. Since she carried an occurrence-based policy, the claim will be covered.

MALPRACTICE LAWSUITS

- Plaintiff: The patient or whoever is acting on behalf of the patient (e.g., the patient's representative) who files the lawsuit claiming injury and/or damage by another party
- Defendant: The party who responds to the lawsuit filed by another party who claims an injury and/or damage (e.g., NP, hospital)

Elements of a Case

The plaintiff must prove that all of the following occurred:

- A duty is owed (a legal duty exists).
- The duty was breached (e.g., not following standard of care, etc.).
- The breach caused an injury (proximate cause).
- Damage occurred.

Phases of a Medical Malpractice Trial

- A lawsuit is filed in the appropriate court.
- The "discovery" phase (requesting of medical records, depositions, expert opinions, etc.) occurs.
- Plaintiff has the "burden of proof."
- Court trial phase (or settle out of court or arbitration) occurs.
- The judgment is given.
- Either the case is dismissed or damages are awarded (physical harm, emotional/mental harm, etc.).

Expert Witnesses

Ideally, the NP who will testify as an expert witness should be someone who practices in the same specialty and geographic area as the NP defendant. For example, an NP who practices in Los Angeles, California, may not be the best choice as an expert witness for an NP who is being sued and who is practicing in Miami, Florida.

REIMBURSEMENT

Budget Reconciliation Act of 1989 (HR 3299)

The first law allowing NPs to be reimbursed directly by Medicare. Prior to this Act, only certified pediatric and family NPs were allowed to be primary providers as long as they practiced in designated "rural" areas.

Balance Budget Act of 1997

Together with the Primary Care Health Practitioner Incentive Act, this law broadened Medicare coverage of NP and clinical nurse specialist services. The Health Insurance Portability and Accountability Act (HIPAA) of 1996 required health providers to have a National Provider Identifier (NPI) number to bill Medicare and Medicaid. NPs can be reimbursed directly by Medicare Part B, Medicaid, Tricare, and some health insurance plans. Medicare will reimburse NPs at 85% of the Medicare Physician Fee Schedule.

NPI Number

The NPI is a unique 10-digit identification number assigned to health care providers (or to any entity that bills Medicare/Medicaid). It is issued by the National Plan and Provider Enumeration System (NPPES). All providers who provide services and bill Medicare must have an NPI number. Individual health care providers may obtain only one NPI for themselves.

To become a Medicare-approved provider, one must first obtain an NPI number online. An individual provider's NPI identifier lasts for his or her lifetime. The identifier does not change regardless of state, group affiliations, or state. Medicare requires the NPI number for financial transactions. Electronic claims submission is required by Medicare and Medicaid. Medicare uses electronic fund transfer (EFT) to reimburse providers.

"Incident to" Billing and Medicare

"Incident to" billing is a way to bill Medicare for outpatient services rendered by a nonphysician health provider (NP, physician assistant [PA]) and receive the 100% physician fee. The location of the services can be at the physician's office, a separate or satellite office, an institution, or in the patient's home.

During the first visit, the physician must evaluate the patient (and write a care plan). Follow-up visits by the NP can be billed as "incident to" so long as the same health problems are being addressed. The physician's NPI number is used to bill for the service. The "incident-to" billing is reimbursed at 100% of the physician rate. But if the same patient is seen for a new problem by the NP (or PA), then the visit is billed under the NP's or PA's NPI number (85% of physician fee).

Medical Coding and Billing

Every time an NP bills Medicare, Medicaid, and/or a health insurance plan, he or she must submit a claim (electronic or paper form). The claim form, or the "superbill," must contain both the *International Classification of Diseases*, 10th edition (*ICD-10*; World Health Organization [WHO], 2016) code(s) or the diagnosis and the Current Procedural Terminology (CPT) code(s). If a bill is missing the CPT code (or *ICD-10* code), then the clinic or hospital will not get paid for the NP's services. If an NP's signature is on the superbill, it is his or her responsibility to make sure that the correct diagnosis (*ICD-10*) and CPT codes are being used. The services rendered must show medical necessity and the appropriateness of diagnostic and/or therapeutic services that were done.

What Is the ICD-10 *Code?*

The *ICD-10* code is used to indicate the patient's diagnosis as determined by the *International Classification of Diseases*, 10th edition (WHO, 2016). Each disease is assigned a specific *ICD-10* code.

What Is an ICD-10 *"Z-Code" (Z00–Z99)?*

ICD-10 uses Z-codes to indicate the reason for each patient encounter. If a procedure is performed, a corresponding CPT code must accompany each Z-code (to justify the procedure, tests, encounter, etc.).

What Is the CPT?

The CPT is a list of standard alphanumeric identifying codes used to identify procedures (e.g., suturing, incision, and drainage) and other medical services. It is maintained by the American Medical Association (AMA).

What Are Evaluation and Management Service (E&M) Codes?

E&M codes are used to bill for patient visits, and are part of the CPT. If a bill is missing an E&M code, the health care provider will not be reimbursed for the time he or she spent with the patient. E&M codes are based on the history, examination, and medical decision making (complexity) that take place. The provider must document that these three components have been met (or exceeded). The complexity and time spent with the patient are assigned codes by the CPT system.

For example, a "problem-focused" visit requires documentation of the chief complaint with a brief history of present illness (HPI), but it does not require a review of systems (ROS) or a past, family, and/or social history.

EXAM TIPS

- **NPs get their "right to practice" from the state legislature.**
- **Identify a problem-focused visit (see example previously noted).**
- **There are various types of nursing leadership.**
- **Claims-based malpractice insurance will cover claims only if the NP is still enrolled with the same insurance company at the time the claim is filed in court.**
- **Occurrence-type malpractice insurance will cover a lawsuit in the future even if you no longer carry the policy so long as you had an active policy during the alleged incident.**
- **The NPI contains 10 numbers/digits.**
- **The *ICD-10* is used for diagnosis codes. The CPT code is used to bill for outpatient office procedures and services. Both the *ICD-10* and CPT codes are required for each bill.**
- **"Incident to" billing is used for Medicare patients and refers to billing of a follow-up visit performed by a nonphysician provider billed under the physician's NPI number (the nonphysician provider is paid 100% vs. the rate of an NP or PA, who receive only 85%).**

28

Culture and Spiritually Related Health Beliefs

CULTURE AND NURSING

Culturally competent care improves patient satisfaction and patient safety (e.g., by reducing medication-related errors). To provide culturally competent care, the advanced practice registered nurse (APRN) must develop knowledge, skills, and positive attitudes about diverse cultures and work individually and within the health care system to promote care that is respectful of all cultures. If a cultural practice has an adverse effect on a patient's health, then the nurse practitioner (NP) needs to explain to the patient in a sensitive manner the reason for not following the practice.

Example: A female patient tells the NP that her shaman/*curandero* "told me not to take my medicine, but to drink herbal tea instead" or "he told me not to drink water for 2 days." The NP respectfully explains to the patient why the practice is harmful to her health.

Leininger's Theory of Cultural Care Diversity and Universality

Madeleine Leininger is recognized as the founder of transcultural nursing and credited with the construct of "culturally congruent care." This theory defines culture as "the specific pattern of behavior that distinguishes any society from others and gives meaning to human expressions of care" (Leininger, 2014). Leininger's Sunrise model is likely the most frequently used to frame culturally competent nursing care and research. The Sunrise model recognizes that care is influenced by many cultural features (i.e., technology, religiosity or spirituality, kinship and social structures, cultural values and beliefs and practices, legal and political systems, economics, and education), all of which shape one's worldview.

CULTURAL AND SPIRITUAL AWARENESS

This is defined as "being knowledgeable about one's own thoughts, feelings, and sensations, as well as the ability to reflect on how these can affect one's interactions with other" (Giger et al., 2007). The following cultural and religious descriptions are generalizations and oversimplifications based on traditional requirements of certain cultures and religion. Consult with the patient and family to understand their unique interpretations and practices.

African Americans

African Americans often use religious coping—typically Christian (e.g., prayer, gospel music, Bible reading, engagement with faith community). Christian pastors and preachers are held in high esteem. Church congregations and religion may be important sources of emotional and tangible support. Some patients may feel that their illness is caused by lack of faith or by sin. Many families have a female head of household (matriarchal).

Latinos/Hispanics

Latino families have a strong matriarchal element, and the mother is an important source of strength and solace in times of illness. People from various Latino cultures may consult folk healers. "Susto" is a cultural illness (*susto* means "fright"). *Mal ojo* (or *mal de ojo*), the "evil eye," is a folk illness (usually of a baby/child). It is caused by an adult who stares with envy at the child. (This is similar to the belief in an "evil eye" among some Muslim and Mediterranean cultures.) The hex can be broken if the person staring at the child touches the child. Another way to break the hex is to pass an egg over the child (with prayers) and then place the egg under the bed overnight. In general, Hispanic families enjoy public affection. Extended family are treated like immediate family. Multigenerational households are common.

Native Americans

There are 562 federally recognized Indian Nations (also known as tribes, villages, bands, pueblos, rancherias, or communities) and Alaskan Native tribes in the United States (National Congress of American Indians, n.d.). These many and varied groups have differing cultural practices and beliefs, but most traditionally view illness as "punishment" by the spirits for wrongful actions. Healing is done by "shamans" using prayers, dance, fasting, smudging, and sometimes ingesting hallucinogenic plants (peyote). Smudging is the ritualistic burning of an herb (with prayer) to help cleanse a person or place. Some groups use medicine pouches, tied to the patient by a string, to help cure the illness.

Note

- American Indian and Alaska Native people have lower health status when compared with other Americans. Their life expectancy is 4.4 years less than the U.S. all-races population. Male life expectancy is 73.7 years, female is 78.1 years (Indian Health Service, 2017).
- Native Americans die at higher rates than other Americans from chronic liver disease/cirrhosis, diabetes, accidents, assault/homicide, self-harm/suicide, and chronic lower respiratory disease. About 16% of persons (all ages) are considered in fair or poor health. The leading cause of death is heart disease (Centers for Disease Control and Prevention, 2017). Among men and women aged 18 years or older, about 20% are smokers.
- Native American women have the highest rates of rape and assault in the United States. They are 2.5 times more likely to experience sexual assault and rape compared with other ethnic groups in the United States (Gilpin, 2016).
- The Indian Health Service, a federal agency, is charged with delivery of health care to this population.

Asians

East Asians (Chinese, Vietnamese, Cambodian, Korean, Japanese) highly value college education and have high regard (respect) for doctors. Listening quietly without questioning is considered a sign of respect. Some think that asking questions (or disagreeing) with the treatment plan shows lack of respect.

Kinship ties are very important. Several generations may live in the same household. Elderly are held in high esteem and their opinion is highly respected. Some Asian cultures have a form of "ancestor veneration" practices. In China, the male child is expected to take care of parents when they age.

Vietnamese

- May stop taking prescription medicine when symptoms resolve or may think that only one visit is needed to "cure" an illness
- Often save large quantities of leftover prescription drugs
- May fear blood tests and surgery because of a belief that blood loss worsens illness
- May believe that Western medicine will put the body out of balance

Buddhists

- Majority come from Asia (Cambodia, Thailand, Bhutan, Japan, Laos, Vietnam, Taiwan, Tibet, etc.)
- Main deity is Buddha; they believe that physical suffering is an inevitable part of life and believe in karma ("good deeds" create happiness and "bad deeds" create pain in the future) and the cycle of rebirth (reincarnation); some dying Buddhists may experience anxiety about being reborn into a lower form or less desirable life
- May be vegetarian
- May practice regular meditation; Buddhists value clarity of mind and may refuse narcotics or medications that alter consciousness

Traditional Chinese Medicine (TCM)

- Practitioners believe life energy (chi or qi) imbalance or blockage is the cause of disease.
- Yin is the female and yang is the male.
- Believe acupuncture and cupping correct energy imbalance.
- Cupping will create large round reddened marks or bruises on back (after 24 hours). Coining is when a coin is rubbed vigorously on skin to create welts. Both of these practices may produce lesions that may be misinterpreted as signs of abuse. The NP should question how a child received such lesions before reporting the lesions as abuse.

Sikhs

Baptized Sikhs (Khalsa) and some others will obey a code of conduct that stipulates one wears five symbols of Sikh identity: uncut hair, a sword, shorts, hair comb, and iron wrist ring. These symbols should not be removed unless negotiated with the patient. Sikhs will not consume meat, alcohol, or stimulants. Adult male Sikhs may wear a large turban-like head covering (usually white color). Most come from southern or Southeast Asia, India, Canada, United Kingdom, and the United States.

Hindus

Spiritual purity is of prime importance and manifested in removing shoes indoors, sprinkling water around a plate of food to symbolize purification, regular bathing, and cleaning mouth and teeth prior to eating. Food may be selected to enhance inner purity (e.g., no meat [especially beef or pork]). May wear a talisman that should not be cut or removed. Countries with highest percentage of Hindus are Nepal, India, and Mauritius.

Muslims

In traditional Muslim families, Sharia law (Islamic law) is followed. Modesty is paramount; garments of adolescent females and women should cover arms, legs, and head. A hijab is a head scarf (hides hair, ears, neck) and the burqa or abaya is the full veil/robe that covers the body. The left hand is reserved for bodily functions (considered unclean). Shake the patient's hand by using your right hand.

Clinicians of same gender preferred. Some male patients may be uncomfortable receiving health care from a female health provider. An unmarried woman needs her father's permission to see a clinician, and a married woman needs her husband's permission. In addition, women are not allowed to be alone or to visit with men who are not family members. If a woman is seen by a male health provider, her husband or another male family member must be present in the room. The female patient may refuse to undress (examine with the gown on).

The Qur'an (Koran) forbids drinking alcohol, eating pork, or eating meat not slaughtered in the "halal" manner. The holy month of Ramadan is observed by 30 days of fasting. It is forbidden to eat or drink fluids/water during the daytime, but one can eat or drink from sunset to before sunrise. If possible, schedule oral medications after sunset. Those who are sick may be exempted (pregnant women, physically or mentally ill people). Children are not expected to fast until puberty.

Sample Test Question

A 22-year-old Muslim woman is seen for a complaint of recurrent abdominal pain. A female NP gives the patient a paper gown with instructions for disrobing and leaves the room. When the NP returns, the patient is still clothed and refuses to undress. The NP's best action is to:

A) Ask the patient whether she prefers to be seen by a male physician
B) Tell the patient what to expect and perform a modified physical exam
C) Instruct the patient to go to the closest ED for an abdominal sonogram
D) Lecture the patient about the importance of performing an abdominal exam without clothing

The correct answer is option B. It is an example of cultural awareness by the NP.

Jews

Orthodox Jews, such as Hasidic Jews, prefer clinicians of the same gender. Male Hasidic Jews may refuse to shake a female clinician's hand. Shabbat (Sabbath) is observed from sundown Friday to sundown Saturday as a holy day that forbids any form of work. Some believe that electricity is a form of work and may stop using light switches or any electronic equipment during Shabbat (may have to turn on the light switch for the patient). Some observant Jews do not drive or use cell phones or other personal electronics at this time. If possible, avoid accessing unnecessary health services on the Sabbath and avoid scheduling follow-up visits or tests on the Sabbath.

Jews may keep kosher dietary laws (kashrut; e.g., not mixing meat and dairy products within specified time frame, eating only meaty foods certified as kosher). Families may have two separate kitchens at home: kosher and nonkosher. Each kitchen has its own utensils, pots, and plates (not allowed to mix because the kosher items will become contaminated).

Jehovah's Witnesses

Jehovah's Witnesses refuse to donate blood, store blood, or accept own blood (autologous transfusion) but accept nonblood plasma expanders and blood components without RBCs (albumin, cryoprecipitate, clotting factors, immunoglobulins). If a blood transfusion is needed to save the life of a child, parents may refuse (may require a court order). Believers do not celebrate civil holidays, birthdays, Christmas, Easter, and others. Health care providers should encourage believers to carry an advanced directive or medical release form that states their convictions; such a card is available from the church. In urban locations, a hospital liaison from the church may be available to support believers with decision making.

Seventh-Day Adventists

Believers are often vegetarian and abstain from tobacco, alcohol, and caffeinated beverages. Adventists believe the human body is a temple of God that deserves care (healthy lifestyle). They observe Sabbath (sundown Friday to sundown Saturday) as a holy day for rest from work/school and spiritual nurturing. If possible, avoid accessing unnecessary health services on the Sabbath.

Amish/Mennonites (Old Order)

Believers do not participate in Medicare or Social Security, or go to war. The individual's community pays for health care (no health insurance). Use of folk practitioners and folk/alternative medicine is common. If surgery or an expensive test is needed, permission from church elders is required. Believers may speak German dialect. They avoid modern technology, such as telephones and electricity, and use horses and buggies for transportation. Large families, traditional roles for women, and agricultural work are characteristic. Amish prefer giving birth (using midwives) and dying at home. These closed communities have higher rates of some genetic diseases such as maple syrup urine disease, Crigler–Najjar syndrome, a type of dwarfism (Ellis–van Creed syndrome), and cystic fibrosis, as well as certain metabolic disorders.

Church of Latter-Day Saints (Mormons)

Mormon churches provide a strong social support network for the ill. The local ward bishop, elders, missionaries, home or visiting teachers, and/or lay people provide spiritual and temporal support. Patients may wear "temple garments" under hospital gown or clothing as a symbol of covenant they made in the temple. Treat such undergarments with respect.

Other Cultural Groups

Lesbian, Gay, Bisexual, Transgender (LGBT) People

Avoid assumptions regarding sexual orientation or gender identity. Facilitate disclosure while remaining respectful of an individual's "coming out" process. Recognize and support the patient's family of choice and use gender-neutral language on forms and during history taking (e.g., "Have you had sex with a male, female, both, or neither?").

Military Veterans

Conditions, such as posttraumatic stress disorder (PTSD) and traumatic brain injury, are prevalent among U.S. veterans. Military personnel are accustomed to self-protect when exposed to certain sounds or experiences (e.g., hide under bed when helicopter is overhead). They are socialized to be stoic about pain or suffering and nonquestioning of authority figures.

FACTORS THAT AFFECT HEALTH CARE

Health Literacy

According to *Healthy People 2020*, health literacy is the "degree to which individuals have the capacity to obtain, process, and understand basic health information and services needed to make appropriate health decisions" (Office of Disease Prevention and Health Promotion, n.d.). It affects the person's ability to learn about how to access health care, complete forms, respond to questions, implement recommended treatments, and so forth. It depends on communication and language, existing knowledge about health, culture, and numerical ability and skills, as well as the demands of the situation and system within which the individual presents.

Language Barriers

Even one misunderstood or misspoken word can affect a patient's decision making or implementation of a treatment. Strategies for communication between patients and health care providers who speak different languages include language access services (virtual, telephonic, or in-person interpreters) and handheld documents at point of service that present clinicians with patient information. Untrained staff and family members should not be used for interpretative services.

Individualistic and Collectivistic Societies

Cultures are often categorized as *individualistic* or *collectivistic*. Individualist societies value the individual above the family, organization, or group. In contrast, collectivist societies consider the rights, needs, and wishes of the family or group over those of individuals. Ways these cultural differences may be observed during clinical encounters are presented in Table 28.1.

Table 28.1 Cultural Differences in Health Care

Individualistic Society Behaviors: United States, Europe, and Australia	Collectivistic Society Behaviors: Asia, Africa, and South America
Clinicians expected to tell patient the truth	Clinicians not expected to tell patient truth; instead share with family
Respect for patient autonomy; patient makes health-related decisions	Family shares (and may ultimately make) health-related decisions; consultation with family is pivotal; decisions will likely conform to family wishes
Needs of younger generations of a family may take precedence over those of elders (e.g., elders are institutionalized in skilled nursing facilities)	Familial piety, or honoring elders by providing the best care possible; against sending elders to long-term care facilities (nursing homes)

Differing Interpretations of Illness

Medical anthropologist and psychiatrist Arthur Kleinman proposed that the culture-infused "illness narrative" is essential for any healing clinician to understand. In other words, things associated with the disease, not the disease itself, are important.

Kleinman offered these questions for assessment:

- What do you think has caused your illness? (Etiology)
- Why do you think it started when it did? (Onset of symptoms)
- What do you think your illness does to you? How does it work? (Pathophysiology)
- How severe is your illness? Will it last a short or long time? (Course of illness)
- What kind of treatment do you think you need? What results do you hope for? (Treatment)
- What are the biggest problems your illness has caused you?
- What do you fear most about your illness?

Noncompliance and other problems are usually explained by a discrepancy between the patient's and professional's interpretation of the illness. When the explanatory models for the illness do not align, the clinician must seek to understand and negotiate them as a "therapeutic ally" with the patient.

EXAM TIPS

- Muslim woman who refuse to wear a gown can be examined through her clothing (modified or partial physical exam). See the example question.
- Jehovah's Witnesses do not accept blood transfusions (including autologous) but some may accept blood components without RBCs (cryoprecipitate, immunoglobins, etc.).
- Prolonged direct eye contact with males or strangers is considered rude by some cultures (Asians, female Muslim).
- Ramadan is a Muslim holiday that lasts for 30 days. Both fluids and food are forbidden from sunrise to sunset.
- Orthodox Jewish patients may refuse to touch anything powered by electricity (e.g., light switch, call light, electronic pumps, cell phones) from sunset Friday to sunset Saturday (Sabbath). Do not schedule visits during the Sabbath. If you call at this time, observant patients will not answer the phone.

CLINICAL PEARLS

- Each person interprets and implements his or her cultural and religious beliefs and practices uniquely; therefore, the clinician should make no assumptions and assess as needed.
- Religious practices often influence behavior around birthing, marriage, child-rearing, illness, death, burial, and mourning.

29

Nursing Research Review

SOURCES OF DATA

Primary Sources (Preferred)

In research, primary sources are preferred. They are the original research from which the data came. Primary sources are factual and not subjected to interpretation by others.

Secondary Sources

Secondary sources are created when the original data (primary data) are interpreted or analyzed by another person (not the original researcher). These are "second-hand" accounts.

ETHICAL ISSUES IN NURSING RESEARCH

Institutional Review Boards (IRBs)

An important duty of the IRB is to ensure the rights, safety, and welfare of human research subjects who are participating in research studies in their institution, hospital, or clinic. According to U.S. Food and Drug Administration (FDA) guidelines, IRBs have the authority to approve or reject research proposals that are submitted to their institution or hospital. If an IRB member has a conflict of interest, "they must absent themselves from deliberation and abstain from voting" (FDA, 2014).

IRB Committee Members

The members of the IRB committee are formally designated to review and monitor research that involves human subjects at their institution. The IRB members are individuals who are affiliated with the institution. Therefore physicians, clinicians, or retail pharmacists who are not affiliated with the institution are generally not included in an IRB committee (unless they are hired as consultants). In addition, experienced staff members, not recent graduates, are preferred. The size of the IRB and the number of members depend on the type of institution.

Vulnerable Populations

Almost all types of biomedical and behavioral research in the United States require informed consent. Groups considered "vulnerable populations" require additional paperwork and consent requirements. The following groups have special protections and have additional informed consent requirements:

- Infants and children younger than 18 years of age
- Pregnant women, fetuses

- Prisoners
- Persons with mental disabilities
- Persons who are economically disadvantaged

Belmont Report

A report that outlines the important ethical principles that should be followed when performing research involving human subjects. The Belmont Report was issued by the National Commission for the Protection of Human Subjects of Biomedical and Behavioral Research (1979).

Tuskegee Syphilis Experiment

The Tuskegee experiment was an infamous study of 600 African American sharecroppers (1932–1972) in Alabama. The men were all tested for syphilis infection, and those who had positive results were never informed or treated. Because of this study, laws were passed that protect human subjects' rights and mandate informed consent.

Informed Consent of Human Subjects

Research subjects must be informed that they have the right to withdraw from the research study at any time without adverse consequences or penalty. There are additional requirements for minors and vulnerable subjects.

- Describe the study. Inform the subject of what he or she is expected to do (e.g., questionnaires, labs).
- Describe the risk or the discomforts of participating in the study in the present and the future (if applicable).
- Describe the benefits of participating in the study in the present and the future (if applicable).
- Discuss the alternatives to the study. Allow enough time for the subject to ask questions.
- Discuss whether there is any compensation or reward for participation.
- Discuss how confidentiality and data will be secured to protect the subject's identity.
- Give the number and/or email address of the contact for the study so that the subject can contact that person if he or she has any concerns or problems with the study.

Minors

Any persons who are younger than 18 years of age.

Emancipated Minor Criteria

- Legal court document declaring that the minor is an "emancipated minor"
- Active duty in the U.S. military
- Legally binding marriage (or divorced from a legally binding marriage)

Consent Versus Assent

Consent may only be given by individuals who are aged 18 years or older. A minor (who is not emancipated) as young as the age of 7 years up to age 17 years can give assent to participate in a research study but cannot give consent legally. The child should be assured that he or she can withdraw from the study after discussing it with his or her parents.

The parent or legal guardian must first consent to the minor's participation in the study. In addition, the researcher needs parental permission to speak with the minor in order to obtain assent (the child signs a separate assent form).

RESEARCH-RELATED TERMS

Statistical Terms

- α: Also known as the significance level or the "*p*-value." It is usually set as either p <.05 or p <.01.
  - A significance level of p <.05 means that there is a 5% probability that study results are due to chance.
  - A significance level of p <.01 means that there is only a 1% probability that the study results are due to chance. Therefore, a α of p <.01 is "better" than an α of p <.05.
- Control group: These are subjects in an experiment who do not receive treatment.
- N: This letter indicates the total size of the sample.
- n: This letter indicates the number of subjects in the group.
- Significance level: Also known as the "α" or a "*p*-value." The *p*-value is usually set at either p <.05 or p <.01. See additional explanation under "α."

Research Terms

Variables

- Any attribute or characteristic that varies and is measurable.
- *Independent variable:* Variable that is being manipulated and is used to influence the dependent variable. In experimental studies, the researcher has control over the independent variable.
- *Dependent variable:* This is the result of the manipulation of the independent variable.
  - *Example*: Manipulation by researcher (independent variable) allows a response to manipulation that can be observed and measured (dependent variable).

Hypothesis

- An idea (or supposition) that can be tested and refuted. When conducting research, an examiner tests a hypothesis (or several hypotheses). He or she can either accept or refute the hypothesis.
- *Null hypothesis:* Null hypothesis (H_0): This is the opposite of the hypothesis being studied.
  - *Example:* If the hypothesis is "corn plants grow faster when expose to sunlight; the null hypotheses is "corn plants will not grow faster when exposed to sunlight." If the research data meets the set p value (p <.01), the results are considered significant (not due to random chance) and the null hypothesis can be rejected. But if the null hypotheses cannot be rejected, it means that there is no relationship between the variables and the results are due to chance.

Normal Curve

- A bell-shaped curve

Measures of Distribution

Mean

- Also known as the average. Calculated by adding all of the scores together and dividing it by the total number.
  Example: 5, 5, 5, 10, 10 (35 ÷ 5 = 7, average is "7")

Median

- The number that is in the middle when values are arranged from lowest to highest (chronological order)
  Example: 1, 3, 4, **5**, 7, 10, 14 (median value is "5")

Mode

- The most common value or frequently occurring value in a set of scores
  Example: 3, 5, **7, 7, 7**, 8, 9, 10, 10 (mode is "7")

Range

- The difference between the largest and smallest values in a distribution
  Example: 2, 3, 5, 7, 10, 15 (15 – 2= 13, range is "13")

RESEARCH DESIGNS

Types of Studies

Prospective

Studies done in the present (to the future). Longitudinal studies are a type of prospective study. Data are obtained in the present, and then periodically measured in the future.

Retrospective

Studies done on events that have already occurred (e.g., chart reviews, recall of events). Another name for this study design is "ex post facto."

Longitudinal

Long-term studies that follow the same group of subjects (or cohort) over many years to observe, measure, and compare the same variables over time. These are observational studies (there is no manipulation or intervention). For example, the Framingham Heart Study has tracked the same research subjects (N = 5,029) from the town of Framingham, Massachusetts. The goal is to study the development and identify the risk factors that are associated with the development of cerebrovascular disease.

Cohort

Cohorts are simply groups of individuals that share some common characteristic such as gender, age, job, ethnicity, and so on. Cohort studies are useful for studying the causative factors or risk factors of a disease(s). For example, the Nurses Health Study is a longitudinal cohort study that examined the effects of oral contraceptive use in nurses over the long term. It has been expanded to study the effect of lifestyle choices on health.

Cross-Sectional

A cross-sectional study compares differences and similarities between two or more groups of people or phenomena and collects data at one point in time.

Case Study

An in-depth investigation of a single person, group, or phenomena.

Descriptive Versus Experimental Studies (Table 29.1)

Descriptive

In these studies researchers observe and collect pertinent information but do not manipulate or change the environment. Also known as *observational studies*.

Correlational

A type of observational study in which the relationship (interrelationships) between at least two variables is evaluated. There are three types of correlations:

- *Positive correlation*: Two variables change together in the same direction. For example, when variable A increases, then variable B also increases.

- *Negative correlation*: An increase in one variable results in a decrease in the other. For example, when variable A increases, this causes variable B to decrease.
- *No correlation*: The variables are not related. For example, a change in variable A does not affect variable B.

Experimental

An important criterion is the use of random sampling and random assignment of research subjects. There is at least one control group and one (or more) intervention or treatment group (manipulation). Causality can be determined (If A + B occur, this will cause C).

Quasi-Experimental

The design is similar to an experimental study except there is no randomization of the research subjects. Instead, recruitment of subjects is by convenience sample.

Deductive Versus Inductive Reasoning

Deductive Reasoning

Involves going from more general to more specific findings. Also known as "top-down" logic. In research, this means starting with a theory (generalization) and then narrowing it down by formulating specific hypotheses (deduction). Quantitative studies use deductive reasoning.

Inductive Reasoning

The opposite of deductive reasoning. Also known as "bottom-up" logic. Involves going from specific findings to generalizations. One starts with specific observations and from these, one may detect a pattern that helps to formulate tentative hypotheses, which may help to generate new theory. Qualitative studies use inductive reasoning.

Table 29.1 Qualitative Versus Quantitative Studies

	Qualitative	Quantitative
Data	Involves words, narratives, subjective opinions	Numerical and measurable data
Number of subjects	Few individuals	May involve large numbers of individuals, databases
Subject recruitment	Small number of subjects, not randomized	Randomization possible if experimental design
Data gathering	In-depth interviews focus groups, observations; audio or video are recorded, data is transcribed	Questionnaires, instruments, measurements, surveys
Logic	Inductive reasoning, specific data can be generalized	Deductive reasoning
Design	May change and evolve to adapt to situation or to subjects	Systematic, design is known before research starts
Statistical testing	Interpretation of common themes and patterns; uses limited statistics such as chi-square	Pearson correlation, paired *t*-test, simple/multiple regression, analysis of variance (ANOVA), etc.
Notes	Researcher is a participant and also an observer (degree of participation varies)	Researcher is an objective observer, declares bias (funding sources)

EXAM TIPS

- **Primary data are the preferred source in research (original study that produced the data).**
- **Experimental studies use randomization with subject selection.**

- Correlational studies search for relationships between a minimum of two variables.
- Deductive logic is used with quantitative studies, and inductive logic is used in qualitative studies.
- Understand the difference between a dependent and an independent variable.
- Know which groups are considered vulnerable populations.
- Know the definition of an IRB. The IRB's most important role is to protect the rights of the human subjects enrolled in a study.
- Know the definition of assent. Assent refers to minors because they legally cannot give consent (unless an emancipated minor).
- Know the definition of N (total number of subjects) versus n (subgroup).
- A normal curve is the "bell curve."

30

Evidence-Based Medicine and Epidemiology

DEFINITION: EVIDENCE-BASED MEDICINE

Evidence-based medicine (EBM) is "the conscientious, explicit and judicious use of current best evidence in making decisions about the care of individual patients" (www.cochrane.org). It is also known as evidence-based practice. There will be several questions on the American Nurses Credentialing Center (ANCC) exam that will test your ability to sort and rate articles by the level of evidence.

HIERARCHY OF RESEARCH EVIDENCE (FIGURE 30.1)

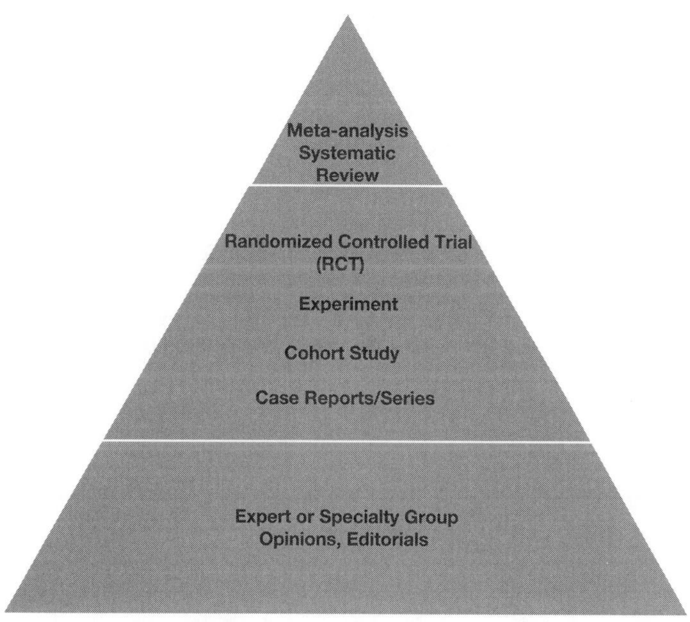

Figure 30.1 Ranking of research evidence. This image can be found in color in the app.

Meta-Analysis

This is a statistical method that combines data from multiple studies (systematic review), resulting in higher statistical power and a single conclusion. This method is considered the gold standard for gathering research evidence for EBM.

Systematic Review

A type of literature review that identifies, selects, and analyzes multiple research articles concerning a health condition, disease, or other health-related practice. Follows specific methodology to identify all the relevant studies on a specific topic. Studies to be included must meet explicit criteria. Studies are ranked from grade A (best evidence) to grade D (poor evidence). After a systematic review is done, the acceptable studies are pooled together and statistical testing of the data (meta-analysis) is performed.

Randomized Controlled Trial (RCT)

Subjects are randomly assigned to either the control group or the treatment group(s). The intervention may be a drug, procedure, or device. Some RCTs use a double-blind design (the intervention is hidden from the patient, clinician, and/or researchers). RCTs are experimental studies.

Experimental Study

In a nutshell, an experiment involves random subject selection, one placebo or control group, and one or more intervention group(s). An RCT is a type of experimental study.

Cohort Study

Cohort studies are a type of research that is used to investigate risk factors for diseases, risk factors for death, and other conditions. The research subjects are observed for a long period. There is no intervention done (not an experiment). The goal is to identify risk factors and associations (not causation) of a disease(s). For example, the Nurses' Health Study is a large cohort study of female RNs aged 30 to 63 years who reside in the state of Massachusetts. A cohort study can be a type of prospective study (present to future).

Case Report

A detailed report of one patient with a disease or an unusual condition that includes demographics, signs and symptoms, diagnosis, response to treatment, and so forth.

Case Series

A series of case reports that involves a series of individuals who are given similar treatment.

Opinions and Editorials

Opinions and editorials can be biased and may not be based on solid evidence. They are the weakest form of evidence.

RESEARCH DATABASES

Cochrane Reviews

The gold standard database and resource for EBM. These are systematic reviews (Cochrane Database of Systematic Reviews). The organization does not accept commercial or conflicted funding. Also known as the Cochrane Collaboration (www.cochrane.org).

MEDLINE

The U.S. National Library of Medicine (NLM) premier database contains more than 23 million journal articles in the life sciences with a concentration in biomedicine. These articles are from 5,600 current biomedical journals from the United States and more than 80 foreign countries.

PubMed

This component of MEDLINE contains over 27 million citations of biomedical, medical, and other life science literature and abstracts.

Cumulative Index to Nursing and Allied Health Literature (CINAHL)

The world's largest source of full-text nursing and allied health journals (>1,300 journals). CINAHL Complete provides indexing of more than 4,000 journals.

GRADES OF RESEARCH EVIDENCE

Research evidence receives a letter grade: A (best evidence), B, C, and D (poor evidence). Well-designed controlled experimental trials (double-blind RCTs) are considered to be grade A (or level 1) evidence.

HOW TO SOLVE EBM QUESTIONS (DRAG-AND-DROP FORMAT)

1. What is the "drag-and-drop" format in the American Nurses Credentialing Center (ANCC) exam?

This is one of the new-format questions. On the left side are three research articles/studies (white boxes are shown here, but they will be yellow on the exam). On the right side are three boxes numbered "1, 2, 3" (black here, but blue on the exam). You must rate the three articles in terms of evidence from best (1), moderate (2), and worst (3).

2. What is the best way to answer this type of question?

The easiest way to answer this type of question is to memorize and understand the highest level of evidence (meta-analysis, systematic review, RCT) and the type of studies that has the lowest level of evidence (opinions, editorials). The leftover study belongs in the middle black box (#2). The first sentence of each article usually gives a clue about the study design. Notice that in option A it is a "meta-analysis," in option B it is a "specialty society opinion," and option C it is an "experimental study."

I teach the following method to my review-course students. These are the steps to follow:

1. Identify the article with the strongest level of evidence (#1 ranking). Look for key words such as "meta-analysis," "systematic review," "RCTs," and the Cochrane, MEDLINE, and/or CINAHL databases.
2. Next, look for the research study that has the weakest evidence (#3 ranking). It has key words such as "expert opinion," "opinion," or "editorial."
3. You are left with one article, which you drag to the middle (#2 ranking).

Example A

A) A meta-analysis using the Cochrane database found 30 RCTs on ginkgo biloba use in patients with early dementia	1.
B) Specialty society editorial in a journal regarding the effectiveness of ginkgo biloba supplementation in dementia	2.
C) In an experimental study of 500 patients with early dementia, one group was given placebo, and the other group was given ginkgo biloba daily for 10 months	3.

Correct Answer With Key Words:
Article A is ranked 1 (key words: *meta-analysis, Cochrane database, RCTs*), Article C is ranked 2 (key words: *experimental study*), and Article B is ranked 3 (key word: *editorial*)

Example B

A) A case report of a 45-year-old woman with Munchausen syndrome by proxy	1.
B) A systematic review of Munchausen syndrome by proxy using MEDLINE and CINAHL found 15 studies	2.
C) An opinion paper written by a psychiatrist who is considered an expert of Munchausen syndrome by proxy that includes treatment recommendations	3.

Correct Answer With Key Words:
Article B is ranked 1(key words: *systematic review, MEDLINE, CINAHL*), Article A is ranked 2 (key words: *case report*), and Article C is ranked 3 (key words: *opinion paper*)

STATISTICAL TERMS (EVIDENCE-BASED MEDICINE)

Absolute Risk Reduction (ARR)

ARR is a measure of the difference between two different treatments in terms of their ability to reduce a particular outcome (i.e., myocardial infarction [MI], stroke).

Relative Risk Reduction (RRR)

RRR is a measure of how much risk is reduced in the experimental group compared with the control group.

Number Needed to Treat (NNT)

This is the number of patients you have to treat to avoid one bad outcome (i.e., MI, stroke). For example, an NNT of seven means that it is necessary to treat seven patients to avoid one bad outcome.

Positive Predictive Value (PPV)

This is the probability that a person with a positive screening test result has the disease.

Negative Predictive Value (NPV)

This is the probability that a person with a negative test result does not have the disease.

EPIDEMIOLOGY TERMS

Active Immunity

Refers to immunity to a disease developed either through vaccination or by infection.

Passive Immunity

Refers to immunity to a disease after receiving antibodies (immunoglobins) from another host. For example, colostrum from breastfeeding gives the neonate antibodies from the mother.

Herd Immunity

Refers to resistance to a disease in a large number of people in the population, which is usually due to immunization programs.

Health

This refers to a state of complete physical, mental, and social well-being.

Horizontal Transmission

Transmission of an infecting agent from one individual to another. For example, horizontal transmission of HIV and other sexually transmitted diseases or infections occurs through sexual intercourse.

Vertical Transmission

Transmission of an infecting agent from mother to infant. Congenital infections from mother to infant can be passed through vertical transmission. Also, an HIV-positive mother who breastfeeds her infant can infect her infant with HIV through vertical transmission.

Endemic

This refers to a baseline level of a particular disease in a population.

Epidemic

Refers to the rapid increase of a disease in a population that involves a large number of people.

Pandemic

This is an epidemic that occurs over a very large area (several countries or continents). It involves a large proportion of the global population.

Morbidity

This refers to an illness or any departure from physical and/or mental health.

Mortality

Death.

Infant Mortality

Refers to infant deaths per 100,000 live births. The leading cause of death in an infant's first year of life is congenital malformations (including chromosomal abnormalities).

Sensitivity

Refers to the ability of a screening test to correctly identify a person *with* the disease.

Specificity

Refers to the ability of a screening test to correctly identify a person *without* the disease.

EXAM TIPS

- **Memorize the definition of sensitivity and specificity.**
- **Learn how to solve EBM "drag-and-drop" format questions (three to four questions). As of fall 2017, only the ANCC exam has this format, although it is possible that the American Academy of Nurse Practitioners Certification Board (AANPCB) may use the question format in future exams.**
- **Learn the difference among endemic, epidemic, and pandemic.**

Practice Questions and Answers

VII

31

Practice Questions

1. A 30-year-old chef complains of pruritic hives over her chest and arms, but denies difficulty swallowing or breathing. She reports a family history of allergic rhinitis and asthma. Which of the following interventions is most appropriate?

A) Obtain a complete and thorough history
B) Recommend an oral antihistamine such as diphenhydramine 25 mg PO QID
C) Give an injection of epinephrine 1:1000 intramuscularly *stat*
D) Call 911

2. Which of the following findings is most likely in young primigravidas with pregnancy-induced hypertension?

A) Abdominal cramping and constipation
B) Edema of the face and the upper extremities
C) Shortness of breath
D) Dysuria and frequency

3. Which of the following symptoms is associated with B_{12} deficiency anemia?

A) Spoon-shaped nails and pica
B) Abnormal neurological exam
C) Vegan diet
D) Tingling and numbness of both feet

4. A second triple screen on a 35-year-old primigravida reveals abnormally low levels of alpha fetoprotein and estriol and high levels of human chorionic gonadotropin. Which of the following interventions is the best choice for this patient?

A) Order an ultrasound
B) Order a computed tomography (CT) scan of the abdomen
C) Order a 24-hour urine for protein clearance
D) Assess for a history of illicit drug or alcohol use

5. All of the following are true statements about diverticula except:

A) Diverticula are located in the colon
B) A low-fiber diet is associated with the condition
C) Most diverticula in the colon are infected with gram-negative bacteria
D) Supplementing with fiber, such as psyllium (Metamucil), is recommended

6. Patients who are diagnosed with gonorrhea should also be treated for which of the following infections?
   A) Chancroid
   B) *Chlamydia trachomatis*
   C) Herpes genitalis
   D) Pelvic inflammatory disease (PID)

7. Kyphosis is a late sign of:
   A) Rheumatoid arthritis
   B) Osteopenia
   C) Osteoporosis
   D) Osteoarthritis

8. A 35-year-old primigravida who is at 18 weeks gestation is expecting twins. What would you would expect her alpha fetoprotein (AFP) values to be?
   A) Normal
   B) Higher than normal
   C) Lower than normal
   D) None of the above

9. Which of the following antihypertensive medications has beneficial effects for an elderly White woman with osteoporosis?
   A) Calcium channel blockers
   B) Angiotensin-converting enzyme (ACE) inhibitors
   C) Beta-blockers
   D) Thiazide diuretics

10. The Lachman maneuver is used to detect which of the following?
    A) Instability of the knee
    B) Nerve damage of the knee due to past knee injuries
    C) Integrity of the patellar tendon
    D) Tears on the meniscus of the knee

11. A 75-year-old woman has been on nifedipine (Procardia XL) 10-mg capsule for many years to control her stage II hypertension. Her blood pressure at this visit is 165/80 mmHg. She is currently complaining of pain at her right hip and in both knees. She has increased her dose of ibuprofen (Motrin) from 400 mg three times daily (TID) to 800 mg TID. She is still in pain and would like something stronger. Which of the following statements is the best explanation of the effects of ibuprofen (Motrin) on her disease?
    A) It increases the chances of adverse effects to her health
    B) It inhibits the effect of renal prostaglandins and blunts the effectiveness of the diuretic
    C) It prolongs the therapeutic effects of hydrochlorothiazide and other diuretics
    D) None of the statements are true

12. All of the following are infections that affect mostly the labia and vagina except:
    A) Bacterial vaginosis
    B) Candidiasis

C) Trichomoniasis
D) *Chlamydia trachomatis*

13. The nurse practitioner would test the obturator and iliopsoas muscle to evaluate for:
    A) Cholecystitis
    B) Acute appendicitis
    C) Inguinal hernia
    D) Gastric ulcer

14. Treatment for mild preeclampsia includes all of the following except:
    A) Bed rest except for bathroom privileges
    B) Close monitoring of weight and blood pressure
    C) Close follow-up of urinary protein, serum creatinine, and platelet count
    D) A prescription of methyldopa (Aldomet) to control blood pressure

15. All of the following services are covered under Medicare Part A except:
    A) Inpatient hospital care
    B) Inpatient psychiatric hospital care
    C) Custodial care
    D) Skilled nursing facility care

16. A 28-year-old student is seen in the school health clinic with complaints of a hacking nonproductive cough, rhinorrhea, pharyngitis, and malaise for the past 2 weeks. He does not take any medications, denies any allergies, and has no significant medical history. Physical examination reveals a low-grade temperature of 99.9°F, respirations of 16 breaths/min, pulse of 90 beats/min, and scattered rales and wheezing of the lungs. The patient does not appear toxic. The total white blood cell count is 10,500/μL. What is the most likely diagnosis?
    A) Bacterial pneumonia
    B) Atypical pneumonia
    C) Acute bronchitis
    D) Pertussis

17. A 39-year-old migrant worker presents to the clinic 2 days after a Mantoux test. What minimum size of induration would be considered positive for this patient?
    A) 3 mm
    B) 5 mm
    C) 10 mm
    D) 15 mm

18. All of the following are correct statements regarding the role of the person named in a durable power of attorney except:
    A) The agent's decisions are legally binding
    B) The agent can make decisions in other areas of the patient's life such as financial issues
    C) The agent can decide for the patient who is on life support when that life support can be terminated
    D) The patient's spouse has a right to override the agent's decisions

19. All of the following are true statements regarding Munchausen syndrome except:

A) It is considered a mental illness
B) The patient has a medical illness that causes an anxiety reaction and denial
C) The patient fakes an illness in order to gain attention from health care providers
D) The patient has an inconsistent medical history along with a past history of frequent hospitalizations

20. Which of the following antihypertensive medications should the nurse practitioner avoid when treating patients with emphysema?

A) Calcium channel blockers
B) Angiotensin-converting enzyme (ACE) inhibitors
C) Beta-blockers
D) Diuretics

21. Which of the following is an accurate description of eliciting Murphy's sign?

A) On deep inspiration by the patient, palpate firmly in the right upper quadrant of the abdomen below the costovertebral angle
B) Bend the patient's hips and knees at 90 degrees, then passively rotate the hip externally, and internally
C) Ask the patient to squat, then place the stethoscope on the apical area
D) Press into the abdomen deeply, then release it suddenly

22. A 28-year-old multipara who is at 32 weeks gestation presents to your office complaining of a sudden onset of small amounts of bright-red vaginal bleeding. She has had several episodes and appears anxious. On exam, her uterus is soft to palpation. Which of the following is most likely?

A) Placenta abruptio
B) Placenta previa
C) Acute cervicitis
D) Molar pregnancy (hydatidiform mole)

23. Epidemiological studies show that Hashimoto's disease occurs most commonly in:

A) Middle-aged to older women
B) Smokers
C) Obese individuals
D) Older men

24. A 48-year-old woman is told by a physician that she is starting menopause. All of the following are possible findings except:

A) Hot flashes
B) Irregular menstrual periods
C) Severe vaginal atrophic changes
D) Cyclic mood swings

25. A 63-year-old patient with a 10-year history of poorly controlled hypertension presents with a cluster of physical exam findings. Which of the following clusters indicates the target organ damage commonly seen in hypertensive patients?

A) Pedal edema, hepatomegaly, and enlarged kidneys
B) Arteriovenous (AV) nicking, left ventricular hypertrophy, and stroke
C) Renal infection, S3 heart sound, neuromuscular abnormalities
D) Glaucoma, jugular vein atrophy, heart failure

26. A 30-year-old primigravida is diagnosed with a possible threatened abortion. The result of the urine pregnancy test is positive. Which of the following statements is true regarding a threatened abortion?

A) Vaginal bleeding and cramping are present, but the cervix remains closed
B) Vaginal bleeding and cramping are present along with a dilated cervix
C) The fetus and placenta are both expelled
D) The products of conception and the placenta remain inside the uterus along with a dilated cervix

27. A 30-year-old woman who is sexually active complains of a large amount of milk-like vaginal discharge for several weeks. A microscopy slide reveals a large number of cells that have blurred margins. Very few white blood cells are seen. The vaginal pH is at 6.0. What is most likely?

A) Trichomonas infection
B) Bacterial vaginosis
C) Candidal infection
D) A normal finding

28. The cytology (Pap smear) result for a 21-year-old sexually active student whose partner uses condoms inconsistently shows a large amount of inflammation. Which of the following is the best follow-up?

A) Call the patient and tell her that she needs to return to the clinic for chlamydia and gonorrhea testing
B) Treat the patient with metronidazole vaginal cream over the phone
C) Call the patient and tell her she will need a repeat Pap smear in 6 months
D) Advise her to use a Betadine douche at H (half strength) × 3 days

29. While performing a Pap smear on a postmenopausal patient, several areas of flat white, irregularly shaped lesions are found on the patient's labia. The skin lesions look thin and atrophic. The patient reports that the lesions are itchy and have been present for several years. Which condition is best described?

A) Chronic scabies infection
B) Lichen sclerosus
C) Chronic candidal vaginitis
D) A physiological variant found in some older women

30. The S2 heart sound is caused by:

A) Closure of the atrioventricular valves
B) Closure of the semilunar valves
C) Opening of the atrioventricular valves
D) Opening of the semilunar valves

31. When an adolescent male's penis grows more in length than width, in which of the following Tanner stages is he classified?

A) Tanner stage II
B) Tanner stage III
C) Tanner stage IV
D) Tanner stage V

32. Fetal TORCH infections can cause microcephaly, mental retardation, hepatosplenomegaly, and intrauterine growth retardation. The acronym TORCH stands for:

A) *Toxoplasma gondii*, other infections, rubella, cytomegalovirus, and herpes
B) Toxic shock syndrome, ocular infections, rubella, cytomegalovirus, and herpes zoster
C) Tetanus, ophthalmic infections, roseola, cancer, and head abnormalities
D) Toxins, other infections, roseola, candidiasis, and head abnormalities

33. Human papillomavirus (HPV) infection of the larynx has been associated with:

A) Laryngeal cancer
B) Esophageal stricture
C) Cervical cancer
D) Metaplasia of the squamous cells

34. A 65-year-old carpenter complains of morning stiffness and pain in both his hands and right knee upon awakening. He feels some relief after warming up. On exam, the nurse practitioner notices the presence of Heberden's nodes. Which of the following is most likely?

A) Osteoporosis
B) Rheumatoid arthritis
C) Osteoarthritis
D) Reiter's syndrome

35. What does a positive posterior drawer sign in a 10-year-old soccer player signify?

A) Normal knee
B) Instability of the knee
C) Swelling on the knee
D) Injury to the meniscus

36. A multigravida who is at 28 weeks gestation has a fundal height of 29 cm. Which of the following is the best recommendation for this patient?

A) Advise the mother that her pregnancy is progressing well
B) Order an ultrasound of the uterus
C) Refer her to an obstetrician for an amniocentesis
D) Recommend bed rest with bathroom privileges

37. A multigravida who is at 34 weeks gestation wants to know at what level her uterine fundus should be. The best answer is to advise the mother that her fundus is:

A) Midway between the umbilicus and the lower ribs
B) At the level of the umbilicus
C) From 33 to 35 cm
D) From 32 to 34 cm

38. Which of the following laboratory tests is a sensitive test for evaluating renal function?

A) Electrolyte panel
B) Estimated glomerular filtration rate (eGFR)
C) Creatinine
D) Blood urea nitrogen (BUN)

39. Which of the following is a true statement regarding acute gastritis?

A) Chronic intake of nonsteroidal anti-inflammatory drugs (NSAIDs) can cause the disorder
B) Chronic lack of dietary fiber is the main cause of the disorder
C) The screening test for the disorder is the barium swallow test
D) The gold standard to evaluate the disorder is a colonoscopy

40. Signs and symptoms of depression include all of the following except:

A) Anhedonia
B) Low self-esteem
C) Apathy
D) Apraxia

41. A mother brings her 4-year-old daughter, who just started attending preschool, to the health clinic. She tells the nurse practitioner that her child is complaining of burning and itching that started in the left eye. Within 2 days it involved both eyes, and the child developed a runny nose and sore throat. During the physical exam, the child's eyes appear injected bilaterally with no purulent discharge. The throat is red, the inferior nasal turbinates are swollen, and lymph nodes are palpable in front of each ear. Which of the following is most likely?

A) Herpes keratitis
B) Corneal ulcer
C) Viral conjunctivitis
D) Bacterial conjunctivitis

42. A 22-year-old sexually active woman is complaining of amenorrhea and new-onset bloody vaginal spotting. On examination, her left adnexa is tender and cervical motion tenderness is positive. Which test should the nurse practitioner order initially?

A) Flat plate of the abdomen
B) Complete blood count (CBC) with white cell differential
C) Urine pregnancy test
D) Pelvic ultrasound

43. A toddler with congenital heart disease is seen for a 1-week history of facial and lower-extremity edema accompanied by shortness of breath. The child's mother reports that the child's appetite has been poor. The chest x-ray reveals that the child has congestive heart failure (CHF). Which of the following heart sounds are found in patients with CHF?

A) S1 and S2
B) S1, S2, and S3
C) S1, S2, and S4
D) Still's murmur and S4

44. A 53-year-old crossing guard complains of twisting his right knee while working that morning. The knee is swollen and tender to palpation. The nurse practitioner diagnoses a grade II sprain. The initial treatment plan includes which of the following?

A) Intermittent application of cold packs the first 24 hours followed by applications of low heat at bedtime
B) Elevation of the affected limb and intermittent applications of cold packs for the next 48 hours
C) Rechecking the knee in 24 hours and encouraging isometric exercises
D) Application of an elastic bandage wrap to the affected knee

45. Erythromycin 200 mg with sulfisoxazole 600 mg suspension (Pediazole) is contraindicated in which of the following conditions?

A) G6PD deficiency anemia
B) Lead poisoning
C) Beta thalassemia minor
D) B_{12} deficiency anemia

46. The mother of an 11-year-old boy with sickle cell anemia calls on the phone because her son woke up with a painful penile erection that will not go away. The nurse practitioner's most appropriate intervention is:

A) Insert a Foley catheter and measure the child's intake and output for the next 24 hours
B) Insert a Foley catheter to obtain a specimen for a urinalysis and urine for C&S (culture and sensitivity)
C) Recommend an increase in the child's fluid intake
D) Recommend immediate referral to the emergency department

47. A positive Coombs test on an Rh-negative pregnant woman means:

A) The mother has autoantibodies against Rh-positive red blood cells (RBCs)
B) The fetus has autoantibodies against Rh-negative red blood cells RBCs
C) The mother does not have Rh factor antibodies
D) The fetus does not have Rh factor antibodies

48. Folic acid supplementation is recommended for women who are planning pregnancy in order to:

A) Prevent renal agenesis
B) Prevent anencephaly
C) Prevent kidney defects
D) Prevent heart defects

49. All of the following are possible causes for secondary hypertension except:

A) Acute pyelonephritis
B) Pheochromocytoma
C) Renovascular stenosis
D) Coarctation of the aorta

50. Fitz-Hugh–Curtis syndrome is associated with which following infection?

A) Syphilis
B) *Chlamydia trachomatis*
C) Herpes genitalis
D) Lymphogranuloma venereum

51. A pelvic exam on a woman who is 12 weeks pregnant would reveal that her uterus is located at which of the following areas?

A) Between the umbilicus and the suprapubic bone
B) Just rising above the suprapubic bone
C) Between the suprapubic bone and the xiphoid process
D) Between the umbilicus and the xiphoid process

52. All of the following are covered under Medicare Part B except:

A) Persons aged 65 years or older
B) Durable medical equipment
C) Mammograms annually starting at age 50
D) Outpatient anesthesiologist's services

53. All of the following patients are at higher risk for suicide except:

A) A 66-year-old White man whose wife of 40 years recently died
B) A high school student with a history of bipolar disorder
C) A depressed 45-year-old woman with family history of suicide
D) A 17-year-old teen who has only one close friend in school

Questions 54 and 55 apply to this case. A 70-year-old male patient complains of a bright-red-colored spot that has been present in his left eye for 2 days. He denies eye pain, visual changes, or headaches. He has a new-onset cough from a recent viral upper respiratory infection. The only medicine he is taking is Bayer aspirin one tablet a day.

54. Which of the following is most likely?

A) Corneal abrasion
B) Acute bacterial conjunctivitis
C) Acute uveitis
D) Subconjunctival hemorrhage

55. Which of the following actions is appropriate follow-up for this 70-year-old patient?

A) Refer the patient to an optometrist
B) Refer the patient to an ophthalmologist
C) Advise the patient that the condition is benign and will resolve spontaneously
D) Prescribe an ophthalmic antibiotic solution

56. An 8-year-old boy with type 1 diabetes is being seen for a 3-day history of urinary frequency and nocturia. He denies flank pain and is afebrile. The urinalysis result is negative for blood and nitrites but is positive for a large amount of leukocytes and ketones. He has a trace amount of protein. Which of the following is the best test to order initially?

A) Urine for culture and sensitivity
B) 24-hour urine for protein and creatinine clearance
C) 24-hour urine for microalbumin
D) Intravenous pyelogram

57. All of the following are complications of severe preeclampsia except:

A) Liver failure
B) Hypertensive encephalopathy
C) Pulmonary edema
D) Placenta previa

58. The best test for diagnosing glaucoma is which of the following?

A) Fluorescein staining
B) Tonometry
C) Snellen vision exam
D) The refractive index

59. Rocky Mountain spotted fever is caused by the bite of a:

A) Mosquito
B) Tick
C) Louse
D) Flea

60. All of the following are false statements about atopic dermatitis except:

A) Contact with cold objects may exacerbate the condition
B) It does not have a linear distribution
C) It is associated with bullae
D) The lesions have vesicles that are full of serous exudate

61. A patient with a history of mitral valve prolapse (MVP) is requesting prophylaxis before her dental surgery. Which of the following would you prescribe this patient?

A) Amoxicillin a half hour before and 2 hours after the procedure
B) Amoxicillin 1 hour before the procedure
C) Amoxicillin 1 hour before and 3 hours after the procedure
D) Prophylaxis is not recommended for this patient

62. Koplik's spots are associated with:

A) Poxvirus infections
B) Rubeola
C) Kawasaki's disease
D) Rubella

63. A 21-year-old new mother reports that she has been feeling irritable and jittery almost daily for the past few months. She complains of frequent palpitations and more frequent bowel movements along with weight loss. Her blood pressure is 160/70 mmHg, pulse is 110 beats/min, and she is afebrile. All of the following conditions should be considered in the differential diagnosis for this patient except:

A) Mitral regurgitation
B) Graves' disease
C) Generalized anxiety disorder
D) Illicit drug use

64. An elderly patient with a productive cough and fever is diagnosed with pneumonia. All of the following organisms are capable of causing community-acquired pneumonia except:

A) *Haemophilus influenzae*
B) *Mycoplasma pneumoniae*
C) *Treponema pallidum*
D) *Streptococcus pneumoniae*

65. Human chorionic gonadotropin (hCG) is produced by the:

A) Placenta
B) Hypothalamus
C) Anterior pituitary
D) Ovaries

66. The majority of serum alpha fetoprotein is produced by the:

A) Fetal liver
B) Maternal liver
C) Placenta
D) Fetal neural tube

67. A middle-aged woman who works in the housekeeping department of a hospital presents to the employee health clinic with a complaint of a needlestick to her left thumb. The needle was in one of the garbage bags from the emergency department. The patient had a little bleeding that stopped spontaneously. Which of the following is the next step?

A) Order an enzyme-linked immunosorbent assay (ELISA) test as soon as possible
B) Recommend a tetanus booster in 1 week
C) Offer the patient hepatitis B immunoglobulin
D) Order a chest x-ray

68. An elderly woman has been taking digoxin (Lanoxin) for 10 years. Her EKG is showing a new onset of atrial fibrillation. Her pulse is 64 beats/min. She denies syncope and dizziness. Which of the following interventions is most appropriate?

A) Order an electrolyte panel and a digoxin level
B) Order a serum thyroid-stimulating hormone (TSH), digoxin level, and an electrolyte panel
C) Order a serum digoxin level and decrease her digoxin dose by half while waiting for results
D) Discontinue the digoxin and order another 12-lead EKG

69. You note the following result on a routine urinalysis of a 37-year-old primigravida who is at 30 weeks gestation. Leukocyte = trace, nitrite = negative, protein = 2+, blood = negative. Her weight has increased by 5 lbs during the past week. Which of the following is most likely?

A) HELLP syndrome
B) Pregnancy-induced hypertension (preeclampsia)
C) Eclampsia of pregnancy
D) Primary hypertension

70. The nurse practitioner who suspects that one of her hypertensive patients has Cushing's syndrome would expect to find which of the following laboratory results?

A) Hyponatremia
B) Hypoglycemia
C) Elevated serum cortisol levels
D) Decreased urine 17-ketosteroids

71. A nursing home resident reports to his physician that his previous roommate was recently started on tuberculosis treatment. A Mantoux test and chest x-ray are ordered for the patient. What is the minimum size of induration considered positive for this patient?

A) 3 mm
B) 5 mm
C) 10 mm
D) 15 mm

72. In small children with acquired immunodeficiency syndrome (AIDS), which of the following vaccines is contraindicated?

A) Diphtheria and tetanus (Td)
B) Hepatitis B and mumps
C) Varicella
D) Td and oral polio

73. A 44-year-old woman who is undergoing treatment for infertility complains of not having had a menstrual period for a few months. The night before, she started spotting and is now having cramp-like pains in her pelvic area. Her blood pressure (BP) is 160/80 mmHg, pulse is 110 beats/min, and she is afebrile. Her labs reveal mild anemia with mild leukocytosis. On pelvic exam, the uterine fundus is noted to be above the symphysis pubis. The cervical os is dilated at 3 cm. Which of the following is most likely?

A) Inevitable abortion
B) Threatened abortion
C) Incomplete abortion
D) Acute pelvic inflammatory disease

74. A 14-year-old girl who is sexually active is brought to the health clinic by her mother for an immunization update. According to the mother, her daughter has had one dose of hepatitis B vaccine. Which of the following vaccines would you administer at this visit?

A) Tdap, hepatitis B, and HPV vaccine
B) DTaP (diphtheria, tetanus, acellular pertussis) and hepatitis B
C) Hepatitis B only
D) MMR (measles, mumps, rubella), Td, and HPV vaccine

75. An Rh-negative pregnant woman with negative rubella titers can be vaccinated at what time in pregnancy?

A) At any time in pregnancy
B) During the second trimester
C) During the third trimester
D) During the postpartum period

76. Medicare Part B will pay for all of the following services except:

A) Outpatient physician visits that are medically necessary
B) Durable medical equipment
C) Outpatient laboratory and radiology tests
D) Eyeglasses and routine dental care

77. Which of the following is used to screen for color blindness in a 7-year-old boy?

A) Snellen chart
B) Ishihara chart
C) Cover/uncover test
D) Red reflex

Questions 78 and 79 apply to this case. A 67-year-old retired clerk presents with complaints of fatigue, shortness of breath, and weight gain over a 2-week period. A nonproductive cough accompanies her symptoms. She reports that climbing up the stairs worsens her dyspnea. The lung exam is positive for fine crackles in the lower lobes with no wheezing. An S3 heart gallop is noted.

78. Which of the following conditions is most likely?

A) Acute exacerbation of asthma
B) Left-sided heart failure
C) Right-sided heart failure
D) Chronic obstructive pulmonary disease

79. Which of the following drugs is most likely to relieve the patient's symptoms?

A) Atenolol (Tenormin)
B) Trimethoprim–sulfamethoxazole (Bactrim DS)
C) Furosemide (Lasix)
D) Hydrocodone/guaifenesin syrup (Hycotuss)

80. A 20-year-old patient has recently been diagnosed with migraines. The nurse practitioner is educating the patient about factors that are known to trigger migraine headaches. Which of the following is incorrect advice?

A) Avoid foods with high tyramine content
B) Avoid foods with high potassium content
C) Get enough sleep
D) Avoid fermented foods

81. Hegar's sign is considered a:

A) Positive sign of pregnancy
B) Probable sign of pregnancy
C) Presumptive sign of pregnancy
D) Problem in pregnancy

82. When palpating a woman who is at 20 weeks gestation, the nurse practitioner should be able to feel the uterine fundus at what level?

A) Just rising above the level of the pubic symphysis
B) Between the pubic symphysis and the umbilicus
C) At the level of the umbilicus
D) Above the level of the umbilicus

83. A 67-year-old woman with a 30-pack-year history of smoking presents for a routine annual physical examination. She complains of being easily short of breath and is frequently fatigued. Physical examination reveals diminished breath sounds, hyperresonance, and hypertrophied respiratory accessory muscles. Her complete blood count (CBC) results reveal that her hematocrit level is elevated. Her pulmonary function test (PFT) results show increased total lung capacity. What is the most likely diagnosis for this patient?

A) Bronchogenic carcinoma
B) Chronic obstructive pulmonary disease (COPD)

C) Chronic bronchitis
D) Congestive heart failure

84. Your female patient of 10 years is concerned about her most recent diagnosis. She was told by her dermatologist that she has an advanced case of actinic keratosis. Which of the following is the best explanation for this patient?

A) It is a benign condition
B) It is a precancerous lesion and needs to be followed up with her dermatologist
C) It will diminish with application of hydrocortisone cream 1% BID for 2 weeks
D) It is important for her to follow up with an oncologist

85. Patient confidentiality is breached when:

A) Medical information is given to a spouse
B) Records are subpoenaed
C) Reports are sent to the public health department
D) Records are released to insurance companies

86. A 25-year-old woman's last menstrual period was 6 weeks ago. She is complaining of nausea with vomiting in the morning and fatigue. Her breasts feel bloated. The nurse practitioner suspects that she is pregnant. Her symptoms would be considered:

A) Positive signs of pregnancy
B) Probable signs of pregnancy
C) Presumptive signs of pregnancy
D) Possible signs of pregnancy

Questions 87 and 88 apply to this case. A 55-year-old male patient describes an episode of chest tightness in his substernal area that radiated to his back while he was jogging. It was relieved immediately when he stopped.

87. The patient's symptoms are highly suggestive of what condition?

A) Angina pectoris
B) Acute myocardial infarction
C) Gastroesophageal reflux disease
D) Acute costochondritis

88. Which of the following would you recommend to this 55-year-old patient?

A) Start an exercise program with walking instead of jogging
B) Consult with a cardiologist for further evaluation
C) Consult with a gastroenterologist to rule out acute cholecystitis
D) Take ibuprofen (Advil) 600 mg for pain every 4 to 6 hours as needed

89. A 73-year-old patient complains of recent episodes of acute-onset left-sided facial asymmetry, slurred speech, weakness, and dizziness, accompanied by weakness of the left arm and left leg. She reports that the episodes occur at random and last from 30 minutes to about 2 hours. Each episode resolved completely. The patient has type 2 diabetes with hyperlipidemia, peripheral arterial disease, hypertension, and osteoporosis. Her symptoms suggest:

A) Benign paroxysmal positional vertigo
B) Ménière's disease
C) Transient ischemic attack (TIA)
D) Cerebrovascular accident (CVA)

90. All of the following measures have been found to help lower the risk of osteoporosis except:

A) Drinking organic orange juice
B) Eating low-fat dairy foods
C) Performing weight-bearing exercises
D) Vitamin D supplementation

91. The first teeth to erupt during infancy are which of the following?

A) First molars
B) Second molars
C) Incisors
D) Canines

92. The positive signs of pregnancy include:

A) Palpation of the fetus and auscultation of the fetal heart tones by the nurse practitioner
B) Palpation of the fetus and a positive quantitative serum pregnancy test
C) Fetal heart tones and a positive quantitative serum pregnancy test
D) Fetal heart tones and feeling of movement of the fetus by the mother

93. Chadwick's sign is characterized by:

A) Softening of the cervix
B) Blue coloration of the cervix and vagina
C) Softening of the uterine isthmus
D) Nausea and vomiting during the first trimester of pregnancy

94. A 21-year-old college student has recently been informed that he has a human papillomavirus (HPV) infection on the shaft of his penis. Which of the following methods can be used to visualize subclinical HPV lesions on the penile skin?

A) Perform a KOH (potassium hydroxide) exam
B) Scrape off some of the affected skin and send it for a culture and sensitivity
C) Apply acetic acid to the penile shaft and look for acetowhite changes
D) Order a serum herpesvirus titer

Questions 95 and 96 apply to this case. A 40-year-old female bank teller has recently been diagnosed with obsessive-compulsive disorder by her therapist.

95. Which of the following symptoms characterize this disorder?

A) Ritualistic behaviors that the patient feels compelled to repeat
B) Increased anxiety when attempting to ignore or suppress the repetitive behaviors
C) Frequent intrusive and repetitive thoughts and impulses
D) All of the above

96. Which of the following medications is indicated for the treatment of obsessive-compulsive disorder?

A) Paroxetine (Paxil CR)
B) Haloperidol (Haldol)
C) Lorazepam (Xanax)
D) Imipramine (Elavil)

97. You would advise an 18-year-old female student who has been given a booster dose of MMR at the college health clinic that:

A) She might have a low-grade fever during the first 24 to 48 hours
B) She should not get pregnant within the next 4 weeks
C) Her arm will be very sore at the injection site for 24 to 48 hours
D) Her arm will have some induration at the injection site in 24 to 48 hours

98. A 68-year-old woman is suspected of having Alzheimer's disease. Which of the following is the best initial method for assessing the condition?

A) CT scan of the brain
B) Folstein Mini-Mental State Exam
C) Patient history obtained from family members and close friends
D) EEG (electroencephalography)

99. A 55-year-old woman who has had type 2 diabetes for 20 years is concerned about her kidneys. She has a history of three urinary tract infections (UTIs) within the past 8 months, but is currently asymptomatic. Which of the following is the best course to follow?

A) Recheck urine during the visit, send a urine specimen for culture and sensitivity, and refer to a nephrologist
B) Order a urinalysis dipstick test to be repeated monthly
C) Order a CT scan of the kidneys
D) Provide empiric treatment for a UTI

100. A nurse practitioner is giving dietary counseling to a 30-year-old male alcoholic who has recently been diagnosed with folic acid deficiency anemia. Which of the following foods should the nurse practitioner recommend to this patient?

A) Tomatoes, oranges, and bananas
B) Cheese, yogurt, and milk
C) Lettuce, beef, and dairy products
D) Spinach, liver, and beans

101. A 14-year-old female adolescent is worried that she has not started to menstruate like most of her friends. During the gynecological examination, the nurse practitioner tells the mother, who is in the room with the patient, that her daughter is starting Tanner stage II. What are the physical exam findings during this stage?

A) Breast buds and some straight pubic hair
B) Fully developed breasts and curly pubic hair
C) Breast tissue with the areola on a separate mound with curly pubic hair
D) No breast tissue and no pubic hair

102. The Phalen test is used to evaluate:

A) Inflammation of the median nerve
B) Rheumatoid arthritis
C) Degenerative joint changes
D) Chronic tenosynovitis

103. Physiological anemia of pregnancy is due to:

A) An increase in the cardiac output at the end of the second trimester
B) A physiological decrease in the production of red blood cells in pregnant women
C) An increase of up to 50% of the plasma volume in pregnant women
D) An increase in the need for dietary iron in pregnancy

104. All of the following are known to cause chronic cough except:

A) Chronic bronchitis
B) Allergic rhinitis
C) Acute viral upper respiratory infection
D) Gastroesophageal reflux disease

105. Which of the following is a true statement about the effect of aspirin on platelet function?

A) The effect on platelets is reversible
B) The effect on platelets is reversible and lasts only 1 week
C) The effect on platelet function is minimal
D) The effect on platelet function is irreversible and lasts 15 to 20 days

106. All of the following agents are used to control the inflammatory changes seen in the lungs of asthmatics except:

A) Albuterol inhaler (Proventil)
B) Triamcinolone (Azmacort)
C) Montelukast (Singulair)
D) Cromolyn sodium inhaler (Intal)

107. Rovsing's sign is associated with which of the following?

A) An acute abdomen, such as during a ruptured appendix
B) Knee instability

C) Damage to the meniscus of the knee
D) Acute cholelithiasis

108. Which of the following is contraindicated in the care of pregnant women with placenta previa?

A) Echocardiogram
B) Intravaginal ultrasound
C) Abdominal ultrasound
D) Pelvic ultrasound

109. A patient is positive for anti-HCV (hepatitis C virus antibody). What is the next step to further evaluate this patient?

A) Refer the patient to a gastroenterologist
B) Order a hepatitis C RNA test
C) Order a hepatitis B comprehensive panel
D) The patient is immune to hepatitis C and no further testing is indicated

110. A 62-year-old woman complains of chronic severe low-back pain. She also reports mild episodes of fecal incontinence and numbness to her lower legs over the past week. You would suspect which of the following?

A) Fracture of the lower spine
B) A herniated disk
C) Cauda equina syndrome
D) Ankylosing spondylitis

111. A 28-year-old male nurse of Hispanic descent reports a history of a cold that resolved 2 weeks ago except for a dry cough and pain over his right cheek that worsens when he bends down. The patient denies fever. He tells the employee health nurse practitioner that he is very allergic to both cephalexin (Keflex) and erythromycin. The patient's vital signs are temperature of 99.2°F, pulse of 72 beats/min, and respirations of 12 breaths/min. Which of the following conditions is most likely?

A) Acute sinusitis
B) Acute bronchitis
C) Fever secondary to the previous viral URI (upper respiratory infection)
D) Hay fever

112. A 38-year-old multigravida who is at 32 weeks gestation calls the family nurse practitioner complaining of vaginal bleeding, abdominal pain, and uterine contractions. There is no watery discharge. She states that her uterus feels hard and is very painful. Which of the following conditions is most likely?

A) Placenta previa
B) Placental abruption
C) Molar pregnancy
D) Ectopic pregnancy

113. The Jarisch–Herxheimer reaction is best described as:

A) An immune-mediated reaction precipitated by the destruction of a large number of spirochetes due to an antibiotic injection
B) Severe chills and elevated blood pressure
C) Caused by infection with either *Chlamydia trachomatis* or gonorrheal infection of the liver capsule
D) Associated with certain viral illnesses

114. During a breast exam of a 30-year-old nulliparous woman, the nurse practitioner palpates several rubbery mobile areas of breast tissue. They are slightly tender to palpation. Both breasts have symmetrical findings. There are no skin changes or any nipple discharge. The patient is expecting her menstrual period in 5 days. Which of the following would you recommend?

A) Referral to a gynecologist for further evaluation
B) Advise the patient to return 1 week after her period so her breasts can be rechecked
C) Advise the patient to return in 6 months to have her breasts rechecked
D) Schedule the patient for a mammogram

115. When evaluating the blood pressure on both the arms and legs of an infant who has a diagnosis of coarctation of the aorta, which of the following is the correct finding?

A) The blood pressure is higher in the arms than in the legs
B) Only the diastolic blood pressure is higher in the legs than in the arms
C) The blood pressure is higher in the legs than the arms
D) The blood pressure is lower in both arms than in the legs

116. Which of the following should you expect to find on a wet-mount slide of a patient diagnosed with bacterial vaginosis?

A) Tzanck cells
B) A large number of leukocytes and squamous epithelial cells
C) A large number of squamous epithelial cells whose surfaces and edges are coated with large numbers of bacteria along with a few leukocytes
D) Epithelial cells and a small amount of blood

117. A 40-year-old woman comes to the medical office complaining of palpitations and some light-headedness for the past 6 months. These are random episodes. The nurse practitioner notices a mid-systolic click with a late systolic murmur that is best heard in the apical area during auscultation of the chest. You would suspect:

A) Atrial fibrillation
B) Sinus arrhythmia
C) Mitral stenosis
D) Mitral valve prolapse

118. Your 35-year-old patient is being worked up for microscopic hematuria. All of the following are differential diagnoses of microscopic hematuria except:

A) Kidney stones
B) Bladder cancer

C) Acute pyelonephritis
D) Renal artery stenosis

119. During a routine physical exam of an elderly woman, a triangular thickening of the bulbar conjunctiva on the temporal side is noted to be encroaching on the cornea. She denies any eye pain or visual changes. Which of the following is most likely?

A) Corneal arcus
B) Pterygium
C) Pinguecula
D) Chalazion

120. A young primigravida reports to you that she is starting to feel the baby's movements in her uterus. This is considered to be which of the following?

A) Presumptive sign
B) Probable sign
C) Positive sign
D) Possible sign

121. Which of the following is recommended treatment for erythema migrans or early Lyme disease?

A) Doxycycline (Vibramycin) 100 mg PO BID × 21 days
B) Ciprofloxacin (Cipro) 250 mg PO BID × 14 days
C) Erythromycin (E-mycin) 333 mg PO TID × 10 days
D) Dicloxacillin (Dynapen) 500 mg PO BID × 10 days

122. Nurse practitioners and clinical nurse specialists derive their legal right to practice from:

A) The nurse practice act in the state where they practice
B) The laws of the state where they practice
C) The Medicare statute
D) The board of nursing in the state where they practice

123. You are checking a 75-year-old woman's breast during an annual gynecological exam. The left nipple and areola are scaly and reddened. The patient denies pain or pruritus. She has noticed this scaliness on her left nipple for the past 8 months. Her dermatologist gave her a potent topical steroid, which she used twice a day for 1 month. The patient never went back for the follow-up. She still has the rash and wants an evaluation. Which of the following is the best intervention for this patient?

A) Prescribe another potent topical steroid and tell the patient to use it twice a day for 4 weeks
B) Order a mammogram and refer the patient to a breast surgeon
C) Advise the patient to stop using soap on her breasts when she bathes to avoid drying up the skin on her areolae and nipples
D) Order a sonogram of the breast and fine-needle biopsy of the breast

124. The following children are considered at higher risk for tuberculosis (TB) except:

A) A child who has recently been diagnosed with leukemia
B) An infant whose family is homeless
C) A child who was born in Japan
D) A Hispanic child with asthma who is using a steroid inhaler

125. During a sports physical exam of a 14-year-old high school athlete, the nurse practitioner notices a split of the S2 component of the heart sound during deep inspiration. She notes that it disappears upon expiration. The heart rate is regular and no murmurs are auscultated. Which of the following is correct?

A) This is an abnormal finding and should be evaluated further by a cardiologist
B) A stress test should be ordered
C) This is a normal finding in some young athletes
D) An echocardiogram should be ordered

126. A 65-year-old man with a body mass index (BMI) of 30 and a history of asthma has hypertension that has been well controlled with hydrochlorothiazide 12.5 mg PO daily. His total cholesterol is 230 g/dL. How many risk factors for coronary artery disease (CAD) does he have?

A) One risk factor
B) Two risk factors
C) Three risk factors
D) Four risk factors

127. A common side effect of metformin (Glucophage) therapy is:

A) Weight gain
B) Lactic acidosis
C) Hypoglycemic episodes
D) Diarrhea

128. While doing a cardiac exam on a 45-year-old man, you note an irregular rhythm with a pulse rate of 110 beats/min. The patient is alert and is not in distress. What is the most likely diagnosis?

A) Atrial fibrillation
B) Ventricular fibrillation
C) Cardiac arrhythmia
D) First-degree right bundle branch block

129. The nurse practitioner is evaluating patients who are at high risk for complications due to urinary tract infections (UTIs). Which of the following patients does not belong in this category?

A) A 38-year-old diabetic patient with an A1C of 7.5%
B) A woman with rheumatoid arthritis who is being treated with methotrexate and low-dose steroids
C) A 21-year-old woman who has a history of irritable bowel syndrome
D) A pregnant woman

130. A 68-year-old woman with hypertension and diabetes is seen by the nurse practitioner for a dry cough that worsens at night when she lies in bed. She has shortness of breath, which worsens when she exerts herself, and has gained 6 lbs during the past 2 months. Her pulse rate is 90 beats/min and regular. She is on a nitroglycerine patch and furosemide daily. The best explanation for her symptoms is:

A) Kidney failure
B) Congestive heart failure
C) ACE inhibitor-induced coughing
D) Thyroid disease

131. A 40-year-old White woman with a body mass index (BMI) of 32 complains of colicky pain in the right upper quadrant of her abdomen that gets worse if she eats fried food. During the physical exam, the nurse practitioner presses deeply on the left lower quadrant of the abdomen. After she releases her hand, the patient complains of pain on the right side of the lower abdomen. What is the name of this finding?

A) Rebound tenderness
B) Rovsing's sign
C) Murphy's sign
D) Psoas test

132. Which of the following viral infections is associated with occasional abnormal forms of lymphocytes during an acute infection?

A) Cytomegalovirus (CMV)
B) Epstein–Barr virus (EBV)
C) Human papillomavirus (HPV)
D) Coxsackievirus

133. A faun tail nevus is a sign of which of the following?

A) Down syndrome
B) Infantile scoliosis
C) Congenital heart disease
D) Spina bifida

134. A 21-year-old woman complains to you of a 1-week episode of dysuria, frequency, and a strong odor to her urine. This is her second episode of the year. The previous urinary tract infection occurred 3 months ago. What is the most appropriate follow-up for this patient?

A) Order a urinalysis and urine for culture and sensitivity (C&S), and treat the patient with antibiotics
B) Order a urine C&S and hold treatment until you get the results from the lab
C) Treat the patient with a 7-day course of antibiotics and order a urine C&S now and after she completes her antibiotics
D) Treat the patient with a stronger drug, such as ofloxacin (Floxin), for 10 days

135. Café-au-lait spots look like tan to light-brown stains that have irregular borders. They can be located anywhere on the body. Which of the following is a correct statement?

A) They are associated with neurofibromatosis or von Recklinghausen's disease
B) They may be identified as precancerous after a biopsy
C) They are more common in children with darker skin
D) They are associated with Wilson's disease

136. During the eye exam of a 50-year-old hypertensive patient who is complaining of an onset of a severe headache, you find that the borders of the disc margins on both eyes are blurred. What is the name of this clinical finding?

A) Normal optic disc
B) Optic neuropathy
C) Papilledema
D) Hypertensive retinopathy

137. A high school teacher complains of a dry cough for the past 6 weeks. It worsens when he is supine. He has episodes of nausea and heartburn, which he self-treats with an over-the-counter (OTC) antacid. He chews mints for his "bad breath." Which of the following is a possible cause for this patient's cough?

A) Asthma
B) Gastroesophageal reflux
C) Pneumonia
D) Chronic postnasal drip

138. The red reflex examination is used to screen for:

A) Cataracts
B) Strabismus
C) Blindness
D) Blinking response

139. A 44-year-old man with Down syndrome starts to develop impaired memory and difficulty with his usual daily routines. He is having problems functioning at the job where he has been employed for the past 10 years. The physical exam and routine labs are all negative. The vital signs are normal. His appetite is normal. The most likely diagnosis is:

A) Tic douloureux
B) Stroke
C) Alzheimer's disease
D) Delirium

140. Which of the following findings is associated with the chronic use of chewing tobacco?

A) Cheilosis and xerostomia
B) Glossitis
C) Geographic tongue
D) Leukoplakia and oral cancer

141. What does a potassium hydroxide (KOH) prep help the nurse practitioner diagnose?

A) Herpes zoster infections
B) Fungal infections
C) Herpes simplex infections
D) Viral infections

142. All of the following are considered selective serotonin reuptake inhibitors (SSRIs) except:

A) Imipramine (Tofranil)
B) Fluoxetine (Prozac)
C) Sertraline (Zoloft)
D) Paroxetine (Paxil CR)

143. All of the following pulmonary tests require the patient's voice to perform correctly except:

A) Egophony
B) Tactile fremitus
C) Whispered pectoriloquy
D) Auscultation

144. While checking for the red reflex on a 3-year-old boy during a well-child visit, the nurse practitioner notes a white reflection on the child's left pupil. Which of the following conditions should be ruled out?

A) Unilateral strabismus
B) Unilateral cataracts
C) Retinoblastoma of the left eye
D) Color blindness of the left eye

145. All of the following infections are reportable diseases except:

A) Lyme disease
B) Gonorrhea
C) Nongonococcal urethritis
D) Syphilis

146. A menopausal woman with osteopenia is attending a dietary education class. Which of the following foods are recommended?

A) Yogurt and sardines
B) Spinach and red meat
C) Cheese and red meat
D) Low-fat cheese and whole grain

147. A patient who has been prescribed warfarin sodium (Coumadin) is advised to avoid eating large amounts of leafy green vegetables because:

A) The high vitamin K levels will decrease the INR
B) They have too much ascorbic acid, which can interact with the medicine
C) The high-fiber content will decrease the absorption of the warfarin (Coumadin)
D) The vitamins in the vegetables will bind with, and inactivate, the warfarin (Coumadin)

Questions 148, 149, and 150 apply to this case. Your patient is a 65-year-old man who has been taking a new prescription of rosuvastatin (Crestor) 40 mg daily for 6 weeks. During a follow-up visit, he reports feeling extremely fatigued and having dark-colored urine. He denies any generalized muscle soreness.

148. Which of the following is the most appropriate treatment plan?

A) Order a CBC with differential
B) Order a liver function profile and CK level
C) Recommend an increase in fluid intake and rest
D) Order a urine culture and sensitivity test

149. Which of the following diagnoses is most likely in this patient?

A) Rhabdomyolysis
B) Acute drug-induced hepatitis
C) Acute mononucleosis
D) A major depressive episode

150. What would you advise him regarding his rosuvastatin (Crestor) prescription?

A) Continue taking the medicine until the lab results are available
B) Take half the usual daily dose until the lab results are available
C) Take the medicine every other day instead of daily until the lab results are available
D) Stop taking the medicine until the lab results are available

151. A nurse practitioner is doing a funduscopic exam on a 35-year-old woman during a routine physical exam. He notices that she has sharp disc margins and a yellowish-orange color in the macular area. The ratio of veins to arteries is 3:2. What is the next most appropriate action?

A) Advise the patient that she had a normal exam
B) Advise the patient that she had an abnormal exam
C) Refer the patient to the emergency room
D) Refer the patient to an ophthalmologist

152. During a sports physical, you note that the vision of an 18-year-old male athlete is 20/30 in both eyes. Which of the following statements is true?

A) The patient can see at 20 ft what a person with normal vision can see at 30 ft
B) The patient can see at 30 ft what a person with normal vision can see at 20 ft
C) The patient cannot engage in contact sports
D) The patient needs to be referred to an ophthalmologist

153. A 30-year-old woman with type 2 diabetes uses regular and NPH (neutral protein Hagedorn) insulin in the morning and in the evening. She denies changes in her diet or any illness, but recently started attending aerobic classes in the afternoon. Her fasting blood glucose level before breakfast is now elevated. Which of the following is best described?

A) Somogyi phenomenon
B) Dawn phenomenon

C) Raynaud's phenomenon
D) Insulin resistance

154. The anti-HCV test of a 60-year-old female patient is positive. Which test is appropriate for follow-up?

A) HCV RNA
B) HCV antibody
C) HCV core antibody
D) HCV surface antigen

155. When the nurse practitioner is evaluating a patient for intermittent claudication, he or she would first:

A) Order a venogram
B) Order TED anti-embolism stockings
C) Check the ankle and brachial blood pressures before and after exercise
D) Check the pedal and posterior tibial pulses

156. All of the following drugs can interact with theophylline (Theo-24) except:

A) Erythromycin (Eryc)
B) Montelukast (Singulair)
C) Phenytoin sodium (Dilantin)
D) Cimetidine (Tagamet)

157. You note a high-pitched and blowing pansystolic murmur while assessing a 70-year-old male patient. It is grade 2/6 and is best heard at the apical area. Which of the following is most likely?

A) Ventricular septal defect
B) Tricuspid regurgitation
C) Mitral regurgitation
D) Mitral stenosis

158. The cover/uncover test is a screening tool for:

A) Color blindness
B) Strabismus
C) Visual acuity
D) Cataracts

159. The mother of a 4-week-old infant is concerned that her infant's eyes are crossed for a few seconds occasionally. The nurse practitioner would:

A) Recommend referral to a pediatric ophthalmologist
B) Advise the mother that this is a normal finding in infants up to 2 months of age
C) Recommend that multivitamin supplements be given to the infant daily
D) Educate the mother on how to patch the infant's eye every 4 hours

160. All of the following are factors important in determining the peak expiratory flow volume except:

A) Weight
B) Height
C) Age
D) Gender

161. You are reviewing a Pap smear result for a 25-year-old woman. Which of the following cells should be obtained in a Pap smear sample to be classified as a satisfactory specimen?

A) Clue cells and endometrial cells
B) Vaginal cells and cervical cells
C) Squamous epithelial cells and endocervical cells
D) Leukocytes and RBCs

162. When assessing a patient suspected of having vertigo, which description provided by the patient is most consistent with the diagnosis?

A) A sensation of imbalance while walking
B) A sensation of spinning or rotating
C) A sensation of "passing out"
D) A sensation of lightheadedness when changing positions from reclining to standing

163. Which of the following statements is false regarding physiological jaundice in newborns?

A) Physiological jaundice is the most common type of jaundice in infants
B) The level of unconjugated bilirubin is increased in the newborn's body
C) Phototherapy is usually indicated for these infants
D) It starts on the second to fourth day of life

164. Koilonychia is associated with which of the following conditions?

A) Lead poisoning
B) Beta thalassemia trait
C) B_{12} deficiency anemia
D) Iron-deficiency anemia

165. Which of the following laboratory tests is positive in a large number of patients with systemic lupus erythematosus?

A) Antinuclear antibody (ANA)
B) Rheumatoid factor
C) Antiparietal antibody
D) Immunoglobulin

166. All of the following are correct statements regarding the S3 component of the heart sound except:

A) It occurs very early in diastole and is sometimes called an *opening snap*
B) It is a normal finding in some children, healthy young adults, and athletes
C) It can be a normal variant if heard in a person aged 40 years or older
D) It signifies congestive heart failure (CHF)

167. A positive straight leg raising test is indicative of which of the following?

A) Myasthenia gravis
B) Inflammation of the sciatic nerve/herniated disk
C) Multiple sclerosis
D) Parkinson's disease

168. Which of the following would you recommend on an annual basis for an elderly patient with type 2 diabetes?

A) Eye exam with an ophthalmologist
B) Follow-up visit with a urologist
C) Periodic visits to an optometrist
D) Colonoscopy

169. A 72-year-old woman complains of a crusty and nonhealing small ulcer on her upper lip that she has had for several years. Which of the following would you recommend?

A) Triamcinolone acetonide (Kenalog) cream BID for 2 weeks
B) Triple antibiotic ointment BID × 2 weeks
C) Hydrocortisone 1% cream BID for 2 weeks
D) The patient needs to be evaluated by a dermatologist

170. All of the following statements about phototherapy are correct except:

A) Light from the blue-to-white spectrum is used
B) It is not always necessary to use a shield for the infant's eyes
C) Unconjugated bilirubin in the skin is converted to a water-soluble nontoxic substance that is excreted in the bile
D) The infant's eyes should be shielded

171. Heberden's nodes are commonly found in which of the following diseases?

A) Rheumatoid arthritis
B) Degenerative joint disease
C) Psoriatic arthritis
D) Septic arthritis

172. The red blood cells in pernicious anemia will show:

A) Microcytic and hypochromic cells
B) Microcytic and normochromic cells
C) Macrocytic and normochromic cells
D) Macrocytic and hypochromic cells

173. All of the following children are within the parameters of normal growth and development for their age group except:

A) A 2-month-old who coos and smiles
B) A 14-month-old who understands complex commands
C) A 20-month-old who can walk without support
D) A 3-year-old who can speak in three- to four-word sentences

174. You are reviewing the bilirubin level of a 3-day-old full-term neonate. You note that it is 10 mg/dL. The infant has a slight yellow color to his skin, mucous membranes, and sclera. The infant is feeding well, is not irritable, and has eight to 10 wet diapers per day. Which of the following is a true statement?

A) Keep monitoring the infant's bilirubin level until it returns to normal in about 1 week
B) Recommend that the infant be treated with phototherapy 10 minutes a day until the bilirubin level is back to a normal range
C) Refer the infant to a neonatologist as soon as possible
D) Refer the infant to the neonatal intensive care unit

175. All of the following statements are correct regarding the Td vaccine except:

A) Fever occurs in up to 80% of the patients
B) A possible side effect is induration on the injection site
C) The Td is given every 10 years
D) The DPT and DT should not be given beyond the seventh birthday

176. Which of the following drugs does the *Eighth Joint National Committee (JNC 8) 2014 Evidence-Based Guideline for the Management of High Blood Pressure in Adult*s recommend for the initial treatment for White adults with microalbuminuria?

A) Angiotensin-converting enzyme (ACE) inhibitors
B) Diuretics
C) Calcium channel blockers
D) Beta-blockers

177. A test called the *visual fields by confrontation* is used to evaluate for:

A) Peripheral vision
B) Central distance vision
C) Narrow-angle glaucoma
D) Accommodation

178. The following skin findings are considered macules except:

A) A freckle
B) Petechiae
C) Acne
D) A flat, 0.5-cm brown birthmark

179. A 20-year-old college student reports to the student health clinic with a laceration of her left hand. She tells the nurse practitioner that she cut her hand while working in her garden. Her last Td booster was 5½ years ago. Which of the following is correct?

A) Administer a booster dose of the Tdap vaccine
B) Administer the Td vaccine and the Td immunoglobulin (HyperTET)
C) Administer Td immunoglobulin (HyperTET) only
D) She does not need any Td immunoglobulin (HyperTET) or a Td booster

180. The apex of the heart is located at:

A) Second intercostal space to the right of the sternal border
B) Second intercostal space to the left of the sternal border
C) The left lower sternal border
D) The left side of the sternum at the fifth intercostal space by the midclavicular line

181. An elderly woman with a history of rheumatoid arthritis reports to the nurse practitioner that she had been taking ibuprofen twice daily for many years. All of the following organ systems are at risk of damage from chronic nonsteroidal anti-inflammatory drug (NSAID) use except:

A) Cardiovascular system
B) Pulmonary system
C) Gastrointestinal system
D) Renal system

182. A 15-year-old boy has just moved into the community and is staying in a foster home temporarily. There is no record of his immunizations. His foster mother wants him to be checked before he enters the local high school. Which of the following immunizations does this patient need?

A) Meningococcal vaccine
B) Measles–mumps–rubella (MMR) vaccine
C) Tdap vaccine
D) All of the above

183. Which cranial nerve (CN) is being evaluated when patients are instructed to shrug their shoulders?

A) CN IX
B) CN X
C) CN XI
D) CN XII

184. An immigrant who is from Southeast Asia has an 11.5-mm area of redness and induration on his left forearm after getting a Mantoux test 72 hours ago. The last test, which was done 12 months ago, was negative. He denies cough, night sweats, and weight loss. What is the next best intervention?

A) Obtain a sputum culture
B) Obtain a chest x-ray
C) Obtain a sputum sample for culture and sensitivity (C&S) and an acid-fast stain
D) Obtain a complete blood count (CBC)

185. Swim therapy (aqua therapy) for a 13-year-old with cerebral palsy is an example of:

A) Primary prevention
B) Secondary prevention
C) Tertiary prevention
D) Health prevention

186. Which of the following individuals is most likely to be at higher risk for osteoporosis?

A) 70-year-old woman of African ancestry who walks daily for exercise
B) 42-year-old obese woman from Cuba who has been taking prednisone 10 mg daily for the past 12 years to control her severe asthma
C) 55-year-old Caucasian woman who is an aerobics instructor
D) 45-year-old Asian woman who has been on high-dose steroids for 1 week

187. What is the primary carbohydrate found in breast milk and commercial infant formulas?

A) Fructose
B) Lactose
C) Glucose
D) Sucrose

188. Which of the following patients is least likely to become an alcoholic?

A) A patient whose father has a history of alcoholism
B) A patient whose wife complains that he drinks too much
C) A patient who drinks one glass of wine nightly with dinner
D) A patient who feels he drinks all the time

189. The following conditions are absolute contraindications for the use of oral contraceptives except:

A) Sexually active patient with amenorrhea
B) History of emboli that resolved with heparin therapy 15 years ago
C) Cigarette smoking at the age of 30 years
D) Hepatitis C infection

190. In the United States, the most common cause of cancer deaths in men is:

A) Lung cancer
B) Prostate cancer
C) Colon cancer
D) Skin cancer

191. You notice a medium-pitched harsh systolic murmur during an episodic examination of a 37-year-old woman. It is best heard at the right upper border of the sternum. What is most likely?

A) Mitral stenosis
B) Aortic stenosis
C) Pulmonic stenosis
D) Tricuspid regurgitation

192. A small abscess on a hair follicle on the eyelid is called:

A) Hordeolum
B) Pterygium
C) Pinguecula
D) Ptosis

193. Which of the following is indicated for the prophylactic treatment of migraine headache?

A) Ibuprofen (Motrin)
B) Naproxen sodium (Anaprox)
C) Propranolol (Inderal)
D) Sumatriptan (Imitrex)

194. A 40-year-old man complains to the nurse practitioner of severe stabbing pains behind his left eye for the past 2 days. They are accompanied by some nasal congestion and rhinorrhea, which is clear in color. The patient denies pharyngitis and fever. Which of the following conditions is most likely?

A) Migraine headache with aura
B) Cluster headache
C) Tic douloureux
D) Cranial neuralgia

195. A male patient has type 2 diabetes mellitus and a "sensitive stomach." Which medication is least likely to cause him gastrointestinal distress?

A) Naproxen sodium (Anaprox)
B) Aspirin (Bayer's aspirin)
C) Erythromycin (E-mycin)
D) Sucralfate (Carafate)

196. All of the following statements are true regarding domestic abuse except:

A) There is no delay in seeking medical treatment
B) The pattern of injuries is inconsistent with the history reported
C) Injuries are usually in the "central" area of the body instead of the extremities
D) Pregnant women have a higher risk of domestic abuse

197. A new mother is breastfeeding her full-term 4-week-old infant. She wants to know whether she should give the infant vitamin supplements. The best advice is:

A) Because she is breastfeeding, the infant does not need any vitamin supplements
B) Breast milk gives the infant all the vitamins he needs until 12 months of age
C) Breastfed infants require vitamin D supplementation beginning in the first few days of life
D) Infant formula can be used to supplement breastfeeding as needed

198. Beta thalassemia minor is considered a:

A) Macrocytic anemia
B) Normocytic anemia
C) Microcytic anemia
D) Hemolytic anemia

199. Potential complications of mitral valve prolapse (MVP) include all of the following except:

A) Severe mitral regurgitation
B) Endocarditis
C) Increased risk of stroke and transient ischemic attack
D) Mitral stenosis

200. A new patient is complaining of severe pruritus that is worse at night. Several family members also have the same symptoms. Upon examination, areas of excoriated papules are noted on some of the interdigital webs of both hands and on the axillae. This finding is most consistent with:

A) Contact dermatitis
B) Impetigo
C) Larva migrans
D) Scabies

201. Which of the following laboratory tests is the most sensitive test for evaluating an active *Helicobacter pylori* infection of the stomach or duodenum:

A) *Helicobacter pylori* titer
B) Fasting gastrin level
C) Upper GI series
D) Urea breath test

202. Which of the following foods would you advise a new mother to introduce to her 6-month-old infant first?

A) Iron-fortified rice cereal
B) Plain rice cereal
C) Iron-fortified pureed chicken meat
D) Plain pureed carrots

203. An obese Asian patient with BMI (body mass index) of 33 complains of fatigue, and excessive thirst and hunger. You suspect type 2 diabetes mellitus. Initial testing to confirm diagnosis can include:

A) Fasting plasma glucose level
B) Glycated hemoglobin level (A1C)
C) Oral glucose tolerance testing
D) All of the above

204. A *bulla* is defined as:

A) A solid nodule less than 1 cm in size
B) A superficial vesicle filled with serous fluid greater than 1 cm in size
C) A maculopapular lesion
D) A shallow ulcer

205. A newborn's mother is discovered to be HBsAg (hepatitis B surface antigen) positive. Which of the following would you recommend for this infant?

A) Give the infant hepatitis B immunoglobulin
B) Give the infant both hepatitis B vaccine and hepatitis B immunoglobulin
C) Give the infant hepatitis B vaccine only
D) Send the infant home because he is not infected

206. All of the following findings are associated with the secondary stage of an infection by the organism *Treponema pallidum* except:

A) Condyloma acuminata
B) Maculopapular rash of the palms and soles
C) Lymphadenopathy
D) Condyloma lata

207. The following are acceptable methods of birth control for breastfeeding mothers except:

A) Diaphragm with spermicidal gel
B) Progesterone-only pills (Micronor)
C) Condoms
D) Low-dose oral contraceptives with at least 20 mcg of estradiol (Alesse, Loestrin)

208. Women with a history of pelvic inflammatory disease (PID) have an increased risk for all of the following complications except:

A) Ectopic pregnancy
B) Scarring of the fallopian tubes
C) Infertility
D) Ovarian cysts

209. The differential diagnosis for genital ulceration includes all of the following except:

A) Syphilis
B) Genital herpes
C) Chancroid
D) Molluscum contagiosum

210. Lead poisoning can cause which type of anemia?

A) Mild macrocytic anemia
B) Normocytic anemia
C) Microcytic anemia
D) Mild hemolytic anemia

211. When evaluating a case of temporal arteritis, the erythrocyte sedimentation rate (ESR) is expected to be:

A) Normal
B) Lower than normal
C) Elevated
D) Indeterminate

212. A 45-year-old woman is complaining of generalized morning stiffness, especially in both her wrist and hands. It is much worse in the morning and lasts for a few hours. She also complains of fatigue and generalized body aches that have been present for the past few months. Which of the following is most likely?

A) Osteoporosis
B) Rheumatoid arthritis
C) Osteoarthritis
D) Gout

213. During a well child visit, a new father wants to know whether he can give fresh whole milk to his 6-month-old son. The nurse practitioner would recommend that:

A) He can start giving whole milk but not skim milk by 6 months of age
B) He should not give whole milk to his son until the boy is at least 12 months of age
C) He can give whole milk to his son at anytime
D) He should not give whole milk to his son without diluting it with water

214. Which of the following drugs is effective therapy for treating pain in patients who are having an acute exacerbation of gout?

A) Acetaminophen (Tylenol)
B) Systemic steroids
C) Indomethacin (Indocin)
D) Allopurinol (Zyloprim)

215. The complications of untreated gout include:

A) Impaired joint mobility and renal damage
B) Impaired joint mobility and liver damage
C) An increased risk of urinary tract infections
D) Bladder cancer

216. A 21-year-old woman who is complaining of random palpitations is diagnosed with mitral valve prolapse (MVP). Her echocardiogram reveals thickened leaflets. You note a grade 3/6 systolic murmur with an ejection click during physical examination. You would advise her that:

A) Endocarditis prophylaxis is recommended for most dental and urological procedures
B) Endocarditis prophylaxis is not necessary
C) She requires lifetime anticoagulation therapy with warfarin sodium
D) Endocarditis prophylaxis is recommended for dental procedures only

217. You note bony nodules located at the proximal interphalangeal joints on both the hands of your 65-year-old female patient. Which of the following is most likely?

A) Bouchard's nodes
B) Heberden's nodes
C) Osteoarthritic nodules
D) Tophi deposits

218. Which chronic illness disproportionately affects the Hispanic population?

A) Diabetes mellitus
B) Hypertension
C) Alcohol abuse
D) Skin cancer

219. A lipid profile for a newly diagnosed hypertensive patient with a BMI (body mass index) of 27 shows a triglyceride level of 950 mg/dL, total cholesterol of 240 mg/dL, LDL (low density lipoprotein) of 145 mg/dL, and HDL (high-density lipoprotein) of 45 mg/dL. What is the best intervention for this patient?

A) Educate the patient about lifestyle changes that will help lower cholesterol levels
B) Initiate a prescription of metformin (Glucophage)
C) Recommend that the patient exercise at least 30 minutes daily
D) Initiate a prescription of fenofibrate (Tricor)

220. Cullen's sign is most commonly associated with which of the following?

A) Acute pancreatitis
B) Myocardial infarction
C) Acute pyelonephritis
D) Preeclampsia

221. A nurse practitioner is evaluating an 80-year-old woman who is a resident of a long-term care facility. She instructs the patient to remember the words *orange, house,* and *world.* A few minutes later, the patient is asked to recall these three words. Which of the following tests is being described?

A) Lachman test
B) Neurological exam
C) Romberg test
D) Mini-Mental State Exam

222. In most states, patients younger than age 18 years may consent to health care without parental or legal guardian consent in all except which of the following cases?

A) Contraception
B) Pregnancy
C) School physical exams
D) Sexually transmitted disease (STD) evaluation and treatment

223. A hypertensive middle-aged man who is Native American has recently been diagnosed with renal insufficiency. He has been on lisinopril (Accupril) for many years. Which of the following laboratory values should be carefully monitored?

A) Hemoglobin, hematocrit, and MCV (mean corpuscular volume)
B) Serum creatinine and estimated GFR (glomerular filtration rate)
C) AST (aspartate aminotransferase) and ALT (alanine aminotransferase)
D) Serum sodium, potassium, and magnesium

224. You suspect an enterobiasis infection in a 6-year-old girl. Which of the following tests would you recommend?

A) Stool culture and sensitivity
B) Stool for ova and parasites
C) The scotch tape test
D) Hemoccult test

225. What is the most common cause of left ventricular hypertrophy in the United States?

A) Chronic atrial fibrillation
B) Chronic hypertension
C) Mitral valve prolapse
D) Pulmonary hypertension

226. An asthmatic exacerbation is characterized by all of the following symptoms except:

A) Tachycardia
B) Severe wheezing
C) Chronic coughing
D) Tachypnea

227. A nurse practitioner's right to practice is regulated under:

A) Medicare regulations
B) The board of medicine
C) The federal government
D) The board of nursing

228. A 10-year-old boy who was recently accepted onto his school's soccer team has a history of exercise-induced asthma. He wants to know when he should use his albuterol inhaler. The nurse practitioner would advise the patient to:

A) Premedicate 10 to 15 minutes before starting exercise
B) Wait until he starts to exercise before using the inhaler
C) Premedicate 30 minutes before starting exercise
D) Wait until he finishes his exercise before using his inhaler

229. Atrophic macular degeneration of the aged (AMD) is the leading cause of blindness in the elderly in the United States. Which of the following statements is correct?

A) It is a slow or sudden painless loss of central vision
B) It is a slow or sudden painless loss of peripheral vision
C) It is an occlusion of the central retinal vein causing degeneration of the macular area
D) It is commonly caused by diabetic retinopathy

230. A 12-year-old girl is complaining of a 2-week history of facial pressure that worsens when she bends over. She complains of tooth pain in her upper molars on the right side of her face. On physical exam, her lung and heart sounds are normal. Which of the following is the most likely diagnosis?

A) An acute dental abscess
B) Chronic sinusitis
C) Acute sinusitis
D) Severe allergic rhinitis

231. Hypovolemic shock would most likely occur with fractures of the:

A) Spine
B) Pelvis
C) Femur
D) Humerus

232. Podagra is associated with which of the following?

A) Rheumatoid arthritis
B) Gout
C) Osteoarthritis
D) Septic arthritis

233. While assessing for a cardiac murmur, the first time that a thrill can be palpated is at:

A) Grade 2
B) Grade 3
C) Grade 4
D) Grade 5

234. A medium-pitched harsh mid-systolic murmur is best heard at the right second intercostal space of the chest. It radiates into the neck. Which of the following is the correct diagnosis?

A) Aortic stenosis
B) Pulmonic stenosis
C) Aortic regurgitation
D) Mitral stenosis

235. Which type of hepatitis virus infection is more likely to result in chronic hepatitis and increased risk of developing hepatocellular carcinoma?

A) Hepatitis A virus
B) Hepatitis B virus
C) Hepatitis C virus
D) Both hepatitis B and hepatitis C

236. What is the caloric content of infant formula and breast milk?

A) 10 kcal/30 mL
B) 15 kcal/30 mL
C) 20 kcal/30 mL
D) 25 kcal/30 mL

237. A 19-year-old woman has recently been diagnosed with acute hepatitis B. She is sexually active and is monogamous. She reports that her partner uses condoms inconsistently. What would you recommend for her male sexual partner who was also tested for hepatitis with the following results: HBsAg (–), anti-HBs (–), anti-HCV (–), anti-HAV (+)?

A) Hepatitis B vaccination
B) Hepatitis B immunoglobulin
C) Hepatitis B vaccination and hepatitis B immunoglobulin
D) No vaccination is needed at this time

238. All of the following conditions are associated with an increased risk of normocytic anemia except:

A) Rheumatoid arthritis
B) Systemic lupus erythematosus
C) Polymyalgia rheumatica
D) Pregnancy

239. You can determine a pulse deficit by counting the:

A) Apical and radial pulses at the same time, then finding the difference between the two
B) Apical pulse first, then the radial pulse, and subtracting to find the difference between the two
C) Apical pulse and the femoral pulse at the same time and finding the difference between the two
D) Radial pulse first, then counting the femoral pulse, and subtracting to find the difference between the two

240. An infant who does not have a history of reactive airway disease and allergy has both inspiratory and expiratory wheezing accompanied by fever and profuse clear nasal discharge. Which of the following is most likely?

A) Tracheobronchitis
B) Bronchiolitis
C) Croup
D) A small foreign body is lodged on the left main bronchus

241. A patient who recently returned from a vacation in Latin America complains of a severe headache and stiff neck that a were accompanied by a high fever for the past 12 hours. While examining the patient, the nurse practitioner flexes both the patient's hips and legs and then tells the patient to straighten them against resistance. The name of this test is:

A) Kernig's maneuver
B) Brudzinski's maneuver
C) Murphy's sign
D) Homan's sign

242. Which of the following groups has been recommended to be screened for thyroid disease?

A) Women aged 50 years or older
B) Adolescent girls
C) Elderly men
D) School-aged children

243. A 65-year-old Hispanic woman has a history of type 2 diabetes. A routine urinalysis reveals a few epithelial cells and is negative for leukocytes, nitrites, and protein. The serum creatinine is 1.5 mg/dL. Which of the following actions would you recommend next?

A) Order a urine test for culture and sensitivity (C&S)
B) Order a spot urine for microalbumin-to-creatinine ratio
C) Because the urinalysis is negative, no further tests are necessary
D) Recommend a screening intravenous pyelogram (IVP)

244. RhoGAM's mechanism of action is:

A) The destruction of Rh-positive fetal RBCs that are present in the mother's circulatory system
B) The destruction of maternal antibodies against Rh-positive fetal RBCs
C) The stimulation of maternal antibodies so that there is a decreased risk of hemolysis
D) The destruction of maternal antibodies against fetal RBCs

245. A chest radiograph shows an area of consolidation on the lower lobe. Which of the following conditions is most likely?

A) Bacterial pneumonia
B) Acute bronchitis
C) Chronic obstructive pulmonary disease (COPD)
D) Atypical pneumonia

246. What type of breath sounds are best heard over the base of the lungs?

A) Fine breath sounds
B) Vesicular breath sounds
C) Bronchial sounds
D) Tracheal breath sounds

247. The most current Eighth Joint National Committee (JNC 8) recommendation for the blood pressure goal in diabetics is:

A) <140/90 mmHg
B) <130/85 mmHg
C) <130/80 mmHg
D) <125/75 mmHg

248. All of the following pharmacological agents are used to treat inflammation in the lungs of asthmatic patients except:

A) Nedocromil sodium (Tilade) two sprays QID
B) Cromolyn sodium inhaler (Intal) two puffs QID
C) Long-acting oral theophylline (Theo-Dur) 200 mg every 12 hours
D) Fluticasone inhaler (Flovent) two puffs BID

249. All of the following clinical findings are considered benign oral findings except:

A) A patch of leukoplakia
B) Fordyce spots
C) Torus palatinus
D) Fishtail uvula

250. The nurse practitioner examines a 4-week-old boy whose mother reports that he has cried for at least 3 hours a day at the same time of day since birth. What is the main goal in the clinical evaluation of this infant?

A) Rule out any physiological cause for the crying spells
B) Make sure that the infant is well clothed
C) Evaluate the environment
D) Order laboratory and diagnostic testing

251. Which of the following findings is associated with thyroid hypofunction?

A) Graves' disease
B) Eye disorder
C) Thyroid storm
D) Myxedema

252. What is the best procedure for evaluating a corneal abrasion?

A) Tonometry
B) Fluorescein stain
C) Visual field test
D) Funduscopy

253. You are examining a patient who has just been diagnosed with Bell's palsy. Bell's palsy is characterized by all of the following except:

A) Drooling
B) Inability to swallow
C) Inability to close the eye on the affected side
D) Drooping of the corner of the mouth on the affected side

254. A new mother who is on her fourth day of breastfeeding complains to the nurse practitioner of sore breasts. The nurse practitioner would:

A) Recommend a decrease in the number of times she breastfeeds her infant per day
B) Recommend that she stop breastfeeding and use infant formula for the next 48 hours
C) Educate the mother that this is normal during the first week or 2 of breastfeeding and the soreness will eventually go away
D) Recommend that she purchase plastic nipple pads for her nursing bra and use them daily

255. A 13-year-old boy's peak expiratory flow results indicate 60% to 80% of the predicted range. How would you classify his asthma?

A) Mild intermittent asthma
B) Mild persistent asthma
C) Moderate persistent asthma
D) Severe asthma

256. Which of the following conditions is associated with a positive Auspitz sign?

A) Contact dermatitis
B) Seborrheic dermatitis
C) Systemic lupus erythematosus
D) Psoriasis

257. Which of the following is used to confirm a diagnosis of Hashimoto's thyroiditis?

A) Serum thyroid-stimulating hormone (TSH)
B) Free T4 test
C) Anti-thyroid peroxidase and anti-thyroglobulin antibodies
D) Thyroid ultrasound

258. A first-grader presents to a school nurse practitioner with a few blisters on one arm and on his face. The child keeps scratching the affected areas. Some of the lesions have ruptured with yellow serous fluid that crusts easily. These findings best describe:

A) Acute cellulitis
B) Herpes zoster
C) Bullous impetigo
D) Erysipelas

259. All of the following statements reflect adequate breast milk production except:

A) Full-term infant is at birth weight by the second week of life
B) Fewer than six wet diapers per day or fewer than four stools per day
C) Infant is nursing fewer than eight times per 24-hour period
D) Weight loss of more than 10% of birth weight

260. The best screening test for both hyperthyroidism and hypothyroidism is:

A) Free T4 (thyroxine)
B) Thyroid-stimulating hormone (TSH)
C) Thyroid profile
D) Palpation of the thyroid gland

261. All of the following are considered benign physiological variants except:

A) Internal tibial torsion
B) Supernumerary nipples
C) Split uvula
D) Cheilosis

262. A 65-year-old woman's bone density result shows severe demineralization of cortical bone. All of the following pharmacological agents are useful in treating this condition except:

A) Raloxifene (Evista)
B) Calcitonin (Miacalcin)
C) Medroxyprogesterone (Depo-Provera)
D) Calcium with vitamin D

263. A fracture on the navicular area of the wrist is usually caused by falling forward and landing on the hands. The affected wrist is hyperextended to break the fall. The nurse practitioner is aware that all of the following statements are true regarding a fracture of the scaphoid bone of the wrist except:

A) It has a higher rate of nonunion compared with the other bones in the wrist when it is fractured
B) The fracture frequently does not show up on an x-ray film when it is taken immediately after the injury
C) The x-ray film will show the fracture if the film is repeated in 2 weeks
D) These fractures always require surgical intervention to stabilize the joint

264. A 10-year-old boy has type 1 diabetes. His late afternoon blood sugars over the past 2 weeks have ranged between 210 mg/dL and 230 mg/dL. He currently injects 10 units of regular insulin and 25 units of NPH in the morning and 15 units of regular insulin and 10 units of NPH insulin in the evening. Which of the following is the best treatment plan for this patient?

A) Increase both types of the morning dose
B) Increase only the NPH insulin in the morning
C) Decrease the afternoon dose of NPH insulin
D) Decrease both NPH and regular insulin doses in the morning

265. The mother of a 13-year-old boy with Down syndrome is in the family nurse practitioner's office and wants to schedule a sports physical for her son. She reports that he wants to join the football team at his school. You would tell the mother that her son:

A) Can play a regular football game as long as he wears maximum protective football gear
B) Cannot play some contact sports because of an increased risk of cervical spine injury
C) Can play certain contact sports after he has been checked for cervical instability
D) None of the above

266. The mother of an 8-year-old boy reports the presence of a round red rash on the child's left lower leg. It appeared 1 week after the child returned from visiting his grandparents, who live in Massachusetts. During the skin exam, the maculopapular rash is noted to have areas of central clearing making it resemble a round target. Which of the following is best described?

A) Erythema migrans
B) Rocky Mountain spotted fever
C) Meningococcemia
D) Larva migrans

267. Some pharmacological agents may cause confusion in the elderly. Which of the following agents is most likely to cause confusion in this population?

A) Cimetidine (Tagamet), digoxin (Lanoxin), diphenhydramine (Benadryl)
B) Acetaminophen (Tylenol), aspirin (Bayer), indomethacin (Indocin)
C) Sucralfate (Carafate), docusate sodium (Surfak), psyllium (Metamucil)
D) Cephalexin (Keflex), amoxicillin (Amoxil), clarithromycin (Biaxin)

268. A 55-year-old woman with a history of migraine headaches has recently been diagnosed with stage II hypertension. Her EKG strips reveal second-degree heart block. The chest x-ray is normal. Which of the following drugs should this patient avoid?

A) Angiotensin-converting enzyme (ACE) inhibitors
B) Angiotensin receptor blockers
C) Diuretics
D) Calcium channel blockers

269. Which of the following cranial nerves (CNs) is evaluated when a wisp of cotton is lightly brushed against the corner of the eye?

A) CN II
B) CN III

C) CN IV
D) CN V

270. When a patient is suspected of having acute pancreatitis, initial testing should include all of the following except:

A) Electrolyte panel
B) Serum amylase level
C) Serum lipase level
D) Barium swallow

271. During a routine physical exam of a 90-year-old woman, a low-pitched diastolic murmur grade 2/6 is auscultated. It is located on the fifth intercostal space (ICS) on the left side of the midclavicular line. Which of the following identifications is correct?

A) Aortic regurgitation
B) Mitral stenosis
C) Mitral regurgitation
D) Tricuspid regurgitation

272. Which of the following situations is considered emergent?

A) A laceration on the lower leg of a patient who has been taking aspirin (Bayer) 81 mg every other day
B) Rapid breathing and tachycardia in a patient with a fever
C) An elderly man with abdominal pain whose vital signs appear stable
D) A 37-year-old male biker with a concussion due to a fall who is slightly agitated and does not appear to understand instructions given by the medical assistant checking his vital signs

273. Which of the following is considered an objective finding in patients who have a case of suppurative otitis media?

A) Erythema of the tympanic membrane
B) Decreased mobility of the tympanic membrane as measured by tympanogram
C) Displacement of the light reflex
D) Bulging of the tympanic membrane

274. Pulsus paradoxus is more likely to be associated with:

A) Sarcoidosis
B) Acute bronchitis
C) Status asthmaticus
D) Bacterial pneumonia

275. A 17-year-old boy reports feeling something on his left scrotum. On palpation, soft and movable blood vessels that feel like a "bag of worms" are noted underneath the scrotal skin. The testicle is not swollen or reddened. The most likely diagnosis is:

A) Chronic orchitis
B) Chronic epididymitis
C) Testicular torsion
D) Varicocele

276. All of the following are true statements regarding elder abuse except:

A) Those aged 80 years or older are at the highest risk for abuse
B) A delay in medical care is a common finding
C) A new onset of a sexually transmitted disease (STD) in an elderly patient may signal sexual abuse
D) Decreased anxiety and depression are common symptoms of abuse in the elderly

277. The S1 heart sound is caused by:

A) Closure of the atrioventricular valves
B) Closure of the semilunar valves
C) Opening of the atrioventricular valves
D) Opening of the semilunar valves

278. Patients with Down syndrome are at higher risk for all of the following except:

A) Atlantoaxial instability
B) Congenital heart disease
C) Early onset of Alzheimer's disease
D) Melanoma

279. All of the following abnormal lab results may be seen in patients with infectious mononucleosis except:

A) Lymphocytosis
B) Positive EBV (Epstein–Barr virus) titers for IgM and IgG
C) Abnormal liver function tests
D) Elevated creatinine level

280. Which of the following is considered an abnormal result on a Weber test?

A) Lateralization to one ear
B) No lateralization in either ear
C) Air conduction lasts longer than bone conduction
D) Bone conduction lasts longer than air conduction

281. The span of the normal adult liver is:

A) 15 to 18 cm in the midclavicular line
B) 6 to 15 cm in midclavicular line
C) 2 to 6 cm in the midsternal line
D) 4 to 8 cm in the midsternal line

282. A patient who is complaining of a new onset of severe headache is being examined. The patient is instructed to lie down on the examining table while the nurse practitioner flexes his head and neck forward to his chest. The patient reacts by quickly flexing his hip and knee. What is the name of this positive finding?

A) Kernig's sign
B) Brudzinski's sign
C) Rovsing's sign
D) Drawer's sign

283. A neighbor's 14-year-old son, who is active in basketball, complains of pain and swelling on both knees. On physical exam, there is tenderness over the tibial tuberosity of both knees. Which of the following is most likely?

A) Chondromalacia patella
B) Left knee sprain
C) Osgood–Schlatter disease
D) Tear of the medial ligament

284. A woman at 32 weeks gestation has a positive throat culture for *Streptococcus pyogenes* (strep throat). She denies allergies but becomes very nauseated with erythromycin. Which of the following is the best choice for this pregnant patient?

A) Clarithromycin (Biaxin)
B) Trimethoprim–sulfamethoxazole (Bactrim DS)
C) Ofloxacin (Floxin)
D) Penicillin (Pen VK)

285. During a sports physical exam, a 16-year-old patient is noted to have a few beats of horizontal nystagmus on extreme lateral gaze that disappear when the eyes move back toward midline. Which statement best describes this clinical finding?

A) It is caused by occult bleeding of the retinal artery
B) This is a normal finding
C) It is a sign of a possible brain mass
D) This is a borderline result and requires further evaluation

286. An urgent care nurse practitioner is assessing a 45-year-old White woman with a body mass index (BMI) of 32 for a complaint of intermittent right upper quadrant abdominal pain over the past few weeks that is precipitated by eating fried foods and peanut butter. On exam, the patient's heart and lungs are normal. There is no pain over the costovertebral angle. During abdominal exam, bowel sounds are present in all quadrants. While the nurse is palpating deeply on the right upper quadrant during deep inspiration, the patient complains of severe sharp pain. Which of the following is best described?

A) Murphy's sign
B) McMurray's sign
C) Rovsing's sign
D) Obturator sign

287. Which of the following drugs is recommended by the Centers for Disease Control and Prevention (CDC) for prophylaxis after exposure to *Bacillus anthracis*?

A) Clindamycin (Cleocin)
B) Azithromycin (Z-Pack)
C) Penicillin G injection
D) Ciprofloxacin (Cipro)

288. A major risk factor for Down syndrome in an infant is:

A) Maternal age younger than 16 years
B) Maternal age older than 35 years
C) A positive family history of Down syndrome
D) A positive family history of genetic disease

289. A new patient who is a 40-year-old female postal worker is being evaluated for complaints of a new-onset erythematous rash on both cheeks and the bridge of the nose, accompanied by fatigue. She reports a history of Hashimoto's thyroiditis and is currently being treated with Synthroid 1.25 mg daily. Which of the following conditions is most likely?

A) Atopic dermatitis
B) Thyroid disease
C) Lupus erythematosus
D) Rosacea

290. A 65-year-old woman comes into the clinic during the first week of November for her annual wellness visit. Her last Td booster was 9 years ago. Which immunization(s) would you recommend for this visit?

A) Influenza vaccine only
B) Tetanus and influenza vaccine
C) Pneumococcal (Pneumovax) and influenza vaccines
D) She does not need any vaccinations to be administered in this visit

291. Which of the following is a true statement regarding pes planus in an infant?

A) It should be evaluated by a pediatric orthopedist if spontaneous correction does not occur by age 12 months
B) The fat pads on an infant's feet can mimic pes planus
C) It is always corrected by wearing special orthotic shoes
D) It is also called *talipes equinovarus*

292. Which of the following statements regarding the rehabilitation of alcoholics is correct?

A) Al-Anon is not designed for family members of alcoholics
B) Disulfiram (Antabuse) is always effective
C) Alcoholics Anonymous is not an effective method for treating this condition
D) Patients should avoid foods or drinks that contain alcohol, such as cough syrups

293. The mother of a 7-year-old boy tells the family nurse practitioner that his teacher has complained to her of her son's frequent episodes of daydreaming. The mother reports that sometimes when her son is at home, he seems not to hear her, seeming to "blank out" for a short period of time. Which of the following is most likely?

A) A partial seizure
B) An absence seizure (petit mal seizure)
C) A grand mal seizure
D) An atonic seizure (drop attack)

294. The Pap smear result for a 20-year-old sexually active college student whose partner uses condoms inconsistently reveals a large number of white blood cells and blood along with inflammatory changes. During the speculum exam, the cervix bled very easily (friable), and a small amount of purulent discharge was present on the cervical surface. No cervical motion tenderness was noted during the bimanual vaginal exam. What is the next step in the management of this patient?

A) Advise the patient to return to the clinic for chlamydia and gonorrhea testing
B) Instruct the patient to use metronidazole vaginal cream
C) Tell the patient she needs a repeat Pap smear in 6 months
D) Advise the patient to use a Betadine douche at bedtime for 3 days

295. A 30-year-old woman complains of having had no period for the last 12 weeks. She is sexually active and her partner has been using condoms inconsistently. The patient has a history of irregular menstrual cycles and severe dysmenorrhea. The urine pregnancy test result is positive. Which of the following is a true statement regarding this pregnancy?

A) The fundus of the uterus should be at the level of the symphysis pubis
B) The cervix should be dilated about 0.5 inches at this time of gestation
C) "Quickening" starts during this period
D) Hegar's sign is present during this period of pregnancy

296. A newborn infant who is small for gestational age is noted to have shortened palpebral fissures and microcephaly with a small jaw. This infant is most likely to be diagnosed with:

A) Down syndrome
B) Fetal alcohol syndrome
C) Growth retardation
D) Hydrocephalus

297. The most common cause of cancer deaths for women in the United States is:

A) Breast cancer
B) Lung cancer
C) Colon cancer
D) Uterine cancer

298. Human papillomavirus infection in women has been associated with the development of:

A) Ectopic pregnancy
B) Infertility
C) Cervical cancer
D) Pelvic inflammatory disease

299. All of the following are included in the criteria used to diagnose patients with AIDS except:

A) Profound fatigue
B) Thrush
C) Kaposi's sarcoma
D) Hairy leukoplakia of the tongue

300. Which of the following conditions is the most common cause of sudden death among young athletes?

A) Brain aneurysm
B) Hypertrophic cardiomyopathy
C) Left ventricular hypertrophy
D) Aortic stenosis

301. The posterior fontanel should be completely closed by:

A) 3 months
B) 4 months
C) 5 months
D) 6 months

302. Which cranial nerve (CN) is being evaluated when Rinne testing is done?

A) CN VII
B) CN VIII
C) CNs IX and X
D) CN XI

303. A middle-aged nurse complains of localized pain on the sole of her left foot, between the third and fourth toes. The pain is aggravated by weight bearing and feels like "a pebble in my shoe." During the physical examination, the nurse practitioner palpates a tender nodule in the metatarsal interspace on the left foot. No redness or swelling is noted. Which of the following conditions is being described?

A) Plantar wart
B) Foreign body
C) Morton's neuroma
D) Metatarsalgia

304. An 18-year-old female patient is being followed up for acne by the nurse practitioner. During the facial exam, papules and pustules are noted mostly on the forehead and the chin areas. The patient has been using over-the-counter topical antibiotic gels and medicated soap daily for 6 months without much improvement. Which of the following would the nurse practitioner recommend next?

A) Isotretinoin (Accutane)
B) Tetracycline (Sumycin)
C) Clindamycin topical solution (Cleocin T)
D) Minoxidil (Rogaine)

305. The following statements are all true regarding herpes zoster except:

A) It is due to reactivation of latent varicella virus
B) The typical lesions are bullae
C) It is usually more severe in immunocompromised individuals
D) Infection of the trigeminal nerve ophthalmic branch can cause corneal blindness

306. A middle-aged Black man complains of a history of outbreaks of painful large nodules and pustules on both his axillae that resolve after treatment with antibiotics. On physical examination, the nurse practitioner notices large red nodules that are tender to palpation. In addition, several pustules are present along with multiple scars on the skin. The nurse practitioner advises the patient that the condition is caused by a bacterial infection of the sweat glands in the axillae. Which of the following conditions is being described?

A) Hidradenitis suppurativa
B) Severe nodular acne
C) Granuloma inguinale
D) Cat scratch fever

307. A possible side effect from the use of nifedipine (Procardia XL) is:

A) Hyperuricemia and hypoglycemia
B) Hyperkalemia and angioedema
C) Edema of the ankles and headache
D) Dry hacking cough

308. Which of the following actions is contraindicated in patients with acute prostatitis?

A) Massaging the infected prostate
B) Serial urine samples
C) Rectal exams
D) Palpation of the epididymis

309. Erysipelas is an infection of the skin most commonly caused by which of the following class of organisms?

A) Streptococci
B) Staphylococci
C) Gram-negative bacteria
D) Fungi

310. What is the first-line class of antibiotics recommended by the American Thoracic Society (ATS) for patients younger than 60 years of age who are diagnosed with community-acquired pneumonia with no comorbidity?

A) First-generation cephalosporins
B) Second-generation cephalosporins
C) Macrolides
D) Beta-lactam antibiotics

311. Acute bronchitis is best characterized by:

A) Fever and wheezing
B) Purulent sputum and fever
C) Paroxysms of coughing that are dry or produce mucoid sputum
D) A gradual onset and fatigue

Questions 312 and 313 apply to this case. The nurse practitioner notices a gray ring on the edge of both irises of an 80-year-old woman. The patient denies visual changes or pain. She reports that she has had the "ring" for many years.

312. Which of the following causes is most likely?

A) Arcus senilis
B) Pinguecula
C) Peripheral cataracts
D) Macular degeneration

313. What is the clinical significance of this finding in a 35-year-old patient?

A) The patient has a higher risk of blindness
B) The patient should be evaluated for hyperlipidemia
C) The patient should be evaluated by an ophthalmologist
D) The patient should be evaluated for acute glaucoma

314. The cones in the retina of the eye are responsible for:

A) Central vision
B) Peripheral vision
C) Night vision
D) Color vision

315. The nurse practitioner would refer patients with all of the following burns to a physician except:

A) Severe facial burns
B) Electrical burns
C) Burns that involve the cartilage of the ear
D) Second-degree burn on the lower arm

316. On auscultation of the chest, a split S2 is best heard at:

A) Second intercostal space, right sternal border
B) Second intercostal space, left sternal border
C) Fifth intercostal space, midclavicular line
D) Fourth intercostal space, left sternal border

317. According to the guidelines outlined in the Eighth Joint National Committee (JNC 8) the target blood pressure goal for hypertensive patients who are aged 60 years or older is:

A) <150/90 mmHg
B) <130/85 mmHg
C) <120/80 mmHg
D) <110/75 mmHg

318. Which of the following would be classified as a second-degree burn?

A) Severe sunburn with blistering
B) Burns that involve the subcutaneous layer of skin
C) Reddened finger after touching a hot iron
D) Burns that involve eschar

319. The mother of a 16-year-old boy is concerned that her son is not developing normally. On physical exam, the patient is noted to have small testes with no pubic or facial hair. What is the most appropriate statement to the mother?

A) Her son is developing normally
B) Her son's physical development is delayed and should be evaluated by a pediatric endocrinologist
C) Her son should be rechecked in 3 months; if he still does not have secondary sexual characteristics, a thorough hormonal workup should be initiated
D) Her son's physiological development is slower than normal but is within the lower limit of normal for his age group

320. The most common type of skin malignancy in the United States is:

A) Squamous cell skin cancer
B) Basal cell carcinoma
C) Melanoma
D) Dysplastic nevi

321. Which cranial nerves (CNs) innervate the extraocular muscles of the eyes?

A) CNs II, III, and VI
B) CNs III, IV, and VI
C) CNs IV, V, and VII
D) CNs V, VI, and VIII

322. Which of the following tests would you recommend to patients to confirm the diagnosis of beta thalassemia or sickle cell anemia?

A) Hemoglobin electrophoresis
B) Bone morrow biopsy
C) Peripheral smear
D) Reticulocyte count

323. All of the following patients have an increased risk of developing adverse effects from metformin (Glucophage) except:

A) Patients with renal disease
B) Patients with hypoxia
C) Obese patients
D) Patients who are alcoholics

324. A middle-aged hypertensive man presents to a public health clinic with complaints of an acute onset of fever, chills, and cough that is productive of rusty-colored sputum. The patient reports episodes of sharp pains on the left side of his back and chest whenever he is coughing. His temperature is 102.2°F, pulse is 100 beats/min, and blood pressure is 130/80 mmHg. The urinalysis does not show leukocytes, nitrites, or blood. These findings are most consistent with:

A) Atypical pneumonia
B) Upper urinary tract infection
C) Bacterial pneumonia
D) Acute pyelonephritis

325. Lifestyle modifications are an important aspect in the treatment of hypertension. Which of the following statements is incorrect?

A) Reduce intake of sodium, potassium, and calcium
B) Reduce intake of sodium and saturated fats
C) Exercise at least three to four times per week
D) Maintain an adequate intake of potassium, magnesium, and calcium

326. Which of the following classes of antihypertensive drugs should a patient be weaned off slowly to avoid the risk of severe rebound hypertension?

A) Diuretics
B) Beta-blockers
C) ACE inhibitors
D) Calcium channel blockers

327. A 70-year-old man with open-angle glaucoma is prescribed Betimol (timolol) ophthalmic drops. All of the following are contraindications to Betimol ophthalmic drops except:

A) Overt heart failure or sinus bradycardia
B) History of asthma
C) Second- or third-degree atrioventricular (AV) block
D) Migraine headaches

328. At what time of the day would you recommend a scotch tape test be done to evaluate for a suspected case of enterobiasis?

A) In the evening after dinner
B) At night before bed
C) Early in the morning
D) It does not matter what time of the day the test is done

329. At what age can a child copy a circle and ride a tricycle?

A) 1 year
B) 2 years
C) 3 years
D) 4 years

330. A 30-year-old male patient with bipolar disorder refuses to take his afternoon dose of pills. The nurse tells him of the possible consequences of his action, but the patient still refuses to cooperate. Which of the following is the best course for the nurse to follow?

A) Document the patient's behavior in his record and the action taken by the nurse
B) Reassure the patient that he will be fine after taking the medicine
C) Document only the patient behavior
D) Document only the nurse's action

331. All of the following are clinical eye findings found in some patients with chronic uncontrolled hypertension. Which is not associated with this disorder?

A) AV nicking
B) Copper wire arterioles
C) Flame-shaped hemorrhages
D) Microaneurysms

332. While reviewing some lab reports, the nurse practitioner notes that one of the results for her teenage male patient is abnormal. The liver function tests are all normal except for a slight elevation in the alkaline phosphatase level. The patient is a member of a soccer team and denies any recent injury. Which of the following statements is true?

A) It is an indication of possible liver damage from alcohol; order a liver ultrasound to rule out fatty liver
B) This is a normal finding due to the skeletal growth spurt in this age group
C) The patient needs to be evaluated further for pancreatic disease
D) The patient needs an ultrasound of the liver to rule out fatty liver and referral to a pediatric rheumatologist

333. Which of the following would be appropriate initial management of a second-degree burn?

A) Irrigate with hydrogen peroxide and apply Silvadene cream BID
B) Irrigate with normal saline and apply Silvadene cream BID
C) Irrigate with tap water and apply Neosporin ointment BID
D) Unroof all intact blisters and apply antibiotic ointment BID

334. When *Molluscum contagiosum* is found on the genital area of children, which of the following is the best explanation?

A) It should raise the suspicion of child sexual abuse
B) It is not considered a sexually transmitted disease
C) It is caused by atypical bacteria
D) It is caused by the poxvirus and will resolve on its own

335. An 80-year-old woman complains about her "thin" and dry skin. Which of the following is the best explanation for her complaint?

A) Genetic predisposition
B) Loss of subcutaneous fat and lower collagen content
C) Atrophy of sebaceous glands
D) Damage from severe sun exposure

336. All of the following statements are correct regarding licensure for nurse practitioners except:

A) It ensures a minimum level of professional competency
B) It grants permission for an individual to practice in a profession
C) It requires verification of educational training from an accredited graduate program
D) It reviews information via a nongovernmental agency

337. Which of the following is the correct statement regarding the size of the arterioles and veins on the fundus of the eye?

A) The veins are larger than the arterioles
B) The arterioles are larger than the veins
C) The arterioles are half the size of the veins
D) The veins and the arterioles are equal in size

338. All of the following factors have been found to increase the risk of atrial fibrillation in predisposed individuals except:

A) Hypertension
B) Excessive alcohol intake
C) Theophylline (Theo-Dur) and pseudoephedrine (Sudafed)
D) Acute esophagitis

339. At what age can a child copy a cross and draw a person with three body parts?

A) 1 year
B) 2 years
C) 3 years
D) 4 years

340. You would associate a positive iliopsoas muscle test result with which of the following conditions?

A) Left cerebral vascular accident
B) Urinary tract infection
C) Heel fractures
D) Acute appendicitis

341. Which of the following classes of drugs is implicated with blunting the signs and symptoms of hypoglycemia in diabetics?

A) Calcium channel blockers
B) Diuretics
C) Beta-blockers
D) Angiotensin receptor blockers (ARBs)

342. All of the following factors increase the risk of mortality for patients diagnosed with bacterial pneumonia except:

A) Alcoholism
B) Very young or old age
C) Multiple lobar involvement
D) Hypertension

343. The bacterium responsible for the highest mortality in patients with community-acquired pneumonia is:

A) *Streptococcus pneumoniae*
B) *Mycoplasma pneumoniae*
C) *Moraxella catarrhalis*
D) *Haemophilus influenzae*

344. A 40-year-old Black man with asthma and hypertension has been following a low-fat, low-sodium diet and walking three times a week for the past 6 months. His blood pressure readings from the past two visits were 160/95 and 170/100 mmHg. On this visit, it is 160/90. What is the most appropriate action for the nurse practitioner to follow at this visit?

A) Continue the lifestyle modifications and recheck his blood pressure again in 4 weeks
B) Initiate a prescription of hydrochlorothiazide 12.5 mg PO daily
C) Initiate a prescription of atenolol (Tenormin) 25 mg PO daily
D) Refer the patient to a cardiologist for a stress EKG

345. When initially treating an adult for acute bronchitis, which of the following should the nurse practitioner be least likely to order?

A) Expectorants
B) Antibiotics
C) Bronchodilators
D) Antitussives

346. All of the following describe normal behavior for a 3-year-old child except:

A) Speaks in three- to four-word sentences that are understood by most strangers
B) Can draw a cross
C) Can draw a circle
D) Can ride a tricycle

347. A woman who has recently been diagnosed with lupus complains that her hands and feet always feel cold even in the summertime. Sometimes her fingertips become numb and turn a blue color. The fingertips eventually turn dark red in color. Which of the following is most likely?

A) Chronic arterial insufficiency
B) This is a normal reaction when one feels very cold
C) Peripheral vascular disease
D) Raynaud's phenomenon

348. A female patient, who has a BMI (body mass index) of 29 has a 20-year history of primary hypertension. She has been taking hydrochlorothiazide 25 mg PO daily with excellent results. On this visit, she complains of feeling thirsty all the time even though she drinks more than 10 glasses of water per day. She reports to the nurse practitioner that she has been having this problem for about 6 months. Upon reading the chart, the nurse practitioner notes that the last two fasting blood glucose levels have been 140 mg/dL and 168 mg/dL. The result of a random blood glucose test is 210 mg/dL. Which of the following is the appropriate action to follow at this visit?

A) Order another random blood glucose test in 2 weeks
B) Initiate a prescription of metformin (Glucophage) 500 mg PO BID
C) Order a 3-hour glucose tolerance test
D) Order an A1C level

349. A middle-aged patient newly diagnosed with type 2 diabetes wants to start an exercise program. All of the following statements are true except:

A) If the patient is unable to eat due to illness, antidiabetic agents can be continued with frequent glucose monitoring
B) Strenuous exercise is contraindicated for most patients with type 2 diabetes because of a higher risk of hypoglycemic episodes
C) Exercise increases the body's ability to metabolize glucose
D) Patients who exercise vigorously in the afternoon may have hypoglycemic episodes in the evening or at night if they do not eat

350. What is the least common pathogen found in community-acquired atypical pneumonia?

A) *Moraxella catarrhalis*
B) *Streptococcus pneumoniae*
C) *Pseudomonas aeruginosa*
D) *Mycoplasma pneumonia*

351. While performing a sports physical on a 16-year-old girl, the nurse practitioner notes a split S2 during inspiration that disappears during expiration. The girl is active and her growth and development have been uneventful. What is the best recommendation for the child's mother?

A) Recommend referral to a pediatric cardiologist
B) Recommend referral for a stress EKG
C) Advise the mother that this is a normal finding
D) Recommend her daughter avoid strenuous physical exertion until further evaluation

352. Patients who are considered mentally competent have a right to consent or refuse medical treatment. What is the legal term for this right?

A) Informed consent
B) Durable power of attorney
C) Competence
D) Advance directives

353. The following statements are true about Wilms' tumor except:

A) The most frequent clinical sign is a palpable abdominal mass
B) It is a congenital tumor of the kidney
C) Microscopic or gross hematuria is sometimes present
D) The tumor commonly crosses the midline of the abdomen when it is discovered

354. At what level of prevention would you classify screening for lung cancer?

A) Primary prevention
B) Secondary prevention
C) Tertiary prevention
D) Screening for lung cancer is not currently recommended

355. Which of the following T-scores is indicative of osteoporosis?

A) T-score of 0 to −1.0
B) T-score of −1.0 to −2.0
C) T-score of −2.5 or less
D) Diagnosis is based on an x-ray series of the spine

356. Which of the following methods is used to diagnose gonorrheal pharyngitis or proctitis?

A) Serum chlamydia titer
B) Gen-Probe
C) Thayer–Martin culture
D) Culture and sensitivity of the purulent discharge

357. The first nurse practitioner program was started by:

A) Alfred Bandura
B) Margaret Sanger
C) Mary Breckinridge
D) Loretta Ford

358. Terazosin (Hytrin), an alpha-blocker, is used to treat which of the following conditions?

A) Benign prostatic hypertrophy and hypertension
B) Chronic prostatitis and atrial fibrillation
C) Urinary tract infections and arrhythmias
D) Benign prostatic hypertrophy and chronic prostatitis

359. A concerned new mother reports to you that her son, who is 3 years of age, is not toilet-trained yet. Which of the following is an appropriate reply?

A) Recommend a referral to a pediatric urologist
B) Advise the mother that her child is developing normally
C) Recommend a bed-wetting alarm
D) Recommend a voiding cystogram

360. Which of the following clinical findings can mimic a case of testicular torsion but is not considered an emergent condition?

A) The "blue dot" sign
B) One swollen testicle with yellow-colored penile discharge
C) Acute onset of dysuria and frequency
D) A varicocele

361. An 18-year-old waitress is diagnosed with pelvic inflammatory disease (PID). The cervical Gen-Probe result is positive for *Neisseria gonorrhoeae* and negative for *Chlamydia trachomatis*. All of the following statements are true regarding the management of this patient except:

A) This patient should be treated for chlamydia even though the Gen-Probe for chlamydia is negative
B) Ceftriaxone 250 mg IM and doxycycline 100 mg PO BID × 14 days are appropriate treatment for this patient
C) Advise the patient to return to the clinic for a follow-up visit within 3 days after treatment
D) Repeat the Gen-Probe test for *Chlamydia trachomatis* to ensure that the previous test was not a false-negative result

362. A girl whose breasts form a secondary mound is at which Tanner stage?

A) Tanner stage II
B) Tanner stage III
C) Tanner stage IV
D) Tanner stage V

363. A 35-year-old smoker is being evaluated for birth control choices. The patient has a history of pelvic inflammatory disease (PID) along with an embolic episode after her last pregnancy. Which of the following methods of birth control would you recommend?

A) Condoms and the vaginal sponge (Today Sponge)
B) Estrogen patches
C) Intrauterine device
D) Depo-Provera (depot medroxyprogesterone)

364. A 21-year-old woman complains of left-sided pelvic pain accompanied by dyspareunia. During the gynecological exam, the nurse practitioner notices green cervical discharge. The patient mentions a new onset of a painful and swollen left knee and denies a history of trauma. This best describes:

A) Septic arthritis
B) Reiter's syndrome
C) Chondromalacia of the patella
D) Disseminated gonorrheal infection

365. You would recommend the pneumococcal vaccine (Pneumovax) to patients with all of the following conditions except:

A) Sickle cell anemia
B) Splenectomy
C) HIV infection
D) G6PD-deficiency anemia

366. A 40-year-old cashier complains of periods of dizziness and palpitations that have a sudden onset. The EKG shows P waves before each QRS complex and a heart rate of 170 beats/min. A carotid massage decreases the heart rate to 80 beats/min. These findings best describe:

A) Ventricular tachycardia
B) Paroxysmal atrial tachycardia

C) Atrial fibrillation
D) Ventricular fibrillation

367. A 25-year-old woman complains of dysuria, severe vaginal pruritus, and a malodorous vaginal discharge. Pelvic examination reveals a strawberry-colored cervix and frothy yellow discharge. Microscopic examination of the discharge reveals mobile organisms that have flagella. The correct pharmacological therapy for the condition is:

A) Oral metronidazole (Flagyl)
B) Ceftriaxone sodium (Rocephin) injection
C) Doxycycline hyclate (Vibramycin)
D) Clotrimazole (Gyne-Lotrimin) cream or suppositories

368. A new mother reports to you that her 6-month-old infant has a cold and has a fever of 99.8°F. The infant is not irritable and is feeding well without problems. The mother wants to know whether it is okay for him to be immunized at this time. Which of the following statements is true?

A) The infant should not be immunized until he is afebrile
B) An infant with a cold can be immunized at any time
C) An infant with a cold can be immunized as long as the infant's temperature is no higher than 100.4°F
D) Because immunization is so important, it should be given to the infant as scheduled

369. Metronidazole (Flagyl) produces the disulfiram (Antabuse) effect when combined with alcoholic drinks or medicine. You would educate the patient that:

A) She should avoid alcoholic drinks during the time she takes the medicine
B) She should avoid alcoholic drinks 1 day before, during therapy, and a few days after therapy
C) She should avoid alcoholic drinks after she takes the medicine
D) There is no need to avoid any food or drink

370. The treatment plan of patients with AIDS who have CD4 counts of less than 200 cells/mm^3 should emphasize:

A) Administer the MMR vaccine
B) Preventive therapy for toxoplasmosis
C) Preventive therapy for PCP
D) Evaluation of the home environment

371. All of the following are true about strawberry hemangiomas found in infants except:

A) Most will involute spontaneously by the age of 18 to 24 months
B) Watchful waiting is the most useful strategy
C) Hemangiomas should be treated with laser therapy if they have not resolved by the age of 12 months
D) Strawberry hemangiomas are benign

372. A 56-year-old mechanic is brought to your office complaining of heavy pressure in the substernal area of his chest that is radiating to his jaw. The pain began while he was lifting up a tire. He now appears pale and is diaphoretic. His blood pressure is 100/60 mmHg, and his pulse is 50 beats/min. What is the most appropriate action?

A) Perform a 12-lead EKG
B) Call 911
C) Administer a morphine injection for pain
D) Observe the patient in the office

373. Which of the following drug classes is indicated for initial treatment of an uncomplicated case of *Helicobacter pylori*-negative peptic ulcer disease?

A) Proton-pump inhibitors
B) H2 receptor antagonists
C) Antibiotics
D) Antacids

374. Erythromycin inhibits the cytochrome P450 (CYP450) system. All of the following drugs should be avoided because of a potential for a drug interaction except:

A) Theophylline (Theo-Dur)
B) Warfarin (Coumadin)
C) Diazepam (Valium)
D) Furosemide (Lasix)

375. If left untreated, Zollinger–Ellison syndrome can cause which of the following?

A) Severe ulceration of the stomach or duodenum
B) Toxic megacolon
C) Chronic diarrhea
D) Malabsorption of fat-soluble vitamins

376. All of the following are considered category X drugs except:

A) Misoprostol (Cytotec)
B) Isotretinoin (Accutane)
C) Finasteride (Proscar)
D) Meperidine (Demerol)

377. During a physical exam of a 6-year-old child, you note some pitting on the fingernails. This finding is correlated with:

A) Iron-deficiency anemia
B) Psoriasis
C) Onychomycosis
D) Vitamin C deficiency

378. Which of the following is correct regarding the best site to listen for mitral regurgitation?

A) It is best heard in the apical area during S2
B) It is best heard at the base during S1

C) It is best heard at the apex during S1
D) It is best heard at the base during S2

379. Extreme tenderness and involuntary guarding at McBurney's point is a significant finding for possible:

A) Acute cholecystitis
B) Acute appendicitis
C) Acute gastroenteritis
D) Acute diverticulitis

380. All of the following may help relieve the symptom(s) of gastroesophageal reflux disease (GERD) except:

A) Losing weight
B) Stopping caffeine intake
C) Chewing breath mints
D) Stopping alcohol intake

381. According to the Centers for Disease Control and Prevention (CDC), which of the following is the recommended treatment for uncomplicated gonorrheal urethritis infection in an adult man?

A) Ceftriaxone (Rocephin) 250 mg IM plus azithromycin 1 g orally
B) Valacyclovir (Valtrex) 500 mg PO BID × 10 days
C) Ceftriaxone (Rocephin) 250 mg IM plus doxycycline 100 mg orally BID for 14 days
D) One dose of oral fluconazole (Diflucan) 150 mg

382. Which of the following is *not* an absolute contraindication for use of oral contraceptive pills?

A) Active hepatitis A infection
B) Thrombosis related to an IV needle
C) Undiagnosed vaginal bleeding
D) Transient ischemic attack (TIA)

383. A nurse practitioner is taking part in a community outreach program for a local hospital. Most of her audience has a diagnosis of hypertension. They are all interested in learning more about a proper diet. When discussing potential sources of potassium and magnesium, which of the following are the best sources for these two minerals?

A) Fruits, leafy greens, and nuts
B) Whole grains, red meat, and dairy
C) Bananas, beef, and yogurt
D) Mushrooms, fermented foods, and vegetables

384. A 35-year-old sexually active man presents with a 1-week history of fever and pain over the left scrotum. It is accompanied by frequency and dysuria. The scrotum is edematous and tender to touch. He denies flank pain, nausea, and vomiting. He reports that the pain is lessened when he uses scrotal-support briefs. The urinalysis shows 2+ blood and a large number of leukocytes. What is the most likely diagnosis?

A) Acute urinary tract infection
B) Acute pyelonephritis
C) Acute orchitis
D) Acute epididymitis

385. A 16-year-old female patient is being treated for her first urinary tract infection. She had an allergic reaction with hives after taking sulfa as a child. Which of the following antibiotics would be contraindicated?

A) Cephalexin (Keflex)
B) Ampicillin (Amoxil)
C) Trimethoprim–sulfamethoxazole (Bactrim)
D) Nitrofurantoin crystals (Macrobid)

386. The mother of a 4-month-old girl calls your office and reports that the infant has a fever of 101.4°F. The infant received her immunizations yesterday. Which of the following is correct?

A) The fever is most likely due to the combination of the MMR and polio vaccines
B) The fever is most likely due to the pertussis component of the DTaP vaccine
C) The infant is probably starting a viral upper respiratory infection
D) The infant had an allergic reaction to one of the vaccines given and should be brought to the emergency department

387. The following statements about benign prostatic hypertrophy are correct except:

A) It occurs in up to 50% of men older than 50 years of age
B) Dribbling and nocturia are common patient complaints
C) Saw palmetto is always effective in reducing symptoms
D) The PSA value is usually slightly elevated

388. *Precocious puberty* is defined as the onset of secondary sexual characteristics before the age of:

A) Age 7 in girls and age 8 in boys
B) Age 8 in girls and age 9 in boys
C) Age 9 in girls and age 10 in boys
D) Age 9 for both girls and boys

389. At what Tanner stage does puberty start?

A) Tanner stage I
B) Tanner stage II

C) Tanner stage III
D) Tanner stage IV

390. Orchitis is caused by which of the following?

A) Mumps virus
B) Measles virus
C) *Chlamydia trachomatis*
D) Chronic urinary tract infections that are not treated adequately

391. A positive obturator sign might signify which of the following conditions?

A) Acute appendicitis
B) Acute pancreatitis
C) Acute cholecystitis
D) Acute hepatitis

392. Spermatogenesis occurs at the:

A) Vas deferens
B) Seminal vesicles
C) Testes
D) Epididymis

393. Prophylaxis for *Pneumocystis jirovecii* pneumonia includes all of the following drugs except:

A) Trimethoprim–sulfamethoxazole
B) Dapsone
C) Aerosolized pentamidine
D) Aerosolized albuterol sulfate (Ventolin)

394. A female patient complains of dizziness when she moves her head. You suspect benign paroxysmal positional vertigo. The diagnosis is supported by the presence of:

A) Tinnitus
B) Horizontal nystagmus with rapid head movement
C) New-onset hearing loss
D) Duration longer than 2 years

395. While performing a routine physical exam on a 60-year-old man, the nurse practitioner notices a soft bruit over the carotid area on the left side of the neck. The patient has a history of hypertension. The patient is at higher risk for:

A) Temporal arteritis and brain aneurysms
B) Dizziness and headaches
C) Abdominal aneurysm and congestive heart failure
D) Stroke and coronary artery disease

396. A kindergarten teacher is diagnosed with acute streptococcal pharyngitis. On exam, her throat is a bright-red color with no tonsillar exudate, and clear mucus is seen on the lower nasal turbinates. The urinalysis shows a large amount of white blood cells and is positive for nitrites. The patient has a sulfa allergy and thinks she is also allergic to penicillins. Which of the following is the best treatment choice?

A) Amoxicillin–clavulanic acid (Augmentin) 500 mg PO BID
B) Levofloxacin (Levaquin) 250 mg PO daily
C) Trimethoprim–sulfamethoxazole (Bactrim DS) 1 tablet PO BID
D) Clarithromycin (Biaxin) 500 mg PO BID

397. All of the following drugs interfere with the metabolism of oral contraceptives except:

A) Tetracycline
B) Rifampin
C) Phenytoin (Dilantin)
D) Ciprofloxacin (Cipro)

398. When starting an elderly patient on a new prescription of levothyroxine (Synthroid), the nurse practitioner should keep in mind that the rationale for beginning with a lower dose in such patients relates to the drug's:

A) Central nervous system effects
B) Cardiac effects
C) Renal effects
D) Hepatic effects

399. It is recommended that women who are pregnant during the winter months ensure which of the following?

A) Increased intake of vitamin C and folate
B) Vaccination against the influenza virus
C) Increased caloric intake of fruits and vegetables
D) Heavier winter clothes to avoid chilling the fetus

400. The earliest age at which the MMR vaccine can be administered is:

A) 4 months
B) 6 months
C) 8 months
D) 12 months

401. The first-line treatment consideration for managing delirium caused by acute alcohol withdrawal includes:

A) Intubation
B) Benzodiazepines
C) Avoidance of physical restraints to decrease agitation
D) Antipsychotics

402. A 5-year old boy is in your office for a school physical. The mother denies a history of chickenpox infection. Which of the following immunizations is indicated at this visit?

A) Tdap, IPV, MMR
B) DTaP, Hib, PCV, IPV
C) MMR, hepatitis B, varicella
D) DTaP, IPV, MMR, varicella

403. All of the following are considered emancipated minors except:

A) 16-year-old who is married
B) 15-year-old who obtained a declaration of emancipation from a state court
C) 17-year-old who is enlisted in the U.S. Army
D) 13-year-old being treated for a sexually transmitted disease

404. Which of the following factors is associated with increased risk of osteopenia in teenage girls?

A) Drinking one glass of low-fat milk daily
B) Anorexia nervosa
C) Participation in sports
D) A normal BMI (body mass index)

405. A 28-year-old male nurse tells the employee health nurse practitioner that he was treated for a urinary tract infection twice the previous year. The patient denies fever, flank pain, or urethral discharge during the visit. Which of the following is the best follow-up for this patient?

A) Refer the patient to a urologist
B) Prescribe the patient ofloxacin (Floxin) for 2 weeks instead of 1 week
C) Advise the patient that he needs to void every 2 hours when awake
D) Refer the patient to the local emergency department, because he has a very high risk of sepsis

Questions 406 and 407 apply to this case. A 50-year-old man complains of marked scalp tenderness accompanied by a bad headache at his left temple. He reports a sudden loss of vision in the left eye for the past several hours. The neurological exam is normal except for the loss of vision in the left eye.

406. Which of the following conditions is most likely?

A) Cluster headache
B) Migraine headache with aura
C) Migraine headache without aura
D) Giant cell arteritis

407. Which of the following diagnostic tests would be most helpful in the diagnosis of this illness?

A) CT scan of the brain
B) Cranial nerve exam
C) Sedimentation rate
D) CBC with differential

408. A postmenopausal woman complains of random episodes of vaginal bleeding for the past 6 months. Which of the following is recommended management for this condition?

A) Cervical biopsy
B) Pap smear
C) Colposcopy
D) Endometrial biopsy

409. Which of the following is not a characteristic of delirium?

A) Sudden onset
B) Patient is coherent
C) Worse in the evenings
D) Brief duration

410. The signs and symptoms of dementia may include all of the following except:

A) Personality changes
B) Difficulty in verbalizing
C) Difficulty in recognizing familiar objects
D) Increase in abstract thinking ability

411. Acute prostatitis can present with all of the following signs and symptoms except:

A) Fever and chills
B) Tenderness of the scrotum on the affected side
C) Perineal pain
D) Slow onset of symptoms

412. Which of the following is the most common cause of nongonococcal urethritis?

A) *Escherichia coli*
B) *Chlamydia trachomatis*
C) *Neisseria gonorrhoeae*
D) *Mycoplasma genitalium*

413. Which of the following is considered a relative contraindication for combined oral contraceptive pills?

A) Undiagnosed vaginal bleeding
B) Hepatoma of the liver
C) Suspected history of transient ischemic attacks (TIAs)
D) Depression

Questions 414 and 415 apply to this case. A 20-year-old Asian man reports pain in his right knee after twisting it while playing soccer. The injured knee locks up when he attempts to straighten his leg.

414. Which of the following conditions is most likely?

A) Injury to the meniscus of the right knee
B) Injury to the patella of the right knee
C) Injury to the ligaments of the right knee
D) Rupture of the quadriceps tendon

415. Which of the following actions is the best course for this patient?

A) Refer him to an orthopedic specialist
B) Refer him to a chiropractor
C) Advise him that the clicking noise will resolve within 2 to 4 weeks
D) Advise him to use an elastic bandage wrap during the first 2 weeks for knee support and to see you again for reevaluation

416. All of the following are correct statements regarding oral contraceptives except:

A) The actual failure rate of oral contraceptives is 3%
B) Desogestrel belongs to the progesterone family of drugs
C) The newer low-dose birth control pills do not require backup during the first 2 weeks of use
D) Oral contraceptives are contraindicated for women 35 years of age or older who smoke

417. A 15-year-old basketball player who is 6 ft tall is seen for complaints of painful lumps on his knees. Upon inspection, the nurse practitioner notes a bonelike growth on the upper tibia midline below the kneecap on both knees. The patient has full range of motion with no joint tenderness, redness, or swelling. Which of the following conditions is best described?

A) Osteosarcoma of the tibia
B) Juvenile rheumatoid arthritis
C) Osgood–Schlatter disease
D) Paget's disease of the bone

418. A cauliflower-like growth with foul-smelling discharge is seen during an otoscopic exam of the left ear of an 8-year-old boy with a history of chronic otitis media. The tympanic membrane and ossicles are not visible, and the patient seems to have difficulty hearing the nurse practitioner's instructions. Which of the following conditions is best described?

A) Chronic perforation of the tympanic membrane with secondary bacterial infection
B) Chronic mastoiditis
C) Cholesteatoma
D) Cancer of the middle ear

419. Sources of legal risk for the nurse practitioner would include all of the following except:

A) Invasive procedures
B) Electronic medical record entries
C) Prescribing medication
D) In-service training

420. The best form of aerobic exercise for a patient with severe rheumatoid arthritis is:

A) Yoga
B) Swimming
C) Riding a bicycle
D) Passive range of motion

421. Which of the following effects are seen in every woman using Depo-Provera (medroxy-progesterone injection) for more than 5 years?

A) Melasma
B) Amenorrhea
C) Weight loss
D) Headache

422. The following measures are used for prophylaxis or treatment of migraine headaches. Which is not considered effective for migraine?

A) Propranolol (Inderal)
B) Resting in a quiet and darkened room
C) Trimethobenzamide (Tigan)
D) Moderate sodium restriction

423. A score of 2 in the Mini-Cog Instrument is highly suggestive of:

A) Delirium
B) Dementia
C) Mild cognitive impairment
D) Normal

424. A 19-year-old male athlete complains of acute knee pain after a football game. The nurse practitioner elicits McMurray's sign, which is positive on the patient's injured knee. This is a test for:

A) Meniscal injury
B) Inflammation of the knee joint
C) Osteophytes of the knee joint
D) Tenosynovitis

425. A 35-year-old man has a history of an upper respiratory viral infection 4 weeks ago. He reports that he started feeling short of breath and now complains of sharp pain in the middle of his chest that seems to worsen when he lies down. The patient's physical exam is within normal limits with the exception of a precordial rub on auscultation. The most likely diagnosis would be:

A) Pulmonary embolism
B) Dissecting aneurysm

C) Pericarditis
D) Esophageal reflux

426. Which type of exercise would you recommend to a 65-year-old arthritic patient who complains of a new onset of a painful, swollen left knee caused by overworking in the garden for 2 days?

A) Quadriceps-strengthening exercises of the left knee followed by the application of cold packs for 20 minutes four times a day
B) Rest the joint and apply cold packs intermittently for the next 48 hours
C) Passive range of motion and cold packs
D) A cool tub bath with warm packs on the knee to avoid stiffening of the joint

427. Symptoms suggestive of ulcerative colitis include all of the following except:

A) Bloody diarrhea mixed with mucus
B) Nausea and vomiting
C) Weight gain
D) Abdominal pain

428. Peak expiratory flow (PEF) meters are used to monitor asthma by using personal best measurements. All of the following factors are used to determine the PEF except:

A) Age
B) Gender
C) Height
D) Weight

429. A red, raised serpiginous-shaped rash is noted by the nurse practitioner on the right foot of a 4-year-old child brought in for a preschool physical by the mother. The child complains of severe itch and keeps scratching the lesion. The mother reports that the child frequently plays in the yard without wearing shoes or sandals. Which of the following is most likely?

A) Larva migrans
B) Erythema migrans
C) Tinea pedis
D) Insect bites

430. All of the following are considered risk factors for urinary tract infections in women except:

A) Diabetes mellitus
B) Diaphragms and spermicide use
C) Pregnancy
D) Intrauterine device

431. You are performing a pelvic exam on a 25-year-old sexually active woman. You palpate a tender and warm cystic mass on the lower edge of the left labia majora, which is red. The most likely diagnosis is:

A) Skene's gland cyst
B) Cystocele
C) Lymphogranuloma venereum
D) Bartholin's gland abscess

432. A 16-year-old girl presents in the school clinic and tells the nurse that she would like birth control pills for contraception because she is sexually active. How should the nurse practitioner proceed?

A) Refuse to see the patient until consent can be obtained from her parent or legal guardian
B) Perform a history and physical exam and, if the patient does not have health contraindications, prescribe birth control pills
C) Speak with the patient about safe sex and have her obtain parental consent for the physical exam
D) Perform a gynecological exam and obtain a Pap smear

433. A patient diagnosed with bacterial vaginosis should be advised that her sexual partner:

A) Needs treatment with ceftriaxone (Rocephin) 250 mg IM with doxycycline 100 mg BID for 14 days
B) Needs treatment with metronidazole (Flagyl) 500 mg PO BID for 7 days and 1 dose of azithromycin (Zithromax)
C) Does not need treatment
D) Needs treatment with clotrimazole cream (Lotrimin) on his penis BID for 1 to 2 weeks

434. Which of the following statements regarding physiological changes found in the elderly is incorrect?

A) There is an increase in the fat-to-lean body ratio
B) There is a decrease in the ability of the liver to metabolize drugs
C) There is an increase in renal function
D) There is a loss of hearing for sounds in the high-frequency range (presbycusis)

435. All of the following clinical signs are seen in patients with Parkinson's disease except:

A) Pill-rolling tremor
B) Difficulty initiating involuntary movement
C) Shuffling gait with cogwheel rigidity
D) Increased facial movements due to tics

436. Which of the following conditions is a possible complication of severe eclampsia?

A) Placenta previa
B) Placenta abruptio
C) Erythroblastosis fetalis
D) Uterine rupture

437. A possible complication of Bell's palsy is:

A) Corneal ulceration
B) Acute glaucoma
C) Inability to swallow
D) Loss of sensation in the affected side

438. Which of the following is most likely to cause delirium?

A) Dehydration
B) Multiple brain infarcts
C) Malnutrition
D) Acute infection

439. A 25-year-old woman presents with severe right-sided pelvic pain that began 48 hours ago. She reports small amounts of vaginal bleeding. The pain is aggravated by jumping or any movement that jars her pelvis. The best initial intervention is which of the following?

A) Follicle-stimulating hormone (FSH) test
B) Urine human chorionic gonadotropin (hCG) test
C) Pelvic ultrasound
D) CBC with white cell differentials

440. Which of the following laboratory values may be elevated on the liver function panel of patients who are alcohol abusers?

A) Serum GGT (gamma glutamyl transaminase)
B) Serum creatinine
C) Serum bilirubin
D) Blood urea nitrogen

Questions 441 and 442 apply to this case. A 10-year-old boy complains of sudden onset of scrotal pain upon awakening that morning. He is also complaining of severe nausea and vomiting. During the physical examination, the nurse practitioner finds a tender, warm, and swollen left scrotum. The cremasteric reflex is negative and the urine dipstick is negative for leukocytes, nitrites, and blood.

441. The most likely diagnosis is:

A) Acute epididymitis
B) Severe *Salmonella* infection
C) Testicular torsion
D) Acute orchitis

442. What type of follow-up should this patient receive?

A) Refer him to a urologist within 48 hours
B) Refer him to the emergency department as soon as possible
C) Prescribe ibuprofen (Advil) 600 mg QID for pain
D) Order a testicular ultrasound for further evaluation

443. Which of the following conditions are possible causes of secondary hypertension?

A) Leukemia and thalassemia major
B) Hashimoto's thyroiditis and polycystic ovaries
C) Renal stenosis and adrenal tumors
D) Myocardial infarction and coronary artery disease

444. You note that your 11-year-old female patient is at Tanner stage II. You would advise her mother that menarche will probably start in:

A) 2 to 3 years
B) 3 to 4 years
C) 5 years
D) It is dependent on the girl's genetic makeup

445. The nurse practitioner does not need to obtain parental consent from all of the following patients except:

A) A 17-year-old who wants to be treated for a sexually transmitted infection
B) A 12-year-old who wants a serum pregnancy test
C) A 15-year-old who wants birth control pills
D) A 14-year-old who wants to be treated for dysmenorrhea

446. There is a higher risk of balanitis in which of the following conditions?

A) Renal insufficiency
B) Diabetes mellitus
C) Graves' disease
D) Asthma

447. Which of the following is useful in primary care when evaluating a patient for possible acute sinusitis or hydrocele?

A) Checking for the cremasteric reflex
B) Transillumination
C) Ultrasound
D) CT scan

448. All of the following are associated with emphysema except:

A) A barrel-shaped chest
B) Pursed-lip breathing
C) A chest radiograph result with infiltrates and flattening of the costovertebral angle
D) Dyspnea when at rest

449. A split S2 heart sound is best heard at which of the following areas?

A) The aortic area
B) The pulmonic area
C) The tricuspid area
D) The mitral area

450. Balanitis is caused by:

A) *Staphylococcus aureus*
B) *Streptococcus pyogenes*
C) *Candida albicans*
D) Trichomonads

451. The sentinel nodes (Virchow's nodes) are found at the:

A) Right axillary area
B) Left supraclavicular area
C) Posterior cervical chain
D) Submandibular chain

452. A 20-year-old White man is being seen for a physical exam by the nurse practitioner. He complains of pruritic macerated areas in his groin that have been present for the past 2 weeks. Which of the following is the most likely?

A) Tinea cruris
B) Tinea corporis
C) Tinea capitis
D) Tinea pedis

453. Cluster headaches are most often seen in:

A) Adolescent girls
B) Middle-aged men
C) Elderly men
D) Postmenopausal women

454. An 18-year-old male patient is found to have a 47,XXY karyotype and is diagnosed with Klinefelter's syndrome. The patient is most likely to have all of the following physical characteristics except:

A) Gynecomastia
B) Long limbs
C) Lack of secondary sexual characteristics
D) Large testes

455. Which of the following drugs can increase the risk of bleeding in patients who are receiving anticoagulation therapy with warfarin sodium (Coumadin)?

A) Trimethoprim–sulfamethoxazole (Bactrim DS)
B) Carafate (Sucralfate)
C) Losartan (Cozaar)
D) Furosemide (Lasix)

456. An adolescent female's areola, nipples, and breast tissue develop and become elevated as one mound. Which of the following is the correct Tanner stage for this phase of breast development?

A) Tanner stage I
B) Tanner stage II
C) Tanner stage III
D) Tanner stage IV

457. About one third of children in the United States are considered obese. Which of the following methods is an appropriate intervention for obese school-aged children?

A) Severe restriction of dietary carbohydrates
B) Increase physical activity and outdoor play
C) Prescribe appetite suppressants
D) Over-the-counter herbal weight-loss pills

458. The cremasteric reflex is elicited by:

A) Asking the patient to open his or her mouth and touching the back of the pharynx with a tongue blade
B) Hitting the biceps tendon briskly with a reflex hammer and watching the lower arm for movement
C) Hitting the patellar tendon briskly with a reflex hammer and watching the lower leg for movement
D) Stroking the inner thigh of a male patient and watching the testicle on the ipsilateral side rise up toward the body

459. You have diagnosed a 30-year-old male patient with contact dermatitis on the left side of the face secondary to poison ivy. You would recommend:

A) Washing with antibacterial soap BID to reduce risk of secondary bacterial infection until it is healed
B) Zanfel poison ivy wash
C) Clotrimazole (Lotrimin) cream BID for 2 weeks
D) Halcinonide (Halog) 1% ointment BID for 2 weeks

460. Pulsus paradoxus is best described as:

A) An increase in systolic blood pressure on inspiration
B) A decrease in diastolic blood pressure on exhalation
C) A decrease in systolic blood pressure on inspiration
D) An increase in diastolic blood pressure on expiration

461. All of the following vaccines are contraindicated in pregnant women except:

A) Influenza
B) Mumps
C) Varicella
D) Rubella

462. Women with polycystic ovary syndrome (PCOS) are at higher risk for the following:

A) Heart disease and endometrial cancer
B) Uterine fibroids and ovarian cancer
C) Premature menopause
D) Pelvic inflammatory disease (PID)

463. A 16-year-old complains of a severe sore throat for 3 days along with a generalized rash and fever. The skin has the texture of fine sandpaper. This constellation of findings best describes:

A) Kawasaki's disease
B) Scarlatina

C) German measles
D) Rubeola

464. A college freshman who is using oral contraceptives calls the nurse practitioner's office asking for advice. She forgot to take her pills 2 days in a row during the second week of the pill cycle and wants to know what to do. What is the best advice?

A) Start a new pack of pills and dispose of the old one
B) Take two pills today and two pills tomorrow, and have your partner use condoms for the rest of the pill cycle
C) Stop taking the pills right away, and start a new pill cycle in 2 weeks
D) Take one pill today and two pills tomorrow, and have your partner use condoms

465. All of the following patients should be screened for diabetes mellitus except:

A) An obese man of Hispanic descent
B) An overweight middle-aged Black woman whose mother has type 2 diabetes
C) A woman who delivered an infant weighing 9.5 lbs
D) A 30-year-old White man with hypertension

466. A 40-year-old nurse complains of new-onset back pain secondary to her job on the medical–surgical floor of a hospital. She reports lifting some obese patients while working the previous night shift. She reports to the worker's compensation clinic where she was referred. She describes the pain as starting in her right buttocks area and radiating down the back of her thigh. It becomes worse when she sits down for long periods. You would suspect:

A) Sciatica
B) Acute muscle spasm
C) Cauda equina syndrome
D) Acute muscle strain

467. A sexually active 22-year-old man is asking to be screened for hepatitis B because his new girlfriend has recently been diagnosed with hepatitis B infection. His lab results are the following: anti-HBV is negative, HBsAg is positive, and HBeAg is negative. Which of the following is true?

A) The patient is immune to the hepatitis B virus
B) The patient is not infected with hepatitis B virus
C) The patient needs hepatitis B vaccine and hepatitis B immunoglobulin
D) The patient needs only hepatitis B immunoglobulin

468. Three of the following are eye findings associated with chronic uncontrolled hypertension. Which one of the following is associated with diabetic retinopathy?

A) AV nicking
B) Copper wire arterioles
C) Flame-shaped hemorrhages
D) Microaneurysms

469. You would advise a patient who is taking a monoamine oxidase inhibitor (MAOI) to avoid foods that contain tyramine. All of the following are foods that contain high levels of tyramine except:

A) Cured meats
B) Beer and red wine
C) Fermented foods
D) Spinach and kale

470. In the majority of children, the first permanent teeth start to erupt at the age of 6 years. Which of the following are the first permanent teeth to erupt in this time period?

A) First molars
B) Second molars
C) Lower or upper incisors
D) Canines

471. A 22-year-old man is brought to an urgent care center by his anxious mother. She reports that her son returned from a camping trip 2 days ago with a high fever and bad headache. Apparently, he had complained to her of a painful and stiff neck along with nausea shortly after he returned. The mother states that her son started breaking out in a rash the day before, parts of which are now turning a dark-red to purple color. During the physical exam, the nurse practitioner evaluates the patient for Kernig's sign, which is positive. Which of the following conditions is most likely?

A) Stevens–Johnson syndrome
B) Meningococcemia
C) Rocky Mountain spotted fever
D) Erythema multiforme

472. Your newly diagnosed diabetic patient reports to you that she had severe hives and swollen lips when she took Bactrim for a bladder infection 2 months ago. Which of the following statements is correct?

A) She cannot take any pills in the sulfonylurea class
B) She can take some of the pills in the sulfonylurea class
C) She can take any of the pills in the sulfonylurea class
D) None of the above

473. Which of the following substances is responsible for the symptoms of dysmenorrhea?

A) Estrogen
B) Human chorionic gonadotropin
C) Prostaglandins
D) Progesterone

474. Which of the following laboratory tests would you order for an older diabetic man with the following complete blood count (CBC) results: hemoglobin = 11 g/dL, hematocrit = 38%, mean corpuscular volume (MCV) = 105 fL, and normal reticulocyte count?

A) Serum ferritin and a peripheral smear
B) Hemoglobin electrophoresis

C) Serum folate acid and B_{12} level
D) Schilling test

475. Auscultation of normal breath sounds of the chest will reveal:

A) Bronchial breath sounds heard at the lower bases
B) High-pitched vesicular breath sounds heard over the upper lobes
C) Vesicular breath sounds heard over the trachea
D) Vesicular breath sounds in the lower lobe

476. The bell of the stethoscope is best used for auscultation of which of the following?

A) S3 and S4 and low-pitched tones
B) S3 and S4 only
C) S1 and S2 and high-pitched tones
D) S1 and S2 only

477. Which of the following is the best method for diagnosing a *Candida albicans* infection of the vagina in the primary care setting?

A) Wet smear
B) Tzanck smear
C) KOH (potassium hydroxide) smear
D) Clinical findings only

478. During a sports physical of a 14-year-old girl, you note her breast development. The areola and the breast tissue are all in one mound. In which Tanner stage is this patient?

A) Tanner stage I
B) Tanner stage II
C) Tanner stage III
D) Tanner stage IV

479. A 13-year-old boy wants to be treated for his acne. He has a large number of closed and open comedones on his face. The patient has been treating himself with over-the-counter benzoyl peroxide and topical salicylic acid products. Which of the following would be recommended next?

A) Isotretinoin (Accutane)
B) Tetracycline
C) Retin-A 0.25% gel
D) Careful face washing with medicated soap at bedtime

480. The Romberg test is done to check for problems with balance. Which area of the brain is responsible for balance?

A) Frontal lobe
B) Temporal lobe
C) Midbrain
D) Cerebellum

481. The major difference between the quasi-experimental design and the experimental design is which of the following?

A) The quasi-experimental design is a type of observational study
B) The quasi-experimental design uses convenience sampling instead of random sampling to recruit subjects
C) The quasi-experimental design is also known as a survey
D) The quasi-experimental design does not have an intervention group

482. A mother brings in her 6-year-old daughter to see the nurse practitioner (NP). She complains that the school nurse found a few nits in her daughter's hair. The mother states that the school has a "no nits" policy regarding head lice and her daughter cannot go back to school until all the nits have been removed. The child was treated with permethrin shampoo (Nix) twice about 3 months ago. During the physical exam, the NP sees a few nits that are about 2 inches away from the scalp. The child denies itchiness on her scalp. Which of the following is the best action for the NP to follow?

A) Prescribe lindane (Kwell) for the child because she may have head lice that are resistant to permethrin
B) Advise the mother to use a nit comb after spraying the child's hair with white distilled vinegar, wait for 15 minutes, and then rinse the hair
C) Advise the mother to retreat the child with permethrin cream instead of shampoo
D) Reassure the mother that the nits will probably drop off after a few weeks

483. What is the pedigree symbol for a diseased male?

A) An empty square
B) An empty circle
C) A filled-in square
D) A filled-in circle

Questions 484 and 485 apply to this case. A 25-year-old man who was involved in a car accident is brought to the local emergency department. He reports wearing a seat belt and was the driver of the vehicle. The patient is complaining of pain on his right lower leg. The right foot is abducted and the ankle is swollen and bruised. There is a small laceration on the ankle. The patient complains of severe right ankle pain when standing.

484. Which of the following tests would be the initial choice for evaluating for possible fractures on the right lower leg?

A) Plain radiographs of the right lower leg, ankle, and foot
B) Ultrasound of the right lower leg
C) MRI of the right ankle
D) Radiograph of the right ankle and knee with special view of the hip

485. In addition to surgical repair of a compound fracture that has broken through the skin, which of the following treatment plans is important to consider in this patient?

A) Application of a topical antibiotic BID until the wound is healed
B) Wound irrigation
C) Use cold packs three times per day
D) Tetanus vaccine and systemic antibiotics

486. Systemic lupus erythematosus (SLE) is more common among patients from all of the following ethnic and racial backgrounds except:

A) African American
B) Asian
C) Hispanic
D) Caucasian

487. Which of the following physical exam findings is most specific for systemic lupus erythematosus (SLE)?

A) Swollen and painful joint involvement
B) Fatigue and myalgia
C) Stiffness and swelling of multiple joints
D) Malar rash

488. An older man is diagnosed with conductive hearing loss in the left ear by the nurse practitioner. Which of the following is the expected result when performing a Rinne test on this patient?

A) AC (air conduction) > BC (bone conduction)
B) Lateralization to the bad ear
C) BC > AC
D) Lateralization to the good ear

489. A physician is referring one of his patients to a nurse practitioner. What type of relationship will exist between the physician and nurse practitioner?

A) Consultative
B) Collaborative
C) Professional
D) Advocate

490. A homeless 47-year-old man with a history of injection drug use and alcohol abuse presents to the public health clinic with a recent history of fever, night sweats, fatigue, and weakness. The patient has recently noticed some thin red streaks on his nailbed and red bumps on some of his fingers that hurt. During the cardiac exam, the nurse practitioner hears a grade 3/6 murmur over the mitral area. The subcutaneous red-purple nodules are tender to palpation. The thin red lines on the nailbeds resemble subungual splinter hemorrhages. Which of the following conditions is most likely?

A) Pericarditis
B) Acute bacterial endocarditis
C) Rheumatic fever
D) Viral cardiomyopathy

491. Which of the following pathogenic bacteria are commonly found in the lungs of older children and adults with cystic fibrosis?

A) *Streptococcus pneumoniae*
B) *Chlamydia pneumoniae*
C) *Pseudomonas aeruginosa*
D) *Staphylococcus aureus*

492. All of the following are physiological changes that occur in the body as we age except:

A) The half-life of some drugs is prolonged
B) There is an increase in cholesterol production by the liver
C) There is a mild increase in renal function
D) There is a slight decrease in the activity of the immune system

493. A 15-month-old who is eating and behaving normally is found to have a high fever. After a few days, the fever resolves and the child breaks out in a maculopapular rash. This is a description of which of the following conditions?

A) Erythema infectiosum
B) Roseola infantum
C) Fifth disease
D) Scarlet fever

494. Which of the following conditions is associated with three stages of rashes?

A) Fifth disease
B) Erythema infectiosum
C) Varicella
D) Rocky Mountain spotted fever

495. Which of the following drug classes is recommended for the treatment of postherpetic neuralgia?

A) Tricyclic antidepressants (TCAs)
B) Selective serotonin reuptake inhibitors (SSRIs)
C) Atypical antidepressants
D) Benzodiazepines

496. A new patient who recently visited a relative in North Carolina complains of an onset of fever and red rashes that started 2 days ago. The rash first appeared on the wrist and the ankles and included the palms of the hands. The patient reports that it is spreading toward his trunk. The patient's eyes are not injected and no enlarged nodes are palpated on his neck. There is no desquamation of the skin. Which of the following is most likely?

A) Kawasaki's disease
B) Meningococcemia
C) Rocky Mountain spotted fever
D) Measles

497. Carpal tunnel syndrome is due to inflammation of the:

A) Ulnar nerve
B) Radial nerve
C) Brachial nerve
D) Median nerve

498. The Somogyi effect is characterized by which of the following?

A) It is a complication of high levels of growth hormone
B) It is the physiological spike of serum blood glucose in the early morning that is caused by secretion of growth hormone

C) It is characterized by high fasting blood glucose in the morning that is caused by the secretion of glucagon by the liver
D) It is a rare phenomenon that only occurs in type 1 diabetic patients

499. The following findings are considered benign lesions of the skin except:

A) Lentigo
B) Seborrheic keratosis
C) Actinic keratosis
D) Rosacea

500. Which of the following is recommended as first-line treatment for essential tremor?

A) Propranolol (Inderal)
B) Phenytoin (Dilantin)
C) Amitriptyline (Elavil)
D) Fluoxetine (Prozac)

501. The atypical antipsychotic drugs have many adverse effects. Which of the following side effects are most likely to be seen with this drug class?

A) Orthostatic hypotension and sedation
B) Malignant hypertension and headache
C) Skin hyperpigmentation and alopecia
D) Severe anxiety and increased appetite

502. A 55-year-old woman who is on a prescription of clindamycin for a dental infection presents to the nurse practitioner with complaints of watery diarrhea for the past 4 days. She complains of abdominal cramping and bloating with diarrheal stools up to 10 times a day. She denies seeing blood or pus in her stool. There is no history of recent travel. The patient has been taking over-the-counter medicine with no relief. The nurse practitioner suspects that the patient has a mild case of *Clostridium difficile* colitis. Which of the following antibiotics is indicated for this infection?

A) Ciprofloxacin (Cipro) 400 mg PO BID × 7 days
B) Metronidazole (Flagyl) 500 mg PO TID × 10 days
C) Levofloxacin (Levaquin) 750 mg PO daily × 7 days
D) Trimethoprim–sulfamethoxazole (Bactrim DS) 1 tablet PO BID × 10 days

503. A 13-year-old girl has a throat culture that is positive for strep throat. She reports that her younger brother was recently diagnosed with strep throat and treated. The patient has a severe allergy to penicillin and reports that erythromycin makes her very nauseated. Which of the following antibiotics is the best choice?

A) Azithromycin (Zithromax)
B) Cephalexin (Keflex)
C) Cefuroxime axetil (Ceftin)
D) Levofloxacin (Levaquin)

504. All of the following groups are classified as "vulnerable populations" and have additional protections as human subjects except:

A) Prisoners
B) Pregnant women, fetuses, and children
C) Elderly
D) Those with intellectual disability

505. A 60-year-old female truck driver presents to the outpatient urgent care clinic of a hospital complaining of the worsening of her low-back pain the past few days. Pain is accompanied by numbness in the perineal area. She describes the pain as "sharp and burning" and points to the left buttock. She reports that the pain started on the mid-buttock of the left leg and recently started to go down the lateral aspect of the leg toward the top of the foot. During the physical exam, the ankle jerk and the knee jerk reflex are 1+ on the affected leg and 2+ on the other leg. The pedal, posterior tibialis, and popliteal pulses are the same on both legs. Which of the following tests should the nurse practitioner consider for this patient?

A) Order an MRI scan of the lumbosacral spine as soon as possible
B) Write a prescription for ibuprofen 800 mg PO QID with a muscle relaxant and advise the patient to follow up with her primary care provider within 3 days
C) Refer the patient to an orthopedic surgeon
D) Ordering an imaging study of the spine is premature because the majority of low back pain cases resolve within 10 to 12 weeks

506. A 70-year-old woman complains of left lower quadrant abdominal pain and fever for 2 days. Her blood pressure of 130/80 mmHg, pulse is 90 beats/min, respirations are 14 breaths/min, and temperature is 100.5°F. During the abdominal exam, the left lower quadrant of the abdomen is tender to palpation. The nurse practitioner (NP) does not palpate a mass; neither is there guarding or rigidity. Rovsing's sign is negative. Bowel sounds are present in all quadrants. The NP is familiar with the patient, who is alert and is asking appropriate questions about her condition. The nurse practitioner suspects that the patient has acute diverticulitis. Which of the following treatment plans is appropriate for this patient?

A) The patient should be referred to the physician as soon as possible
B) The patient has a mild case of acute diverticulitis and can be treated with antibiotics in the outpatient setting with close follow-up
C) This patient has a moderate to severe case of acute diverticulitis and needs to be admitted to the hospital for IV antibiotics
D) The patient should be referred to the emergency department as soon as possible

507. What is the name of the physiologically active compound that is derived from soybeans?

A) Isoflavones
B) Estrogen
C) Progesterone
D) Resveratrol

508. All of the following conditions are contraindications for bupropion (Wellbutrin, Zyban) except:

A) Anorexia nervosa and bulimia
B) Seizure disorders

C) Peripheral neuropathy
D) Brain injury

509. The nurse practitioner is educating a new patient with Raynaud's phenomenon about lifestyle recommendations to decrease exacerbations of the disorder. Which of the following lifestyle changes would not be useful for this patient?

A) Increasing consumption of caffeine-containing drinks and foods such as chocolate
B) Wearing gloves or mittens during cold weather and being careful when handling frozen foods
C) Smoking and exercising at least three times a week
D) Decreasing emotional stress and lifestyle stressors

510. The Health Insurance Portability and Accountability Act (HIPAA) was passed by Congress in 2003. All of the following statements about HIPAA are correct except:

A) It provides federal protections for personal health information
B) It is applicable to all health care providers and payers who bill electronically and transmit health information over the Internet
C) Patients have the right to view their mental health and psychotherapy-related health information
D) It gives patients the right to view and correct errors in their medical records

511. Which of the following is involved with sensorineural hearing loss?

A) Outer ear
B) Middle ear
C) Inner ear
D) Cranial nerve VIII

512. A 13-year-old adolescent girl is brought to the health clinic by her mother for a sports physical. The mother reports that the teen's last vaccines were given at the age of 6 years. Which of the following vaccines is recommended by the Centers for Disease Control and Prevention (CDC) for this patient?

A) Td and HPV vaccines
B) Tdap, MCV4, and the HPV vaccines
C) DTap and the flu vaccine
D) DT and MCV4 vaccines

513. An 87-year-old man is being seen at the health clinic. He tells the nurse practitioner that his grandson locks him in the bedroom when the grandson goes out of the house and sometimes withholds food from him if he does not give the grandson spending money. The patient appears frail, with poor grooming, and has a strong odor of urine on his clothing. Which of the following is the best action for the nurse practitioner to take?

A) Report the patient's grandson for elder abuse to the state protective health services
B) Speak to the grandson and educate him about the importance of proper grooming for his grandfather
C) Advise the grandson that if the patient has the same complaints the next time he is seen, the grandson will be reported for elder abuse to the state authorities
D) Advise the patient that he should call his son as soon as possible to tell him about the grandson's actions

514. A patient with chronic obstructive pulmonary disease (COPD) is referred for pulmonary function testing. All of the following results are characteristic of pulmonary function tests in patients with COPD except:

A) Increase in the TLC (total lung capacity)
B) Dyspnea
C) Increase in the RV (residual volume)
D) Reduction of the FEV1 (forced expiratory volume in 1 second)

515. The nurse practitioner is evaluating a middle-aged woman who has experienced gradual weight gain, lack of energy, dry hair, and an irregular period for the past 8 months. Routine annual laboratory testing showed a thyroid-stimulating hormone (TSH) level of 10 mU/L. The nurse practitioner decides to order a thyroid profile. Results show that TSH is 8.50 mU/L and serum free T4 is decreased. During the physical exam, the patient's body mass index (BMI) is 28. The heart and lung exams are both normal. Which of the following is the best treatment plan for this patient?

A) Advise the patient that the decreased thyroid-stimulating hormone (TSH) level means her thyroid problem has resolved
B) Start the patient on levothyroxine (Synthroid) 0.25 mcg PO daily
C) Start the patient on Armour thyroid
D) Refer the patient to an endocrinologist

516. A 75-year-old patient has a history of benign prostatic hyperplasia (BPH). Which of the following clinical findings is expected during the prostatic exam of this patient?

A) Prostate feels rubbery and uniformly enlarged
B) Prostate feels boggy and warm
C) Prostate feels hard and indurated
D) Presence of tender nodules on the lateral edge of the gland

517. A 55-year-old woman brings her mother, who is 82 years of age, to the emergency department of a local hospital. She reports she found her mother on the floor when she checked on her that morning. Her mother was awake and oriented, but needed help getting up. Her mother states that she thinks she passed out. She is being evaluated by a physician who orders an EKG and x-rays of both hips. Regarding laboratory testing, which of the following tests is important to perform initially?

A) Urinalysis
B) Serum electrolytes
C) Blood glucose
D) Hemoglobin and hematocrit

518. All of the following clinical signs and symptoms are seen early in testicular torsion except:

A) Nausea and vomiting
B) Absence of the cremasteric reflex
C) Affected testicle is elevated compared with the normal testicle
D) Affected testicle is swollen and feels cold to touch

519. The research term/symbol that is used to indicate the "total population" in a research study is stated as:

A) n
B) N
C) p
D) P

520. A 22-year-old man presents to the urgent care clinic with burns caused by a hot-oil spill while frying food. He denies facial involvement, dyspnea, or weakness. During the physical exam, the nurse practitioner notices bright-red skin with numerous bullae on the right arm and hand and bright-red skin on the right thigh and the right lower leg. On a pain scale of 1 to 10, he reports the pain as 8. Based on the rule of nines, what is the total body surface areas (TBSA) of this patient's burns?

A) 36%
B) 27%
C) 18%
D) 9%

521. What is the significance of a positive Lachman sign?

A) Instability of the knee caused by damage to the anterior cruciate ligament of the knee
B) Posterior cruciate ligament laxity which may cause locking of the knee
C) Achilles tendon rupture
D) Patellar tendon rupture

522. A positive Chvostek's sign is associated with:

A) Hypocalcemia
B) Hypernatremia
C) Hypokalemia
D) Hyperkalemia

523. The nurse practitioner calls a patient to discuss the results of routine laboratory tests, which are all normal. She calls the patient twice and each time the call goes to voicemail. Which of the following is the most appropriate action to take?

A) Because the results are normal, the nurse practitioner can leave a voicemail message describing the laboratory results
B) When the nurse practitioner is unable to speak with the patient directly, she should leave a message with her name and telephone number and instruct the patient to call back
C) The clinic policy may not require the nurse practitioner to call patients if their laboratory results are normal
D) It is up to the physician to determine whether a laboratory result can be discussed with a patient over the telephone

524. Which of the following drugs that are used to treat attention deficit hyperactivity disorder (ADHD) is not classified as an amphetamine/stimulant?

A) Dexmethylphenidate (Focalin XR)
B) Mixed salts of amphetamine (Adderall)
C) Methylphenidate (Ritalin)
D) Atomoxetine (Strattera)

525. A 25-year-old man with schizophrenia comes in for a routine annual physical. He is a heavy smoker and has a body mass index (BMI) of 28. The patient has been on olanzapine (Zyprexa) for 10 years. Regarding the patient's prescription, which of the following laboratory tests is recommended for monitoring the adverse effects of atypical antipsychotics?

A) Fasting blood glucose, fasting lipid profile, and weight
B) Urinalysis, serum creatinine, 24-hour urine for protein and creatinine clearance
C) Liver function tests only
D) CBC with differential, liver function tests, and weight

526. Native Americans view illness or disease as being caused by which of the following?

A) Poor blood circulation in the body
B) A punishment by the "spirits" for wrongful actions against others or for failure to follow spiritual rules
C) An imbalance of the flow of energy in the body
D) An imbalance of the hot and cold energy forces in the body

527. A 74-year-old man presents with recurrent abdominal cramping and pain associated with diarrhea that occurs from four to five times per day. He reports that currently he is having an exacerbation. The stools are bloody with mucus and pus. The patient reports that he has lost weight and is always fatigued. The patient denies recent travel or outdoor camping. Which of the following conditions is most likely?

A) Giardiasis
B) Irritable bowel syndrome (IBS)
C) Diverticulitis
D) Ulcerative colitis

528. A middle-aged man who is homeless reports to the local public health clinic complaining of a painless and shallow ulcer on the penile shaft for the past 2 weeks. He is sexually active and had unprotected intercourse with two male partners over the past few months. The patient is tested for HIV, syphilis, gonorrhea, hepatitis B, and herpes types 1 and 2. The syphilis and HIV tests are both positive. The gonorrhea, hepatitis B, and herpes tests are negative. The nurse practitioner is aware of the nationally notifiable infectious conditions. Which of the following is true regarding reporting of any of these sexually transmitted infections?

A) Health care providers must obtain the patient's permission before reporting the positive HIV and syphilis test results to the local public health department
B) The nurse practitioner should obtain the patient's and sexual partner's permission before reporting the positive test results to the local health department
C) Health care providers are mandated by law to report certain types of diseases to the local health department even if the patient does not give permission
D) The nurse practitioner should consult with the supervising physician about this issue

529. A medical assistant is calling out the names of patients who are in the waiting room. The medical assistant is following the HIPAA Privacy Rule if she performs which of the following actions?

A) Calls patients by using their full name to show respect
B) Calls patients by using their last name or surname
C) Calls patients by using their preferred nicknames
D) Calls patients by using their first name only

530. A 14-year-old girl with amenorrhea is tested for pregnancy and has a positive result. The patient tells the nurse practitioner (NP) that she is seriously considering terminating the pregnancy. She tells the NP that she wants to be referred to a Planned Parenthood clinic. The NP's personal beliefs and religious beliefs are pro-life. Which of the following is the best action for the NP?

A) The NP should tell the patient about her personal beliefs and advise her against getting an abortion
B) The NP should advise the patient that a peer who is working with the NP can help answer the patient's questions more thoroughly
C) The NP should excuse herself from the case
D) The NP should refer the patient to an obstetrician

531. During the physical exam of a 60-year-old adult, the nurse practitioner performs an abdominal exam. The nurse practitioner is checking the left upper quadrant of the abdomen. During percussion, an area of dullness is noted beneath the lower left ribcage. Which of the following is a true statement regarding the spleen?

A) The spleen is not palpable in the majority of healthy adults
B) The spleen is 8 to 10 cm in the left midaxillary line at its longest axis
C) The spleen is 2 to 6 cm between the 9th and 11th ribs on the left midaxillary line
D) The splenic size varies depending on the patient's gender

532. All of the following drug classes are approved for treating hypertension. Which of the following antihypertensive drug classes is associated with the largest number of research studies?

A) Angiotensin-converting enzyme (ACE) inhibitors
B) Angiotensin receptor blockers (ARBs)
C) Thiazide diuretics
D) Calcium channel blockers (CCBs)

533. When a domestic dog is suspected of being infected with the rabies virus, it can either be killed for a brain biopsy or it can be quarantined. What is the minimum number of days a dog suspected of rabies must be quarantined?

A) 4 weeks
B) 21 days
C) 14 days
D) 10 days

534. Thiazide diuretics have been shown to have a beneficial effect on the bones, making them a desirable treatment option in hypertensive women with osteopenia or osteoporosis. What is the mechanism of action for their effect on the bones?

A) Thiazide diuretics decrease calcium excretion by the kidneys and stimulate osteoclast production
B) Thiazide diuretics increase both calcium and magnesium retention by the kidneys
C) Thiazide diuretics increase bone mineral density (BMD)
D) Thiazide diuretics influence electrolyte excretion by the kidneys

535. What is the best description of a variable?

A) It is an important part of every research study
B) It is the probability that a factor is important for the research data
C) It is the value or number that occurs the most frequently
D) It is a condition, characteristic, or factor that is being measured

536. A 30-year-old man with a history of gout is walking to the examination room and the nurse practitioner (NP) notices that he is limping. When the patient sits down, the NP notes that the metatarsophalangeal joint of the great toe is very swollen and is bright red. The patient reports that he attended a party the night before and hand "one too many" drinks. He requests a prescription to treat his painful toe. The NP prescribes indomethacin (Indocin) 50 mg TID PRN and colchicine for the patient. Regarding colchicine, which of the following instructions is correct?

A) Take one pill every 1 to 2 hours until relief is obtained or adverse gastrointestinal effects occur, such as abdominal pain, nausea, or diarrhea
B) Take one pill every hour until relief is obtained up to 24 hours
C) Take one pill every 4 to 6 hours until the pain is relieved
D) Take two to three pills QID until relief is obtained or adverse gastrointestinal effects occur, such as abdominal pain, nausea, or diarrhea

537. What type of testing is recommended before starting a patient on a prescription of hydroxychloroquine (Plaquenil)?

A) Complete blood count (CBC)
B) Serum creatinine and urine for microalbumin
C) Liver function tests
D) Comprehensive eye exam

538. The result of a postmenopausal woman's dual-energy x-ray absorption (DXA) scan shows osteopenia. Which of the following T-scores is indicative of osteopenia?

A) T-score of −1.0 or higher
B) T-score between −1. 0 to −2.5
C) T-score of less than −2.5
D) T-score of −2.50 to −3.50
E) Normal results

539. An adult patient was recently discharged from the hospital with a prescription of clindamycin. The patient reports that he took his last dose yesterday. He presents in the primary care clinic with complaints of the recent onset of watery diarrhea from 10 to 15 times a day with abdominal cramping. He denies fever and chills. Which of the following conditions is most likely in this patient?

A) *Clostridium difficile*-associated diarrhea
B) Giardiasis
C) Pseudomembranous colitis
D) Irritable bowel syndrome

540. Which of the following individuals is more likely to be affected by alpha thalassemia anemia?

A) 53-year-old Greek patient
B) 25-year-old Chinese patient
C) 62-year-old Russian patient
D) 38-year-old African American patient

541. What is the most common cause of infertility among women in the United States?

A) Fallopian tube scarring due to pelvic inflammatory disease (PID)
B) Ovulation disorders
C) Age older than 35 years
D) Endometriosis

542. A 65-year-old man presents to the clinic complaining of random recurrent episodes of dizziness with nausea. The patient describes it as the sensation of the room moving or of the room spinning. It is worsened by sudden head movement. During the episodes, he becomes very nauseated. He also has tinnitus with hearing loss in his right ear. The patient has type 2 diabetes and is on a prescription of metformin 500 mg PO BID and an angiotensin-converting enzyme (ACE) inhibitor. The blood glucose level during his visit is 80 mg/dL. Which of the following conditions is most likely?

A) Vasovagal presyncopal episode
B) Ménière's disease
C) Atypical migraine
D) Hypoglycemia

543. All of the following physiological changes are present in the lungs of the elderly except:

A) Decreased forced expiratory volume (FEV1)
B) Slightly increased residual volume (RV)
C) Increased lung compliance
D) Earlier airway collapse with shallow breathing

544. A 50-year-old woman of Irish descent presents with history of lethargy, feeling weak, nausea, anorexia with diarrhea and abdominal pain. The woman's skin appears tanned, but she denies prolonged sun exposure. During physical exam, the nurse practitioner notes hyperpigmentation of the nipple area, the gums, and the lips. The electrolyte panel reveals hyperkalemia and hyponatremia. She reports craving salty foods. Which of the following is most likely?

A) Addison's disease
B) Cushing's disease
C) Metabolic syndrome
D) Cutaneous drug reaction

545. A female adult patient presents with complaints of "bad burns" that are very painful. A large pot of boiling water tipped over and spilled on her arms and her anterior chest and abdomen. During the physical exam, the nurse practitioner notices bright-red skin with numerous bullae on the left arm and hand and large patches of bright-red skin on the anterior chest and abdominal area. On a pain scale of 1 to 10, she reports the pain as 9. Her vital signs are stable with tachycardia (pulse is 100 beats/min). She does not appear to be in shock. Using the rule of nines, what are the total body surface area (TBSA) and the depth of the burns in this patient?

A) The patient has a TBSA of 15% with full-thickness burns of the left arm and left hand, and partial-thickness burns of the anterior chest and abdominal area
B) The patient has a TBSA of 20% with partial-thickness burns on the left arm, left hand, and mild burns on the anterior chest and abdominal area
C) The patient has a TBSA of 27% with partial-thickness burns on the left arm and left hand, and superficial burns on the anterior chest and abdominal area
D) The patient has a TBSA of 18% with full-thickness burns of the left arm and left hand, and superficial burns on the anterior chest

546. Some nurse practitioners bill directly for their services. Regarding reimbursement, who is considered a third-party payer?

A) The patient
B) The health care provider
C) The health insurance companies, health plans, Medicare, and Medicaid
D) The federal government

547. A 14-year-old boy is brought in by his mother who reports that her son has been complaining for several months of recurrent bloating, stomach upset, and occasional loose stools. She reports that he has difficulty gaining weight and is short for his age. She has noticed that his symptoms are worse after eating large amounts of crackers, cookies, and breads. She denies seeing blood in the boy's stool. Which of the following conditions is most likely?

A) Amebiasis
B) Malabsorption
C) Crohn's colitis
D) Celiac disease

548. Which of the following pharmacological agents is the best choice for an elderly patient with insomnia?

A) Diazepam (Valium)
B) Zolpidem (Ambien)
C) Temazepam (Restoril)
D) Diphenhydramine (Benadryl)

549. An elderly Hispanic man has been taking finasteride (Proscar) for several months. The nurse practitioner decides to check the prostate specific antigen (PSA) value. The PSA result is 10 ng/mL. The patient's baseline PSA was 30 ng/mL. Which of the following actions is the next step?

A) Add the baseline PSA value to the treatment PSA value
B) The treatment PSA value is the correct value
C) Multiply the treatment PSA value by 2
D) Divide the baseline PSA value by the treatment PSA value

550. An adult patient is being evaluated for tuberculosis infection with a Mantoux test. The PPD result is 10.5 mm. The patient denies weight loss, cough, and night sweats, and the results of a chest x-ray are negative. The patient reports that he is in the United States illegally and is fearful about discovery. What is the most appropriate action for the nurse practitioner?

A) The nurse practitioner has a legal duty to report the patient to the local federal agency responsible for illegal migrants
B) The nurse practitioner is legally mandated to report illegal migrants to state authorities
C) The nurse practitioner should call the state health department to report that the patient has a tuberculosis infection
D) The nurse practitioner has an ethical duty to provide quality health care to patients

551. A 22-year-old woman is going on a 5-day cruise for her honeymoon. She reports a history of severe motion sickness. Which of the following medicines can be prescribed for motion sickness?

A) Dimenhydrinate (Dramamine)
B) Metoclopramide (Reglan)
C) Ondansetron (Zofran)
D) Scopolamine patch (Transderm Scop)

552. Which of the following is considered by Latinos/Hispanics to be a spiritual illness that can cause symptoms such as loss of appetite, crying, diarrhea, and weakness or death among infants and small children?

A) *Mal ojo* or *mal de ojo*
B) Chronic nightmares
C) *Trabajo*
D) *Malo*

553. A 45-year-old man fell asleep while smoking in his bedroom and started a fire. According to the patient, he refused to go to the emergency department because he had only minor burns. About 12 hours later, he presents to a walk-in urgent care center complaining of a new cough that is productive of saliva with clear mucus containing small carbonaceous black particles. His brows appear singed. Which of the following is the priority when evaluating this patient?

A) Perform a medical history, including prescription, over-the-counter, and herbal medicines
B) Assess the patient for respiratory distress
C) Evaluate the patient for asthma and atopy
D) Use the rule of nines to evaluate the total body surface area (TBSA)

554. Which of the following benzodiazepines has the shortest half-life?

A) Lorazepam (Ativan)
B) Alprazolam (Xanax)
C) Triazolam (Halcion)
D) Clonazepam (Klonopin)

555. Multiple myeloma is a malignancy of the:

A) White blood cells (WBC)
B) Red blood cells (RBC)
C) Plasma cells
D) Platelets

556. A 62-year-old man with chronic obstructive pulmonary disease (COPD) complains to the nurse practitioner that his prescription for ipratropium bromide (Atrovent) is not working. He reports that he still feels short of breath even after using it four times a day for 3 months. Which of the following actions is the next step for the nurse practitioner?

A) Increase the patient's dose of ipratropium bromide (Atrovent) to three inhalations QID
B) Continue the ipratropium bromide and start the patient on oxygen by nasal cannula
C) Continue ipratropium bromide (Atrovent) and add two inhalations of an albuterol (Ventolin) inhaler QID
D) Start the patient on oxygen by nasal cannula at bedtime and PRN during the daytime

557. A co-worker calls the nurse practitioner and wants to know about a patient's progress. She tells the NP that they are neighbors and she is worried about the patient's health status. The co-worker works in the same facility, but is not directly involved with this patient's care. Which of the following actions is the most appropriate?

A) Share with the co-worker the patient's health status
B) Advise the co-worker to call the patient right away and ask her for verbal permission
C) Inform the co-worker that you cannot release any information about this patient because the co-worker is not directly involved in the patient's care
D) Reassure the co-worker that the patient is doing fine and is getting better quickly

558. What is the name of the immune process that is responsible for anaphylactic reactions?

A) IgE-mediated reaction
B) IgG-mediated reaction
C) Antibody reaction
D) Atopic reaction

559. A 76-year-old woman reports that for the previous 4 months, she has noticed severe stiffness and aching in her neck and both shoulders and hips that is worsened by movement. She reports having a difficult time getting out of bed because of the severe stiffness and pain. It is difficult for her to put on a jacket or blouse or to fasten her bra. Along with these symptoms, she also has a low-grade fever, fatigue, loss of appetite, and weight loss. Starting yesterday, the vision in her right eye has progressively worsened. She has annual eye exams and denies that she has glaucoma. Which of the following conditions is most likely?

A) Rheumatoid arthritis (RA)
B) Degenerative joint disease
C) Polymyalgia rheumatica (PMR)
D) Fibromyalgia

560. The most important job of an institutional review board (IRB) is:

A) Protecting the interests of the hospital or the research institution
B) Protecting the rights of the human subjects who participate in research done at the institution
C) Protecting the researcher and research team from lawsuits
D) Evaluating research protocols and methodology for appropriateness and safety

561. The nurse practitioner orders an ankle–brachial index (ABI) test for a patient. Which of the following disorders is the ABI test used for?

A) Venous insufficiency
B) Osteoarthritis of the arm or the ankle
C) Peripheral arterial disease
D) Rheumatoid arthritis

562. A college student is seen as a walk-in appointment in a college health clinic. She complains of the abrupt onset of sore throat, nasal congestion, runny nose, and malaise. Vital signs are a temperature of 99.8°F, pulse of 84 beats/min, and respirations of 14 breaths/min. The physical exam reveals an erythematous throat, swollen nasal turbinates, and rhinitis. The nurse practitioner suspects viral upper respiratory infection. All of the following treatments are appropriate except:

A) Saline nasal spray (Ocean nasal spray)
B) Pseudoephedrine (Sudafed)
C) Ibuprofen (Advil)
D) Oral prednisone (Medrol Dose Pack)

563. All of the following foods are best avoided by individuals with celiac sprue except:

A) Rice cereal
B) Blueberry muffins
C) Organic wheat bread
D) Rye bread

564. Medicare Part A will pay for all of the following services except:

A) Minor surgery in a walk-in surgical center
B) Plastic surgery to repair facial damage from a burn
C) Kidney transplantation
D) Medical supplies and drugs that are used while the patient is in the hospital

565. A male 16-year-old with a recent history of a cat bite is brought to the walk-in clinic by his mother. The bite occurred about 2 hours before the visit. The nurse practitioner evaluates the wound and notes two small puncture wounds. There is no redness or purulent discharge. The mother reports that the teenager received a tetanus booster when he was 12 years old. Which of the following is the correct action to take?

A) Clean the wound with soap and water and apply a topical antibiotic and a bandage
B) Because the wound is clean and does not appear infected, there is no need for antibiotics
C) Give the patient a tetanus booster using the Tdap form of the vaccine
D) Clean the wound with soap and water and prescribe amoxicillin–clavulanate (Augmentin) 500 mg PO BID × 10 days

566. A White 15-year-old male is brought by his father for a physical exam. The father is concerned that his son is "too short" for his age. The father reports that when he was the same age, he was much taller. His son wants to try out for the football team, but the father is concerned because his son might be "too short" to join. Which of the following physical exam findings is worrisome?

A) Small, smooth testicles with no pubic or facial hair
B) Smooth testicles with rugated scrotum that is a darker color than the patient's normal skin color
C) Smooth testicles with coarse and curly pubic hair
D) Straight pubic and axillary hair with a long thin penis

567. What is the best diagnostic test for thalassemia?

A) CBC
B) MCV
C) Hemoglobin electrophoresis
D) Bone marrow biopsy

568. An elderly female patient who is a retired nurse was recently discharged from the hospital. A few days later, she started having random and recurrent episodes of dizziness, which prompted today's health care visit. She denies passing out, but describes the sensation of the room spinning or moving, which is worsened by sudden head movement. During the episodes, she is nauseated and sometimes vomits. The patient reports that she was given IV antibiotics and one of them was tobramycin. Which of the following medications is helpful in treating her symptom of dizziness?

A) Scopolamine patch (Transderm Scop)
B) Meclizine (Antivert)
C) Dimenhydrinate (Dramamine)
D) Duloxetine (Cymbalta)

569. A 17-year-old high school student is considering her birth control options. She wants to know more about Seasonale. Which of the following statements is false?

A) Taking Seasonale results in only four periods per year
B) Her period will occur within the 7 days when she is on the inert pills
C) It is a progesterone-only method of birth control and does not contain estrogen
D) Take one tablet daily for 84 consecutive days followed by 7 days of inert pills

570. Which of the following diseases is associated with a high risk of giant cell arteritis?

A) History of transient ischemia attacks (TIA)
B) Frequent migraine headaches with focal neurological findings
C) Polymyalgia rheumatica (PMR)
D) Systemic lupus erythematosus (SLE)

571. *Candidal intertrigo* is the name for an infection that is caused by the yeast *Candida albicans.* What is the location of this type of candida infection?

A) Scalp
B) Flexor areas of the elbows and the knees
C) Body areas where skin rubs together, such as under breasts or in groin area
D) Hands

572. A nurse practitioner is teaching a 54-year-old woman with stress urinary incontinence about Kegel exercises. The patient is instructed to tighten her pelvic floor muscles for a count of 10 and then to relax them for a count of 10. The nurse practitioner instructs the patient that Kegel exercises should be done consistently every day at what frequency?

A) Perform 30 exercises each time in the morning and the evening
B) Perform 20 exercises each time two times a day
C) Perform 15 exercises each time three to four times a day
D) Perform 10 exercises each time three times a day

573. A 19-year-old student who is on a prescription of combined oral contraceptive pills is being seen for an annual gynecological exam in the college health center. The nurse practitioner has obtained the Pap smear and is about to perform the bimanual exam. She gently removes the plastic speculum from the vagina. While the NP is performing the bimanual vaginal exam, the patient complains of slight discomfort during deep palpation of the ovaries. Which of the following is a true statement?

A) The uterus and the ovaries are both very sensitive to any type of palpation
B) The fallopian tubes and ovaries are not sensitive to light or deep palpation
C) The ovaries are sensitive to deep palpation but they should not be painful
D) The uterus and the ovaries are not important organs of reproduction

574. All of the following statements about common health beliefs of many traditional Asian cultures are true except:

A) An imbalance of the hot and cold (yin/yang) vital forces can cause illness, and treating a hot disease with a "cold" treatment (i.e., certain foods/herbs) can help to restore balance and cure the illness
B) If the patient is very ill or dying, immediate family and extended family members will visit the patient daily in shifts to provide emotional support
C) Infants and small children may wear an amulet such as a red string on the wrist or a piece of cloth on the neck or the wrist
D) Surgical procedures are regarded as important treatment for many illnesses

575. A 45-year-old gardener is seen as a walk-in patient in a private clinic. He reports stepping on a nail that morning. His last tetanus vaccine was 7 years ago. Which of the following vaccines is recommended?

A) DTaP
B) DT
C) Td
D) Tdap

576. Acanthosis nigricans is associated with all of the following disorders except:

A) Obesity
B) Diabetes
C) Colon cancer
D) Tinea versicolor

577. The nurse practitioner suspects that a middle-aged woman may have systemic lupus erythematosus (SLE). Which of the following laboratory tests is most specific for this disease?

A) Erythrocyte sedimentation rate (ESR)
B) C-reactive protein (CRP)
C) Antinuclear antibody (ANA)
D) IgG antibody

578. An elderly Hmong patient, who is originally from Thailand, is seen by the nurse practitioner for a follow-up visit. He is accompanied by his eldest daughter. The patient presented 6 weeks ago with complaints of the recent onset of morning headaches. He was diagnosed with stage 2 hypertension and prescribed hydrochlorothiazide, one 25-mg tablet daily. On this visit, he tells the nurse practitioner that the new medicine cured the headache, so he stopped taking it. What is the best plan to follow during this visit?

A) Educate the patient about hypertension, how the medicine works on his body, and the importance of taking his pill daily
B) Reassure the patient that he can resume his prescription medicine again the next morning
C) Tell the patient that you will lower the dosage of hydrochlorothiazide to 12.5 mg daily
D) Speak to the patient in a loud voice and confront him about his behavior

579. A 68-year-old woman has recently been diagnosed with polymyalgia rheumatica. The nurse practitioner is discussing the treatment options with the patient. Which of the following medications is the first-line treatment for this condition?

A) Etanercept (Enbrel)
B) Oral prednisone
C) Indomethacin
D) Methotrexate

580. Which of the following is a true statement regarding the first-pass metabolism process?

A) Drugs that are administered by intramuscular injection all go through the process of first-pass metabolism
B) After being swallowed, oral drugs are absorbed by the GI tract and metabolized by the bacteria in the small intestines before being released into the general circulation
C) Drugs administered through the skin (patches) are metabolized by the dermis of the skin
D) After a drug is taken by the oral route, it is absorbed in the small intestines and enters the liver through the portal circulation, where it is metabolized before being released into the general circulation

581. What is the best description of Cullen's sign?

A) The onset of hyperactive bowel sound before the onset of ileus
B) A reddish-purple discoloration that is located on the flank area
C) A bluish discoloration or bruising that is located on the umbilical area
D) The acute onset of subcutaneous bleeding seen during acute pancreatitis

582. Glucosamine sulfate is a natural supplement that is used for which of the following conditions?

A) Rheumatoid arthritis
B) Osteoarthritis
C) Osteoporosis
D) Metabolic syndrome

583. A charitable foundation plans to build a community youth center in a large urban area with a history of gang violence. What type of health prevention activity is being done in this area?

A) Primary prevention
B) Secondary prevention
C) Tertiary prevention
D) Health prevention

584. The bacillus Calmette-Guérin (BCG) vaccine is used to immunize a person against which of the following?

A) Enterobiasis
B) Tuberculosis
C) Anthrax
D) Smallpox

585. A 13-year-old girl is brought by her mother to the health clinic because the girl is complaining of vaginal discharge and pain. The mother tells the nurse practitioner that her daughter is not sexually active yet. The mother is divorced, lives with her boyfriend, and works full time. During the exam, the nurse practitioner notes that the vaginal introitus is red, with tears and a torn hymen. The cervix is covered with green discharge. The nurse practitioner suspects that the child has been sexually abused by the mother's boyfriend. What is the best action for the nurse practitioner to take?

A) Ask the mother questions about her boyfriend's behaviors
B) Advise the mother to watch how her boyfriend interacts with her daughter and to call within 1 week to discuss his behavior with her
C) Advise the mother that you suspect that her daughter has been sexually abused
D) Report the child abuse to the department of child protective services

586. A 75-year-old woman presents complaining of a soft lump on her abdomen that is located on the periumbilical area. She tells the nurse practitioner that she does not know how long she has had the lump or whether it has changed in size or shape. She denies abdominal pain, problems with defecation, loss of appetite, weight loss, or trauma. When performing an abdominal exam, what is the best method to differentiate an abdominal wall mass from an intra-abdominal mass?

A) Palpate the abdominal wall while the patient is relaxed
B) Instruct the patient to lift her head off the table while tensing her abdominal muscles to visualize any masses and then palpate the abdominal wall
C) Instruct the patient to lie still for a few seconds while you palpate the abdominal wall
D) Palpate the abdomen deeply, then release the palpating hand quickly

587. Which of the following structures of the eyes is responsible for color vision?

A) Rods
B) Macula
C) Cones
D) Pupils

588. A new patient is being interviewed by the nurse practitioner. The patient reports that she had a gastrectomy procedure 5 years ago to treat severe obesity. Currently, her body mass index (BMI) is 25 and the patient denies complications from the procedure. The nurse practitioner is aware that the patient is at higher risk for which of the following disorders?

A) Folate deficiency anemia
B) B_{12}-deficiency anemia
C) Iron-deficiency anemia
D) Normocytic anemia

589. Which of the following is a precursor lesion of squamous cell skin cancer?

A) Basal cell skin cancer
B) Squamous cell skin cancer
C) Melanoma
D) Actinic keratosis

590. What is the median?

A) It is the number that occurs most frequently
B) It is the middle number in a group of numbers
C) It is the average number in a group of numbers
D) It a measure of central tendency

591. Which of the following is a good example of how the "utilitarian" principle is applied?

A) Helping a patient decide the type of treatment that he or she wants
B) Using limited societal financial resources on programs that will positively affect the largest number of people and have the lowest possible negative outcomes
C) Minimizing the bad outcome when offering treatment choices to a patient
D) Being more careful when using health care financial resources for any purpose

592. All of the following clinical findings are major or minor criteria for pelvic inflammatory disease (PID). Which of the following is classified as a minor criterion that is not required for diagnosis of PID?

A) Cervical motion tenderness
B) Adnexal tenderness
C) Uterine tenderness
D) Oral temperature >101°F (>38°C)

593. Which structure of the eye is responsible for 20/20 vision (sharpest vision)?

A) Rods
B) Cones
C) Optic disc
D) Fovea of the macula

594. A nurse practitioner, who is a recent graduate, is asking an experienced nurse practitioner's opinion about managing a patient who has multiple health problems. What type of relationship exists between the nurse practitioners?

A) Collaborative relationship
B) Consultative relationship
C) Referral relationship
D) Formal relationship

595. A 15-year-old girl who attends a public school is referred to the nurse practitioner by one of her teachers. The teen's parents are recently divorced. The teen has been missing school and is falling behind in her schoolwork. After closing the exam room door, the nurse practitioner starts to interview the teen, asking about her moods, her appetite, her sleep, whether she has any plan of hurting herself or others, and other questions. In what type of health prevention activity is the nurse practitioner engaging?

A) Primary prevention
B) Secondary prevention
C) Tertiary prevention
D) Dropout prevention program

596. All of the following signs and symptoms are present with an anticholinergic drug overdose except:

A) Dilated pupils
B) Flushing and tachycardia
C) Hypertension
D) Confusion

597. A woman who is in the third trimester of pregnancy presents to the nurse practitioner for a physical exam. During the physical exam, the nurse practitioner finds all of the following cardiac changes associated with pregnancy except:

A) Systolic ejection murmur
B) Diastolic murmur
C) Displaced apical impulse
D) Louder S1 and S2

598. An 80-year-old man with hypertension and hyperlipidemia presents with complaints of the rapid onset of severe low-back pain accompanied by abdominal pain that is gradually worsening. The patient appears pale and complains that he does not feel well. During the abdominal exam, the nurse practitioner detects a soft pulsatile mass just above the umbilicus as she palpates this area with her hand. Which of the following conditions is most likely?

A) Abdominal aortic aneurysm
B) Cauda equina syndrome
C) Acute diverticulitis
D) Adenocarcinoma of the colon

599. What is the pedigree symbol for a diseased or affected female?

A) An empty square
B) An empty circle
C) A filled-in square
D) A filled-in circle

600. The gold-standard test for visualizing a torn meniscus or joint abnormalities is the:

A) Computed tomography (CT) scan
B) Magnetic resonance imaging (MRI) scan
C) X-ray with special views of the affected knee
D) Lachman's maneuver

601. A research participant tells the nurse practitioner that he wants to withdraw from the study. Regarding this case, the nurse practitioner is aware that all research study consent forms should contain which of the following information?

A) The patient's demographic information
B) The possible risks of the study
C) Information that a research subject can voluntarily withdraw from the study at any time without any penalties or adverse consequences
D) The benefits from the study

602. All of the following factors are associated with a higher risk of osteopenia and osteoporosis except:

A) Excessive alcohol intake and cigarette smoking
B) Asian or Caucasian ancestry
C) Obesity
D) Older age

603. A skilled nursing facility (SNF) can provide all of the following except:

A) Physical therapy and other types of rehabilitation
B) Skilled nursing care and medical care
C) Reimbursement by Medicare
D) Provision of custodial care

604. All of the following are classified as activities of daily living (ADL) except:

A) Ability to feed self (self-feeding)
B) Ability to manage bladder and bowel elimination
C) Personal hygiene and grooming
D) Grocery shopping

605. A positive psoas and obturator sign is highly suggestive of which of the following conditions?

A) Ectopic pregnancy
B) Acute appendicitis
C) Peritonitis
D) Abdominal aortic aneurysm

606. All of the following are true statements about sexuality in the older adult except:

A) Erectile dysfunction is very common
B) It may take longer to become aroused
C) The elderly are no longer interested in sexuality
D) Dyspareunia is a common symptom of atrophic vaginitis

607. Which of the following drugs is most likely to cause sexual dysfunction in males?

A) Selective serotonin reuptake inhibitors (SSRIs)
B) Angiotensin-converting enzyme (ACE) inhibitors
C) Amphetamines
D) Atypical antidepressants

608. Which of the following drugs is classified as a 5-alpha reductase inhibitor?

A) Terazosin (Hytrin)
B) Tamsulosin (Flomax)
C) Finasteride (Proscar)
D) Sildenafil (Viagra)

609. One of the developmental milestones for this age group is the ability to draw a stick-figure "person" with six separate body parts. What is the age group that this finding is associated with?

A) 3-year-olds
B) 4-year-olds
C) 5-year-olds
D) 6-year-olds

610. When does an infant triple its birth weight?

A) 3 months
B) 6 months
C) 12 months
D) 15 months

611. Grey–Turner's sign is highly suggestive of which of the following conditions?

A) Acute pancreatitis
B) Acute appendicitis
C) Acute diverticulitis
D) Gastric cancer

612. A nurse practitioner is writing a referral for a middle-aged diabetic who has an A1C of 8.5% despite being on three antidiabetic medications. She is referring the patient to an endocrinologist. What type of relationship exists between the nurse practitioner and the endocrinologist?

A) Consultative relationship
B) Collaborative relationship
C) Referral relationship
D) Formal relationship

613. Which bacterium is the most common pathogen seen in otitis externa infections?

A) *Pseudomonas aeruginosa*
B) *Streptococcus pyogenes*
C) *Haemophilus influenzae*
D) *Moraxella catarrhalis*

614. The Patient Protection and Affordable Care Act, enacted into law under President Obama, sought to expand health insurance coverage for Americans. All of the following are true statements about this law except:

A) Preexisting health conditions cannot be used to exclude individuals from obtaining coverage
B) The health plan ensures that all Americans have health insurance coverage
C) Young adults up to the age of 26 years who live with their parents are covered under their parents' health insurance plan
D) Employers who choose not to participate in the national health insurance plan are fined

615. All of the following are considered instrumental activities of daily living (IADL) except:

A) Grocery shopping
B) Managing one's finances
C) Grooming and hygiene
D) Using a telephone and a computer

616. The Rinne and the Weber tests are used to assess which of the following cranial nerves (CNs)?

A) CNs III, IV, and VI
B) CN VII
C) CN VIII
D) CNs IX and X

617. A 68-year-old woman complains of leaking a small amount of urine whenever she sneezes, laughs, and/or strains. The problem has been present for many months. The patient denies dysuria, frequency, and nocturia. The urine dipstick test is negative for white blood cells, red blood cells, ketones, and urobilinogen. What is the name of this condition?

A) Urge incontinence
B) Overflow incontinence
C) Urinary incontinence
D) Stress incontinence

618. Medicare Part D reimburses for which of the following services?

A) Preventive health care such as routine Pap smears and physical exams
B) Prescription drugs
C) Alcohol misuse/abuse counseling
D) Over-the-counter drugs and vitamins

619. A 35-year-old woman is complaining of gradual weight gain, lack of energy, and amenorrhea. The urine pregnancy test is negative. A complete blood count (CBC) shows hemoglobin of 13.5 g/dL and mean corpuscular volume (MCV) of 84 fL. The nurse practitioner suspects that the patient may have hypothyroidism. The thyroid-stimulating hormone (TSH) level is 10 mU/L. Which of the following is the next step in the evaluation?

A) Check the thyroid profile
B) Check the total T3 level
C) Check the FSH level
D) Recheck the TSH in 4 to 6 months

620. During a routine physical exam of an 82-year-old woman, the nurse practitioner palpates an irregular mass on the midabdomen that is not tender and is about 2 cm in size. Which of the following is the best initial imaging test to further evaluate the abdominal mass?

A) CT scan of the abdomen
B) KUB study
C) Abdominal ultrasound
D) MRI of the abdomen

621. A male adolescent presents to the nurse practitioner for a wellness exam. The patient's face is long and narrow with a prominent forehead and chin, and he has large ears. The mother reports that her son has intellectual disabilities and autistic disorder. Which of the following conditions is being described?

A) Fragile X disorder
B) Marfan's syndrome
C) Turner's syndrome
D) Down syndrome

622. A chest radiograph is included in this question. What condition is associated with the findings in this radiograph?

A) Atypical pneumonia
B) Tuberculosis
C) Bacterial pneumonia
D) Viral pneumonia

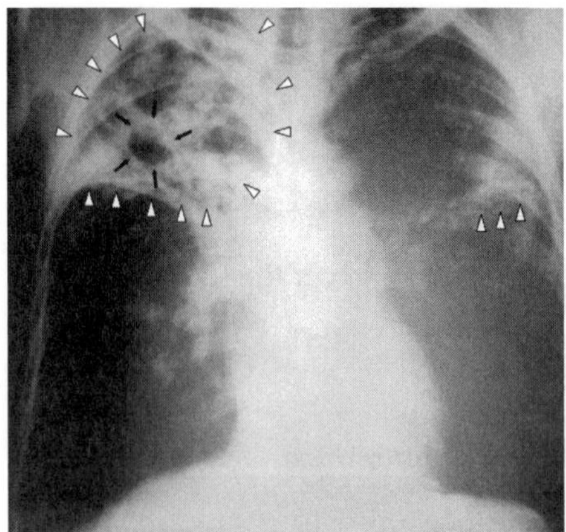

Source: Centers for Disease Control and Prevention.

623. Which area of the lung is the most common location of a *Mycobacterium tuberculosis* infection?

A) Lower lobes
B) Left lower lobe
C) Right middle lobe
D) Upper lobes

624. An 18-year-old college student, who is sexually active, wants to start taking birth control pills. The nurse practitioner at the college health clinic explains the risks and benefits of combined oral contraceptives to the patient. All of the following are appropriate laboratory tests for this patient except:

A) Chlamydia test
B) Gonorrhea test
C) HIV test
D) Pap smear

625. A 40-year-old female nurse is seen in the employee health office for an employment physical exam. She is a recent immigrant and reports a history of bacillus Calmette-Guérin (BCG) vaccination. Which of the following is recommended by the Centers for Disease Control and Prevention for tuberculosis testing of persons with a history of BCG vaccination?

A) Purified protein derivative (PPD) test
B) Mantoux test
C) Serum interferon-gamma release assay (IGRA)
D) Chest radiograph

626. Thiazolidinediones are contraindicated in which of the following patient populations?

A) Alcoholic patients
B) Heart failure patients
C) Obese patients
D) Elderly patients

627. According to the U.S. Preventive Services Task Force, which of the following tests should be used to screen for lung cancer?

A) Chest radiograph
B) Bronchoscopy with biopsy
C) Low-dose computed tomography (LDCT)
D) Sputum for cytology

628. Which of the following laboratory test results meet the diagnostic criteria for prediabetes?

A) Fasting plasma glucose of 79 mg/dL
B) A1C of 5.9%
C) Random blood glucose of 200 mg/dL with polyuria, polydipsia, and polyphagia
D) Random blood glucose of 200 mg/dL

629. A 38-year-old male veteran is diagnosed with posttraumatic stress disorder (PTSD). He attends group therapy sessions once per week, but reports that his symptoms remain the same. He is requesting treatment for his condition. Which of the following is the first-line medication for PTSD?

A) Selective serotonin reuptake inhibitors (SSRIs)
B) Benzodiazepines
C) Tricyclic antidepressants (TCAs)
D) Selective norepinephrine reuptake inhibitors (SNRIs)

630. While performing a funduscopic exam, the nurse practitioner notices arteriovenous (AV) nicking on the patient's retina. What causes AV nicking?

A) It is caused by an arteriole crossing a venule, which compresses the venule and causes it to bulge on each side
B) It is associated with diabetic retinopathy
C) It is caused by a copper wire arteriole that becomes distended
D) It occurs when the optic disc becomes ischemic

631. A new mother is planning to breastfeed her newborn infant for at least 6 months. She wants to know whether she should give the infant vitamins. Which of the following vitamin supplements is recommended by the American Academy of Pediatrics (APA) during the first few days of life?

A) Vitamin D drops
B) Vitamin E drops
C) It is not necessary to give breastfed infants vitamin supplements because breast milk contains enough vitamins and minerals that are necessary for the infant's growth and development
D) Folic acid drops

632. A sexually active 16-year-old girl is brought by her mother for a physical exam. During the exam, the nurse practitioner notices some bruises on both breasts. All of the following are important areas to evaluate in this patient during this visit except:

A) Depression
B) Tanner stage
C) Sexual history
D) Sexually transmitted diseases (STDs)

633. The mother of a 12-month-old infant reports to the nurse practitioner that her child had a high fever for several days, which spontaneously resolved. After the fever resolved, the child developed a maculopapular rash. Which of the following is the most likely diagnosis?

A) Fifth disease (erythema infectiosum)
B) Roseola infantum (exanthema subitum)
C) Varicella
D) Infantile maculopapular rashes

634. A 13-year-old boy is brought in by his mother for a physical exam. During the genital exam, the nurse practitioner notices that the patient is at Tanner stage II. Which of the following is the best description of this Tanner stage?

A) The penis is growing more in length than in width and the testicles become larger with darker scrotal skin and the pubic hair is starting to curl
B) The penis is growing more in width than in length with darker scrotal skin and more numerous pubic hairs that are darker, curly, and more coarse
C) The testicles become larger and the skin of the scrotum starts to become darker with straight, fine, countable hairs on the genitals and the axilla
D) The testicles and penile width and length are developing quickly

635. An 8-year-old child is seen as a walk-in appointment by the nurse practitioner. The mother reports that her child has been febrile for 2 days and is not eating well due to painful sores inside the mouth. The child's temperature is 101°F, pulse is 88 beats/min, and respirations are 14 breaths/min. During the physical exam, the nurse practitioner notices several small blisters and shallow ulcers on the child's pharynx and the oral mucosa. The child has small round red rashes on both palms and soles. Which of the following conditions is most likely?

A) Herpes simplex infection
B) Hand, foot, and mouth disease (HFMD)
C) Varicella infection
D) Secondary syphilis infection

636. According to Erik Erikson, adolescents are at what psychosocial developmental stage?

A) Autonomy versus shame
B) Industry versus inferiority
C) Identity versus role confusion
D) Intimacy versus isolation

637. At what age can a child ride a bicycle?

A) 2 to 3 years of age
B) 3 to 4 years of age
C) 4 to 5 years of age
D) 5 to 6 years of age

638. When an infant is found to have tufts of fine dark hair on the sacrum, which of the following tests is recommended?

A) Ultrasound of the sacrum
B) Plain radiograph of the lumbar sacral spine
C) No imaging test is necessary
D) Genetic testing

639. All of the following are true statements about the human papillomavirus vaccine (Gardasil) except:

A) The Centers for Disease Control and Prevention (CDC) recommends the first dose at age 11 to 12 years
B) The CDC does not recommend the HPV vaccine for males
C) For children younger than age 14 years, only two doses of the vaccine are needed
D) The minimum age at which the vaccine can be given is 9 years

640. According to *Diagnostic and Statistical Manual of Mental Disorders* (*DSM-5*), some of the following criteria must be present to diagnose a child with autistic disorder. Which criterion is incorrect?

A) Onset of symptoms before age 3 years
B) Lack of social interaction or social reciprocity
C) Stereotyped and repetitive movements such as hand flapping
D) Depressed affect

641. A middle-aged male smoker with chronic gastroesophageal reflux disease (GERD) was diagnosed with Barrett's esophagus 5 years ago. He is being seen by the nurse practitioner for a physical exam. The patient reports that he ran out of his proton-pump inhibitor (PPI) medication and he has not taken it for 5 days. He is complaining of severe episodes of daily heartburn. His gastroenterologist is out of town for 1 week. Which of the following is the best plan to follow during this visit?

A) Write a prescription for the same PPI and give a 1-week supply without refills
B) Give the patient free samples of an H2 blocker
C) Prescribe another PPI because worsening of symptoms is a sign that the previously prescribed PPI is not effective
D) Advise the patient to take over-the-counter antacids PRN

642. Which of the following murmurs can radiate to the neck?

A) Mitral stenosis
B) Mitral regurgitation
C) Aortic regurgitation
D) Aortic stenosis

643. What is the most common type of cancer in young children?

A) Acute lymphoblastic leukemia
B) Multiple myeloma
C) Aplastic anemia
D) Non-Hodgkin's lymphoma

644. A 4-week–old boy is seen in the family practice clinic for a complaint of forceful vomiting that occurs immediately after feeding. The vomitus is composed of infant formula and is not bilious. The infant is bottle-fed with infant formula that was recommended by the pediatrician. The mother reports that the infant seems hungry and sucks on the bottle without any problems. His birth weight was 7 lbs, 5 oz (3.4 kg). The current weight is 7 lbs (3.2 kg). Which of the following clinical findings is an important clue regarding the possible cause of the infant's vomiting?

A) Irritable and crying infant
B) Sunken anterior fontanel and dry lips
C) Positive rooting reflex
D) Round olive-like mass located in the right upper quadrant of the abdomen

645. What is the most powerful known risk factor for the development of active tuberculosis?

A) Asthma
B) HIV infection
C) Chronic obstructive pulmonary disease
D) Chronic bronchitis

646. The Ishihara chart is useful for evaluating which of the following conditions?

A) Nystagmus
B) Esodeviation
C) Color blindness
D) Strabismus

647. At what level is the uterine fundus at 12 weeks gestation?

A) At the height of the symphysis pubis
B) Between the symphysis pubis and the umbilicus
C) At the level of the umbilicus
D) It depends on the size of the fetus

648. Which of the following medications is associated with the highest incidence of erectile dysfunction?

A) Lamotrigine (Lamictal)
B) Clonazepam (Klonopin)
C) Paroxetine (Paxil)
D) Doxepin (Sinequan)

649. All of the following signs and/or symptoms are seen in patients with rhabdomyolysis except:

A) Myalgias and generalized weakness
B) Bone pain
C) Muscles that are tender on palpation
D) Dark-colored urine

650. Which condition is caused by trauma to the blood vessels located in Kiesselbach's triangle?

A) Posterior epistaxis
B) Subdural hematoma
C) Anterior epistaxis
D) Stroke

651. Infection of the skin and mucous membranes with human papillomavirus (HPV) is associated with an increased risk of certain types of cancers. All of the following cancers are associated with HPV infection except:

A) Oropharyngeal cancer
B) Anal cancer
C) Basal cell carcinoma
D) Penile cancer

652. A 78-year-old woman's dual-energy x-ray absorptiometry (DEXA) scan yields a T-score of −2.8. Which of the following pharmacological options is preferred for treating this condition?

A) Selective estrogen receptor modulators (SERMs)
B) Bisphosphonates
C) Hormone replacement therapy
D) Calcium with vitamin D

653. What type of infection is caused by the human parvovirus B19?

A) Fifth disease
B) Roseola infantum
C) Condyloma acuminata
D) Scarlet fever

654. All of the following viruses can infect the fetus and/or the mother during pregnancy. Which of the following viruses is not associated with serious sequelae?

A) Human parvovirus B19
B) Varicella
C) Rubella
D) Rhinovirus

655. Which of the following is the preferred treatment for an enterobiasis infection?

A) Wash clothes and bedsheets with hot water
B) Strict handwashing after using the toilet
C) Albendazole (Albenza)
D) Fluconazole (Diflucan) oral

656. Which of the following human papillomavirus (HPV) strains is associated with cervical cancer?

A) HPV subtypes 12 and 14
B) HPV subtypes 16 and 18
C) HPV subtypes 20 and 26
D) HPV subtype 30

657. A 6-year-old girl who attends preschool part time is brought to the clinic by her mother as a walk-in patient. The mother reports that her daughter has recently begun swim lessons. The symptoms began as redness on the left eye and spread to the second eye within 2 days. The child's eyes are watery and crusted in the morning when she wakes up. Her vital signs are temperature of 98.8°F, pulse of 90 beats/min, and respirations of 16 breaths/min. The eye exam reveals bilateral injected conjunctiva. When the lower eyelid is examined, the nurse practitioner notes that it is pink with a cobblestone appearance. There is ipsilateral preauricular adenopathy. All of the following treatment measures are appropriate except:

A) Prescribe a topical ophthalmic vasoconstrictor to be used two times per day as needed for up to 3 days to reduce redness
B) Write a note excusing the child from school because she should not attend until the symptoms resolve
C) Prescribe ophthalmic topical antibiotic eye drops, two to three drops to be applied in each eye QID for 7 days
D) Advise use of cool compress over closed eyes as needed for comfort, washing hands often with soap and water, and to avoid rubbing eyes or sharing towels

658. All of the following physiological changes may occur in the third trimester of pregnancy except:

A) Chadwick's sign
B) S3 heart sound
C) Mild edema of ankles and hands
D) Increase in urinary frequency

659. Which of the following drug classes is associated with rhabdomyolysis?

A) Biguanides
B) Thiazolidinediones
C) Tetracyclines
D) HMG-CoA reductase inhibitors

660. What type of murmur can radiate to the left axilla?

A) Aortic regurgitation
B) Aortic stenosis
C) Mitral stenosis
D) Mitral regurgitation

661. A middle-aged man with a body mass index (BMI) of 28 is complaining of sharp burning pain that starts at the middle of the right buttock and radiates down the posterior aspect of the thigh and lower leg. He is complaining of weakness of the ankle and foot that is interfering with walking. The pain started 3 months ago and is becoming more frequent and severe. It is aggravated by prolonged sitting, which is interfering with his job as a truck driver. His past medical history is positive for hypertension and metabolic syndrome. The patient is taking lisinopril–hydrochlorothiazide (Zestoretic) 10 mg/12.5 mg once a day. Which of the following tests is appropriate to further evaluate the patient's symptoms?

A) Straight leg raising test
B) McMurray test
C) Lachman test
D) Markle test

662. A 16-year-old male patient with psoriasis is scratching and rubbing one of the psoriatic plaques located on his right elbow. Fine silvery scales with pinpoint areas of bleeding are noted on the plaque. What is the name of this clinical finding?

A) Erosion
B) Lichenification
C) Auspitz sign
D) Koebner phenomenon

663. A 36-year–old woman complains of fatigue and headaches accompanied by widespread muscle and joint pain that started 6 months ago. She reports insomnia and feeling tired even with adequate sleep. She was diagnosed with major depression 1 year ago and is currently on escitalopram (Lexapro) 20 mg PO daily. She is also taking B-complex vitamins and melatonin at bedtime for sleep. During the physical exam, the nurse practitioner notes bilateral areas of tender points on the neck, jaw, shoulders, chest, upper back, and greater trochanter. The symptoms and physical exam findings are highly suggestive of which condition?

A) Rheumatoid arthritis
B) Osteoarthritis
C) Fatigue syndrome
D) Fibromyalgia

664. Which of the following conditions is considered a radiculopathy?

A) Polymyalgia rheumatica
B) Sciatica
C) Stroke
D) Dementia

665. An adult man with a large subungual hematoma on one of his big toes presents as a walk-in patient. What is the best method of treating this condition?

A) Cold pack to the area three to four times daily for the next 24 to 48 hours
B) Naproxen sodium (Aleve) one to two tablets PO twice per day
C) Trephination using a large paperclip or 18-gauge needle
D) Cryotherapy of the affected area

666. A 42-year-old obese White man presents to the clinic with a history of recurrent heartburn. He is diagnosed by the nurse practitioner with gastroesophageal reflux disease (GERD). Which of the following drug classes is preferred initially to treat symptoms of GERD?

A) Histamine-2 receptor antagonist
B) Proton-pump inhibitor
C) Antibiotic
D) Antiviral

667. Which of the following symptoms in an older male patient with a history of gastroesophageal reflux disease is most worrisome?

A) Chronic heartburn
B) Recurrent regurgitation of sour-tasting food
C) Hoarseness and sore throat
D) Odynophagia and early satiety

668. A 4-year-old boy diagnosed with acute otitis media returns in 48 hours with a possible rupture of the tympanic membrane (TM) of the right ear. The mother reports seeing pus and a small amount of blood on the pillow that morning. The child states that his ear is no longer painful. During the ear exam, the otoscope is used to visualize the TM, which has a perforation on the lower edge that is draining a small amount of purulent discharge. All of the following topical ear medications should be avoided in patients with perforation of the TM except:

A) Gentamycin ear drops
B) Ofloxacin ear drops
C) Tobramycin ear drops
D) Neomycin sulfate ear drops

669. A preschool girl who is homeschooled is brought by her mother to the walk-in clinic because of acute onset of fever, runny nose, cough, sore throat, and red eyes with a morbilliform rash. The mother reports that her daughter has never been immunized. The family recently returned from a vacation. Which of the following conditions is the most likely?

A) Rubella
B) Varicella

C) Fifth disease
D) Rubeola

670. Abrupt loss of consciousness accompanied by generalized tonic–clonic seizures followed by a postictal period characterize what type of seizure disorder?

A) Absence seizure
B) Grand mal seizure
C) Atonic seizure
D) Myoclonic seizure

671. A 22-year-old woman who is a member of the track team is seen by the nurse practitioner in the college health clinic with a complaint of "shin splints." She states that she has recurrent localized pain on the anterior aspect of the left shin that is aggravated by running and jumping. She recently increased the intensity of her training schedule because she is planning to participate in a local marathon. During the physical examination, the nurse notes a focal area of tenderness on the anterior medial aspect of the left tibia. Which of the following conditions is most likely?

A) Medial tibial stress fracture
B) Morton's neuroma
C) Acute tendinitis
D) Osgood–Schlatter disease

672. What type of cast is used to stabilize a fracture of the scaphoid bone?

A) Long arm cast
B) Thumb spica cast
C) Short leg cast
D) Leg cylinder cast

673. A plain chest radiograph is included in this question. What is your diagnosis?

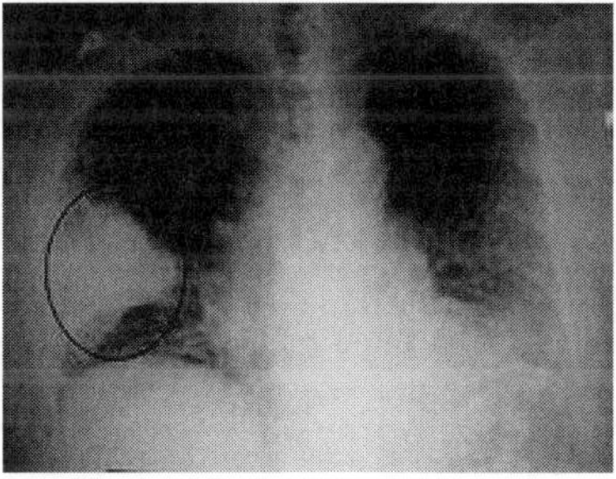

Source: Wikimedia. James Heilman.

A) Right lobe atelectasis
B) Right upper lobe pneumonia
C) Right middle lobe pneumonia
D) Right lower lobe pneumonia

674. A 36-year-old woman is seen by the nurse practitioner for a Pap smear and gynecological exam. The patient is of Ashkenazi Jewish ethnicity. Her mother died of breast cancer at age 50 years. Her 57-year-old sister has recently been diagnosed with breast cancer. The breast exam is negative for a dominant mass and the axillae do not contain any masses. All of the following are appropriate measures for this patient except:

A) Mammogram and MRI of the breast
B) Referral to a breast specialist
C) Check serum carcinoembryonic antigen (CEA) and cancer antigen (CA) 125 levels
D) Genetic counseling and *BRCA* testing

675. A 20-year-old woman reports that for several years, she has had random episodes of palpitations and shortness of breath that resolve spontaneously. She denies chest pain, arm pain, and syncope. Her past medical and family histories are negative for coronary artery disease, stroke, or lung disease. During the cardiac exam, the nurse practitioner notices a grade 3/6 murmur that is accompanied by a mid-systolic click, which is heard best heard at the apical area. The apical pulse is 78 beats/min, blood pressure is 120/60 mmHg, and temperature is 98.6°F. The cardiac exam is highly suggestive of which of the following conditions?

A) Mitral valve prolapse
B) Aortic stenosis
C) Atrial septal defect
D) Pulmonary regurgitation

Questions 676 and 677 apply to this case. A 17-year-old high school student is diagnosed by the nurse practitioner with serous otitis media of the left ear. He states that his nose is always congested because of dust mite allergy. His medical history includes allergic rhinitis and asthma.

676. What is the expected result of the Rinne test in patients who have serous otitis media of the left ear?

A) Air conduction (AC) > bone conduction (BC)
B) Bone conduction (BC) > air conduction (AC)
C) Lateralization to the left ear
D) Sound is heard by both ears

677. The student reports a history of chronic nasal congestion. He occasionally has fits of sneezing when he is in a dusty room. The nurse practitioner is using an otoscope to examine his nasal tissue. The inferior nasal turbinates appear swollen and pale. Which of the following medications is considered first-line treatment for allergic rhinitis?

A) Azelastine (Astelin) one to two sprays in each nostril twice a day
B) Saline nasal spray one to two sprays in each nostril four times a day as needed
C) Cetirizine (Zyrtec) one 5-mg tablet PO at bedtime
D) Budesonide (Rhinocort) one to two sprays in each nostril twice a day

678. All of the following medications can cause insomnia except:

A) Sertraline (Zoloft)
B) Pseudoephedrine (Sudafed)
C) Theophylline (Theo-Dur)
D) Alprazolam (Xanax)

679. Which of the following is the best method to diagnose a vaginal trichomonas infection?

A) Whiff test
B) Potassium hydroxide (KOH) test
C) Wet smear with microscopy
D) Culture

680. All of the following conditions are more common in the geriatric population except:

A) Macular degeneration
B) Osteoporosis
C) Parkinson's disease
D) Acute otitis media

681. All of the following medications have drug interactions with levothyroxine (Synthroid) except:

A) Antacids
B) Tricyclic antidepressants
C) Anticoagulants
D) Penicillins

682. Which of the following is considered an abnormal finding?

A) A "clunk" sound heard while performing the Ortolani maneuver
B) A 6-month-old infant who starts to babble
C) A 10-year-old boy with aching pain on the front of the thighs that starts in late afternoon or at night
D) A 12-month-old who is "cruising"

683. An obese middle-aged man with type 2 diabetes is diagnosed with familial hypercholesterolemia. During the physical exam, the nurse practitioner notices that the patient has raised, sharply demarcated yellowish patches on the inner canthi of both eyes and on the upper and lower eyelids that are symmetrical and nontender. Which of the following conditions is being described?

A) Psoriasis
B) Warts
C) Xerosis cutis
D) Xanthelasma

684. Bouchard's nodes are associated with which of the following conditions?

A) Osteoarthritis and rheumatoid arthritis
B) Osteoporosis and osteopenia
C) Degenerative joint disease
D) Autoimmune disorders

685. Which is a true statement regarding occurrence-based malpractice insurance policies?

A) If the insurance company's lawyer finds the nurse practitioner negligent, it is the nurse's responsibility to pay for the claim
B) Claims against the nurse practitioner are covered as long as the nurse had an active malpractice policy at the time of the incident
C) Claims against the nurse practitioner are usually paid if the nurse is found not to be negligent
D) Claims against the nurse practitioner are covered if the malpractice insurance is in effect when the lawsuit is filed

686. According to Maslow's hierarchy of needs, an 80-year-old grandmother who is knitting scarves for her grandchildren would be fulfilling which of the following needs?

A) Safety and security
B) Self-actualization
C) Self-esteem
D) Love and belonging

687. An 88-year-old woman with a history of hypertension, osteoarthritis, and high cholesterol complains to the nurse practitioner of an episode of weakness in her left arm that slowly progressed to her left leg. It was accompanied by dizziness and slurred speech. She has had the same symptoms before, and each time they resolved within several hours. Which of the following conditions is most likely?

A) Cerebrovascular accident (CVA)
B) Acute vertigo
C) Multiple sclerosis (MS)
D) Transient ischemic attack (TIA)

688. Which of the following regimens is known as "triple therapy" for treating a *Helicobacter pylori* infection?

A) Metronidazole (Flagyl) BID, doxycycline BID, and omeprazole (Prilosec) daily
B) Bismuth subsalicylate (Pepto-Bismol) tablets QID, metronidazole (Flagyl) QID, azithromycin (Zithromax), and cimetidine (Tagamet) daily
C) Amoxicillin BID, sulfamethoxazole–trimethoprim (Bactrim DS) BID, and ranitidine (Zantac) daily
D) Clarithromycin (Biaxin) BID, amoxicillin BID, and omeprazole (Prilosec) daily

689. A 90-year-old woman is diagnosed with isolated systolic hypertension of the elderly. Which of the following antihypertensive medications are preferred for the treatment of this condition?

A) Calcium channel blockers and thiazide diuretics
B) Angiotensin-converting enzyme inhibitors and loop diuretics
C) Beta-blockers and potassium-sparing diuretics
D) Alpha-blockers and calcium channel blockers

690. A photograph of a skin lesion is included in this question. (This image can be found in color in the app.) What is the patient's diagnosis?

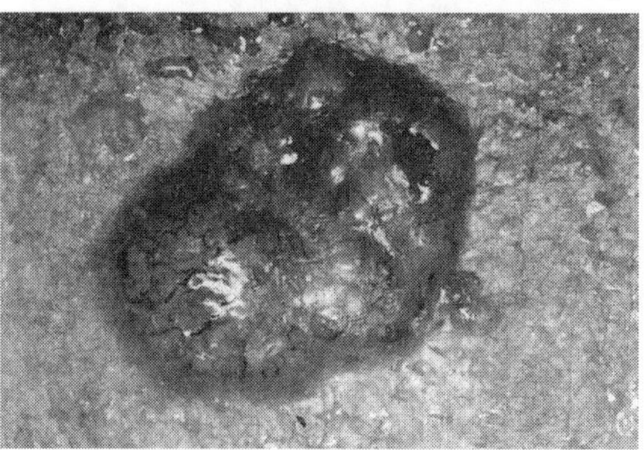

Source: Courtesy of John Hendrix.

A) Nevus
B) Melanoma
C) Basal cell carcinoma
D) Squamous cell carcinoma

691. The cytology (Pap smear) results for a 35-year-old woman reveal a high-grade squamous intraepithelial lesion (HSIL) of the cervix. The human papillomavirus (HPV) test is positive for the type 16 strain. Rate the three actions to take in chronological order, from first to last, using the numbers 1, 2, and 3.

A) ___ Colposcopy
B) ___ Loop electrosurgical excision procedure (LEEP)
C) ___ Cervical biopsy

692. A photograph of a skin lesion is included in this question. (This image can be found in color in the app.) What is the diagnosis?

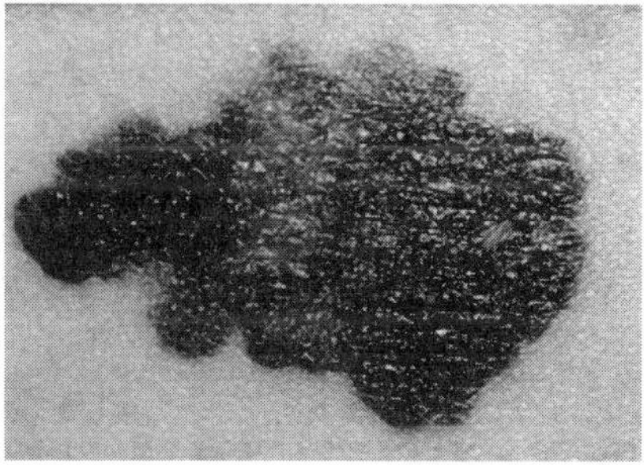

Source: National Cancer Institute. Retrieved from https://visualsonline.cancer.gov/details.cfm?imageid=9186

A) Basal cell carcinoma
B) Squamous cell carcinoma
C) Nevus
D) Melanoma

693. A 28-year-old woman with a history of hypothyroidism presents to an urgent care clinic complaining of numbness and tingling in the fingertips of both her hands for several hours. On examination, both radial pulses are at +2 and equal bilaterally. The patient reports that over the past few months she has had identical episodes, each lasting several hours. During these episodes, the skin changes color from blue to white, and then to dark red. Eventually, it returns to normal and the tingling and numbness disappear. Which of the following conditions is best described?

A) Hashimoto's disease
B) Raynaud's phenomenon
C) Peripheral neuropathy
D) Vitamin B_{12} deficiency anemia

694. What is the gold-standard test for alpha thalassemia minor and sickle cell anemia?

A) Ferritin
B) Hemoglobin electrophoresis
C) Total iron-binding capacity (TIBC)
D) Folate level

695. A 55-year-old woman with rheumatoid arthritis sees the nurse practitioner for an episodic visit. She has been taking ibuprofen twice daily for many years. All of the following organ systems are at risk for damage from chronic nonsteroidal anti-inflammatory drug (NSAID) use except:

A) Cardiovascular system
B) Musculoskeletal system
C) Gastrointestinal system
D) Renal system

696. Which of the following eye findings is seen in patients with diabetic neuropathy?

A) Arteriovenous nicking
B) Copper wire arterioles
C) Flame hemorrhages
D) Neovascularization

697. Which of the following findings are seen in a patient with folate-deficiency anemia?

A) Microcytic and hypochromic red blood cells
B) Microcytic and normochromic red blood cells
C) Normal size and color of the red blood cells
D) Macrocytic and normocytic red blood cells

698. All the following signs and symptoms are associated with irritable bowel syndrome except:

A) Diarrhea with blood mixed in the stool
B) Diarrhea and/or constipation
C) Abdominal pain relief after defecation
D) Mucus with stools

699. An 8-month-old girl is brought by her grandmother to see the nurse practitioner because of intermittent, random episodes of vomiting, abdominal bloating, currant jelly stools, and irritability with poor appetite. The infant is trending in the 10th percentile on the growth chart and appears lethargic. During the abdominal exam, a sausage-like mass is palpated on the right side of the abdomen. The infant's presentation is highly suggestive of which condition?

A) Lactic intolerance
B) Intussusception
C) Inflammatory bowel disease
D) Irritable bowel syndrome

700. A 36-year-old man presents to the nurse practitioner complaining of a history of cervical and upper back pain for many months. On examination, the range of motion of the patient's spine is limited, especially with lateral flexion. The other joints in the patient's body are normal. Only the spine seems to be affected. The patient reports that a laboratory test from a previous doctor showed increased ESR (erythrocyte sedimentation rate), negative antinuclear antigen (ANA), and negative rheumatoid factor. Which of the following is best described?

A) Rheumatoid arthritis
B) Lupus erythematosus
C) Degenerative joint disease of the spine
D) Ankylosing spondylitis

701. A postmenopausal woman who has been on low-dose estrogen and progesterone replacement hormone therapy for her severe vasomotor symptoms complains to the nurse practitioner that over the past 4 months she has had a few episodes of small amounts of vaginal bleeding that seem to occur at random. She denies uterine cramping and dyspareunia. Which of the following is the best treatment plan for this patient?

A) Recommend a dilation and curettage (D&C) procedure, which is very helpful in cases of postmenopausal bleeding
B) Schedule the patient for uterine ultrasound and endometrial biopsy
C) Prescribe a 13-day course of progesterone pills to induce uterine shedding of the thickened endometrial lining at the end of the month
D) Refer the patient to a gynecologist for further evaluation

702. Which of the following is a sensitive screening test for human immunodeficiency virus (HIV)?

A) Combination HIV-1 and HIV-2 antibody immunoassay with p24 antigen
B) Western blot test
C) ELISA test
D) HIV antibody test

703. All of the following findings are associated with labyrinthitis or vestibular neuritis except:

A) Acoustic nerve damage
B) Symptoms provoked by changes in head position
C) Vertigo with nausea and vomiting
D) Nystagmus

704. Which of the following is a true statement regarding the beliefs of most patients who are Jehovah's Witnesses?

A) Transfusion of blood is prohibited even in cases of emergency
B) Consumption of pork products is strictly prohibited
C) Transfusion of blood is allowed in certain medical conditions
D) Consumption of alcohol products is strictly prohibited

705. Transillumination is useful in helping to diagnose which of the following conditions?

A) Sinusitis and hydrocele
B) Testicular tumor and acute otitis media
C) Nasal masses and other tumors in the facial region
D) Hydrocephalus and epididymitis

706. A middle-aged woman has been experiencing low-back pain that recently started to radiate to both buttocks and down her legs. She complains of leg weakness and problems with walking. Along with these symptoms she reports new onset of urinary incontinence, in which she leaks a small amount of urine at random. She also reports numbness on her perineal area, which is new. She denies trauma but reports that she recently moved to a new apartment and has been lifting and moving furniture. Which of the following is best described?

A) Sciatica
B) Acute muscle spasm
C) Cauda equina syndrome
D) Acute muscle strain

707. An adult patient who was recently discharged from the hospital was prescribed clindamycin. The patient reports that he took his last dose yesterday. He presents in the primary care clinic with a complaint of recent onset of watery diarrhea from 10 to 15 times a day with abdominal cramping. He denies fever and chills. Which of the following conditions is most likely in this patient?

A) *Clostridium difficile*-associated diarrhea (CDAD)
B) Giardiasis
C) Pseudomembranous colitis
D) Irritable bowel syndrome

708. Which of the following is the treatment for nongonococcal urethritis?

A) Ceftriaxone (Rocephin) 250 mg IM
B) Azithromycin 1 g PO in a single dose
C) Doxycycline 100 mg PO BID × 14 days
D) Treatment is not necessary

709. Which of the following infections can cause a "barky" cough?

A) Epiglottitis
B) Croup
C) Bronchiolitis
D) Common cold

710. A 30-year-old woman with mild persistent asthma and allergic rhinitis is seen in an urgent care clinic for complaints of shortness of breath and wheezing. She reports using her albuterol inhaler two to three times per day for 4 days the previous week. She reports waking up for 3 nights due to wheezing the past week. She had previously been prescribed low-dose flunisolide (AeroBid), two inhalations twice per day. Vital signs reveal a temperature of 99.0°F, pulse of 88 beats/min, and respiratory rate of 14 breaths/min. Which of the following actions is the next step?

A) Administer nebulized albuterol treatment
B) Prescribe a Medrol dose pack
C) Use the spirometer to assess severity of symptoms
D) Add a long-acting beta-agonist inhaler

711. What is the preferred treatment for hypertensive patients with a history of heart failure?

A) Beta-blockers or calcium channel blockers
B) Angiotensin-converting enzyme (ACE) inhibitors or angiotensin receptor blockers (ARBs)
C) Calcium channel blockers or angiotensin receptor blockers (ARBs)
D) Alpha-blockers or beta-blockers

712. The 2013 American College of Cardiology/American Heart Association (ACC/AHA) Arteriosclerotic Cardiovascular Disease (ASCVD) risk calculator measures the risk of a cardiovascular event within 10 years after measurement. What is the cutoff value when treatment for hyperlipidemia is recommended?

A) 6.5% or higher
B) 7.5% or higher
C) 8% or higher
D) 10 % or higher

713. A 55-year-old male patient with a body mass index (BMI) of 30 has a history of angina and type 2 diabetes. His lipid profile results are total cholesterol of 280 mg/dL, low-density lipoprotein (LDL) of 195 mg/dL, and high-density lipoprotein (HDL) of 25 mg/dL. The nurse practitioner diagnoses him with hyperlipidemia and wants to start him on statin therapy. What intensity of treatment is recommended for this patient?

A) Low-intensity statin
B) Moderate-intensity statin
C) High-intensity statin
D) Very high-intensity statin

714. All of the following are considered overarching goals in *Healthy People 2020* except:

A) Achieve health equity, eliminate health disparities, and improve health of all groups
B) Create social and physical environments that promote good health for all
C) Promote quality of life, healthy development, and healthy behaviors across all life stages
D) Encourage sexual abstinence and condom use

715. An asthmatic 20-year-old woman who was seen for a viral upper respiratory infection 2 weeks ago presents to the nurse practitioner's office complaining of a recent onset of shortness of breath, inspiratory and expiratory wheezing, and chest tightness. She has been using her albuterol inhaler four to six times a day with poor relief. She is unable to speak in full sentences. When the nurse practitioner quickly evaluates the patient, she notices that the patient is pale, diaphoretic, fatigued, and using her sternocleidomastoid accessory muscles for respiration. Her respiratory rate is 32 breaths/min and pulse is 130 beats/min. Which of the following interventions is not indicated?

A) Administer oxygen by nasal cannula
B) Give the patient a nebulized short-acting beta 2 agonist
C) Quickly assess the patient with the pulse oximeter and check breath sounds
D) Initiate cardiopulmonary resuscitation (CPR) immediately

716. The ELISA and Western blot tests are used to detect which of the following?

A) HIV RNA
B) HIV DNA
C) HIV antibodies
D) HIV antigen

717. A 65-year-old man has been on atorvastatin (Lipitor) 60 mg daily for the past 3 months. Two weeks ago he started taking a high-dose B-complex vitamin. He complains of feeling very fatigued lately and denies lack of sleep. He has noticed that he has a loss of appetite and his urine has been a darker color for the past 2 weeks. He denies dysuria, frequency, and nocturia. The nurse practitioner notices that the patient's sclera has a slight yellow tinge. You would:

A) Discontinue atorvastatin (Lipitor) and order a liver function profile
B) Continue the atorvastatin (Lipitor) but on half the dose
C) Schedule him for a complete physical examination
D) Schedule him for a liver function profile

718. What is the second most common type of dementia in the United States?

A) Alzheimer's disease
B) Parkinson's disease
C) Dementia with Lewy bodies
D) Vascular dementia

719. A 56-year-old man complains of several episodes of severe lacerating pain that shoots up his right cheek and is precipitated by drinking cold drinks or chewing. The episodes start suddenly and end spontaneously after a few seconds with several episodes per day. He denies any trauma, facial weakness, or difficulty swallowing. He has stopped drinking cold drinks because of the pain. Which of the following is most likely?

A) Trigeminal neuralgia
B) Cluster headache
C) Acute sinusitis
D) Sinus headache

720. An 18-year-old male who recently returned from a camping vacation is complaining of abrupt onset of fever, abdominal cramps, watery diarrhea, foul flatus, vomiting, and anorexia for 2 days. He has explosive diarrhea with a very strong "foul" odor. He reports that he remembers swallowing lake water a few times while swimming. Which of the following conditions is most likely?

A) Giardiasis
B) Irritable bowel syndrome
C) Crohn's disease
D) Celiac disease

721. According to evidence-based medicine (EBM) experts, which of the following types of research has the lowest ranking?

A) Randomized controlled trial
B) Experiment
C) Cohort study
D) Expert opinion

722. According to evidence-based medicine (EBM) experts, which of the following types of research has the highest ranking?

A) Meta-analysis
B) Randomized controlled trial
C) Cohort study
D) Expert opinion

723. A 4-month-old infant has an anterior fontanel that has fused. Which of the following is the best plan for this infant?

A) Tell the mother that it is normal in some infants to have early closure of the anterior fontanel
B) Order an MRI of the head
C) Advise the mother to return in 4 weeks for a recheck
D) Refer the infant to a pediatric neurosurgeon

724. A positive anterior drawer sign of the knee is highly suggestive of?

A) Meniscus damage
B) Posterior cruciate ligament damage
C) Anterior cruciate ligament damage
D) Medial collateral ligament damage

725. A 33-year-old man is diagnosed with a mild case of *Clostridium difficile* infection of the colon. The patient reports a history of hospitalization the previous month. Which of the following regimens is the preferred treatment?

A) Metronidazole (Flagyl) 500 mg orally TID × 10 to 14 days
B) Azithromycin 250 mg orally once daily × 5 days (Z-Pack)
C) Vancomycin 125 mg orally QID × 10 to 14 days
D) Treatment with antibiotics is not recommended

32

Answers With Rationales

1. **A) Obtain a complete and thorough history** Before prescribing medications, a thorough history must be obtained to determine possible causes of hives. The patient denied difficulty with swallowing and breathing, so there was no medical emergency that would require calling 911.

2. **B) Edema of the face and the upper extremities** Common signs and symptoms of pregnancy-induced hypertension include edema of the face and the upper extremities, weight gain, blurred vision, elevated blood pressure, proteinuria, and headaches.

3. **D) Tingling and numbness of both feet** Vitamin B_{12} deficiency anemia can cause nerve cell damage if not treated. Symptoms of B_{12} deficiency anemia may include tingling or numbness in fingers and toes, difficulty walking, mood changes or depression, memory loss, disorientation, and dementia.

4. **A) Order an ultrasound** Abnormally low levels of alpha fetoprotein and estriol and high levels of human chorionic gonadotropin are abnormal during pregnancy. An ultrasound should be ordered to further evaluate the fetus for characteristics of Down syndrome and/or fetal demise.

5. **C) Most diverticula in the colon are infected with gram-negative bacteria** Diverticula in the colon can be infected with both gram-negative and gram-positive bacteria.

6. **B) *Chlamydia trachomatis*** When diagnosed with gonorrhea, the patient should also be treated for *Chlamydia trachomatis.*

7. **C) Osteoporosis** Kyphosis is a curvature of the spine that causes a rounding of the back, which leads to a slouching posture. Severe thinning of the bones (osteoporosis) contributes to this curvature in the spine. Symptoms that may occur with severe cases of kyphosis include difficulty breathing, fatigue, and back pain.

8. **B) Higher than normal** Alpha fetoprotein (AFP) is produced in the fetal and maternal liver. Higher levels of AFP are commonly seen in multiple gestations due to the growing liver in each fetus, which cumulatively lead to higher AFP levels.

9. **D) Thiazide diuretics** Thiazide diuretics have a favorable effect in patients with osteopenia and osteoporosis by slowing down the kidney's excretion of calcium and increasing distal tubule calcium reabsorption. This results in decreased bone demineralization.

Thiazide diuretics are a good choice of therapy for this population because they treat hypertension and slow bone loss.

10. **A) Instability of the knee** The Lachman maneuver is a test performed to assess for knee instability (i.e., damage to the motion of anterior translation [laxity] of the anterior cruciate ligament [ACL]) or tear of the ACL. The maneuver should be tested on *both* knees, comparing the injured and the opposite knee, the uninjured knee is used as the "control." The test is positive if the injured knee slips back further (laxity). Perform the test by bending the knee 30 degrees. Stabilize the femur with one hand. Place the other hand under the proximal tibia at the level of the joint line and then pull forward. The laxity is graded on a 0 (normal)-to-3 scale (1.0–1.5 cm of translation).

11. **B) It inhibits the effect of renal prostaglandins and blunts the effectiveness of the diuretic** Nonsteroidal anti-inflammatory drugs (NSAIDs) and acetylsalicylic acid (ASA) inhibit the vasodilatory effects of prostaglandins, which predisposes the kidney to ischemia. NSAIDs can cause acute kidney injury by decreasing renal blood flow. Nonselective NSAIDs can adversely affect the kidneys, GI tract, liver, cardiovascular system, and the lungs (bronchospasm).

12. **D) *Chlamydia trachomatis*** Infections that commonly affect the labia and vagina include bacterial vaginosis, candidiasis, and trichomoniasis. *Chlamydia trachomatis* commonly affects the cervix, endometrial lining, fallopian tubes, and pelvic cavity.

13. **B) Acute appendicitis** Signs and symptoms of an acute abdomen include involuntary guarding, rebound tenderness, boardlike abdomen, and a positive obturator and psoas sign. A positive obturator sign occurs when pain is elicted by internal rotation of the right hip from 90 degrees hip/knee flexion. The psoas sign is positive when pain occurs with passive extension of the thigh while the patient is lying on his or her side with knees extended, or when pain occurs with active flexion of the thigh at the hip.

14. **D) A prescription of methyldopa (Aldomet) to control blood pressure** Recommended care for women diagnosed with preeclampsia includes bed rest with bathroom privileges, weight and blood pressure monitoring, and closely following urine protein and serum protein, creatinine, and platelet counts. Oral medications are not used as first-line treatment.

15. **C) Custodial care** Medicare Parts A and B do not cover custodial care or nursing home care (help with bathing, dressing, using bathroom, and eating). Medicare Part A coverage includes inpatient hospitalization, inpatient psychiatric hospitalization, and skilled care given in a certified skilled nursing facility (SNF).

16. **B) Atypical pneumonia** The most common organism causing community-acquired atypical pneumonia is *Mycoplasma pneumoniae,* an atypical bacterium. The populations with the highest infection rates are college students, school-aged children, and military recruits. Respiratory symptoms (cough) are accompanied by pharyngitis, rhinorrhea, and sometimes ear pain. It is easily spread from aerosol droplets.

17. **C) 10 mm** The Mantoux tuberculin skin test is administered on the volar aspect of the lower arm (nondominant arm preferred) and read 48 to 72 hours after the test is given. An induration of 10 mm or larger is considered as positive among recent immigrants (<5 years) from high-prevalence countries. If the site has erythema but no induration, the result would be negative. Color is not important.

18. **B) The agent can make decisions in other areas of the patient's life such as financial issues** The person named in a durable power of attorney (the agent or proxy) is designated by the patient to make all medical decisions, as well as any decisions regarding the patient's private affairs in the event that the patient becomes incompetent and unable to make his or her own decisions. This is dependent on the type of power of attorney that is instituted. B) is the right answer only if so stated in the power of attorney. Generally, a spouse cannot override the power of attorney. Do not confuse with the durable power of attorney for health care, who legally can only make health-related decisions for the patient.

19. **B) The patient has a medical illness that causes an anxiety reaction and denial** Munchausen syndrome is a psychiatric disorder in which the patient fakes a medical illness or disorder to gain attention from health care providers. These patients often use the emergency department to gain attention.

20. **C) Beta-blockers** Beta-blockers should be avoided in patients with a history of emphysema. Studies have shown evidence of a reduction in forced expiratory volume in 1 second (FEV1), increased airway hyperresponsiveness, and inhibition of bronchodilator response to beta agonists in patients receiving beta-blockers.

21. **A) On deep inspiration by the patient, palpate firmly in the right upper quadrant of the abdomen below the costovertebral angle** Murphy's sign is tested during an abdominal examination for biliary disorders. As the patient breathes in, the abdominal contents are pushed downward as the diaphragm moves down and the lungs expand. As the patient stops/hold the breath, the gallbladder comes in contact with the examiner's fingers and may elicit pain. To be considered positive, the same maneuver must not elicit pain when performed on the left side. A negative Murphy's test in the elderly is not useful for ruling out cholecystitis if history and other tests suggest the diagnosis.

22. **B) Placenta previa** Placenta previa occurs when the placenta implants abnormally, partially, or wholly, in the lower segment of the uterus or over the internal os. A classic presentation is painless bright-red vaginal bleeding in the second and/or third trimester. Do not perform digital cervical in any pregnant women with bleeding until the position of the uterus is known (abdominal ultrasound). Avoid vaginal exam, sexual intercourse, or rectal exam if placenta previa is suspected.

23. **A) Middle-aged to older women** Hashimoto's disease (Hashimoto's thyroiditis, or chronic lymphocytic thyroiditis) is an autoimmune disease. An enlarged thyroid is most often the first sign of the disease. Hashimoto's disease is about seven times more common in women than in men. It can occur in teens and young women, but is more common in middle age.

24. **C) Severe vaginal atrophic changes** As women reach menopause, changes that may occur include hot flashes, irregular menstrual periods, and cyclic mood swings. Vaginal changes, such as dryness and thinning, may also begin to occur. Vaginal atrophy (atrophic vaginitis) is the thinning and inflammation of the vaginal walls due to a decline in estrogen. Vaginal atrophy occurs most often after menopause and worsens as women get older.

25. **B) Arteriovenous (AV) nicking, left ventricular hypertrophy, and stroke** AV nicking and copper wire/silver wire arterioles are signs of hypertensive retinopathy, left

ventricular hypertrophy affects the heart, and stroke damages the brain. These are all examples of target organ damage.

26. **A) Vaginal bleeding and cramping are present, but the cervix remains closed** *Threatened abortion* is defined as vaginal bleeding and cramping without the presence of cervical dilation.

27. **B) Bacterial vaginosis** In bacterial vaginosis (BV), the normal hydrogen peroxide-producing lactobacilli are replaced by an overgrowth of anaerobic bacteria. BV is a vaginosis (does not cause inflammation) rather than a vaginitis. No symptoms may be present or the patient's history may include strong vaginal odor ("fishy" odor) and increased vaginal discharge (milky white, thin, adherent discharge or dull gray discharge). Findings include alkaline pH greater than 4.5, the presence of clue cells (wet smear using microscopy), and positive "whiff test" (a strong "fishy" odor when vaginal discharge is mixed with one drop of potassium hydroxide [KOH]). Clue cells are squamous epithelial cells dotted with large numbers of bacteria that obscure borders.

28. **A) Call the patient and tell her that she needs to return to the clinic for chlamydia and gonorrhea testing** The patient may have cervicitis and needs to be screened for gonorrhea and chlamydia infection.

29. **B) Lichen sclerosus** Lichen sclerosus is more common in older women. It is a chronic condition that causes thin, white patches of skin usually in the genital area in women. The lesions appear as small white spots early in the disease and grow into bigger patches. Itching is very common; however, other symptoms include discomfort, bleeding from skin tears, and blisters. A skin biopsy allows for differentiation from other dermatological conditions.

30. **B) Closure of the semilunar valves** A heart valve normally allows blood to flow in only one direction. A heart valve opens or closes incumbent upon differential blood pressure on each side. A form of heart disease occurs when a valve malfunctions and allows some blood to flow in the wrong direction. The S2 sound results from reverberation within the blood associated with the sudden block of flow reversal.

31. **B) Tanner stage III** In Tanner stage III in males, the testicular volume increases, the scrotum enlarges, and the penis begins to lengthen. *Tanner stages* are: Tanner I: Prepubertal small penis. Tanner II: The penis length remains unchanged. Tanner III: Penis begins to lengthen. Tanner IV: Penis increases in length *and* circumference. Tanner V: Scrotum and penis are mature size.

32. **A) *Toxoplasma gondii*, other infections, rubella, cytomegalovirus, and herpes** The acronym TORCH stands for *Toxoplasma gondii*, *o*ther infections, *r*ubella, *c*ytomegalovirus, and *h*erpes. Although several of the conditions listed in the other answer options can also cause fetal problems, they do not comprise the TORCH disorders.

33. **A) Laryngeal cancer** Human papillomavirus (HPV) exposure is a risk factor in laryngeal cancer. HPV DNA transforms the moist membranes of epithelial cells (cervix, anus, mouth, and throat). The juvenile type is related to vertical transmission and the adult

type to orogenital contact. HPV subtype 16 accounts for the majority of oral tumors, oropharynx cancers, and laryngeal cases.

34. **C) Osteoarthritis** Signs of osteoarthritis (OA) include stiffness of joints, especially in the morning and after sitting for long periods. Visible signs of OA are an element in the diagnosis. (Rheumatoid arthritis and gout often rely more heavily on lab tests.) Heberden's nodes (bony overgrowths) are classic signs of OA. They are located at the distal interphalangeal joints. They are felt as hard, nontender nodules usually 2 to 3 cm in diameter but sometimes encompass the entire joint. Enlargement of the middle joint of a finger is called a *Bouchard's node*.

35. **B) Instability of the knee** The drawer test is used to identify mediolateral or anteroposterior plane instability of the knee. The test is performed on the unaffected and affected knee for comparison. The anterior drawer test evaluates the anterior cruciate ligament (ACL). To perform the test, the patient lies supine and the knee is placed at 90-degree flexion. Grasp the posterior aspect of the tibia over the upper calf muscle; then, with a steady force, try to push the lower leg forward and backward. Anterior or posterior movement of the knee is positive. With the leg extended, stabilize the femur with one hand and the ankle with the other. Try to abduct and adduct the knee. There should be no medial or lateral movement.

36. **A) Advise the mother that her pregnancy is progressing well** Between 20 and 35 weeks, the fundal height is equal to the number of weeks of gestation plus or minus 2 cm. Fundal height is measured as the distance between the pubic bone and the uterine fundus. For example, a woman who is at 30 weeks of gestation who has a fundal height of 29 cm is within normal limits. But if the fundal height is 27 cm (3 cm difference), it is abnormal. Next step is to order a fetal ultrasound.

37. **C) From 33 to 35 cm** After 20 weeks gestation, fundal height in centimeters should measure approximately the same as the number of weeks of gestation.

38. **B) Estimated glomerular filtration rate (eGFR)** The estimated glomerular filtration rate (GFR) is a sensitive test used to measure and monitor kidney function and evaluate chronic kidney disease (CKD). GFR can be estimated from serum creatinine. The estimated GFR calculation uses serum creatinine along with age and values assigned for gender and race. The National Kidney Foundation has determined different stages of CKD based on the value of estimated GFR.

39. **A) Chronic intake of nonsteroidal anti-inflammatory drugs (NSAIDs) can cause the disorder** Signs and symptoms of gastritis are nausea/vomiting, upset stomach, loss of appetite, and burning/aching or gnawing pain located in the epigastric area. Nonselective NSAIDs (aspirin, ibuprofen, naproxen, others) have adverse effects on the gastrointestinal (GI) tract, kidneys, central nervous system, and cardiovascular effects, and decrease platelet aggregation (aspirin). Chronic use of nonselective NSAIDs disrupts the production of prostaglandins, which involves cycloxygenase-1 (COX-1) and COX-2. The GI mucosa uses COX-1 to produce mucosal protective factors. Blocking COX-1 decreases these protective factors and increases risk of gastritis, ulcers, and GI bleeding. Selective NSAIDs, such as celecoxib (Celebrex), do less damage to the GI tract because they block only COX-2, which is responsible for pain and inflammation.

40. **D) Apraxia** Apraxia is characterized by loss of the ability to execute or carry out learned purposeful movements despite the desire and the physical ability to perform the movements. Apraxia is not a sign or symptom of depression; it is a disorder of motor planning caused by damage to specific areas of the cerebrum. Common signs of depression include anhedonia (loss of interest in activities that the patient finds pleasurable), unintentional weight loss or gain, fatigue, change in appetite, insomnia or hypersomnia, feelings of guilt and worthlessness, and recurrent thoughts of suicide.

41. **C) Viral conjunctivitis** The causative organisms of viral conjunctivitis (pink eye) include adenovirus and other virus types. It can present with or without cold symptoms. Patient complains of itchy red eyes and may have clear discharge accompanied by preauricular lymphadenopathy. Does not affect vision. If a contact lens wearer, assume bacterial infection and obtain culture of eye discharge.

42. **C) Urine pregnancy test** The patient's history of amenorrhea and new onset of bloody vaginal spotting combined with positive physical findings of left adnexal tenderness and cervical motion tenderness are highly suggestive of an ectopic pregnancy rather than pelvic inflammatory disease (PID). Refer this patient to the emergency department if ectopic pregnancy is suspected. The presence of amenorrhea should be treated as a pregnancy until proven otherwise.

43. **B) S1, S2, and S3** Congestive heart failure (CHF) is the inability of the heart to pump a sufficient amount of blood to the organs to meet the body's requirements. It is common to hear S1, S2, and S3 heart sounds on exam. Common signs and symptoms of CHF include fatigue, shortness of breath with activity, and edema of lower extremities.

44. **B) Elevation of the affected limb and intermittent applications of cold packs for the next 48 hours** Elevation of the injured knee above the heart will reduce the amount of swelling that can occur. Use of ice packs immediately after the injury is most effective and will reduce swelling in the tissue. Ice the affected area for 15 to 20 minutes at a time intermittently to prevent frostbite and further damage to tissue. Allowing 30 to 45 minutes between icing of the limb is recommended.

45. **A) G6PD deficiency anemia** Glucose-6-phosphate dehydrogenase (G6PD) deficiency is a hereditary condition that occurs when the red blood cells break down, causing hemolysis, due to absence or lack of sufficient G6PD, an enzyme that is needed to help the red blood cells work efficiently. Certain foods and medications may trigger this reaction. Some of the medications include antimalarial drugs, aspirin, nitrofurantoin, nonsteroidal anti-inflammatory drugs (NSAIDs), quinidine, quinine, and sulfa medications.

46. **D) Recommend immediate referral to the emergency department** Priapism (painful penile erection not related to sexual activity) is a true urological emergency that may lead to permanent erectile dysfunction and penile necrosis if not treated appropriately. It can be associated with a number of medical conditions (sickle cell anemia, leukemia, or spinal cord injury) and/or some pharmacological agents.

47. **A) The mother has autoantibodies against Rh-positive red blood cells (RBCs)** The mother's autoantibodies can attack the fetus's Rh-positive RBCs and cause destruction of these cells, which can cause severe anemia and complications in the fetus. Today this

is preventable with the administration of anti-RhD immunoglobulin (Rho[D] immune globulin) to an Rh-negative mother at 28 weeks gestation and after birth if the newborn is Rh positive.

48. B) Prevent anencephaly Folic acid (B vitamin) supplementation has been shown to decrease the incidence of neural tube defects (NTDs), including spina bifida and anencephaly. Folic acid supplementation should begin preconception and continue during pregnancy. Folic acid prevents some NTDs by correcting abnormal homocysteine metabolism. Women need to take 0.4 mg/day during their childbearing years. There is an increased incidence of NTDs in diabetics, who require a higher dose to be therapeutic.

49. A) Acute pyelonephritis Acute pyelonephritis does not involve any vascular change; however, *chronic* pyelonephritis (reflux nephropathy) is a factor for secondary hypertension. Pheochromocytoma is a rare tumor of the adrenal glands that results in a release of too much epinephrine and norepinephrine, hormones that control heart rate, metabolism, and blood pressure. Renovascular stenosis is a narrowing of one or both arteries leading to the kidneys. It can cause severe hypertension and irreversible kidney damage. Coarctation of the aorta is a congenital heart defect of the aorta; it is a narrowing of the aorta that causes the heart to work harder to get blood to flow through the narrow aortic passageway to other organs, which, in turn, causes an increase in blood pressure.

50. B) *Chlamydia trachomatis* Fitz-Hugh–Curtis syndrome (or perihepatitis) is a complication of pelvic inflammatory disease (PID). It is more common with chlamydial PID, but it can also occur with gonorrheal PID infection. It is caused by inflammation of the liver capsule, which leads to scarring. Signs and symptoms include sharp pain on the right upper quadrant (pleuritic-like) with PID symptoms. Like PID, it is treated with antibiotics.

51. B) Just rising above the suprapubic bone At 12 weeks gestation, the uterus is approximately the size of a grapefruit and would be felt just above the suprapubic bone on bimanual exam.

52. D) Outpatient anesthesiologist's services According to the Medicare.gov website, Medicare Part A covers anesthesia that is received while in an inpatient hospital. Medicare Part B covers outpatient care, durable medical equipment, home health services, and other medical services, including some preventive services such as annual physical exams, and mammograms (baseline age 50 years).

53. D) A 17-year-old teen who has only one close friend in school Risk factors for suicide include (a) elderly White men (especially after the death of a spouse); (b) past history of suicide; (c) family history of suicide; (d) plans for use of a lethal weapon such as a gun or knife; (e) gender (higher attempt rate in females, but higher success rate in males); and (f) personal history of bipolar disorder or depression.

54. D) Subconjunctival hemorrhage Bright-red blood in a sharply defined area surrounded by normal-appearing conjunctiva indicates subconjunctival hemorrhage. The blood stays red because of direct diffusion of oxygen through the conjunctiva. Risk factors include diabetes, hypertension, illnesses that cause severe coughing or sneezing, blood-thinning medications and aspirin, and herbal supplements such as ginkgo.

55. **C) Advise the patient that the condition is benign and will resolve spontaneously** Subconjunctival hemorrhages do not require any treatment. The blood in the eye will be absorbed within 10 to 14 days.

56. **A) Urine for culture and sensitivity** An 8-year-old male patient with the diagnosis of diabetes has a high risk of urinary tract infections (UTIs). A large amount of leukocytes in the urinalysis is abnormal, and he has been having symptoms of frequency and nocturia for the past 3 days. The urine culture would be ordered because he has a high risk of infection. The urine culture and sensitivity (C&S) is the best evaluation for diagnosing a UTI.

57. **D) Placenta previa** Severe preeclampsia can cause placental abruption, but not placenta previa (placenta implants over internal os). Serious complications include hypertensive encephalopathy, liver failure, kidney failure, pulmonary edema, seizures, retinal detachment, disseminated intravascular coagulation, and death.

58. **B) Tonometry** A tonometer is used to measure the intraocular pressure (IOP) of the eye to screen for glaucoma. Normal range IOP is 10 to 22 mmHg.

59. **B) Tick** Rocky Mountain spotted fever is caused by a bite from a tick infected with the parasite *Rickettsia rickettsii*. The mortality rate is 1% to 7% if left untreated.

60. **B) It does not have a linear distribution** Atopic dermatitis, also known as *eczema*, is a skin condition in which the lesions occur in a linear fashion. They may have many different stages, including erythematous papules and vesicles, with weeping, drainage, and/or crusting. Lesions are commonly pruritic and are found on the scalp, face, forearms, wrists, elbows, and backs of the knees.

61. **D) Prophylaxis is not recommended for this patient** Current American Heart Association guidelines (2017) do not recommend endocarditis prophylaxis for most patients with aortic or mitral valve disease, including those with mitral valve prolapse with regurgitation or for patients with hypertrophic cardiomyopathy. Patients at highest risk for infective endocarditis (IE) are those with prosthetic heart valves, including mechanical, bioprosthetic, and homograft valves; prior history of IE; unrepaired cyanotic congenital heart disease; prosthetic material used for valvular repair; repaired congenital heart disease with residual shunts or with catheter-based intervention; and others. The high-risk procedures are dental work with manipulation of tissue, tooth extractions, and certain respiratory tract procedures.

62. **B) Rubeola** Rubeola is the Latin name for measles. Signs and symptoms of measles infection include fever over 101°F, coryza, cough, conjunctivitis, rash, and Koplik's spots on the buccal mucosa. Do not confuse rubeola with rubella (German measles or 3-day measles).

63. **A) Mitral regurgitation** Signs and symptoms of mitral regurgitation do not include frequent bowel movements with weight loss.

64. **C) *Treponema pallidum*** *Treponema pallidum* is a gram-negative spirochete bacterium that causes syphilis.

65. **A) Placenta** Human chorionic gonadotropin (hCG) is a hormone produced by the placenta after implantation. It can also be produced in gestational trophoblastic disease or hydatidiform mole (molar pregnancy).

66. **A) Fetal liver** Alpha fetoprotein (AFP) is produced mainly by the growing fetal liver. A small amount comes from the mother's liver, but by the end of the first trimester, most of the AFP is produced by the fetal liver.

67. **A) Order an enzyme-linked immunosorbent assay (ELISA) test as soon as possible** Employee health clinic protocols for needlesticks recommend ordering an ELISA test as soon as possible to establish baseline blood work for the employee.

68. **B) Order a serum thyroid-stimulating hormone (TSH), digoxin level, and an electrolyte panel** Obtaining baseline blood work to evaluate for causes of new-onset atrial fibrillation is recommended before decreasing or stopping medications. Thyroid disease is a common cause of new-onset atrial fibrillation.

69. **B) Pregnancy-induced hypertension (preeclampsia)** This patient is manifesting the classic triad of symptoms of preeclampsia: hypertension, edema (weight gain), and proteinuria.

70. **C) Elevated serum cortisol levels** Elevated serum cortisol levels are seen in patients with Cushing's syndrome.

71. **B) 5 mm** Tuberculin skin tests are tests of delayed hypersensitivity. Purified protein derivative (PPD) tuberculin antigen is injected intradermally to form a 6-mm to 10-mm wheal. The skin test is read within 48 to 72 hours, when the induration is most evident. Erythema without induration is generally considered to be of no significance. An induration that is 5 mm or more in diameter indicates a positive reaction and the need for treatment of latent tuberculosis infection in high-risk groups.

72. **C) Varicella** The data regarding efficacy of the varicella vaccine are insufficient; therefore, varicella vaccine is contraindicated in HIV-infected individuals.

73. **A) Inevitable abortion** Inevitable abortion is defined as vaginal bleeding with pain, cervical dilation, and/or cervical effacement. Threatened abortion is defined as vaginal bleeding with absent or minimal pain and a closed, long, and thick cervix. Incomplete abortion involves moderate to diffuse vaginal bleeding, with the passage of tissue and painful uterine cramping or contractions. Acute pelvic inflammatory disease is a sudden onset of inflammation and pain that affects the pelvic area, cervix, uterus, and ovaries, and is caused by infection.

74. **A) Tdap, hepatitis B, and HPV vaccine** There are two types of HPV vaccine. Gardasil can be used for both girls and boys, but Cervarix can only be used for females. HPV vaccine is recommended for preteen boys and girls at age 11 or 12 years. Young women can get HPV vaccine until age 27 years and men can get the HPV vaccine until age 22 years.

75. **D) During the postpartum period** The measles, mumps, and rubella (MMR) vaccine is contraindicated in pregnancy. The Advisory Committee on Immunization Practices

recommends that pregnancy be avoided for 4 weeks after vaccination, that women who become pregnant within that period be advised of the theoretical risk to the fetus (congenital rubella syndrome), and that vaccination during pregnancy is generally not a reason to terminate the pregnancy.

76. **D) Eyeglasses and routine dental care** Medicare Part B covers medically necessary services (i.e., service or supplies that are needed to diagnose or treat a medical condition that meets acceptable standards of medical practice) and preventive services such as flu shots. This includes (a) outpatient physician visits, labs, x-rays; (b) durable medical equipment; (c) annual mammograms/colonoscopy after age 50 years; and (d) rehabilitation. It does not cover eyeglasses or routine dental care.

77. **B) Ishihara chart** The Ishihara chart (or Ishihara Color Test) is used to evaluate color blindness and can be used in patients ranging from school-aged children to adults. It displays colored numbers with different colored dots on the background. A pediatric color vision test for preschool children (3–6 years of age) uses shapes instead of numbers.

78. **B) Left-sided heart failure** During left-sided heart failure, the left ventricle cannot pump with enough force to push the blood into the lungs and circulation. Signs and symptoms of left-sided heart failure include dyspnea on exertion, fatigue at rest or with minimal exertion, generalized weakness, orthopnea, and paroxysmal nocturnal dyspnea, cough, and edema. If pulmonary edema occurs, frothy or pink sputum with cough may be seen.

79. **C) Furosemide (Lasix)** Loop diuretics, such as furosemide (Lasix), are used to help remove the extra fluid load in hemodynamically stable patients (contraindicated if systolic blood pressure <90 mmHg, severe hyponatremia, acidosis).

80. **B) Avoid foods with high potassium content** Foods that are high in potassium are not associated with migraines. Each of the other responses—foods high in tyramine content (blue cheese, smoked meats, salami, beer, soy, fava beans), change in sleep patterns, and fermented foods—are all possible migraine triggers. Other triggers include skipping meals/fasting, hormonal fluctuation, environmental factors, stress, overexertion, visual triggers such as eyestrain/bright glaring lights, and others.

81. **B) Probable sign of pregnancy** Hegar's sign is softening of the lower portion of the uterus and is considered a probable sign of pregnancy.

82. **C) At the level of the umbilicus** At 12 weeks gestation the uterine fundus should be palpable just above the symphysis pubis; at 20 weeks gestation it is at the level of the umbilicus. After this, measurements in centimeters should approximately equal the number of weeks of gestation.

83. **B) Chronic obstructive pulmonary disease (COPD)** Chronic obstructive pulmonary disease (COPD) is a progressive lung disease that includes emphysema and chronic bronchitis. The most common risk factor for COPD is long-term cigarette smoking (80%–90%). Another cause is alpha-1 antitrypsin deficiency and chronic fume exposure. COPD is now the third leading cause of death in the United States. The three cardinal symptoms of COPD are dyspnea, chronic cough, and sputum production. The lungs

are hyperinflated, which changes the shape of the chest and diaphragm, making the mechanics of breathing more difficult. Excess mucus and obstructed airflow from progressive thickening and stiffening of the airways diminish breath sounds. COPD creates a high hematocrit percentage due to chronic hypoxemia.

84. **B) It is a precancerous lesion and needs to be followed up with her dermatologist** Actinic keratoses are small, raised skin lesions that result from extended sun exposure. Some actinic keratoses may develop into skin cancer; therefore, further evaluation is needed to determine if removal is required.

85. **A) Medical information is given to a spouse** Patient confidentiality is breached when medical information is given to a spouse or any other individual without consent of the patient.

86. **C) Presumptive signs of pregnancy** Presumptive signs of pregnancy are symptoms experienced by the woman, such as amenorrhea, breast tenderness, nausea/vomiting, fatigue, and increased urinary frequency.

87. **A) Angina pectoris** The classic pain of angina is described as discomfort, pressure, tightness, or heaviness on the center or left side of the chest that is precipitated by exertion and relieved by rest. The pain can be referred to the back, shoulders, neck, or jaw. The pain is not sharp, knife-like, or stabbing in nature. Angina is caused by transient myocardial ischemia. The most common cause of angina is coronary artery disease. If the angina worsens, is not relieved by rest, or lasts more than 20 minutes, it may be due to acute myocardial infarction (MI). If acute MI is suspected, call 911.

88. **B) Consult with a cardiologist for further evaluation** Blood tests that indicate tissue damage to the heart include troponin and creatine phosphokinase (CPK). Testing ordered should include EKG, nuclear stress test/stress echocardiogram, and coronary angiography. The patient would need a cardiology consultation for abnormal and/or invasive tests.

89. **C) Transient ischemic attack (TIA)** Transient ischemic attack (TIA) is a transient episode of ischemia in the brain, retina, or spinal cord without acute infarction. About 10% to 20% of patients with TIA will have a stroke within 90 days. TIA signs and symptoms are acute onset of facial asymmetry, slurred speech, weakness, monocular visual loss, headache, and hemiplegia that resolves within minutes to several hours. TIA is a neurological emergency; should undergo brain imaging (MRI preferred) within 24 hours of onset.

90. **A) Drinking organic orange juice** Commercial orange juice is fortified with calcium and vitamin D. But organic products usually do not have any additives such as calcium. Vitamin D levels must be sufficient for the body to absorb calcium. Eating foods high in vitamin D and calcium along with calcium and vitamin D supplements is advised to protect the bones and prevent bone loss. Performing weight-bearing exercises daily also increases bone strength.

91. **C) Incisors** The incisors are the first teeth to erupt during infancy.

92. **A) Palpation of the fetus and auscultation of the fetal heart tones by the nurse practitioner** Presumptive signs of pregnancy are symptoms experienced by the woman, such as amenorrhea, breast tenderness, nausea/vomiting, fatigue, and increased urinary frequency. Probable signs of pregnancy are signs detected by the examiner, such as an enlarged uterus. Positive signs of pregnancy are direct evidence of pregnancy such as audible fetal heart tones or cardiac activity on ultrasound.

93. **B) Blue coloration of the cervix and vagina** Chadwick's sign is defined by a bluish discoloration of the cervix and vagina. These changes are caused by the increased vascularity and congestion in the pelvic area during pregnancy.

94. **C) Apply acetic acid to the penile shaft and look for acetowhite changes** Lesions of human papillomavirus (HPV) infection will turn white with application of acetic acid. Routine use of this procedure to detect mucosal changes due to HPV is not recommended because results do not influence clinical management (CDC, 2015). Condoms may lower the risk of HPV infection and might decrease the time to clear in women with HPV infection.

95. **D) All of the above** Obsessive-compulsive disorder is an anxiety disorder in which people have unwanted and repeated thoughts, feelings, ideas, sensations (obsessions), or behaviors that make them feel driven to do something (compulsions). Often the person carries out the behaviors to get rid of the obsessive thoughts, but this only provides temporary relief. Not performing the obsessive rituals can cause great anxiety. Signs and symptoms of obsessive-compulsive disorder include ritualistic behaviors that are repeated, increased anxiety when the patient attempts to ignore repetitive behaviors, and frequent intrusive and repetitive thoughts and impulses.

96. **A) Paroxetine (Paxil CR)** The first medication usually considered is a type of antidepressant called a *selective serotonin reuptake inhibitor (SSRI)*. Paroxetine (Paxil CR) is in the SSRI drug class. Haloperidol (Haldol) is an antipsychotic, alprazolam (Xanax) is a benzodiazepine, and doxepin (Sinequan) is a tricyclic antidepressant.

97. **B) She should not get pregnant within the next 4 weeks** MMR should not be administered to women known to be pregnant. In addition, women should be counseled to avoid becoming pregnant for 28 days following vaccination.

98. **C) Patient history obtained from family members and close friends** To assess a patient for dementia, the first step is obtaining a thorough history of the patient's behavior, medical history, and medications. There are questionnaires to assess for dementia. The Folstein Mini-Mental State Exam is probably one the most common tools used to assess for dementia.

99. **A) Recheck urine during the visit, send a urine specimen for culture and sensitivity, and refer to a nephrologist** Although the patient is currently asymptomatic, her history of three urinary tract infections (UTIs) in 8 months warrants testing while she is in the office. A UTI is defined as the presence of 100,000 organisms per milliliter of urine in asymptomatic patients or greater than 100 organisms per milliliter of urine with pyuria (>7 WBCs/mL) in a symptomatic patient. Diabetic patients are at higher risk for UTIs and over time may develop bladder damage (cystopathy) and nephropathy. A nephrology consult is prudent.

100. **D) Spinach, liver, and beans** Folic acid deficiency is associated with excessive alcohol intake and malnutrition. Folate is a water-soluble B vitamin (vitamin B9). Folate is present in the following foods: liver, dark leafy vegetables (spinach, turnip, broccoli), beans (soy, lentils, peas), pasta, breads, and cereals.

101. **A) Breast buds and some straight pubic hair** Tanner stage II in females is noted for breast and papilla elevated as a small mound and increased areola diameter (breast buds). Tanner II pubic hair for females is sparse, lightly pigmented straight hair along the medial border of the labia.

102. **A) Inflammation of the median nerve** The Phalen maneuver is a diagnostic test for carpal tunnel syndrome. The test is performed by pushing the back of the hands together for 1 minute. This compresses the median nerve within the carpal tunnel. Characteristic symptoms (burning; tingling; numbness over the thumb, index, middle, and ring fingers) convey a positive test result.

103. **C) An increase of up to 50% of the plasma volume in pregnant women** Physiological anemia of pregnancy is caused by the increased volume of plasma during pregnancy when compared to the production of red blood cells.

104. **C) Acute viral upper respiratory infection** Chronic cough can be caused by chronic bronchitis, allergic rhinitis, and gastroesophageal reflux disease (GERD). The cough associated with a viral URI is a mild to moderate hacking cough. The cough is usually dry (no sputum). With postnasal drip, the cough may bring up some nasal secretions. The cough abates with the viral illness.

105. **D) The effect on platelet function is irreversible and lasts 15 to 20 days** The use of aspirin affects platelet function, is irreversible, and can last up to 15 to 20 days.

106. **A) Albuterol inhaler (Proventil)** Albuterol is a short-acting bronchodilator that is used for immediate relief of shortness of breath in patients with asthma. It works by opening the air passages but does not have any steroidal/anti-inflammatory effect such as triamcinolone (Azmacort), nor an effect such as a leukotriene blocker (Singulair). Steroids and leukotrienes help the inflamed channels to remain open and clear but take longer to get into the system to work.

107. **A) An acute abdomen, such as during a ruptured appendix** Rovsing's sign identifies an acute abdomen, such as occurs in acute appendicitis. With the patient in the supine position, the examiner palpates deep into the left lower quadrant of the abdomen. The maneuver is positive if pain is referred to the right lower quadrant.

108. **B) Intravaginal ultrasound** No type of vaginal exam should be performed in patients diagnosed with placenta previa. Intravaginal ultrasound and pelvic exams are contraindicated.

109. **B) Order a hepatitis C RNA test** When a patient tests positive for anti-HCV (hepatitis C virus antibody), the follow-up test recommended by the CDC is the hepatitis C RNA test. The majority of patients with hepatitis C infection have chronic infection.

110. **C) Cauda equina syndrome** Cauda equina is a serious condition caused by compression of the lumbar, sacral, or coccygeal nerve roots in the lower portion of the spinal cord. It is considered a surgical emergency. If left untreated, acute pressure causes ischemia and can lead to permanent nerve damage, including loss of bowel and bladder control and paralysis of the legs. Signs and symptoms include a change in bowel and bladder control (incontinence), saddle-pattern anesthesia (perineum), sciatica, low-back pain, and loss of sensation or movement below level of the lesion. Causes include disk herniation, abscess, tumor, inflammation, and others.

111. **A) Acute sinusitis** Acute sinusitis symptoms include cough, facial pain, and low-grade fever.

112. **B) Placental abruption** Symptoms of placental abruption are bright-red vaginal bleeding, board-like uterus on palpation, and pain. However, there can be concealed hemorrhage, and the patient may not have vaginal bleeding. Placenta previa is painless bleeding. Ectopic and molar pregnancy would not progress to 32 weeks gestation.

113. **A) An immune-mediated reaction precipitated by the destruction of a large number of spirochetes due to an antibiotic injection** The dying bacteria release antigens that cause a host reaction. Herxheimer reaction, or Jarisch–Herxheimer reaction, may occur with infections caused by spirochete bacteria such as syphilis and Lyme disease. It is more commonly seen after treatment of early-stage syphilis. It usually occurs in the first 24 hours after therapy. Signs and symptoms are headache, myalgias, rigors, sweating, hypotension, and worsening of rash (if present). No treatment is needed, as it usually resolves within 12 to 24 hours.

114. **B) Advise the patient to return 1 week after her period so her breasts can be rechecked** Symptoms of fibrocystic breast disease include cyclic tenderness with prominent breast tissue that is present in both breasts. The symptoms are worse about 1 week before menses. A few days after menses starts, the bloating and breast tenderness resolve. Symptoms are caused by elevated hormone levels (progesterone). Fibrocystic disease is differentiated from breast cancer by the lack of a dominant mass or other symptoms such as peau d'orange, dimpling, retraction, or eczema-like rash on the nipples and areola.

115. **A) The blood pressure is higher in the arms than in the legs** In coarctation of the aorta, blood pressure is higher in the arms than in the legs due to the narrowing in the aorta. Blood pressure must rise to get adequate blood flow to the lower extremities; therefore, the blood pressure above the coarctation rises to compensate for this.

116. **C) A large number of squamous epithelial cells whose surfaces and edges are coated with large numbers of bacteria along with a few leukocytes** Diagnosis of bacterial vaginosis includes three of four Amsel criteria: (1) white, thick adherent discharge; (2) pH greater than 4.5; (3) positive whiff test (amine odor mixed with 10% potassium hydroxide [KOH]); (4) clue cells greater than 20% on a wet mount (epithelial cells dotted with large numbers of bacteria that obscure cell borders).

117. **D) Mitral valve prolapse** Mitral valve prolapse (MVP) occurs when the mitral valve does not close all the way, causing a late systolic murmur heard best in the apical area

during auscultation of the chest. Following a normal S1 and briefly quiet systole, the valve suddenly prolapses, resulting in a mid-systolic click. The click is so characteristic of MVP that even without a subsequent murmur, its presence alone is enough for the diagnosis. Immediately after the click, a brief crescendo–decrescendo murmur is heard, usually best at the apex. Symptoms patients may experience at times include palpitations and dizziness.

118. D) Renal artery stenosis Renal artery stenosis refers to narrowing of the kidney arteries. It is commonly noted in individuals older than 50 years of age and is associated with atherosclerosis and hypertension. Hematuria is not associated with renal artery stenosis. Evidence of blood in the urine can be seen with kidney stones, bladder cancer, and acute pyelonephritis.

119. B) Pterygium Pterygium is a triangular growth on the white part of the eye that also extends onto the cornea. Corneal arcus is a white- to greyish-colored ring around the edge of the cornea of both eyes. Chalazion is a stye in the eye that may cause pain and swelling. Pinguecula is a benign growth on the conjunctiva caused by the degeneration of its collagen fibers. Thick, yellow fibers may be seen.

120. A) Presumptive sign Presumptive signs are sensations that are felt by the mother, but they could also be caused by other conditions. They are some of the earliest symptoms of pregnancy, such as nausea, fatigue, breast tenderness, amenorrhea, and quickening (16 to 20 weeks).

121. A) Doxycycline (Vibramycin) 100 mg PO BID × 21 days Erythema migrans is the rash characteristic of Lyme disease and it usually appears 7 to 10 days after a tick bite. Lyme disease is caused by *Borrelia burgdorferi,* a spirochete. The rash appears either as a single expanding red patch or a central spot surrounded by clear skin that is in turn ringed by an expanded red rash (bull's eye). The choice of antibiotic depends on bacterial sensitivity. Doxycycline 100 mg BID for 14 to 21 days is the recommended treatment of adults.

122. A) The nurse practice act in the state where they practice The nurse practice act is a statute enacted by the legislature of each state. The act delineates the legal scope of the practice of nursing within the geographic boundaries of the jurisdiction. The purpose of the act is to protect the public. The state board of nursing is the agency that enforces the nurse practice act. The Medicare statute provides the funds for paying for health services at the age of 65 years and older.

123. B) Order a mammogram and refer the patient to a breast surgeon A scaly, reddened rash on the breast that does not resolve after a few weeks of medical treatment may indicate breast cancer. She should have a mammogram performed and see a breast surgeon for evaluation and treatment. Paget's disease of the breast is a rare type of cancer involving the skin of the nipple and, usually, the areola. It may be misdiagnosed at first because its early symptoms are similar to those caused by some benign skin conditions. Most patients with Paget's disease of the breast also have one or more tumors inside the same breast, either ductal carcinoma in situ or invasive breast cancer.

124. C) A child who was born in Japan Japan is not considered a high-risk country for tuberculosis (TB) infection; other Asian countries, such as India, Bangladesh, Pakistan,

China, and the Philippines, have a higher incidence. Other high-risk areas are Africa, the Western Pacific, and Europe (Russia). Additional risk factors for TB are immunocompromised status (HIV, steroid therapy), homelessness, injection drug users, and working or residing with people at high risk for TB.

125. **C) This is a normal finding in some young athletes** It is common to hear a split S2 heart sound over the pulmonic area of the heart with inspiration. As long as it disappears with expiration, with no other abnormal symptoms, this is a normal finding. The sound is caused by splitting of the aortic and pulmonic components.

126. **D) Four risk factors** The risk factors for coronary artery disease for this patient are (1) 65-year-old male, (2) overweight (body mass index [BMI] of 30), (3) hypertension, and (4) total cholesterol 230 g/dL.

127. **D) Diarrhea** Common side effects of metformin (Glucophage) include diarrhea, stomach pain, nausea, and flatulence.

128. **A) Atrial fibrillation** Atrial fibrillation is chaotic electrical activity of the heart, caused by several ectopic foci in the atria without any signs of distress. There are three pathological irregular rhythms: (1) ectopic beats (may be atrial, junctional, or ventricular), (2) atrial fibrillation, and (3) second-degree heart block. All are confirmed by EKG.

129. **C) A 21-year-old woman who has a history of irritable bowel syndrome** Irritable bowel syndrome is not associated with higher risk for urinary tract infection (UTI). Risk factors for UTI are gender (female), pregnancy, spermicide use during the past year, having a mother with history of UTIs, having a new sex partner during the past year, urinary incontinence, and cystocele.

130. **B) Congestive heart failure** In congestive heart failure (CHF), the heart's ventricular function is inadequate. Symptoms include fatigue, diminished exercise capacity, shortness of breath, hemoptysis, cough, orthopnea, hypertension, nocturnal dyspnea, and edema. The kidneys begin to lose their normal ability to excrete sodium and water, leading to fluid retention. Lung congestion/pulmonary edema causes shortness of breath and a decreased ability to tolerate exercise.

131. **B) Rovsing's sign** The Rovsing sign is right lower quadrant pain intensified by left lower quadrant abdominal pressure (i.e., pain referred to the opposite side of the abdomen after release of palpation). It is associated with peritoneal irritation and appendicitis.

132. **B) Epstein–Barr virus (EBV)** EBV is a member of the herpesvirus family and one of the most common viruses. During adolescence, EBV causes infectious mononucleosis. In most cases of infectious mono, the clinical diagnosis can be made from the triad of fever, pharyngitis, and lymphadenopathy lasting 1 to 4 weeks. Serology tests show normal to moderately elevated white blood cells and increased numbers of lymphocytes, greater than 10% atypical lymphocytes, and a positive reaction to a mono spot test. The antibody response in primary EBV infection appears to be quite rapid.

133. **D) Spina bifida** A faun tail nevus is an abnormal tuft of hair in the lumbosacral area, which can be a sign of spina bifida. If found, order an ultrasound of the lesion to rule out an opening in the lower spine (spina bifida).

134. **A) Order a urinalysis and urine for culture and sensitivity (C&S), and treat the patient with antibiotics** Because this is the second urinary tract infection for the year and the last episode was 3 months ago, the best action is to order the urinalysis and urine C&S to identify the organism causing the infection. Antimicrobial-resistant strains are increasing. Start empiric treatment with an antibiotic for 7-day duration (do not use 3-day regimen).

135. **A) They are associated with neurofibromatosis or von Recklinghausen's disease** Café-au-lait spots are caused by an increase in melanin content, often with the presence of giant melanosomes. They have irregular borders and vary in color from light to dark brown. Neurofibromatosis causes tumors to grow in the nervous system, and these tumors commonly cause skin changes.

136. **C) Papilledema** The funduscopic examination visualizes vessels and assesses intracranial tension and is recommended in new-onset headaches. Papilledema is optic disc swelling cause by increased intracranial pressure. The swelling is usually bilateral. Signs include venous engorgement, loss of venous pulsation, hemorrhages over and/or adjacent to the optic disc, blurring of optic margins, and elevation of the optic disc. On visual field exam there may be an enlarged blind spot.

137. **B) Gastroesophageal reflux** Classic signs of gastroesophageal reflux disease (GERD) include acid reflux (regurgitation) into the esophagus, heartburn, and nausea. Complications include ulcers, esophageal strictures, Barrett's esophagus, cough, asthma, and throat or laryngeal inflammation. Risk factors include obesity, pregnancy, smoking, and alcohol use.

138. **A) Cataracts** Instruct patient to look straight ahead and avoid moving the eyes. Use a direct ophthalmoscope (set at "0"), stand about 18 inches from the patient and shine the light directly on the eyes. Examine each eye, and then both eyes. A normal red reflex exam will show an orange to red color and round shape, with both eyes symmetrical. If the red reflex test of an infant shows white-colored reflection, rule out retinoblastoma or congenital cataract. Refer any patient with an abnormal light reflex to an ophthalmologist (American Academy of Pediatrics, 2008).

139. **C) Alzheimer's disease** Delirium is an acute decline in mental status and is temporary. Common causes are fever, shock, drugs, alcohol, and dehydration. Alzheimer's disease involves a permanent change to the brain that causes short-term memory loss, agnosia, apraxia, and aphasia. In this case, the patient's physical exam is normal; however, he is having memory loss and difficulty working and carrying out his normal tasks.

140. **D) Leukoplakia and oral cancer** The chronic use of tobacco increases the risk of oral cancer and leukoplakia. Cheilosis is skin fissures/maceration in the corner of the mouth, most commonly caused by anemia, bacterial infection, vitamin deficiencies, or oversalivation.

141. **B) Fungal infections** The potassium hydroxide (KOH) prep test is performed to evaluate for tinea or candida (yeast) infection of the skin. In vaginal discharge, the yeast organism is outside the skin cells, so KOH is not needed to visualize it. But for skin cells, yeast is not visible unless the skin cell walls are destroyed by KOH. The test involves placing a sample of skin on a glass slide, with one to two drops of KOH (causes lysis of

skin cells) and a coverslip on top. If done correctly, you can visualize the budding spores and pseudohyphae.

142. **A) Imipramine (Tofranil)** Imipramine (Tofranil) is a tricyclic antidepressant (TCA). Fluoxetine (Prozac), sertraline (Zoloft), and paroxetine (Paxil CR) are selective serotonin reuptake inhibitors (SSRIs).

143. **D) Auscultation** Auscultation is a technique used to evaluate lung sounds, whereas tactile maneuvers use the hands. Fremitus occurs as a result of vibration of the chest wall when a person speaks and is heard through a stethoscope. Tactile fremitus is a type of vocal fremitus found over the area of secretions. Tactile fremitus is evaluated using the surface of both hands over the back/lungs. In bronchophony (the ability to hear increased loudness of the spoken sounds), even a whisper can be heard through the stethoscope.

144. **C) Retinoblastoma of the left eye** Retinoblastoma is a congenital tumor of the retina. It usually affects only one eye (rarely both eyes are involved). During infancy, the tumor is a small size and it continues to grow with the child. This rare cancer is diagnosed by noting a pupil that appears white or has white spots on it. One or both eyes may be affected. It is often first noted in photographs, because a white glow is present in the eye instead of the usual "red eye" that results from the flash.

145. **C) Nongonococcal urethritis** A number of communicable diseases are required to be reported to the state public health department. They include Lyme disease, gonorrhea, and syphilis. Statistics of reportable diseases are kept in each state, and a subset is then reportable to the Centers for Disease Control and Prevention (CDC). The most common bacterial cause of nongonococcal urethritis (NGU) is *Chlamydia trachomatis,* but it may also be caused by *Ureaplasma urealyticum, Haemophilus vaginalis,* or *Mycoplasma genitalium.* Viral causes include herpes simplex and adenovirus; rarely, a *Trichomonas vaginalis* (parasite) may cause NGU. It can also be caused by a mechanical injury such as a catheter or cystoscopy.

146. **A) Yogurt and sardines** Postmenopausal women are advised to increase their dietary intake of calcium and vitamin D to help protect their bones from osteopenia and osteoporosis. Good sources of calcium include low-fat dairy products (yogurt), dark leafy vegetables, canned salmon or sardines with bones, soy products, and calcium-fortified cereals and orange juice. Just 3 ounces of canned sardines, including bones, drained of oil, provides 324 mg of calcium.

147. **A) The high vitamin K levels will decrease the INR** Green leafy vegetables have high levels of vitamin K, which can bind with the blood-clotting cascade and decrease the bleeding time. Vitamin K and warfarin sodium (Coumadin) have opposing effects. Vitamin K helps to decrease bleeding time; Coumadin helps to increase bleeding time. Leafy green vegetables high in vitamin K would normally decrease the bleeding time. In a patient who is taking Coumadin, the high vitamin K would interfere with the desired effect of the Coumadin (which would be to prolong or increase clotting time) and, in fact, would have the opposite effect, which would be to shorten or decrease the clotting time.

148. **B) Order a liver function profile and CK level** Statin medications, such as rosuvastatin (Crestor), can affect liver function and increase liver enzymes as well as cause the patient to feel weak, fatigued, and have muscle aches. Therefore, checking the liver function profile is recommended.

149. **B) Acute drug-induced hepatitis** Liver enzymes, such as ALT, AST, and CK levels, can be elevated with the use of medications such as statins. High liver enzymes can cause an acute drug-induced hepatitis.

150. **D) Stop taking the medicine until the lab results are available** This patient's symptoms suggest liver involvement; have the patient stop the statin until the lab results are back, then the patient and the clinician can make informed decisions.

151. **A) Advise the patient that she had a normal exam** The optic disc of a normal examination has sharp margins, a yellowish-orange to a creamy pink color, and round or oval shape. To test, have the patient look at a distant fixed point and direct the light of the ophthalmoscope at the fundus. The ophthalmoscope (set at +8 to +10) should be close to your eyes; your head and scope move together. Check for the red reflex, then adjust the diopter setting; approach more closely to inspect the optic disc, veins, arteries, and the macula. The veins are darker in color and larger than the arterioles (3:2 ratio).

152. **A) The patient can see at 20 ft what a person with normal vision can see at 30 ft** The Snellen factions, 20/20, 20/30, and so forth, are a measure of sharpness (acuity) of sight. The numerator (top number) represents the test distance, 20 ft. The denominator (bottom number) represents the distance at which the average eye can see the letters on a certain line of the eye chart. When vision results are 20/30 in both eyes, this means that the patient can see at 20 ft what a person with normal vision can see at 30 ft.

153. **A) Somogyi phenomenon** This is caused by too much insulin (or missing a meal or snack) in the evening, which results in hypoglycemia in the early morning (2 a.m. to 3 a.m.). The body compensates by secreting glucagon (from the liver) and epinephrine, which results in high blood glucose levels in the morning. The Somogyi phenomenon (or Somogyi effect) is also known as the *rebound effect*.

154. **A) HCV RNA** The anti-HCV test detects the presence of antibodies to the hepatitis C virus, indicating exposure to HCV. The anti-HCV test cannot distinguish between someone with active or previous HCV infection (reported as positive or negative). The HCV RNA test is qualitative and used to distinguish between a current or past infection. It is reported as "negative" or "not detected." It may also be ordered after treatment is complete to see whether the virus has been eliminated.

155. **C) Check the ankle and brachial blood pressures before and after exercise** Initial evaluation for intermittent claudication would include checking the ankle and brachial blood pressures before and after exercise.

156. **B) Montelukast (Singulair)** Montelukast is a leukotriene modifier used in the treatment of asthma, asthma maintenance, bronchospasm prophylaxis, and chronic obstructive pulmonary disease (COPD). It is an asthma controller functioning as a chemical mediator in inflammation. Theophylline is methylxanthine used to treat asthma, acute asthma, and for maintenance as a bronchodilator. There is no

contraindication/drug interaction of these two drugs/classes. Medications that are contraindicated with theophylline include erythromycin, phenytoin sodium, and cimetidine.

157. **C) Mitral regurgitation** Mitral regurgitation is best heard at the apical area, and manifests as a high-pitched, blowing pansystolic murmur. It occurs when the mitral valve does not close properly. It is the abnormal leaking of blood from the left ventricle, through the mitral valve, and into the left atrium. When the ventricle contracts, there is backflow (regurgitation) of blood into the left atrium. Mitral regurgitation is the most common form of valvular heart disease. Murmurs are graded (classified) depending on how loud they sound with a stethoscope. The scale is 1 to 6 on loudness. A grade 2/6 is a grade 2 on the 6-point scale.

158. **B) Strabismus** The cover/uncover test screens for strabismus. Color blindness is evaluated by using the Ishihara tool. To use the Ishihara chart, the child must be familiar with reading numbers and be able to follow instructions. Visual acuity (distance vision) is evaluated using the Snellen chart. Cataracts are screened by using the red reflex test. Use the direct ophthalmoscope (set at "0") and shine the light into both the eyes at about 18 inches away from the patient. Instruct the patient to stare in one direction forward (and avoid moving the eyes). Turn off the room light. In someone with advanced cataracts, the red reflex will show a white reflection instead of the normal orange to red color.

159. **B) Advise the mother that this is a normal finding in infants up to 2 months of age** Infants' eyes commonly cross over at times, and this is a normal finding up to 2 months of age.

160. **A) Weight** Peak expiratory flow volume is determined by using height, gender, and age.

161. **C) Squamous epithelial cells and endocervical cells** An optimal Pap smear sample contains sufficient mature and metaplastic squamous cells to indicate adequate sampling from the transformation zone and sufficient endocervical cells to indicate that the upper limit of the transformation zone was sampled, and to provide a sample for screening for adenocarcinoma and its precursors.

162. **B) A sensation of spinning or rotating** *Vertigo* is defined as having a sensation of spinning or rotating.

163. **C) Phototherapy is usually indicated for these infants** The majority of infants with physiological jaundice do not need phototherapy. This form of jaundice is caused by the buildup of unconjugated bilirubin because the infant's immature liver cannot metabolize and excrete it quickly enough.

164. **D) Iron-deficiency anemia** Koilonychia is also known as *spoon-shaped nails*. The finger nails are thin and have a concave shape. Koilonychia is associated with severe iron-deficiency anemia.

165. **Antinuclear antibody (ANA)** Screening tests for systemic lupus erythematosus include ANA. The rheumatoid factor test is performed to diagnose rheumatoid arthritis. Antiparietal antibody testing is done to evaluate for antibodies against the parietal cells. The parietal cells make a substance that the body needs to absorb vitamin

BImmunoglobulin testing is done to assess for the amount of antibodies in the blood for a specific disease.

166. **C) It can be a normal variant if heard in a person aged 40 years or older** The S3 heart sound occurs early in diastole and is sometimes referred to as an *opening snap*. It is a normal variant in children, healthy young adults, and athletes. Bibasilar crackles in lung bases and the presence of S3 heart sounds are classic findings of congestive heart failure (CHF).

167. **B) Macrocytic and normochromic cells/herniated disk** To perform the straight leg test, have the patient lie supine on an exam table. Lift the patient's leg toward his or her head while the knee is straight. If the patient experiences sciatic pain when the straight leg is at an angle between 30 and 70 degrees, then the test is positive and a herniated disk is likely to be the cause of the pain. The straight leg test should be done on the pain-free side first to find out which range of movement is normal and to enable the patient to distinguish between "normal" stretching of muscles and a different sort of pain.

168. **A) Eye exam with an ophthalmologist** Elderly patients with type 2 diabetes should have a dilated eye exam done annually by an ophthalmologist. They should also see a podiatrist once or twice a year. Preventive care also includes receiving a flu shot annually, receiving a Pneumovax vaccine if older than 60 years of age, and taking a 81-mg baby aspirin each day.

169. **D) The patient needs to be evaluated by a dermatologist** Nonhealing ulcers of the skin are a risk for skin cancer and should be evaluated by a dermatologist for treatment.

170. **B) It is not always necessary to use a shield for the infant's eyes** When using phototherapy, the eyes should always be protected by using a shield or goggles to prevent damage to the eyes.

171. **B) Degenerative joint disease** Heberden's nodes are bony nodules on the distal interphalangeal joints, commonly seen in degenerative joint disease.

172. **C) Macrocytic and normochromic cells** Anemias resulting from vitamin B_{12} or folate deficiency are sometimes referred to as *macrocytic* or *megaloblastic* anemia because red blood cells are larger than normal. A diagnosis of pernicious anemia first requires demonstration of megaloblastic anemia with a complete blood count (CBC) with differential that evaluates the mean corpuscular volume (MCV), as well the mean corpuscular hemoglobin concentration (MCHC). Pernicious anemia is identified with a high MCV (macrocytic) and a normal MCHC (normochromic).

173. **B) A 14-month-old who understands complex commands** A 14-month-old child should developmentally be able to say "mama" and "dada," know his own name, and know at least two to four words. A 2-year-old is able to understand simple commands.

174. **A) Keep monitoring the infant's bilirubin level until it returns to normal in about 1 week** Bilirubin is excreted through the urine and feces. Increased fluids and wetting eight to 10 diapers a day is sufficient fluid intake/excretion to help bring down the bilirubin level. Levels should continue to be monitored and should improve in approximately 1 week.

175. **A) Fever occurs in up to 80% of the patients** Side effects of the Td vaccine include induration at the injection site. Td is given in adults every 10 years. The DPT and DT should not be given beyond 7 years of age. Fever may occur, but studies do not support 80% of patients having fever.

176. **A) Angiotensin-converting enzyme (ACE) inhibitors** According to the Eighth Joint National Committee (JNC 8; James et al., 2014), non-Black and Black hypertensive patients with chronic kidney disease (i.e., microalbuminuria) with or without diabetes can be treated with either angiotensin-converting enzyme (ACE) inhibitors or an angiotensin receptor blocker (ARB), alone or in combination with another drug class. The blood pressure goal for adults and older adults from this risk group is blood pressure less than 140/90 mmHg.

177. **A) Peripheral vision** The visual fields by confrontation test is used to evaluate peripheral vision. The Snellen chart is used to measure central distance vision. A tonometer is used to assess for glaucoma. The ophthalmoscope is used to assess for cataracts.

178. **C) Acne** A macule is a flat, nonraised lesion on the skin. Acne lesions are papules because they consist of raised, erythemic lesions on the skin. A freckle, petechiae, and a flat birthmark are all considered macules.

179. **A) Administer a booster dose of the Tdap vaccine** The Centers for Disease Control and Prevention (CDC) recommends the Tdap for teens or adults who need a Td booster (once in a lifetime). A tetanus vaccine booster is recommended for recent injuries if it has been more than 5 years since the last dose.

180. **D) The left side of the sternum at the fifth intercostal space by the midclavicular line** The apex of the heart is directed downward, forward, and to the left. The apex is overlapped by the left lung and pleura. The apex lies behind the fifth left intercostal space, slightly medial to the midclavicular line.

181. **B) Pulmonary system** Chronic use of nonsteroidal anti-inflammatory drugs (NSAIDs) is associated with increased risk of ulcers, perforation, and bleeding of the gastrointestinal tract, heart attacks, cardiovascular damage, strokes, acute interstitial nephritis and kidney injury, and liver damage. It does not affect the lungs or the pulmonary system.

182. **D) All of the above** This 15-year-old teenage patient will follow the Centers for Disease Control and Prevention (CDC) "catch-up" schedule (CDC, 2017) and needs the meningococcal vaccine, MMR vaccine, and Tdap vaccine. In addition to these three vaccines, this patient needs the hepatitis B vaccine, human papillomavirus (HPV) vaccine, and varicella vaccine (if no history of chickenpox).

183. **C) CN XI** Cranial nerves (CNs) IX through XII are the glossopharyngeal, vagal, spinal accessory, and hypoglossal, respectively. CN XI tests for spinal accessory. The procedure to test trapezius muscle strength is to have the patient shrug the shoulders against resistance. To test sternocleidomastoid muscle strength, have the patient turn the head to each side with resistance.

184. **B) Obtain a chest x-ray** A Mantoux result greater than 10 mm is positive for recent immigrants (<5 years) from high high-prevalence countries such as parts of Asia (Pakistan,

India, Philippines, China, etc.), Africa (Congo, Kenya, Nigeria, Ethiopia, etc.), Eastern Europe (including Russia), Latin America (Mexico, Guatemala, etc.), and the Caribbean (Haiti).

185. C) Tertiary prevention Tertiary prevention is any type of rehabilitation for a particular condition. Examples include physical rehab (swimming), cardiac rehab, and/or speech therapy.

186. B) 42-year-old obese woman from Cuba who has been taking prednisone 10 mg daily for the past 12 years to control her severe asthma Risk factors for osteoporosis include postmenopause, early menopause, use of chronic steroids, smoking, excessive use of alcohol, sedentary lifestyle, insufficient intake of calcium and vitamin D in the diet, and being an Asian or Caucasian female.

187. B) Lactose Lactose is the primary carbohydrate found in breast milk and formula.

188. C) A patient who drinks one glass of wine nightly with dinner Excessive use or exposure to alcohol increases the risk of becoming an alcoholic. A patient who drinks one glass of wine at dinner has a lower risk of becoming an alcoholic than someone who has been exposed to alcohol while growing up, one who drinks all the time, or one whose family believes he is drinking excessively.

189. C) Cigarette smoking at the age of 30 years Cigarette smoking at age 30 years is considered a relative—not absolute—contraindication. However, in a patient aged 35 years or older, smoking is an absolute contraindication. Pregnancy or suspected pregnancy is another absolute contraindication (sexually active woman who presents with amenorrhea). Liver tumors or impaired liver function is also an absolute contraindication (hepatitis C infection).

190. A) Lung cancer Lung cancer is the most common cause of cancer deaths in men (Centers for Disease Control and Prevention, 2017). Prostate cancer and colon cancer are the second and third causes of cancer death in men.

191. B) Aortic stenosis One of the most frequent pathological systolic murmurs is due to aortic stenosis. The murmur of aortic stenosis is typically a mid-systolic ejection murmur, heard best over the "aortic area" or right second intercostal space, with radiation into the right neck. It has a harsh quality and may be associated with a palpably slow rise of the carotid upstroke. Additional heart sounds, such as an S4, may be heard secondary to hypertrophy of the left ventricle, which is caused by the greatly increased work required to pump blood through the stenotic valve.

192. A) Hordeolum Hordeolum is a common, painful, acute bacterial infection of the hair follicle on the eyelid. It is a focal infection (usually staphylococcal) involving either the glands of Zeis (external hordeola or styes) or, less frequent the meibomian glands (internal hordeola). Histologically, hordeola represent focal collections of polymorphonuclear leukocytes and necrotic debris (i.e., abscesses). Pinguecula is a thickening of the bulbar conjunctiva, located on the inner and outer margins of the cornea. Pterygium is a thickening of the conjunctiva located on the nasal or temporal cornea. Pinguecula and pterygium are both caused by the UV light of long-term sun exposure. Sunglasses with

UV protection are recommended to prevent damage to the conjunctiva. Ptosis is the drooping of the upper eyelid.

193. **C) Propranolol (Inderal)** Propranolol (Inderal) is a beta-blocker. Sufficient evidence and consensus exist to recommend propranolol, timolol, amitriptyline, divalproex, sodium valproate, and topiramate as first-line agents for migraine *prevention*. The goal of preventive therapy is to improve patients' quality of life by reducing migraine frequency, severity, and duration, and by increasing the responsiveness of acute migraines to treatment. A full therapeutic trial may take 2 to 6 months. Ibuprofen (Motrin), naproxen sodium (Anaprox), and sumatriptan (Imitrex) are all medications used to treat symptoms of migraine headache.

194. **B) Cluster headache** Cluster headaches' cardinal symptoms are an excruciating, unilateral, orbital, supraorbital, and/or temporal pain. The attack ranges from 15 minutes to 3 hours or more. Autonomic symptoms include ptosis (drooping eyelid), miosis (pupil constriction), lacrimation (tearing), and rhinorrhea in the nostril on the affected side of the face. Migraine headaches with aura include visual changes, such as blind spots or flashing lights, that appear before the onset of the headache. Trigeminal neuralgia (tic douloureux) is a unilateral headache from compression or inflammation of the trigeminal nerve (cranial nerve V).

195. **D) Sucralfate (Carafate)** Naproxen sodium, aspirin, and erythromycin all have gastrointestinal side effects. Sucralfate is used to protect the stomach lining by building a protective layer over the stomach lining; it allows healing to occur.

196. **A) There is no delay in seeking medical treatment** When assessing for domestic abuse, the most common body area that is abused is the "swimsuit" area, which is usually covered by clothing. Suspect abusive relationships when the history is inconsistent with the injury. Due to shame and the secrecy of domestic violence, most victims do not seek medical attention until after several episodes of violence. The violent partner may refuse to let the partner out of his or her "control." Studies have shown that the incidence of battery escalates during pregnancy.

197. **C) Breastfed infants require vitamin D supplementation beginning in the first few days of life** The American Academy of Pediatrics (2010) recommends vitamin D 400 IU/day supplementation starting at the first few days of life for all breastfed infants to decrease the risk of rickets. It can be given as part of a multivitamin infant supplement or in a vitamin D supplement. Both are over the counter. Breastmilk alone does not provide infants with an adequate intake of vitamin D (CDC, 2015).

198. **C) Microcytic anemia** Beta thalassemia minor is a genetic disorder in which the bone marrow produces small, pale, red blood cells in which mild hypochromic, microcytic anemia occurs.

199. **D) Mitral stenosis** Complications of mitral valve prolapse (MVP) include mitral regurgitation, endocarditis, and increased risk of stroke and transient ischemic attacks. The most common complication of mitral valve prolapse (MVP) is mitral valve regurgitation (mitral insufficiency). An abnormal mitral valve increases the chance of developing endocarditis from bacteria, which can further damage the mitral valve. Doctors used

to recommend that people with MVP take antibiotics before certain dental or medical procedures to prevent endocarditis (not a current practice). Stroke is a very rare complication of MVP.

200. D) Scabies Scabies is a parasitic disease (infestation) of the skin caused by the human itch mite *Sarcoptes scabiei.* The rash is generally characterized as red, raised excoriated papules. The scabies mite is generally transmitted from one person to another by direct contact with the skin of the infested person and can also be acquired by wearing an infested person's clothing (fomites), such as sweaters, coats, or scarves. Following the incubation period, the infested person will complain of pruritus (itching), which intensifies at bedtime under the warmth of the blankets. Common sites of infection are the webs of fingers, wrists, flexors of the arms, the axillae, lower abdomen, genitalia, buttocks, and feet.

201. D) Urea breath test The urea breath test is a very sensitive test used to evaluate a patient for an active *Helicobacter pylori* infection. It can also be used to document treatment response after a treatment regimen of antibiotics (14 days) and proton-pump inhibitor (PPI) therapy.

202. A) Iron-fortified rice cereal At 6 months of age, it is recommended that the infant be fed iron-fortified rice cereal. Introducing only one new food at a time is recommended; in case an allergy does develop, you will be able to identify which food caused the allergy.

203. D) All of the above Type 2 diabetes mellitus screening tests include fasting plasma glucose level (>126 mg/dL), random plasma glucose level (>200 mg/dL), and oral glucose tolerance testing (2-hour blood glucose level >200 mg/dL) with a 75-g glucose load. Normal A1C levels are less than 6%.

204. B) A superficial vesicle filled with serous fluid greater than 1 cm in size This is a blister—a circumscribed, fluid-containing, elevated lesion of the skin, usually more than 5 mm in diameter.

205. B) Give the infant both hepatitis B vaccine and hepatitis B immunoglobulin For a mother who tests positive for HBsAg, the newborn infant should be given hepatitis B vaccine and hepatitis B immunoglobulin for protection.

206. A) Condyloma acuminata Findings consistent with the diagnosis of syphilis, caused by the *Treponema pallidum* organism, include painless chancre, maculopapular rash of the palms and soles, lymphadenopathy, and condyloma lata. Condyloma acuminata (genital warts) are caused by the human papillomavirus (HPV) and spread to others by skin-to-skin contact.

207. D) Low-dose oral contraceptives with at least 20 mcg of estradiol (Alesse, Lo-estrin) Low-dose oral contraceptives that contain estradiol are contraindicated for breastfeeding mothers. Estrogen is an FDA pregnancy category X drug and it should not be given to pregnant, suspect pregnant, or breastfeeding women. Breastfeeding women may use progestin-only pills (POP), but they are not as effective as combined oral contraceptives. They are more effective if breastfeeding (100%). Mechanical forms of birth control (condoms, diaphragms) and the IUD are other options of birth control for this population.

208. D) Ovarian cysts Women with a history of pelvic inflammatory disease (PID) have a higher risk of ectopic pregnancy, scarring of the fallopian tubes, and infertility due to the scarring of the fallopian tube(s).

209. D) Molluscum contagiosum Genital ulcers may occur with syphilis, genital herpes, and chancroid. Molluscum contagiosum is a viral skin infection. In adults, molluscum contagiosum appears on the face, neck, armpits, arms, and hands. Other common places include the genitals, abdomen, and inner thigh. Lesions often begin as small, firm, dome-shaped growths; have a surface that feels smooth, waxy, or pearly; are flesh-colored or pink; have a dimple in the center (may be filled with a thick, white substance that is cheesy or waxy); and are painless but itch. Scratching or picking can spread the virus.

210. C) Microcytic anemia Anemias can be classified according to the mean corpuscular volume (MCV) into microcytic, normocytic, and macrocytic anemias. A microcytic anemia is defined by an MCV of less than 80 fL. The differential diagnosis of a microcytic anemia includes iron-deficiency anemia (IDA), thalassemias; anemia of chronic disease (ACD); and sideroblastic anemias, including lead poisoning. Lead causes anemia by mimicking healthful minerals such as calcium, iron, and zinc. It is absorbed by the bones, where it interferes with the production of red blood cells. This absorption can also interfere with calcium absorption, which is needed to keep the bones healthy.

211. C) Elevated Headache is the most common chief complaint and presents in more than two thirds of patients with temporal arteritis. The headache tends to be new or different in character than previous headaches and is typically sudden in onset, localizing to the temporal region. Any new headache in patients older than 50 years warrants a consideration of temporal arteritis. Erythrocyte sedimentation rate (ESR) greater than 50 mm/hr is suspect. The normal ESR for males is 0 to 15 mm/hr, and for females is 0 to 20 mm/hr. The ESR can be slightly more elevated in the elderly.

212. B) Rheumatoid arthritis When rheumatoid arthritis is active, symptoms can include fatigue, loss of energy, depression, low-grade fever, muscle and joint aches, and stiffness. Muscle and joint stiffness are usually most notable in the morning and after periods of inactivity. During flares, joints frequently become red, swollen, painful, and tender. This occurs because the lining of the tissue of the joint (synovium) becomes inflamed, resulting in the production of excessive joint fluid (synovitis).

213. B) He should not give whole milk to his son until the boy is at least 12 months of age The American Academy of Pediatrics does not recommend offering whole milk to children younger than 12 months of age.

214. C) Indomethacin (Indocin) Nonsteroidal anti-inflammatory drugs (NSAIDs), such as indomethacin (Indocin), have been used for the treatment of *acute gout*. Colchicine may be added to the NSAIDs if relief is not obtained. Maintenance therapy consists of allopurinol and/or probenecid. Allopurinol is used to prevent gout attacks, not to treat them once they occur. It may take several months or longer before the full benefit of allopurinol is felt. Allopurinol may increase the number of gout attacks during the first few months that it is taken, although it will eventually prevent attacks.

215. **A) Impaired joint mobility and renal damage** Left untreated, gout can develop into a painful and disabling chronic disorder. Persistent gout can destroy cartilage and bone, causing irreversible joint deformities and loss of motion. High urate levels can deposit in the kidney and also lead to kidney stones.

216. **B) Endocarditis prophylaxis is not necessary** Prophylaxis treatment for endocarditis is no longer recommended for patients with mitral valve prolapse (MVP).

217. **A) Bouchard's nodes** Bony nodules at the proximal interphalangeal joints of the hands are called *Bouchard's nodes*. Heberden's nodes are nodules on the distal interphalangeal joints. Tophi deposits are seen with gout, in which high levels of uric acid occur in the blood and cause nodules in the joint that can eventually destroy the bone. Osteoarthritic nodules develop in the joints of the hands.

218. **A) Diabetes mellitus** The risk of diabetes mellitus is two to three times higher in Mexican Americans than in non-Hispanic Americans.

219. **D) Initiate a prescription of fenofibrate (Tricor)** A triglyceride level above 800 mg/dL is considered to be "very high"; there is an increased risk of acute pancreatitis, especially if the patient also drinks alcohol. Two fibrate drugs have been approved for use in the United States: fenofibrate (Tricor) and gemfibrozil (Lopid). Another option is nicotinic acid, but fibrates are more potent and better tolerated. In addition, lifestyle changes are important; these include avoiding foods with concentrated sugars, alcohol, weight loss if overweight or obese, and regular, moderate to intense aerobic exercise.

220. **A) Acute pancreatitis** Cullen's sign is commonly seen in acute pancreatitis. It refers to a yellowish-blue skin color change around the umbilicus. It is thought to occur due to the pancreatic enzymes that run along the ligament and subcutaneous tissues around the umbilicus.

221. **D) Mini-Mental State Exam** The Lachman test is performed on the knee; a positive result is indicative of anterior cruciate ligament damage or rupture. The Romberg test is for assessment of the cerebellum. The Mini-Mental State Exam (MMSE), also known as *Folstein Mini-Mental State Exam,* is performed to assess for cognitive impairment and dementia. It is also used to estimate the severity of cognitive impairment at a specific time and to follow the course of cognitive changes in an individual over time, thus making it an effective way to document an individual's response to treatment. Requiring about 10 minutes to complete, the MMSE samples several cognitive functions, including arithmetic, memory, and orientation.

222. **C) School physical exams** Any student younger than 18 years of age must have parental permission to have a school physical exam done.

223. **B) Serum creatinine and estimated GFR (glomerular filtration rate)** One of the best tests for assessing renal function is the estimated GFR, which requires the creatinine

value so that it can be calculated using a mathematical formula (Cockcroft–Gault equation, others). Native Americans/Alaska Natives have the highest rate of diabetes of any group in the United States. Aspartate aminotransferase (AST) and alanine aminotransferase (ALT) are used to evaluate liver function. Electrolytes are not used to evaluate renal function.

224. C) The scotch tape test Enterobiasis infection (pinworms) is caused by small worms that infect the intestines. Symptoms include itching around the anus, which is usually worse at night. The scotch tape test is done by applying the scotch tape on the anal area at bedtime; the worms commonly come out at night and will stick to the tape, which is used for diagnosis.

225. B) Chronic hypertension Left ventricular hypertrophy develops in response to some factor, such as high blood pressure, that requires the left ventricle to work harder. As the workload increases, the walls of the chamber grow thicker, lose elasticity, and eventually may fail to pump with as much force as a healthy heart. High blood pressure, a blood pressure reading greater than 140/90 mmHg, is the greatest risk factor.

226. C) Chronic coughing A patient experiencing respiratory distress from an asthmatic exacerbation presents with tachypnea (>20 breaths/min), tachycardia or bradycardia, cyanosis, and anxiety. The patient appears exhausted, fatigued, and diaphoretic and uses accessory muscles to help with breathing. Physical exam reveals cyanosis and "quiet" lungs with no wheezing or breath sounds audible. A "chronic" cough is not a symptom of an acute exacerbation but is commonly present in people with asthma Although cough usually accompanies dyspnea and wheezing, it may present in isolation as a precursor of typical asthmatic symptoms, or it may remain the predominant or sole symptom of asthma. Cough-variant asthma is a type of asthma in which the main symptom is a dry, nonproductive cough.

227. D) The board of nursing Advanced practice registered nursing (APRN) practice is typically defined by the state nurse practice act and governed by the state board of nursing, but other laws and regulations may affect practice, and other boards may play a role. For instance, in some states nurse-midwives are regulated by a board of midwifery or public health. In other states, both the board of medicine and the board of nursing regulate nursing practice.

228. A) Premedicate 10 to 15 minutes before starting exercise Exercise-induced asthma is best controlled by using the Proventil inhaler (bronchodilator) approximately 10 to 15 minutes before exercise, to prevent vasospasm of the bronchioles and shortness of breath with exercise. The effects of these bronchodilators usually last approximately 4 hours. They also work quickly to open up the bronchioles if an acute attack/shortness of breath occurs.

229. A) It is a slow or sudden painless loss of central vision Atrophic macular degeneration (AMD) occurs when the macula—the central portion of the retina that is important for reading and color vision—becomes damaged. This portion contains the fovea, with the largest number of cones in the eye, responsible for color vision and visual acuity. AMD is a single disease, but it can take two different forms: dry and wet. The atrophic or dry form of macular degeneration is the most common. There is a gradual withering of the visual cells and the blood vessels of the choroid (the vascular layer of tissue behind the retina). Usually the atrophic form results in only moderate loss of central vision. Although there is no medical or surgical treatment for the dry form of macular degeneration, eyesight may be helped somewhat by low-vision aids. These devices include magnifying lenses, brighter light for reading, or an electronic magnifier using a TV screen.

230. **C) Acute sinusitis** Signs and symptoms of acute sinusitis include headache, facial pain that worsens with bending over, eye/ear pressure and pain, aching in upper jaw/teeth, reduced smell and taste, cough (especially at night due to the nasal drainage), sore throat, bad breath, and fatigue.

231. **B) Pelvis** Hemorrhagic (hypovolemic) shock is due to acute blood or body fluid loss. Hypovolemic shock can occur from a fractured pelvis secondary to internal bleeding from a fractured bone fragment that lacerates an artery or vein. The amount of blood loss after trauma is often difficult to determine; consequently, hemorrhage after blunt trauma is often underestimated. A femoral closed fracture, for example, may lose 1 to 2 liters of blood, a pelvic fracture can lose more than 2 liters of blood, whereas a simple rib fracture can lose up to 125 mL. The abdominal cavity can accommodate a large amount of blood without distension; initially the blood does not irritate the peritoneum, making the diagnosis of hemoperitoneum difficult to establish.

232. **B) Gout** Gout (also known as *podagra* when it involves the big toe) is characterized by recurrent attacks of acute inflammatory arthritis—a red, tender, hot, swollen joint. The metatarsal–phalangeal joint at the base of the big toe is the most commonly affected (approximately 50% of cases). Pain occurs due to the accumulation of uric acid and salts in the joint.

233. **C) Grade 4** A fine vibration, felt by an examiner's hand on a patient's body over the site of an aneurysm or on the precordium, results from turmoil in the flow of blood and indicates the presence of an organic murmur of grade 4 or greater intensity. A thrill can also be felt over the carotids if a bruit is present and over an arteriovenous fistula in the patient undergoing hemodialysis.

234. **A) Aortic stenosis** The murmur associated with aortic stenosis can be auscultated as harsh and high pitched in the right second intercostal space. It typically radiates to the carotid arteries and apex.

235. **D) Both hepatitis B and hepatitis C** Of the primary hepatitis viruses, only B and C are associated with hepatocellular cancer. Chronic hepatitis B and C infection often results in cirrhosis of the liver, which increases the risk of liver cancer.

236. **C) 20 kcal/30 mL** The caloric content of infant formula and breast milk is 20k cal/30 mL.

237. **C) Hepatitis B vaccination and hepatitis B immunoglobulin** Hepatitis B surface antigen (HBsAg) is a marker of *infectivity*. If positive, it indicates either an acute or a chronic hepatitis B infection. Antibody to hepatitis B surface antigen (anti-HBs) is a marker of *immunity*. Antibody to hepatitis B core antigen (anti-HBc) is a marker of acute, chronic,

or resolved hepatitis B virus (HBV) infection; it may be used in prevaccination testing to determine *previous exposure to HBV*. The hepatitis B panel results for the individual in this question (negative HBsAg, anti-HBc, and anti-HBs) indicates the partner is *susceptible* (not immune), has not been infected, and is still at risk of future infection—and thus *needs vaccine.* Interpretation of the negative hepatitis C anti-HCV screening test indicates that the partner is not infected. Hepatitis B immunoglobulin contains antibodies that provide "instant" immunity against hepatitis B, but its action lasts for several days, only. It is not a vaccine. It is given to infants and others who are at high risk of becoming infected and are not immune. The hepatitis B vaccine stimulates the body to make its own antibodies, which are permanent. A total of three doses are needed to gain full immunity against hepatitis B.

238. **D) Pregnancy** Mild normocytic anemia is associated with chronic autoimmune or inflammatory disorders and chronic infection. Its exact mechanism is unknown. Pregnancy does not cause normocytic anemia, but it may cause several other types of anemia: iron-deficiency anemia (microcytic anemia, which can develop in some women who have very low ferritin levels), folate-deficiency anemia (macrocytic anemia), and vitamin B_{12} deficiency (also a macrocytic anemia).

239. **A) Apical and radial pulses at the same time, then finding the difference between the two** The pulse deficit is the difference between the apical pulse and the radial pulse. These should be taken at the same time, which will require that two people take the pulse: one with a stethoscope and one at the wrist. Count for 1 full minute. Then subtract the radial from the apical.

240. **B) Bronchiolitis** Symptoms of tracheobronchitis include prominent dry, nonproductive cough; later, coughing up phlegm is common. Bronchiolitis is a viral infection caused by respiratory syncytial virus (RSV), which is commonly seen during the winter/spring months in infants and young children. Typical signs/symptoms include fever and inspiratory/expiratory wheezing with clear drainage. Croup is a viral infection with a classic "barking" cough; the patient may have a runny nose, but typically no fever. When a child swallows a foreign object, choking, wheezing, and shortness of breath may occur, but no fever or clear drainage are present.

241. **A) Kernig's maneuver** Kernig's maneuver is performed by having the patient flex both hips and legs and then straighten the legs against resistance, testing for meningeal and spinal inflammation. Flexion of hip and knees is a positive sign for meningitis. Brudzinski's maneuver is performed by placing the patient's hands behind his or her head, and gently tucking chin to chest. Murphy's sign is elicited by having the patient inspire with the tips of the examiner's fingers placed on the right upper quadrant, at the liver border, under the ribs. Pain on inspiration is suggestive of cholecystitis. Homan's sign is flexion of the foot, causing pain in the posterior calf area, suggestive of a deep vein thrombosis.

242. **A) Women aged 50 years or older** Women have a greater risk of developing thyroid disease than men. Being age 50 or older increases the risk of thyroid disease for both men and women. Screening for thyroid disease is therefore recommended for women 50 years of age and older.

243. **B) Order a spot urine for microalbumin-to-creatinine ratio** The American Diabetes Association (ADA) now prefers a spot urine for the microalbumin-to-creatinine ratio (ACR) test instead of a urine albumin test. Use the first morning void sample. The ACR has high predictive value for albuminuria and early kidney disease in patients with prediabetes, diabetes, and hypertension (McCulloch & Bakris, 2016). Because the patient has type 2 diabetes, both an annual urinalysis and an annual ACR test are recommended. Regarding the urinalysis result, a few epithelial cells is within normal limits.

244. **A) The destruction of Rh-positive fetal RBCs that are present in the mother's circulatory system** Rh_o(D) immune globulin (RhoGAM) is used to prevent the immunological condition known as *rhesus disease* or *hemolytic disease of the newborn*. RhoGAM is a solution of IgG anti-D (anti-RhD) antibodies that suppresses the mother's immune system from attacking Rh-positive blood cells that have entered the maternal bloodstream from fetal circulation. In an Rh-negative mother, RhoGAM can prevent temporary sensitization of the maternal immune system to RhD antigens, which can cause Rh disease in the current or subsequent pregnancies.

245. **A) Bacterial pneumonia** Pneumonia is an inflammatory condition of the lung especially affecting the alveoli. It is associated with fever, chest symptoms, and consolidation on a chest x-ray. Infectious agents include bacteria, viruses, fungi, and parasites. Consolidation is not present in the lungs with bronchitis, chronic obstructive pulmonary disease (COPD), or atypical pneumonia.

246. **B) Vesicular breath sounds** Vesicular breath sounds are heard best over the base of the lungs. Vesicular sounds are soft and/or blowing, heard throughout inspiration, and fade away with expiration. Bronchial sounds are heard over the bronchi, the largest tubes in the anterior chest. Sounds are loud and high pitched. Tracheal breath sounds are heard over the trachea. These sound harsh and similar to air being blown through a pipe. Vesicular breath sounds are heard best over the base of the lungs. Vesicular sounds are soft and/or blowing, heard throughout inspiration, and fade away with expiration. Bronchial sounds are heard over the bronchi, the largest tubes in the anterior chest. Sounds are loud and high pitched. Tracheal breath sounds are heard over the trachea. These sound harsh and similar to air being blown through a pipe.

247. **A) <140/90 mmHg** The Eighth Joint National Committee (JNC 8) blood pressure goal for adults and older adults 60 years of age or older who have diabetes (with or without chronic kidney disease) is blood pressure less than 140/90. In addition, all patients with hypertension should have lifestyle intervention (i.e., weight loss, smoking cessation, healthy diet), which should be continued throughout treatment.

248. **C) Long-acting oral theophylline (Theo-Dur) 200 mg every 12 hours** Theophylline is used to control inflammation of the lungs. Nedocromil sodium (Tilade), cromolyn sodium (Intal), and fluticasone inhaler (Flovent) help to treat inflammation.

249. **A) A patch of leukoplakia** Leukoplakia mainly affects the mucous membranes of the mouth. It is thought to be caused by irritation. Leukoplakia are patches on the tongue, in the mouth, or on the inside of the cheek that occur in response to long-term irritation,

including smoking, holding chewing tobacco or snuff in the mouth for a long period, or other tobacco use, especially pipes (smoker's keratosis). Leukoplakia on the tongue is also an early sign of HIV.

250. **A) Rule out any physiological cause for the crying spells** For infants who cry for several hours during the day, ruling out a physiological problem that may be causing the distress is recommended.

251. **D) Myxedema** Myxedema (or myxedema) is seen in patients with severe hypothyroidism. It refers to the skin changes (thickened skin) seen in chronic severe hypothyroidism. Myxedema coma is a medical emergency with mortality rates exceeding 20%. It is treated with very high doses of thyroid hormone. A thyroid storm occurs when there is extreme elevation of thyroid hormones. Thyroid storm is life-threatening; untreated, the mortality rate is about 90%. Call 911 if suspected.

252. **B) Fluorescein stain** Fluorescein stain is an eye stain used to detect abrasions or foreign objects in the cornea of the eye. Orange dye (fluorescein) is used to stain the eye and a blue light is used to detect/visualize any foreign bodies or abrasions in the eye. Visual field test assesses vision. Tonometry measures the pressure inside the eye. The funduscopic exam is performed with an ophthalmoscope to visualize the inside of the eye.

253. **B) Inability to swallow** Bell's palsy (acute idiopathic facial nerve palsy) is caused by inflammation of cranial nerve VII (facial nerve). CN VII does not innervate the throat, so swallowing is not affected. Signs and symptoms of Bell's palsy come on suddenly and may include rapid onset of mild weakness to total paralysis on one side of the face occurring within hours to days, making it difficult to smile or close the eye on the affected side. Other symptoms are facial droop and difficulty making facial expressions, pain around the jaw or in or behind the ear on the affected side, increased sensitivity to sound on the affected side, headache, a decrease in ability to taste, and changes in the amount of tears and saliva produced. In rare cases, Bell's palsy can affect the nerves on both sides of the face. Early treatment with oral glucocorticoids (prednisone) is recommended. If herpes simplex 1 infection is suspected, use combined therapy with valacyclovir (Valtrex) and prednisone for 1 week.

254. **C) Educate the mother that this is normal during the first week or 2 of breastfeeding and the soreness will eventually go away** Nursing during the first 2 weeks after delivery may cause tenderness and soreness of the nipples and usually resolves after this. The mother should continue to breastfeed as she has been advised, and she should make sure the infant is latching on appropriately.

255. **C) Moderate persistent asthma** The Global Initiative for Asthma has four clinical classifications of severity: intermittent (normal FEV1 between exacerbations, FEV1 >80%), mild persistent (FEV1 >80%), moderate persistent (FEV1 60%–80%), and severe persistent (FEV1 <60%). Daily symptoms with more than one nighttime episode of symptoms per week, 60% to 80% FEV1, and greater than 30% FEV1 variability and need for short-acting beta-2 agonist for symptom control, are classified as moderate persistent severity in patients older than 12 years of age.

256. **D) Psoriasis** The Auspitz sign is simply bleeding that occurs after psoriasis scales have been removed. It occurs because the capillaries run very close to the surface of the skin under a psoriasis lesion, and removing the scale essentially pulls the tops off the

capillaries, causing bleeding. Auspitz sign is also found in other scaling disorders such as actinic keratoses.

257. C) Anti-thyroid peroxidase and anti-thyroglobulin antibodies These are the two types of antibodies that are positive in Hashimoto's thyroiditis. Anti-thyroid peroxidase antibody is also known as *antimicrosomal antibody*. Hashimoto's thyroiditis is the most common cause of hypothyroidism in the United States. The serum TSH and free T4 test are tests for hypothyroidism, but they are not specific for Hashimoto's thyroiditis, an autoimmune disease.

258. C) Bullous impetigo Bullous impetigo is an infection of the skin caused by *Staphylococcus aureus*, which produces exfoliative toxin A. The infection is more common in young children. It is characterized by flaccid large blisters filled with serous fluid. When the bullae rupture, the serous fluid dries up and resembles honey-colored crusts. If the child has a limited number of skin lesions, topical therapy with mupirocin (Bactroban) is effective. But if lesions are extensive, systemic antibiotics, such as Dicloxacillin and cephalexin, are the treatment of choice.

259. A) Full-term infant is at birth weight by the second week of life The full-term infant should be back to birth weight at 2 weeks of age. The infant should be nursing every 2 to 4 hours and should wet six to 10 diapers per day (24-hour period).

260. B) Thyroid-stimulating hormone (TSH) The best screening test for both hypothyroidism and hyperthyroidism is TSH level. A normal TSH rules out primary hypothyroidism in asymptomatic patients. Abnormal TSH should be followed by determination of thyroid hormone levels. *Overt hypothyroidism* is defined as a clinical syndrome of hypothyroidism associated with elevated TSH and decreased serum levels of T4 or T3. *Subclinical hypothyroidism* is defined as a condition without typical symptoms of hypothyroidism, elevated TSH (>5 µU/mL), and normal circulating thyroid hormone. *Overt thyrotoxicosis* is defined as the syndrome of hyperthyroidism associated with suppressed TSH and elevated serum levels T4 or T3. Subclinical thyrotoxicosis is devoid of symptoms, but TSH is suppressed, although there are normal circulating levels of thyroid hormone.

261. D) Cheilosis Cheilosis or angular cheilosis (perleche) is an acute or chronic inflammation of the labial mucosa and adjacent skin due to excessive moisture and/or salivation. The corners of the mouth are macerated with fissures and painful reddened skin. Risk factors are dentures, poor oral hygiene, drooling, dry mouth (sicca symptoms), oral fungal infection, immunodeficiency, and vitamin deficiency.

262. C) Medroxyprogesterone (Depo-Provera) Long-term use (>3 years) of medroxyprogesterone (Depo-Provera) increases risk of bone loss. Avoid with osteopenia, osteoporosis, long-term amenorrhea, or in underweight women with anorexia. First-line treatment of osteoporosis is the biphosphanates. Lifestyle measures are weight-bearing exercises and adequate calcium and vitamin D intake.

263. D) These fractures always require surgical intervention to stabilize the joint Common signs and symptoms of a fracture of the navicular area include pain, swelling, and tenderness over the thumb side of the wrist, and "crunchiness" and pain with gripping motions. Immediately following the injury, the fracture may not be found on x-ray, leading to misdiagnosis as a sprain. This fracture may be more accurately diagnosed with a bone scan if it does not appear on an x-ray. However, fracture is usually visible if the x-ray is repeated in 2 weeks. Treatment depends largely on the severity and shape of the fracture line. Fractures that are not displaced (those where the break line is small) are immobilized (casting). Nondisplaced fractures that do not heal after 3 to 4 months often require surgical intervention, and the use of other modalities, such as electrical stimulation.

264. B) Increase only the NPH insulin in the morning Regular insulin is rapid/short-acting insulin. Depending on the type of regular insulin, the onset is 10 to 15 minutes and peaks within an average of 1.5 hours, with a duration of 3 to 5 hours. NPH insulin is an intermediate-acting insulin. Depending on the type of NPH insulin, the onset is 1.5 to 3 hours. NPH peaks in 4 to 12 hours, and the duration is from 18 to 24 hours. By increasing the morning NPH, the peak will occur in the afternoon, bringing down the blood glucose.

265. C) Her son can participate in some sports after he has been checked for cervical instability Atlantoaxial instability (AAI) denotes increased mobility at the articulation of the first and second cervical vertebrae (atlantoaxial joint). The American Academy of Pediatrics issued a position statement in 1984 on AAI and Down syndrome (DS): All children with DS who wish to participate in sports should have cervical spine x-rays. Repeated x-rays are not indicated for children with DS who have had a previously normal neck x-ray. Persons with DS who have no evidence of AAI may participate in all sports.

266. A) Erythema migrans Erythema migrans is a symptom of early Lyme disease. It is an annular lesion that slowly enlarges with time (days to weeks) and has central clearing. It is caused by a bite from an infected (*Borrelia burgdorferi*) blacklegged tick. If untreated, infection will spread to joints, nervous system, and heart. Most cases of Lyme disease occur in the Northeast, mid-Atlantic states, Wisconsin, Minnesota, and northern California.

267. A) Cimetidine (Tagamet), digoxin (Lanoxin), diphenhydramine (Benadryl) These medications are included in the Beers criteria, a list of medications that are inappropriate for (or should be used with caution in) the elderly. Cimetidine, digoxin, and diphenhydramine have many adverse effects. Elderly patients taking cimetidine are at risk for neuropsychiatric changes, which may be temporarily reversed by physostigmine. Older patients are also more likely to develop toxicity, and diagnosis of digoxin toxicity can be difficult in this group. Benadryl can worsen glaucoma, a consideration for elderly individuals. Thick oral secretions are also a side effect, making the medication unsafe for the elderly with lung disease. It can also cause high blood pressure, a common ailment associated with aging.

268. D) Calcium channel blockers Common side effects of calcium channel blockers include headaches, edema of the lower extremities, and heart block or bradycardia. Contraindications for calcium channel blockers include second- or third-degree atrioventricular (AV) block, bradycardia, and congestive heart failure.

269. D) CN V Cranial nerves (CNs) are assessed as follows: CN II (optic)—distance vision, near vision; CNs III, IV, VI (oculomotor, trochlear, abducens)—extraocular movements

(EOMs), visual fields of gaze; CN V (trigeminal; three branches are V_1 [ophthalmic], V_2 [maxillary], V_3 [mandibular])—motor portion, clench jaws; sensory portion, corneal reflex/facial sensation. The procedure to test CN V includes inspection for muscle atrophy and tremors, palpation of jaw muscles for tone and strength when the patient clenches teeth, testing of superficial pain and touch sensation in each branch, and testing of temperature sensation if there are unexpected findings to pain or touch. A wisp of cotton is used to test the corneal reflex.

270. **D) Barium swallow** When a patient has acute abdominal pain, initial labs performed are serum electrolytes, amylase, and lipase. Barium swallow would not be performed initially.

271. **B) Mitral stenosis** The low-frequency rumbling murmur of mitral stenosis is mid-diastolic and with severity from a short decrescendo murmur to a longer crescendo murmur. It is best heard at the fifth intercostal space, 8 to 9 cm from the midsternal line, slightly medial to the midclavicular line, and does not radiate. Because it is low pitched, it is heard best with the bell of the stethoscope. Aortic regurgitation is a high-pitched diastolic murmur, heard at the second ICS to the right of the sternum. Mitral regurgitation is a pansystolic murmur that radiates to the axilla, and is loud and high pitched when auscultated.

272. **D) A 37-year-old male biker with a concussion due to a fall who is slightly agitated and does not appear to understand instructions given by the medical assistant checking his vital signs** The biker who has the concussion is the emergent situation due to his agitation and his inability to follow directions, which could mean he has some type of brain trauma. A concussion is a traumatic brain injury (TBI) that may result in a bad headache, altered levels of alertness, or unconsciousness. The following are emergency symptoms for which immediate medical care should be sought: changes in alertness and consciousness, seizures, muscle weakness on one or both sides, persistent confusion, repeated vomiting, unequal pupils, unusual eye movements, problems with walking, or coma. The patient on aspirin who has a laceration can be treated with pressure to stop the bleeding until help arrives. The elderly man with abdominal pain has apparently normal vital signs. Tachycardia is common in patients with fever.

273. **B) Decreased mobility of the tympanic membrane as measured by tympanogram** Acute suppurative otitis media is an acute infection affecting the mucosal lining of the middle ear and the mastoid air system. Suppurative stage: The tympanic membrane bulges and ruptures spontaneously through a small perforation in the pars tensa. Ear discharge is usually present. Diagnosis is usually made simply by looking at the eardrum through an otoscope. The eardrum will appear red and swollen, and may appear either abnormally drawn inward or bulging outward. Using the tympanogram with the otoscope allows a puff of air to be blown lightly into the ear. Normally, this should cause movement of the eardrum. In an infection, or when there is fluid behind the eardrum, this movement may be decreased or absent.

274. **C) Status asthmaticus** Pulsus paradoxus is most likely to be seen with status asthmaticus. With inspiration, systolic pressure drops due to the increased pressure (positive pressure). Some pulmonary risks of having increased pressure include asthma and emphysema. Cardiac causes for pulsus paradoxus include tamponade, pericarditis, and cardiac effusion.

275. D) Varicocele Palpation of varicose veins, described as a "bag of worms," in the scrotum is a classic symptom of a *varicocele*, an abnormal tortuosity and dilation of the veins of the pampiniform plexus within the spermatic cord. It is most common on the left side and may be associated with pain. It occurs in boys and young men and is associated with reduced fertility. The condition is often visible only when the patient is standing. Chronic epididymitis and chronic orchitis are caused by a bacterial infection and commonly cause burning, urinary frequency, and pain. Testicular torsion is an emergent condition in which the testicle becomes twisted, interrupting the blood supply to the testis; to avoid damage, the condition must be corrected within 6 hours.

276. D) Decreased anxiety and depression are common symptoms of abuse in the elderly In an abusive situation, the patient may experience increased anxiety, may not want the nurse practitioner to see his or her unclothed body, may not speak in front of the abuser, and may exhibit depression and despair. A new onset of a sexually transmitted disease (STD) may indicate signs of sexual abuse. These patients commonly delay treatment for acute and chronic conditions.

277. A) Closure of the atrioventricular valves A heart valve normally allows blood to flow in only one direction. A heart valve opens or closes incumbent upon differential blood pressure on each side. A form of heart disease occurs when a valve malfunctions and allows some blood to flow in the wrong direction. The S1 heart sound is caused by turbulence caused by the closure of mitral and tricuspid valves at the start of systole.

278. D) Melanoma Patients with Down syndrome are at higher risk for atlantoaxial instability, congenital heart defects, and early onset of Alzheimer's disease. Children with Down syndrome who participate in certain sports activities must be carefully examined for an unstable neck and heart disease prior to participation to prevent injury.

279. D) Elevated creatinine level Infectious mononucleosis is caused by Epstein–Barr virus (EBV). Symptoms consist of lymphadenopathy, fever, hepatosplenomegaly, malaise, and abdominal discomfort in adolescents and young adults. Host immune response to the viral infection includes CD8+ T lymphocytes with suppressor and cytotoxic functions, the characteristic atypical lymphocytes found in the peripheral blood. EBV antibodies may be ordered when symptoms suggest mononucleosis, but a mono test is negative. A positive test for IgM antibodies is most likely a current, or a very recent, EBV infection. With a positive IgG concentration, it is highly likely that the patient recently had an EBV infection. EBV infection does not infect the kidneys; therefore, the serum creatinine is not affected. But EBV can infect the brain/nerves, bone marrow, liver, and other organs. It is also associated with certain cancers.

280. A) Lateralization to one ear The Weber test is a quick screening test for hearing. It can detect unilateral conductive hearing loss (middle ear hearing loss) and unilateral sensorineural hearing loss (inner ear hearing loss). In the Weber test, a vibrating tuning fork is placed in the middle of the forehead, above the upper lip, under the nose, over the teeth, or on top of the head equidistant from the patient's ears on top of thin skin in contact with the bone. In a normal patient, the Weber tuning fork sound is heard equally loud in both ears, with no one ear hearing the sound louder than the other (lateralization). In a patient with hearing loss (otitis media, cerumenosis), the Weber tuning fork sound is heard louder in one ear (lateralization) than the other (the "bad" ear).

281. B) 6 to 15 cm in the midclavicular line This range is generally less than 12 cm, but 6 to 15 cm is considered normal for adults.

282. B) Brudzinski's sign Brudzinski's sign is positive for meningitis when a patient spontaneously flexes his or her hips and knees after lying down and having his or her head and neck flexed forward to the chest.

283. C) Osgood–Schlatter disease Osgood–Schlatter disease is characterized by bilateral pain over the tibial tuberosity upon palpation, along with knee pain and edema with exercise.

284. D) Penicillin (Pen VK) Pen VK is safe to use for strep throat during pregnancy. Pen VK is an FDA category B medication and it can be used during pregnancy and lactation.

285. B) This is a normal finding Horizontal nystagmus is a normal variation on physical exam. Full movement of the eyes is controlled by the integrated function of cranial nerves III (oculomotor), IV (trochlear), and VI (abducens). Holding the patient's chin to prevent movement of the head, ask the patient to watch your finger as it moves through the six cardinal fields of gaze. Then ask the patient to look to the extreme lateral (temporal) positions. A few horizontal nystagmic beats are within normal limits (WNL).

286. A) Murphy's sign Murphy's sign is suggestive of acute cholecystitis and gallbladder disease. It is elicited by palpating the subcostal region on the right upper abdomen; in response, the patient abruptly stops inspiration because of the severe pain.

287. D) Ciprofloxacin (Cipro) Ciprofloxacin is the preferred drug for anthrax (*Bacillus anthracis*) prophylaxis. The other option is levofloxacin (Levaquin). The CDC-recommended prophylaxis for persons known or suspected to have been exposed to a substantial inoculum of spores from a deliberate-release scenario is antibiotic therapy for 60 days and administration of anthrax vaccine adsorbed (BioThrax).

288. B) Maternal age older than 35 years The risk factor of having an infant with Down syndrome is increased when the mother is older than 35 years of age.

289. C) Lupus erythematosus Classic symptoms of lupus erythematosus are butterfly rash across both cheeks and the bridge of the nose, and fatigue. Risk factors also include being female and 40 years old. Rosacea also has a similar rash but usually not associated with fatigue.

290. C) Pneumococcal (Pneumovax) and influenza vaccines The tetanus (Td) immunization is good for about 10 years. October/November is the beginning window of the flu season, and annual influenza vaccination is recommended. The pneumococcal (pneumonia) vaccine is indicated for patients older than 65 years.

291. B) The fat pads on an infant's feet can mimic pes planus The fat pads on an infant's feet can resemble pes planus, or flat feet.

292. **D) Patients should avoid foods or drinks that contain alcohol, such as cough syrups** The intake of foods and medications that contain alcohol must be avoided because it can precipitate a relapse in a recovering alcoholic. This includes everyday products that contain alcohol, such as mouthwashes and cough syrups. Al-Anon (for adults) and Alateen (for teens) are 12-step programs for families and friends of alcoholics. Antabuse is effective for some patients. Alcoholics Anonymous (AA) is a 12-step program that is designed to help alcoholics.

293. **B) An absence seizure (petit mal seizure)** A petit mal seizure is a brief seizure that usually lasts less than 15 seconds. During the seizure, the child may appear not to be listening, to have "blanked out," or to be daydreaming.

294. **A) Advise the patient to return to the clinic for chlamydia and gonorrhea testing** The patient has signs and symptoms of mucopurulent cervicitis (friable cervix, purulent discharge) and should be tested for chlamydia and gonorrhea. Empiric treatment for mucopurulent cervicitis should be started (doxycycline BID for 7 days) even if these tests are negative, but the patient's cervix appears infected. Douching increases the risk of pelvic inflammatory disease (PID) and is not recommended.

295. **A) The fundus of the uterus should be at the level of the symphysis pubis** At 12 weeks gestation, the fundus of the uterus should be located approximately at the symphysis pubis.

296. **B) Fetal alcohol syndrome** Classic symptoms of fetal alcohol syndrome include small palpebral fissures and microcephaly with a small jaw.

297. **B) Lung cancer** Lung cancer is the most common cause of cancer deaths in women as well as men (U.S. Cancer Statistics Working Group, 2017).

298. **C) Cervical cancer** There are more than 30 types of human papillomavirus (HPV). HPV types in the anogenital region have been strongly associated with low-grade and high-grade cervical change, cervical neoplasia, as well as anogenital and other cancers. An HPV vaccine is recommended for girls and boys between the ages of 15 and 21 years of age to help prevent four strains of this virus.

299. **A) Profound fatigue** Criteria used to diagnose AIDS include hairy leukoplakia of the tongue, Kaposi's sarcoma, and thrush.

300. **B) Hypertrophic cardiomyopathy** Congenital cardiovascular disease is the leading cause of nontraumatic sudden athletic death, with hypertrophic cardiomyopathy being the most common cause. Despite public perception to the contrary, sudden death in young athletes is exceedingly rare. It most commonly occurs in male athletes, who have estimated death rates nearly fivefold greater than the rates of female athletes.

301. **A) 3 months** The posterior fontanel normally closes by 3 months of age. The anterior fontanelle closes between 12 and 18 months of age.

302. **B) CN VIII** The acoustic nerve, cranial nerve VIII, is being evaluated when the Rinne test is performed. The Rinne test is performed by placing the base of a vibrating tuning fork against the patient's mastoid bone to evaluate bone conduction. Ask the patient to tell

you when the sound is no longer heard. Then place the tuning fork in the front of the ear to evaluate air conduction. The air conduction should be twice as long as *bone conduction*.

303. C) Morton's neuroma Morton's neuroma is characterized by pain, burning, or numbness between two adjacent toes with weight bearing. Some patients describe the sensation as feeling as if they are walking on a pebble.

304. B) Tetracycline (Sumycin) First-line treatment for acne vulgaris includes over-the-counter medicated soap and water with topical antibiotic gels. The next step in treatment would be the initiation of oral tetracycline.

305. B) The typical lesions are bullae Herpes zoster (shingles) occurs secondary to reactivation of the varicella-zoster (VZV) virus. This infection can be more severe in immunocompromised patients due to their inability to fight infection. Shingles rash starts as small blisters on a red base, with new blisters continuing to form for 3 to 5 days. The rash is painful, and commonly appears in clusters, following one dermatome on one side of the body. When the trigeminal nerve is involved, there is an increased risk of corneal blindness.

306. A) Hidradenitis suppurativa Hidradenitis suppurativa is a chronic skin condition, commonly found in the apocrine glands in the axilla and/or groin, that causes painful nodules under the skin. These abscesses tend to open and drain fluid and pus. Significant scarring of the skin may result from these outbreaks.

307. C) Edema of the ankles and headache Common side effects of calcium channel blockers, such as Procardia, include edema of the ankles, dizziness, headaches, flushing, and weakness. Angiotensin-converting enzyme (ACE) inhibitors tend to have the side effects of angioedema and a dry hacking cough. Diuretics can cause hyperkalemia and hyperuricemia.

308. A) Massaging the infected prostate Massaging the infected prostate is contraindicated for acute prostatitis because the massage can spread the bacteria from the prostate into the bloodstream and lead to sepsis.

309. A) Streptococci Erysipelas is a skin infection commonly caused by group A beta-hemolytic streptococci. This infection is usually more superficial than other bacterial infections of the skin, such as cellulitis.

310. C) Macrolides The American Thoracic Society recommends azithromycin or clarithromycin (macrolides) as the first line of therapy for community-acquired pneumonia without comorbidity.

311. C) Paroxysms of coughing that are dry or produce mucoid sputum A cough is the main symptom of acute bronchitis. It may be dry at first (does not produce mucus) and after a few days may bring up mucus from the lungs (productive cough). The mucus may be clear, yellow, or green. Small streaks of blood may be present.

312. A) Arcus senilis Arcus senilis (*arcus senilis corneae*) is a white, gray, or blue opaque ring in the corneal margin (peripheral corneal opacity), or white ring in front of the periphery of the iris. It is present at birth, but then fades; however, it is commonly present in older adults. It can also appear earlier in life as a result of hypercholesterolemia. It does not affect vision. Unilateral arcus is a sign of decreased blood flow to the unaffected eye due to carotid artery disease or ocular hypotony.

313. B) The patient should be evaluated for hyperlipidemia Arcus senilis is caused by lipid deposits deep in the edge of the cornea and is quite commonly present in the elderly. However, it can also appear earlier in life as a result of hypercholesterolemia.

314. D) Color vision There are two types of photoreceptors in the human retina: rods and cones. Cones are active at higher light levels (photopic vision), and are capable of color vision and night vision, as well as high spatial acuity. The central fovea is populated exclusively by cones. There are three types of cones referred to as *short-wavelength sensitive cones, middle-wavelength sensitive cones,* and *long-wavelength sensitive cones—S-cones, M-cones,* and *L-cones* for short. Rods are responsible for vision at low light levels (scotopic vision). They do not mediate color vision, and have a low spatial acuity.

315. D) Second-degree burn on the lower arm Burns are described according to the depth of injury to the dermis and are loosely classified into first, second, third, and fourth degrees. A second-degree (superficial partial-thickness) burn extends into the superficial (papillary) dermis. It appears red with clear blisters, blanches with pressure, has a moist texture, and is painful to sensation. A second-degree burn takes 2 to 3 weeks to heal. First- and second-degree burns are appropriately treated by a nurse practitioner. Third-degree burns should be referred to a physician. Examples of third-degree burns include electrical burns, severe burns on the face, and burns involving cartilage, such as the ear and nose.

316. B) Second intercostal space, left sternal border The S2 heart sound results from closure of the aortic and pulmonic valves. The right ventricular systolic ejection time is longer than the left, so the pulmonic valve closes slightly later than the aortic valve. The slightly different closing times of the valves make the S2 heart sound. It is heard best using the diaphragm of the stethoscope.

317. A) <150/90 mmHg For the general population (no diabetes or chronic kidney disease) the recommended systolic blood pressure (SBP) goal at age 60 years or older goes up by 10 mmHg to blood pressure less than 150/But if the patient is a diabetic and/or has chronic kidney disease, then the blood pressure goal does not change and continues at blood pressure less than 140/90.

318. A) Severe sunburn with blistering Burns are described according to the depth of injury to the dermis: First degree—erythema without blistering, painful; second degree—red skin with superficial blisters, painful; third degree—entire skin layering, involving the subcutaneous tissue and may include soft tissue facia, painless.

319. B) Her son's physical development is delayed and should be evaluated by a pediatric endocrinologist Puberty may be delayed for several years and still occur normally, in which case it is considered constitutional delay, a variation of healthy physical development. Delay of puberty may also occur due to malnutrition, many forms of systemic disease, or to defects of the reproductive system (hypogonadism) or the body's responsiveness to sex hormones. Hypogonadism occurs when the sex glands produce little or no hormones. In men, these glands (gonads) are the testes. A 16-year-old male without secondary sexual characteristics should be referred to an endocrinologist. If there is no testicular development by 14 years of age, an endocrinology consult is warranted.

320. B) Basal cell carcinoma Basal cell carcinoma (BCC) is the most common type of skin cancer diagnosed in the United States each year. More than one out of every three new cancers are skin cancers, and the vast majority are BCCs. BCCs are abnormal, uncontrolled growths or lesions that arise in the skin's basal cells, which line the deepest layer of the epidermis. Initially appearing as a dome-shaped waxy lesion with telangiectasia, it enlarges with raised "pearly" edges and telangiectasia and the center may ulcerate. BCCs can also look like open sores, red patches, pink growths, or scars. Usually caused by a combination of cumulative UV exposure and intense, occasional UV exposure, BCC can be highly disfiguring if allowed to grow, but almost never metastasizes beyond the original tumor site.

321. B) CNs III, IV, and VI Cranial nerves III (oculomotor), IV (trochlear), and VI (abducens) innervate the extraocular muscles. They are tested by inspecting the eyelids for drooping, and inspecting pupil size for equality and their direct and consensual response to light and accommodation.

322. A) Hemoglobin electrophoresis Patients with the diagnosis of beta thalassemia and/or sickle cell anemia would be screened using hemoglobin electrophoresis to identify the blood disorder.

323. C) Obese patients Metformin is used for initial therapy for type 2 diabetes. In patients who are obese, it can help with weight loss. The starting dose is 500 mg once a day. Maximum dose is 2 g or 2,000 mg/day. Titrate dose slowly to minimize side effects (flatus, bloating, and diarrhea). Contraindications to the use of metformin include significant renal and hepatic disease, alcoholism, conditions associated with hypoxia (cardiac/pulmonary problems), sepsis, dehydration, and advanced age.

324. C) Bacterial pneumonia The most common cause of bacterial pneumonia is *Streptococcus pneumoniae. Haemophilus influenzae, Chlamydia pneumoniae, Mycoplasma pneumoniae,* and *Legionella pneumophila* are other important bacteria that cause pneumonia. Typically, pneumonia comes on very quickly; the patient has high fever/chills, productive cough with yellow or brown sputum, shortness of breath, and may have chest pain with breathing/coughing. The gold standard for diagnosing bacterial pneumonia is the chest x-ray, which shows infiltrates and/or lobar consolidation Older people can have confusion or a change in their mental abilities. In patients with bacterial pneumonia, it is important to determine whether bacteria are present in the urine, in order to identify appropriate antibiotics to treat the bacteria.

325. A) Reduce intake of sodium, potassium, and calcium Lifestyle modifications for hypertension include exercise three to four times a week, diet modifications of reduced intake of sodium and saturated fats, and adequate dietary intake of potassium, magnesium, and calcium.

326. **B) Beta-blockers** Reverse rebound hypertension can occur if beta-blockers are abruptly stopped. Recommendations include weaning off the beta-blockers when changing medications.

327. **D) Migraine headaches** Migraines are not a contraindication to Betimol (timolol). Contraindications include bronchial asthma, asthma history, severe COPD, uncompensated heart failure, second- or third-degree AV block, sinus bradycardia, and cardiogenic shock. Caution should be used if the following conditions are present: closed-angle glaucoma, peripheral vascular disease, bronchospastic disease, diabetes, hyperthyroidism, and myasthenia gravis.

328. **C) Early in the morning** The scotch tape test is best done in the morning for several days in a row. The female pinworms do not lay eggs every day; therefore, testing over the course of several days will be more accurate.

329. **C) 3 years** Developmental stages in children include the following: 1 year—walk; 2 years—walks up steps with the same foot; 3 years—pedals a tricycle and copies a circle; 4 years—copies a cross and draws a person with 3 parts.

330. **A) Document the patient's behavior in his record and the action taken by the nurse** Patients have the right to refuse their medications. Bipolar disorder tends to worsen if it is not treated. Explain that there is a good chance that manic and depressive episodes will become more frequent and severe over time. If a patient is noncompliant, the patient behavior and the actions taken by the nurse both must be documented.

331. **D) Microaneurysms** Keith Wagener Barker (KWB) grades for uncontrolled hypertension are as follows: Grade 1—generalized arteriolar constriction seen as "silver wiring" and vascular tortuousities; grade 2—grade 1 plus irregularly located, tight constrictions known as *AV nicking* or *AV nipping*; grade 3—grade 2 plus cotton wool spots and flame-shaped hemorrhages; and grade 4—grade 3, but with swelling of the optic disc (papilledema). Microaneurysms occur with diabetic retinopathy.

332. **B) This is a normal finding due to the skeletal growth spurt in this age group** Alkaline phosphatase is part of a group of related enzymes. The bone form of the enzyme creates the alkaline conditions it requires to be most active with a chemical reaction involving the osteoblasts. The rapid bone growth and increased deposit of calcium during growth spurts and adolescence elevates the alkaline phosphatase level.

333. **B) Irrigate with normal saline and apply Silvadene cream BID** Burns should be cleansed with saline solution and Silvadene (silver sulfadiazine) cream applied BID to the site. Hydrogen peroxide is no longer recommended. Intact blisters should not be unroofed.

334. **A) It should raise the suspicion of child sexual abuse** *Molluscum contagiosum* is spread by direct skin-to-skin contact. Lesions found in the genital area of young children should be evaluated for suspicion of child sexual abuse.

335. **B) Loss of subcutaneous fat and lower collagen content** Thinning of the skin in older women is due to the loss of subcutaneous fat and lower collagen content.

336. D) It reviews information via a nongovernmental agency The state board of nursing (SBON) is a regulatory agency created by the state government and is devoted to monitoring nurses' personal and professional behaviors. SBONs have the legislative power to initiate, regulate, and enforce provisions of the nurse practice act.

337. A) The veins are larger than the arterioles The fundus of the eye is opposite the lens, and includes the retina, optic disc, macula and fovea, and posterior pole. The eye's fundus is the only part of the human body where the microcirculation can be observed directly. The retinal arteries and veins emerge from the nasal side (left) of the optic disc. Vessels directed temporally have an arching course; those directed nasally have a radial course. Arteries are brighter red and narrower than veins.

338. D) Acute esophagitis Factors that influence the risk of atrial fibrillation include hypertension, excessive alcohol consumption, and medications such as Theo-Dur and Sudafed.

339. D) 4 years Developmental stages in children include the following: 1 year—walk; 2 years—walks up steps with the same foot; 3 years—pedals a tricycle and copies a circle; 4 years—copies a cross and draws a person with three body parts.

340. D) Acute appendicitis A positive iliopsoas muscle test may be seen with acute appendicitis. The right iliopsoas muscle lies under the appendix, This test is performed by asking the patient to actively flex the thigh at the hip. A "positive psoas sign" is noted when the patient exhibits pain in the right lower quadrant due to the inflamed tissue.

341. C) Beta-blockers Beta-blockers are known to blunt the signs and symptoms of hypoglycemia in patients with diabetes.

342. D) Hypertension Hypertension is not associated with an increase in mortality with pneumonia. But patients with multiple lobar involvement, infants, the elderly, those with chronic illnesses (including cirrhosis of the liver, congestive heart failure), individuals without a functioning spleen, and those who have other diseases that result in a weakened immune system experience complications. Patients with immune disorders or various types of cancer, transplant patients, and AIDS patients also experience complications. An alcohol-impaired pulmonary immune system is no defense against pneumonia-producing bacteria.

343. A) *Streptococcus pneumoniae* Community-acquired pneumonia (CAP) is the sixth most common cause of death in the United States and the leading cause of death from infectious diseases. It is associated with significant morbidity and mortality, and poses a major economic burden to the health care system. *S. pneumoniae* is the leading cause of CAP.

344. B) Initiate a prescription of hydrochlorothiazide 12.5 mg PO daily The Eighth Joint National Committee (JNC 8)-recommended pharmacological treatment for Black adult hypertensive patients (without chronic kidney disease or diabetes) is a thiazide-type diuretic or calcium channel blocker (CCB), used alone or in combination. For White adults, the JNC 8 recommends a thiazide-type diuretic or angiotensin-converting enzyme (ACE) inhibitor or an angiotensin receptor blocker (ARB) or a CCB, used alone or in combination. Do not combine an ACE inhibitor with an ARB. Although unusual, a serious adverse effect from these two drug classes is angioedema. Beta-blockers should be avoided in patients with chronic lung disease, such as asthma and chronic obstructive pulmonary disease (COPD), because they can cause bronchoconstriction.

345. **B) Antibiotics** Acute bronchitis is normally a viral infection, so expectorants, bronchodilators, and antitussives would be prescribed for the cough. Antibiotics are not effective against viral infections.

346. **B) Can draw a cross** Developmental stages in children include the following: 1 year—walk; 2 years—walks up steps with the same foot; 3 years—pedals a tricycle and copies a circle; 4 years—copies a cross and draws a person with three parts.

347. **D) Raynaud's phenomenon** Raynaud's phenomenon occurs from vasospasms of the blood vessels, leading to decreased blood supply to the hands and feet, which causes bluish discoloration, with fingertips turning a dark-red color if severe. Stress and cold weather are classic triggers for this syndrome.

348. **D) Order an A1C level.** The next step is to check the A1C level. The treatment goal is an A1C less than 7%. But if the patient is frail or has frequent hypoglycemic episodes, the American Diabetes Association allows a goal of up to 8%. If the A1C level is 6.5 or higher, the patient has type 2 diabetes.

349. **B) Strenuous exercise is contraindicated for most patients with type 2 diabetes because of a higher risk of hypoglycemic episodes** Exercise is recommended because exercise helps to use the glucose stores and reduce blood sugar. When exercising, the patient should monitor blood sugar closely, especially if using insulin, to avoid hypoglycemia.

350. **C) *Pseudomonas aeruginosa*** *P. aeruginosa* is an uncommon cause of community-acquired pneumonia. It is more common in patients with cystic fibrosis and hospitalized patients. In mild cases, it can be treated with ciprofloxacin (Cipro) or levofloxacin (Levaquin), which are fluoroquinolones. *P. aeruginosa* is resistant to several antibiotics and it can be tricky to treat. Many patients need hospitalization.

351. **C) Advise the mother that this is a normal finding** Explain to the mother that in healthy adolescents, a split S2 during inspiration that disappears during expiration is a normal variation.

352. **C) Competence** Competence refers to having the ability to make one's own decisions regarding one's own course of health care, as long as one is documented as being mentally capable. Informed consent is giving permission to perform a particular procedure, understanding the purpose of the procedure/treatment, success/failure rate, other alternatives to the procedure, risks and benefits of the procedure, prognosis, and success rate. To give informed consent, the patient must be 18 years of age or older. Durable power of attorney is the legal document giving one person the authority to make decisions regarding another person's health care and personal affairs on that person's behalf. Advance directives are written instructions to be performed in the event the patient is not mentally competent and not able to make decisions for himself or herself. The living will is an example of an advance directive.

353. **D) The tumor commonly crosses the midline of the abdomen when it is discovered** A Wilms' tumor is a congenital tumor of the kidney that should never be palpated, once diagnosed, to avoid spread of the tumor cells. Microscopic or gross hematuria may be present.

354. **D) Screening for lung cancer is not currently recommended** Primary prevention involves methods to avoid occurrence of disease in the general population. Secondary prevention involves screening, diagnosis, and treatment of existing disease in early stages before it causes significant morbidity. Tertiary prevention involves methods to reduce the negative impact of an existing disease by restoring function and reducing disease-related complications. Screening for lung cancer is not currently recommended for the general population.

355. **C) T-score of −2.5 or less** Osteoporosis is defined as having a T-score of −2.5 or less. Risk factors should also be considered when interpreting T-scores for diagnosis.

356. **C) Thayer–Martin culture** Thayer–Martin selective agar is an enriched medium for the selective isolation of *Neisseria* species. *N. gonorrhoeae* is a gram-negative bacteria that can infect the genitourinary and reproductive tracts, throat, eyes (infants), and rectum. Thayer–Martin culture is recommended for screening to diagnose gonorrheal pharyngitis or proctitis.

357. **D) Loretta Ford** Loretta Ford, PhD, RN, FAAN, is considered the founder of the nurse practitioner (NP) movement, and has received many awards for her work. Ford has graduate degrees in nursing, a doctorate from the University of Colorado, and was certified as a public health nurse. In the early 1960s, she and pediatrician Henry K. Silver were colleagues at the University of Colorado. With a regional shortage of family care physicians and pediatricians hampering health care delivery to rural and underserved areas, they saw that innovation was needed to solve the problem. Using a small grant from the university, in 1965 they created a demonstration project focusing on extending the nurse's role in the community. They published their findings and developed an educational curriculum for NPs. Other schools followed and started their own NP programs.

358. **A) Benign prostatic hypertrophy (BPH) and hypertension** Terazosin (Hytrin) is a treatment option for men with BPH and hypertension. Symptoms of BPH include difficulty urinating (hesitation, dribbling, weak stream, and incomplete bladder emptying), painful urination, and urinary frequency and urgency. Terazosin is in a class of medications called *alpha-blockers*. It relieves the symptoms of BPH by relaxing the muscles of the bladder and prostate. It lowers blood pressure by relaxing the blood vessels so that blood can flow more easily through the body.

359. **B) Advise the mother that her child is developing normally** Toilet-training begins at approximately 2 years of age and may take 1 to 2 years to complete. Boys who are not toilet-trained by 3 years of age may still be developing normally.

360. **A) The "blue dot" sign** The blue dot sign describes a tender nodule located underneath the skin of the testicle that appears as a round, blue-to-purple mass. Also known

as *torsion of testicular appendage*, it is not an emergent condition. It is the most common cause of testicular area pain in younger boys. Treatment is symptomatic.

361. **D) Repeat the Gen-Probe test for *Chlamydia trachomatis* to ensure that the previous test was not a false-negative result** Treatment for both gonorrhea and chlamydia is recommended for the diagnosis of pelvic inflammatory disease (PID), regardless of whether the chlamydia test (or gonorrhea test) was negative. Repeating the Gen-Probe test (or another nucleic acid amplification test [NAAT]) for chlamydia is not recommended. Pelvic inflammatory disease (PID) is a clinical diagnosis. The Centers for Disease Control and Prevention (CDC) states that an internal vaginal swab specimen is equivalent to a cervical specimen when using the newer NAATs. Self-collected vaginal swabs are equivalent in sensitivity/specificity to those collected by a clinician. Treatment should be initiated as soon as the presumptive diagnosis has been made because prevention of long-term sequelae is dependent on early administration of appropriate antibiotics. All regimens used to treat PID should also be effective against *N. gonorrhoeae* and *C. trachomatis* because negative endocervical screening for these organisms does not rule out upper reproductive tract infection.

362. **C) Tanner stage IV** The breast bud stage is Tanner stage II. In Tanner stage IV, the areola and papilla form a secondary mound. Tanner stages for breast development are I, prepuberty; II, breast bud; III, breast and areola one mound; IV, breast and areola secondary mound; and V, adult pattern.

363. **A) Condoms and the vaginal sponge (Today Sponge)** Contraindications for hormonal contraception include migraine headaches; cigarette smoking or obesity in women older than 35 years; history of thromboembolic disease; hypertension or vascular disease if older than 35 years of age; systemic lupus erythematosus with vascular disease, nephritis, or antiphospholipid antibodies; breastfeeding (may use progestin-only pills); hypertriglyceridemia; coronary artery disease; congestive heart failure; and strokes.

364. **D) Disseminated gonorrheal infection** Symptoms of pelvic inflammatory disease (PID) with painful, swollen joints of extremities indicate disseminated gonorrheal infection. Untreated disseminated gonorrhea can lead to septic arthritis. Symptoms may be mild, ranging from slight joint pain and no fever to severe joint pain with high fever. PID symptoms do not occur with septic arthritis, Reiter's syndrome, or chondromalacia of the patella.

365. **D) G6PD-deficiency anemia** Pneumococcal vaccine is not indicated for glucose-6-phosphate dehydrogenase (G6PD)-deficiency anemia. There two types of pneumonia vaccine for adults: PPSV23 (Pneumovax 23) and PCV13 (Prevnar 13). Pneumococcal vaccine is recommended for individuals beginning at age 65 years, but the two types should not be given together. The Centers for Disease Control and Prevention (CDC) recommends administering Prevnar 13 first, then waiting at least 1 year (12 months) and giving the Pneumovax. The immunogenic response is better using this method. Prevnar 13 is recommended for all infants and children younger than 2 years of age, all adults aged 65 years or older, and people (2 to 64 years old) with certain medical conditions that increase risk of pneumococcal disease, such as functional or anatomic asplenia (sickle cell), HIV infection, chronic renal failure, leukemia, heart failure, cyanotic congenital

heart disease, chronic lung disease (asthma, chronic obstructive pulmonary disease [COPD]), diabetes, and others.

366. **B) Paroxysmal atrial tachycardia** Signs and symptoms of paroxysmal atrial tachycardia include a rapid, regular heart rate that begins and ends very quickly. The atria are beating at a very fast rate, but it is not life-threatening. Ventricular tachycardia is usually associated with heart disease, occurs when the ventricles are beating rapidly and inefficiently, and can lead to death if not treated. Atrial fibrillation is an irregular heartbeat that can be life-threatening if not treated. Ventricular fibrillation occurs when the heartbeat is rapid and chaotic, and death will occur if the condition is not treated.

367. **A) Oral metronidazole (Flagyl)** Trichomoniasis symptoms include dysuria, severe vaginal pruritus, and malodorous vaginal discharge. Wet prep microscopic examination should show trichomonads that are pear-shaped and have several flagella (whiplike tails) at one end. The Centers for Disease Control and Prevention (CDC) recommendation for treatment is metronidazole. A single dose is effective treatment in most cases of *Trichomonas* infections.

368. **C) Immunization is acceptable as long as the temperature is not higher than 100.4°F** An infant with a cold can be immunized as long as the infant's temperature is no higher than 100.4°F.

369. **B) She should avoid alcoholic drinks 1 day before, during therapy, and a few days after therapy** The patient should avoid alcoholic drinks during and for at least 3 days after therapy with metronidazole (Flagyl). Flagyl and alcohol together cause severe nausea and vomiting, flushing, fast heartbeat (tachycardia), and shortness of breath. The reaction has been described as being similar to the effects of Antabuse.

370. **C) Preventive therapy for *Pneumocystis carinii* pneumonia (PCP)** *Pneumocystis jirovecii* pneumonia (previously known as *Pneumocystis carinii* pneumonia, or PCP) can be life-threatening in patients with AIDS with a low CD4 count. HIV-infected adults and adolescents, including pregnant women and those on antiretroviral therapy (ART), should receive prophylaxis if their CD4 counts <200 cells/mm^3. Trimethoprim-sulfaxazole (Bactrim DS), one tablet daily, is the preferred regimen. It also offers cross protection against toxoplasmosis. If CD4 count is >200 cells/mm^3 for more than 3 months (in response to ART), PCP prophylaxis can be discontinued.

371. **C) Hemangiomas should be treated with laser therapy if they have not resolved by the age of 12 months** True strawberry hemangiomas will eventually resolve by the time the child goes to kindergarten. Most will reduce or disappear in the first 2 years. Laser treatment is rarely needed.

372. **B) Call 911** Heavy chest pressure in the substernal area radiating to the jaw, diaphoresis, low blood pressure, and bradycardia are signs of cardiac distress. This patient is exhibiting classic symptoms of a myocardial infarction and needs immediate treatment. Call 911 immediately and transfer the patient to the emergency department.

373. **B) H2 receptor antagonists** Because the ulcer is not infected with *Helicobacter pylori*, antibiotics are not recommended. The first-line treatment option are H2 receptor

antagonists (also known as *H2 blockers*) such as ranitidine (Zantac), famotidine (Pepcid), or nizatidine (Axid). Other causes of peptic ulcer disease are nonsteroidal anti-inflammatory drugs (NSAIDs); the patient should be educated to avoid use of these agents.

374. D) Furosemide (Lasix) Many medications are contraindicated with the cytochrome P450 system. Lasix is one medication that can be used.

375. A) Severe ulceration of the stomach or duodenum Zollinger–Ellison syndrome occurs when tumors (gastrinomas) in the intestine, pancreas, or lymph nodes near the pancreas produce excessive amounts of gastrin, which, in turn, increases the amount of acid produced by the stomach. High amounts of acid in the stomach produce ulcers of the stomach or duodenum. Untreated Zollinger–Ellison syndrome can lead to severe ulceration of the stomach or duodenum.

376. D) Meperidine (Demerol) Demerol is an FDA category C drug. It is a controlled drug under Schedule II. It cannot be called into the pharmacy and it cannot be refilled by phone. The prescription script (paper) of the drug is required by the pharmacy before it can be filled.

377. B) Psoriasis Fingernail pitting is correlated with psoriasis. Psoriasis can cause pitting on all finger and toenails, along with thickening and an irregular shape of the nail.

378. C) It is best heard at the apex during S1 Mitral regurgitation results from damage to the mitral valve (mitral valve prolapse [MVP], rheumatic heart disease, infective endocarditis). Most patients are initially asymptomatic. The best ausculatory area is the apex or mitral area of the chest. Mitral regurgitation is a systolic (S1) murmur. It may be associated with a midsystolic click if the patient has concurrent MVP. The click is so characteristic of MVP that even without a subsequent murmur, its presence alone is enough for the diagnosis. Immediately after the click, a brief crescendo–decrescendo murmur is heard, usually at the apex. The best imaging test for identifying mitral regurgitation is transthoracic echocardiography.

379. B) Acute appendicitis Symptoms of an acute abdomen, such as appendicitis, include extreme tenderness and involuntary guarding at McBurney's point. McBurney's point is the name given to the point over the right side of the abdomen that is one third of the distance (approximately 2 inches) from the anterior superior iliac spine to the umbilicus. This point roughly corresponds to the most common location of the base of the appendix where it is attached to the cecum. (During pregnancy the location of the appendix changes as the uterus grows.)

380. C) Chewing breath mints Gastroesophageal reflux disease (GERD) is a condition in which food comes up the esophagus from the stomach because of a weak sphincter. The reflux is usually worsened by lying down, and can cause a cough and esophageal irritation if not treated. Effective treatment may include weight loss, decreased caffeine intake, and avoidance of alcohol.

381. A) Ceftriaxone (Rocephin) 250 mg IM plus azithromycin 1 g orally Drug therapy is based on the 2015 Centers for Disease Control and Prevention (CDC; 2015) sexually transmitted disease guidelines. In patients with gonorrheal infection, always co-treat for chlamydia.

382. **B) Thrombosis related to an IV needle** Thrombosis related to either a known trauma or an IV needle does not represent a contraindication for use of oral contraceptives.

383. **A) Fruits, leafy greens, and nuts** The best sources of both potassium and magnesium are fruits (bananas, cantaloupe, papaya, kiwi), leafy greens (spinach, kale, chard), and nuts (cashews, almonds, walnuts, peanuts).

384. **D) Acute epididymitis** Acute epididymitis is the infection presented here. Scrotal edema and pain with palpation do not occur in urinary tract infection or pyelonephritis. Acute orchitis symptoms include testicular pain and edema, are usually associated with the mumps, but do not have frequency and dysuria.

385. **C) Trimethoprim–sulfamethoxazole (Bactrim)** With the allergic history to a sulfa drug, it would be safest to avoid Bactrim.

386. **B) The fever is most likely due to the pertussis component of the DTaP vaccine** The pertussis component of the vaccine is most likely the cause of the fever.

387. **C) Saw palmetto is always effective in reducing symptoms** Research does not support the theory that saw palmetto reduces the symptoms of benign prostatic hyperplasia in all cases. The word "always" in the option choice is a clue that it is the wrong answer.

388. **B) Age 8 in girls and age 9 in boys** *Precocious puberty* is defined as onset of secondary-sexual characteristics by the age of 8 years in girls and 9 years in boys.

389. **B) Tanner stage II** *Puberty* is defined as the period in life when secondary sexual characteristics begin to develop, identified as Tanner stage II for boys and girls.

390. **A) Mumps virus** Orchitis (infection of the testicle) is caused by the mumps virus. It can cause sterility in males.

391. **A) Acute appendicitis** A positive obturator sign may indicate acute appendicitis. The test is performed with the patient supine. The examiner rotates the hip, using full range of motion. The test is positive if pain is experienced with movement or flexion of the hip.

392. **C) Testes** Spermatogenesis takes place within several structures of the male reproductive system. The initial stages occur within the testes and progress to the epididymis, where the developing gametes mature and are stored until ejaculation. New sperm take 2 to 3 months to fully mature.

393. **D) Aerosolized albuterol sulfate (Ventolin)** Prophylaxis for *Pneumocystis jirovecii* pneumonia (previously known as *Pneumocystis carinii* pneumonia, or PCP) includes the use of trimethoprim-sulfamethoxazole (Bactrim), dapsone, and aerosolized pentamidine. Aerosolized pentamidine is an antimicrobial treatment for prevention, along with Bactrim and dapsone, which are antibacterial medications.

394. **B) Horizontal nystagmus with rapid head movement** Symptoms of benign paroxysmal positional vertigo include horizontal nystagmus with rapid head movement. Performing the Dix–Hallpike maneuver and/or the roll test will cause the symptoms of vertigo to appear.

395. D) Stroke and coronary artery disease Carotid stenosis puts the patient at risk for stroke and coronary artery disease. A bruit is a murmur heard over the carotid artery in the neck, suggesting arterial narrowing and atherosclerosis. It may increase risk of cerebrovascular disease. Bruits at the bifurcation of the common carotid artery are best heard high up under the angle of the jaw. At this level the common carotid artery bifurcates and gives rise to its internal branch. If one hears a bruit only in the base of the neck, or along the course of the common carotid artery, it is referred to as *diffuse*. Diffuse bruits are not a very specific indicator of internal carotid artery disease. Bruits heard only at the bifurcation are more specific for internal carotid artery origin stenosis.

396. B) Levofloxacin (Levaquin) 250 mg PO daily Streptococcal pharyngitis and urinary tract infection are both covered by using Levaquin, which is a fluoroquinolone. Amoxicillin–clavulanic acid (Augmentin) and trimethoprim–sulfamethoxazole (Bactrim) would not be used because of the patient's allergies. Fluoroquinolones can be used in patients aged 18 years or older.

397. D) Ciprofloxacin (Cipro) Cipro is the only medication listed that will not interfere with the metabolism and absorption of oral contraceptives.

398. B) Cardiac effects Levothyroxine (Synthroid) should be started on the lowest dose in elderly patients due to the severe side effects that can occur. These include palpitations, tachycardia, anxiety, irritability, elevated blood pressure, flushing, and insomnia.

399. B) Vaccination against the influenza virus Influenza vaccine is recommended as a preventative for all pregnant patients because of decreased maternal immune status during pregnancy. The vaccine is safe for use during pregnancy.

400. D) 12 months The earliest age at which MMR vaccination should be given is 12 months. Giving the vaccine any earlier may be less effective because the infant still has antibodies from the mother, which may interfere with the production of the antibodies stimulated by the vaccine.

401. B) Benzodiazepines Acute alcohol withdrawal delirium is managed with benzodiazepines.

402. D) DTaP, IPV, MMR, varicella The best clue is that the mother denies a history of chickenpox infection; therefore, this child requires the varicella vaccine. Only two answer options include varicella. The child does not need hepatitis B vaccination.

403. D) 13-year-old being treated for a sexually transmitted disease There are three primary ways for a minor to become emancipated: marriage, court order, and military service. A minor can be treated for a sexually transmitted disease without parental permission in most states.

404. B) Anorexia nervosa Anorexia nervosa increases the risk for osteopenia in teenage girls as a result of the poor intake of foods high in calcium and vitamin D.

405. A) Refer the patient to a urologist Urinary tract infections (UTIs) are relatively rare in young men with normal urinary tracts. Urethritis can mimic a UTI; rule out gonorrhea and chlamydia. A urine culture before initiating antibiotics and a test of cure is recommended for this group. Therefore, they should be referred to a urologist for evaluation and treatment. Additional tests that should be conducted may include intravenous pyelography, renal ultrasound, CT scan, or cystoscopy.

406. D) Giant cell arteritis Loss of vision does not occur with headaches. Loss of vision, along with marked scalp tenderness and a bad headache at the left temple, are symptoms of giant cell arteritis. Inflammation of the arteries of the head at the temple area causes the symptoms.

407. C) Sedimentation rate Sedimentation rate is used to assess for inflammation in the body, which is elevated in giant cell arteritis. Giant cell arteritis can cause blindness if it is not treated (high-dosed steroid). Refer to emergency department as soon as possible. Signs and symptoms include fever, fatigue, headache, jaw claudication, and transient visual loss (amaurosis fugax) to permanent blindness. Patients with history of polymyalgia rheumatica are at very high risk for giant cell arteritis.

408. D) Endometrial biopsy Random episodes of vaginal bleeding in a postmenopausal woman are not normal. Endometrial biopsy is needed to evaluate a specimen of the endometrial lining for abnormal cells, which may indicate cancer.

409. B) Patient is coherent Characteristics of delirium include an acute and dramatic onset of symptoms that are temporary, and usually worsen in the evening. Symptoms may last hours to days, and the patient is incoherent and disoriented. Delirium is usually brought on by fever, shock, drugs, alcohol, or dehydration.

410. D) Increase in abstract thinking ability Characteristics of dementia include irreversible symptoms with a gradual onset. Short-term memory loss is an early sign of dementia. As symptoms progress, the patient may become incoherent, unable to talk, walk, feed self, or perform self-care.

411. D) Slow onset of symptoms Acute prostatitis symptoms include fever, chills, tenderness of the scrotum on the affected side, and abrupt onset of symptoms.

412. B) *Chlamydia trachomatis* The most common cause of nongonococcal urethritis is *Chlamydia trachomatis*, but it can also be caused by *Ureaplasma urealyticum, Haemophilus vaginalis*, and *Mycoplasma genitalium*.

413. D) Depression Depression is a relative contraindication for combined oral contraceptive pills (OCPs) due to their hormonal effects, which can affect mood. Absolute contraindications include hepatoma of the liver, history of embolic episode, history of transient ischemic attacks (TIAs), and undiagnosed vaginal bleeding. OCPs should not be considered for patients with a history of these problems due to the potential health risks.

414. **A) Injury to the meniscus of the right knee** Pain in the knee with "locking up" while attempting to straighten the leg is highly suggestive of injury to the meniscus. The best imaging test for meniscus injury is the MRI.

415. **A) Refer him to an orthopedic specialist** Referral to orthopedics is advised for evaluation of the need for treatment and surgery (arthroscopic repair). If the tear is minor and the pain and other symptoms resolve quickly, muscle-strengthening exercises may be all that is needed to recover fully. In this case, a patient is usually referred to physical therapy. A large meniscus tear that causes symptoms or mechanical problems with the function of the knee joint may require arthroscopic surgery for repair.

416. **C) The newer low-dose birth control pills do not require backup during the first 2 weeks of use** All forms of oral contraceptive pills require a second backup method of contraception during the first 2 weeks of use. It is possible to have "breakthrough" ovulation in the first week when taking birth control pills for the first time; therefore, a second backup (condoms) is recommended.

417. **C) Osgood–Schlatter disease** Osgood–Schlatter disease is characterized by pain over the tibial tuberosity with palpation of a bony mass over the anterior tubercle of one or both knees. Exercise worsens the pain.

418. **C) Cholesteatoma** An abnormal skin growth in the middle ear behind the eardrum is called cholesteatoma. Repeated infections and/or a tear or pulling inward of the eardrum can allow skin into the middle ear. Cholesteatomas often develop as cysts or pouches that shed layers of old skin, which build up inside the middle ear. Over time, the cholesteatoma can increase in size and destroy the surrounding delicate bones of the middle ear, leading to hearing loss that surgery can often improve. Permanent hearing loss, dizziness, and facial muscle paralysis are rare, but can result from continued cholesteatoma growth.

419. **D) In-service training** Legal risks for the nurse practitioner include invasive procedures, electronic medical record entries, and prescribing of medications. In-service training does not directly affect the patient; therefore, legal risks are not a problem.

420. **B) Swimming** The American College of Rheumatology states that exercise is beneficial for everyone, including those with rheumatoid arthritis, and currently recommends 150 minutes of moderate-intensity aerobic activity each week. Safe forms of aerobic exercise, such as walking and aquatic exercise, help arthritis patients to control weight, and improve sleep, mood, and overall health.

421. **B) Amenorrhea** Depo-Provera (contraceptive injection) is a progesterone hormone that causes cessation of periods. One common side effect seen in women who have been taking Depo-Provera for more than 5 years is amenorrhea. As women continue using Depo-Provera, fewer experience irregular bleeding and more experience amenorrhea. By month 12, amenorrhea was reported by 55% of women, and by month 24, amenorrhea was reported by 68% of women.

422. **D) Moderate sodium restriction** Regarding migraine headaches, sodium restriction is not effective. But propranolol (migraine prophylaxis), trimethobenzamide (nausea),

and resting in a quiet and darkened room are helpful. Pain relief medications, such as analgesics, NSAIDs, caffeine, ergots, and "triptans," can be effective treatment.

423. B) Dementia The Mini-Cog (Mini-Cognitive Assessment Test) consists of a three-item word recall and a clock drawing test. A score of 0 to 2 is suggestive of dementia. A score of 3 to 5 means a low likelihood of dementia.

424. A) Meniscal injury With an acute knee injury, the knee should be assessed using McMurray's sign. A positive McMurray's sign indicates a meniscal injury. Inflammation of the knee, osteophytes, and tenosynovitis would not elicit a positive McMurray's sign.

425. C) Pericarditis Pericarditis is inflammation of the sac around the heart. Common signs and symptoms include chest pain over the center/left side of the chest; shortness of breath, especially with lying down; low-grade fever; weakness; fatigue; dry cough; and abdominal or leg swelling. Pericardial rub may be auscultated.

426. B) Rest the joint and apply cold packs intermittently for the next 48 hours New onset of a painful, swollen left knee (inflammation) should be treated using RICE: Rest the knee/joint, use alternating ice packs for the first 24 to 48 hours, use compression if knee feels unstable, and elevate the limb to decrease swelling.

427. C) Weight gain Symptoms of ulcerative colitis include bloody diarrhea mixed with mucus, nausea/vomiting, abdominal pain, and possible weight loss with long-term diarrhea.

428. D) Weight Peak expiratory flow volume is determined by using height, gender, and age. Weight is not used in the formula.

429. A) Larva migrans Larva migrans results from infection with the eggs of parasites (worms) that are commonly found in the intestines of dogs and cats. Children are at high risk of developing this infection if they come in contact with dirt that is contaminated with dog or cat feces. Eating foods that are grown in contaminated soil and/or raw liver are other means of transferring the infection. After the eggs hatch, the parasite can migrate to other organs of the body if left untreated.

430. D) Intrauterine device An intrauterine device (IUD) is not a risk factor for urinary tract infections (UTIs). In addition to causing increased urine glucose, diabetes may increase the risk of UTIs through mechanisms that include impaired immune cell delivery, inefficient white blood cells, and inhibition of bladder contractions that allow urine to remain stagnant in the bladder. Diaphragms are associated with an increased risk of UTIs. Urinating before inserting the diaphragm and also after intercourse may reduce this risk. Hormonal and mechanical changes increase the risk of urinary stasis and vesicoureteral reflux. These changes, along with an already short urethra (approximately 3–4 cm in females) and difficulty with hygiene due to a distended pregnant belly, increase the frequency of UTIs in pregnant women. Indeed, UTIs are among the most common bacterial infections during pregnancy.

431. **D) Bartholin's gland abscess** Bartholin's glands are located in the base of the labia minora at about the 4 o'clock and 8 o'clock positions. Their function is to provide moisture for the vestibule. They are small (about pea sized) unless they become clogged or infected. If this occurs, an abscess may form and glands will enlarge and become painful.

432. **B) Perform a history and physical exam and, if the patient does not have health contraindications, prescribe birth control pills** In the United States, the majority of states grant minors the right to privacy to obtain contraceptives (such as birth control pills), pregnancy testing, and testing for sexually transmitted infection (Guttmacher Institute, n.d.). To safely prescribe birth control pills, it is necessary to obtain a history and perform a physical exam to rule out health contraindications, rule out pregnancy, and evaluate the patient's decision-making skills and ability to follow instructions. Contraceptive options and safe sex education are also part of the first visit. It is not necessary to obtain a Pap smear to prescribe birth control pills. The U.S. Preventive Services Task Force does not recommend a Pap smear for woman younger than age 21 years.

433. **C) Does not need treatment** Bacterial vaginosis is a bacterial infection, but is not considered a sexually transmitted disease for which the partner needs treatment. Studies show that men rarely carry this infection.

434. **C) There is an increase in renal function** Physiological changes in the elderly include increase in the fat-to-lean body ratio, decrease in the ability of the liver to metabolize drugs, loss of hearing for sounds in the high-frequency range, and a *decrease* in renal function.

435. **D) Increased facial movements** Clinical signs of Parkinson's disease include pill-rolling tremors, difficulty initiating involuntary movements, and shuffling gait with cogwheel rigidity. Facial movement decreases, resulting in generalized rigidity with masked facies.

436. **B) Placenta abruptio** Abruptio placenta is a possible complication of severe eclampsia. With elevated blood pressure, the placenta can pull away from the uterine lining, which causes painful, bright red bleeding.

437. **A) Corneal ulceration** Due to the paralysis caused by the seventh cranial nerve damage, the eyelid on the affected side may not close voluntarily. This leads to dryness, which, in turn, can result in ulceration.

438. **D) Acute infection** Delirium is an acute decline in mental status and is temporary. Common causes are fever, shock, drugs, alcohol, severe dehydration, and acute infection.

439. **B) Urine human chorionic gonadotropin (hCG) test** Severe right-sided pain with vaginal bleeding in a 25-year-old patient requires an evaluation for pregnancy by initially performing a urine hCG test, which can be done quickly in the primary care clinic. A serum hCG test can also be drawn at the same visit. If a ruptured ectopic pregnancy is suspected, call 911.

440. **A) Serum GGT (gamma glutamyl transaminase)** The serum gamma glutamyl transaminase may become elevated in patients who are alcohol abusers. It can be used to screen for chronic alcohol abuse and occult alcoholism. The GGT can become elevated in liver disease and bile duct obstruction. It is a sensitive test for detecting obstructive jaundice, cholangitis, and cholecystitis.

441. **C) Testicular torsion** Signs and symptoms of testicular torsion include sudden onset of unilateral scrotal pain, nausea, vomiting, and abdominal pain. Acute epididymitis causes fever, chills, nausea, and unilateral pain and is most commonly seen in sexually active men. Unilateral scrotal pain does not occur with *Salmonella* infection. Acute orchitis is often based on having a recent mumps infection (parotitis) with testicular edema.

442. **B) Refer him to the emergency department as soon as possible** Immediate referral to the emergency department is required to prevent irreversible ischemia. Success of treatment is usually 100% if treated within the first 6 hours and 0% if treated after 24 hours. The diagnosis of testicular torsion is often made clinically, but if it is in doubt, an ultrasound is helpful in evaluating the condition. Emergency diagnosis and treatment are usually required within 4 to 6 hours to prevent necrosis.

443. **C) Renal stenosis and adrenal tumors** Secondary hypertension is most likely seen following renal stenosis and adrenal tumors. Renal stenosis causes secondary hypertension by plaque formation in the arteries, causing damage to coronary arteries (atherosclerosis). Adrenal tumors initiate secondary hypertension by releasing a large amount of aldosterone, which causes water and salt retention and loss of too much potassium.

444. **A) 2 to 3 years** Menarche normally begins approximately 2 to 3 years following Tanner stage II (breast budding). Median age of menarche in the United States is 12.43 years. It usually occurs within 2 to 3 years after breast budding (American College of Obstetricians and Gynecologists, 2015).

445. **D) A 14-year-old who wants to be treated for dysmenorrhea** Treatment for teenagers may be done without parental consent for sexually transmitted infections, pregnancy testing, and contraception counseling and treatment. Parental consent is required for any type of physical exam or for other problems that require more invasive testing.

446. **B) Diabetes mellitus** Balanitis is a yeast infection of the glans of the penis. Men who are not circumcised and who have diabetes mellitus are at higher risk for developing balanitis.

447. **B) Transillumination** Transillumination is a technique used with a light source, such as the otoscope, to visualize fluid below the skin surface, which will appear as a "glow." Ultrasound and CT scan are not readily available in the primary care setting; the patient must be sent to radiology for these tests to be performed.

448. **C) A chest radiograph result with infiltrates and flattening of the costovertebral angle** Emphysema is characterized by having a barrel-shaped chest, pursed-lip breathing, and dyspnea when at rest. Infiltrates on an x-ray indicate bacterial infection, such as pneumonia.

449. **B) The pulmonic area** The S2 heart sound is physiologically split in about 90% of people. The second heart sound is produced by the closure of the aortic and pulmonic valves. The sound produced by the closure of the aortic valve is termed *A2*, and the sound produced by the closure of the pulmonic valve is termed *P2*. The A2 sound is normally much louder than the P2 due to higher pressures in the left side of the heart; thus, A2 radiates to all cardiac listening posts (loudest at the right upper sternal border) and P2 is usually only heard at the left upper sternal border.

450. **C) *Candida albicans*** Balanitis is a yeast infection of the glans of the penis. *Candida albicans* is the causative source. *Staphylococcus aureus* and *Streptococcus pyogenes* are bacterial infections. Trichomonads are protozoans that cause infection.

451. **B) Left supraclavicular area** The sentinel nodes are found at the supraclavicular area of the chest. They are the first lymph nodes that a cancer lesion will drain into. Therefore, when cancer is diagnosed, these nodes are biopsied to see whether the cancer has spread into the lymph system.

452. **A) Tinea cruris** Tinea cruris (jock itch) is a common skin infection that is caused by a type of fungus called *tinea*. The fungus thrives in warm, moist areas of the body and, as a result, infection can affect the genitals, inner thighs, and buttocks. Infections occur more frequently in the summer or in warm, wet climates. Tinea cruris appears as a red, itchy rash that is often ring shaped. Tinea corporis involves the body, tinea capitis involves the head, and tinea pedis involves the feet.

453. **B) Middle-aged men** The most prominent feature of cluster headache is severe pain that is almost always on only one side of the head, accompanied by tearing, rhinorrhea, ptosis (drooping of upper eyelid), and miosis (constriction of the pupil). Cluster headaches occur periodically; spontaneous remissions interrupt active periods of pain. The cause of the condition is currently unknown. It affects approximately 0.1% of the population, and men are more commonly affected than women. The headaches typically start before age 30.

454. **D) Large testes** Signs and symptoms of Klinefelter's syndrome include gynecomastia, long limbs, and lack of secondary sexual characteristics. Testes are usually small. Infertility is a major concern for these boys. If treated early, they may have a normal sexual/reproductive system in the future.

455. **A) Trimethoprim–sulfamethoxazole (Bactrim DS)** Warfarin sodium (Coumadin) interacts with Bactrim and will increase the risk of bleeding; therefore, concurrent use is contraindicated.

456. **C) Tanner stage III** During Tanner stage III, the breast and areola and nipples grow together in one mound. There is no separation yet. At Tanner stage IV, the areola and the nipple separate to form a distinct mound. The most important clue is "secondary mound."

457. **B) Increase physical activity and outdoor play** Lifestyle changes, such as increasing physical activity and spending more time outdoors, are appropriate recommendations for children. Consider referral to a registered dietician for dietary recommendations and counseling. Participation in an exercise program designed for children (if available) is

also appropriate. Severe caloric and/or carbohydrate restriction is not recommended for this age group.

458. D) Stroking the inner thigh of a male patient and watching the testicle on the ipsilateral side rise up toward the body The cremasteric reflex is elicited by stroking the inner thigh (proximal to distal) with a blunt instrument such as a handle of the reflex hammer. The testicle and scrotum should rise on the stroked (ipsilateral) side.

459. B) Zanfel poison ivy wash Zanfel is a soap-like product (OTC) that removes urushiol oil from poison ivy, poison sumac, and poison oak. It will relieve the itch and pain quickly. A topical steroid can be used to speed up healing. For rashes, hydrocortisone cream 1% BID (OTC) is helpful.

460. C) A decrease in systolic blood pressure on inspiration In patients with pulsus paradoxus, systolic pressure drops on inspiration due to the increased pressure (positive pressure). Some pulmonary risks of having increased pressure include asthma and emphysema.

461. A) Influenza Not all vaccinations are safe to get during pregnancy. However, the flu vaccine can be given before, during, and after pregnancy. The other vaccines are live viruses and are contraindicated during pregnancy.

462. A) Heart disease and endometrial cancer Chronic anovulation results in high levels of estrogen and androgens in the body. The risk of heart attack is four to seven times higher in women with polycystic ovary syndrome (PCOS) than women of the same age without PCOS. Women with PCOS are at greater risk of having high blood pressure and have high levels of low-density lipoprotein (LDL) and low levels of high-density lipoprotein (HDL) cholesterol. Lack of ovulation is usually the reason for fertility problems in women with PCOS. More than 50% of women with PCOS have diabetes or prediabetes (impaired glucose tolerance) before the age of 40. Women with PCOS are also at risk for endometrial cancer. Irregular menstrual periods and the lack of ovulation cause women to produce the hormone estrogen, but not progesterone. Without progesterone, the endometrium becomes thick, which can cause heavy or irregular bleeding. Over time, this can lead to endometrial hyperplasia and cancer.

463. B) Scarlatina Scarlatina (scarlet fever) is a rash that usually first appears on the neck and chest, then spreads over the body. It is described as "sandpapery" in feel. The texture of the rash is more important than the appearance in confirming the diagnosis. The rash can last for more than a week. As the rash fades, peeling (desquamation) may occur around the fingertips, toes, and groin area. Another sign is a bright red tongue with a "strawberry" appearance.

464. B) Take two pills today and two pills tomorrow, and have your partner use condoms for the rest of the pill cycle When forgetting to take the birth control pill on 2 consecutive days, it is recommended to take two pills immediately and two pills the next day, then continue the rest of the pack. Stress the importance of the use of condoms for protection against pregnancy and STIs.

465. D) A 30-year-old White man with hypertension The 30-year-old White man with hypertension would be the last patient to be screened for diabetes. Not having any information about him also puts him lower on the list. Obesity, ethnicity (Hispanic/Latino Americans, African Americans, Native Americans, Asian Americans, Pacific Islanders, and Alaska natives), family history of diabetes, and gestational diabetes (mother of the infant weighing 9.5 lbs) are all risk factors. These were present in all of the other selections. Other risk factors for diabetes include impaired glucose tolerance test, sedentary lifestyle, polycystic ovary syndrome (PCOS), and hypertension.

466. A) Sciatica Sciatica is defined as pain that begins in the buttock area and radiates down one leg. Other symptoms include weakness and tingling sensation. Acute muscle spasm and strain do not cause tingling down the leg. Cauda equina syndrome is an emergent issue, in which there is neurological involvement and the patient complains of weakness and loss of bladder and bowel control.

467. C) The patient needs hepatitis B vaccine and hepatitis B immunoglobulin Because he is HBsAg positive, and anti-HBV and HBeAg negative, he needs hepatitis B immunoglobulin and hepatitis B vaccine.

468. D) Microaneurysms Microaneurysms are seen with diabetic retinopathy. Arteriovenous (AV) nicking, copper wire arterioles, and flame hemorrhages are seen with uncontrolled hypertension.

469. D) Spinach and kale These two foods are high in potassium, vitamin K, and other vitamins. They do not contain tyramine. Tyramine levels increase in food when they are aged or fermented. A hypertensive crisis can develop in patients if monoamine oxidase inhibitor (MAOI) drugs are mixed with high-tyramine foods.

470. A) First molars The first molars are the first permanent teeth to develop; they appear at approximately 6 years of age.

471. B) Meningococcemia Kernig's maneuver is performed by flexing both hips and legs and having the patient straighten the legs against resistance, testing for meningitis. A positive test indicates meningitis. Other characteristics of meningitis include high fever, headache, stiff neck, and nausea/vomiting.

472. C) She can take any of the pills in the sulfonylurea class The patient can take sulfonylureas. The sulfonamide component in the typical sulfa antibiotics is of a slightly different molecular structure than that in sulfonylureas. Although cross-reactivity is technically possible, current literature does not consider this likely, and sulfonylureas are typically well tolerated in patients with a sulfa allergy.

473. C) Prostaglandins Prostaglandins are hormones the body produces prior to menses; they eventually cause the uterus to contract to shed the endometrial lining. Contractions cause pain. The greater the amount of prostaglandins that are released, the more pain one will experience. Contractions of the uterus cause vasoconstriction of blood supply to the uterus, which, in turn, will cause pain.

474. C) Serum folate acid and B_{12} level The patient has macrocytic anemia (MCV 102). The differential diagnoses are B_{12} deficiency and folate deficiency anemia. Initial test is the serum folate and B_{12} level. Other tests for macrocytic/megaloblastic anemias are the peripheral smear, methylmalonic acid, and homocysteine level. If B_{12} deficiency, order anti-parietal antibodies to check for pernicious anemia.

475. D) Vesicular breath sounds in the lower lobe Normal sounds of the chest wall include vesicular breath sounds in the lower lobes. Bronchial breath sounds are heard best at the second and third intercostal spaces. Tracheal breath sounds are heard over the trachea.

476. A) S3 and S4 and low-pitched tones The bell is most useful for picking up low-pitched sounds; for example, S3, S4, and mitral stenosis. The diaphragm is most useful for picking up high-pitched sounds; for example, S1, S2, aortic or mitral regurgitation, and pericardial friction rubs.

477. A) Wet smear The wet smear or wet prep is best used to diagnose *Candida albicans* infection of the vagina (candidiasis) in the primary care setting. To perform the wet smear or wet prep, a small amount of vaginal discharge is obtained and smeared on a slide, then one to two drops of normal saline solution is applied. *Candida albicans* is a type of yeast organism (fungi). *Candida* viewed under the microscope will have pseudohyphae and spores. The specimen may also include white blood cells because *Candida* causes an inflammatory reaction in the vagina.

478. C) Tanner stage III Tanner stages for breast development: I, prepuberty; II, breast bud; III, breast and areola one mound; IV, breast and areola secondary mound; V, adult pattern.

479. C) Retin-A 0.25% gel Topical agents are the first-line treatment for acne vulgaris. Retin-A 0.25% gel would be the next step. Oral preparations (tetracycline) would then be offered, and Accutane would be the final step.

480. D) Cerebellum The Romberg test evaluates the cerebellum and the vestibular system (inner ear), which are responsible for balance. This test is performed by having the client stand up straight with feet together and with arms straight down the side of the body. Next the patient is instructed to close his or her eyes and stand still for at least 20 seconds. The test is positive if patient cannot maintain balance with eyes closed.

481. B) The quasi-experimental design uses convenience sampling instead of random sampling to recruit subjects The quasi-experimental design uses an intervention (it is not an observational study or a survey). It has many similarities to an experimental study except that the human subjects are recruited by convenience and not at random (as in an experimental study).

482. B) Advise the mother to use a nit comb after spraying the child's hair with white distilled vinegar, wait for 15 minutes, and then rinse the hair According to the Centers for Disease Control and Prevention (CDC), nits that are more than ¼ inch from the scalp are usually not viable. The child also does not have an itchy scalp. One method of removal is to soak the patient's head with distilled vinegar (and then rinse after), which will break down the protein of the nit casings, making it easy to comb them out of the hair.

483. C) A filled-in square A filled-in square is a diseased or affected male and a filled-in circle is a diseased or affected female. An empty square is a healthy male and an empty circle is a healthy female.

484. A) Plain radiographs of the right lower leg, ankle, and foot Plain radiographs or x-rays are the first exam ordered for suspected or obvious bony fractures. Severe pain on weight bearing and bruising of the right ankle is highly suggestive of a fracture. MRI scan is not an initial test because it is very expensive. MRIs are preferred for joints and soft tissue.

485. D) Tetanus vaccine and systemic antibiotics A break in the skin with a compound fracture is an indication for use of a tetanus vaccine (if last dose is more than 5 years ago) and systemic antibiotics.

486. D) Caucasian Lupus is two to three times more prevalent among women of African American, Asian, Hispanic, and Native American backgrounds than in Caucasian women.

487. D) Malar rash A malar rash is the butterfly-shaped rash on the middle of the face that is caused by a type of photosensitivity reaction. It is associated with systemic lupus erythematosus (SLE). The other answer options are found with diseases such as rheumatoid arthritis, polymyalgia rheumatica, and others.

488. C) BC>AC A normal result in the Rinne test is air conduction (AC) greater than bone conduction (BC). When there is a conductive hearing loss (i.e., ceruminosis, otitis media), the result will be BC greater than AC. The reason is that the sound waves are blocked (i.e., cerumen, fluid in middle ear). Therefore, the patient cannot hear them as well as through bone conduction.

489. B) Collaborative A collaborative relationship exists when a health caregiver refers a patient to others (physicians, specialists, physical therapy, etc.) to help with patient treatment and management. Consult reports and progress reports are sent to the primary caregiver to report the patient's progress. Consultative relationships are informal, such as talking to a colleague about a patient's treatment.

490. B) Acute bacterial endocarditis Bacterial endocarditis is also known as *infective endocarditis* (*IC*). It is a serious bacterial infection of the heart valves and the endocardial surface. The bacteria most commonly involved are *Staphylococcus* and *Streptococcus* species. Subcutaneous red painful nodules on the finger pads are called *Osler's nodes*. Subungual splinter hemorrhages on the nailbeds are caused by microemboli. Janeway's lesions are caused by bleeding under the skin (usually located on the palms and the soles) and are painless red papules and macules. Other findings are conjunctival hemorrhages, petechiae, cardiac friction rubs, arrhythmias, murmurs, and others. Three blood cultures obtained at separate sites 1 hour apart are used to identify the causative organism. Some of the risk factors are damaged prosthetic valves, history of rheumatic fever, and injection drug use.

491. C) *Pseudomonas aeruginosa* *P. aeruginosa* is a common chronic lung infection seen in older children and adults with cystic fibrosis. This infection is difficult to eliminate and sometimes is the cause of death.

492. C) There is a mild increase in renal function Physiological changes that occur in the elderly include decrease in renal function, increased half-life of some medications, increase in cholesterol production by the liver, and slight decrease in the immune system.

493. B) Roseola infantum Roseola infantum is caused by herpes virus 6 (HHV-6). The signs and symptoms of roseola infantum include high fever for a few days with a maculopapular rash occurring after the fever breaks. Febrile seizures occur in up to 15% of infants. Fifth disease (erythema infectiosum) is caused by parvovirus B_{19}. It causes a red facial rash or "slapped cheek" appearance; in a few days a lacy-appearing rash appears on the trunk, arms, and legs. Erythema infectiosum is the same as fifth disease. Scarlet fever is a red rash that feels like sandpaper that usually begins on the neck and trunk and spreads to the extremities. Patients with scarlet fever have other symptoms such as fever, sore throat, and beefy red tongue. Scarlet fever is caused by the group A Streptococcus bacterium.

494. A) Fifth disease Fifth disease has three stages. The prodromal stage begins with symptoms of an upper respiratory infection, such as low-grade fever, headache, chills, and malaise. In the second stage, a red rash appears on the cheeks, known as the "slapped cheek" rash. This usually resolves in 2 to 3 days. In the third stage, the rash moves to the arms and legs and becomes a lacy-appearing rash that is flat and appears purple; this may last for a few weeks.

495. A) Tricyclic antidepressants (TCAs) TCAs and anticonvulsants are recommended for postherpetic neuralgia. These medications may help with the neuropathic pain.

496. C) Rocky Mountain spotted fever Given the location in the East, Rocky Mountain spotted fever is most likely the infection causing symptoms of fever and a rash on ankles and wrists, moving to the palms of the hands and the trunk. Rocky Mountain spotted fever is caused by the bacterium *Rickettsia rickettsii*, which is transmitted by a bite from an infected tick.

497. D) Median nerve Compression of the median nerve within the carpal tunnel produces characteristic symptoms—burning; tingling; numbness over the thumb, index, middle, and ring fingers. The Phalen maneuver is a diagnostic test for carpal tunnel syndrome. It is performed by pushing the back of the hands together for 1 minute. Eliciting carpal tunnel symptoms indicates a positive result for the test.

498. C) It is characterized by high fasting blood glucose in the morning that is caused by the secretion of glucagon by the liver The Somogyi phenomenon or Somogyi effect occurs when nocturnal hypoglycemia (2 a.m.–3 a.m.) stimulates the liver to produce glucagon, which causes the fasting blood glucose to become elevated. It is also known as the "rebound effect."

499. C) Actinic keratosis Actinic keratoses are small, raised lesions on skin that has been in the sun for a long period of time, although they are pre-cancerous lesions. These lesions are usually benign but can develop into skin cancer; therefore, further evaluation is needed to determine whether removal is required.

500. A) Propranolol (Inderal) Propranolol (Inderal) is approved for management of essential tremor to help control symptoms. Essential tremors are permanent and cannot be cured. Before prescribing propranolol, order an EKG. Do not use beta-blockers if a patient has second- or third-degree heart block or chronic lung disease.

501. A) Orthostatic hypotension and sedation Orthostatic hypotension and sedation are common side effects of atypical antipsychotics such as olanzapine (Zyprexa), quetiapine (Seroquel), and risperidone (Risperdal). It is also a common side effect of the older antipsychotics like haloperidol (Haldol). Antipsychotics do not cause severe anxiety and hyperphagia (increased appetite). They lower anxiety and cause sedation, sleepiness, anorexia, and hypotension, and increase the risk of sudden death in frail elders.

502. B) Metronidazole (Flagyl) 500 mg PO TID × 10 days First-line treatment for a mild case of *Clostridium difficile* colitis is metronidazole (Flagyl) 500 mg PO TID for 10 days. Discontinuation of the offending antibiotic (if possible) or switching to another antibiotic class is recommended. The role of probiotic supplementation is controversial. Complications are pseudomembranous colitis, toxic megacolon, and fulminant colitis.

503. A) Azithromycin (Zithromax) If the patient has a severe penicillin allergy, there is a 10% chance of cross-reactivity to cephalosporins (especially first generation). Because the patient is a child, the levofloxacin is contraindicated. Nausea is a common adverse reaction to erythromycin (it is not an allergic reaction). The best option is to use azithromycin because of its minimal GI adverse effects. Azithromycin has fewer drug interactions compared with other macrolides.

504. C) Elderly Elderly who are mentally competent are not considered a vulnerable population group.

505. A) Order an MRI scan of the spine as soon as possible The patient has new-onset numbness of the perineal area (saddle anesthesia), the sciatica is worsening, and the deep tendon reflexes of the lower extremity are decreased on the affected side. Rule out cauda equine syndrome and order an MRI (preferred test). The MRI can detect nerve root compression, herniated disk, cancer, and spinal stenosis (narrowing of the spinal canal). In addition, the patient needs to follow up with a neurologist as soon as possible.

506. B) The patient has a mild case of acute diverticulitis and can be treated with antibiotics in the outpatient setting with close follow-up The patient has a mild case of acute diverticulitis and can be treated as an outpatient with antibiotics and a clear fluid diet. If outpatient treatment is selected, close follow-up (within 24–48 hours) is very important. Instruct patients to go to the hospital if symptoms get worse, if fever increases, if unable to tolerate PO treatment, and if pain worsens. Order a complete blood count (to check for leukocytosis, neutrophils, and possible shift to the left), chemistry profile, and urinalysis (to rule out renal causes).

507. A) Isoflavones Soy isoflavones (phytoestrogens) mimic the action of estrogen in the body. They are derived from soybeans and soybean products (soy milk, tofu). Supplementation with isoflavones may help some women with menopausal hot flashes.

508. C) Peripheral neuropathy Bupropion increases the risk of seizures. Contraindications are seizures, anorexia nervosa, and bulimia. Avoid with any condition that increases seizures, such as after abrupt withdrawal of alcohol or sedatives and with certain head injuries. For peripheral neuropathy, treatment options are an SNRI (duloxetine/ Cymbalta), tricyclic antidepressants, anticonvulsants, topical capsaicin cream, and others.

509. A) Increasing consumption of caffeine-containing drinks and foods such as chocolate Lifestyle changes associated with decreasing exacerbations are wearing gloves or mittens during cold weather, taking care when handling frozen foods (wear gloves), and avoiding vasoconstricting agents (caffeine, smoking, cocaine, amphetamines) and emotional stress. Exercise and reducing lifestyle stress are recommended. Raynaud's disease usually involves the fingers and/or toes due to severe arteriolar vasospasm causing ischemia. During an exacerbation, the fingers change color becoming white, blue, and red (think of the American flag as a reminder). Raynaud's is classified either as primary (Raynaud's disease) or secondary (Raynaud's phenomenon). Individuals with secondary Raynaud's have a higher risk of autoimmune disorders such as scleroderma, Sjögren's syndrome, and systemic lupus erythematosus. The disorder affects mostly young women (ages 15–30 years).

510. C) Patients have the right to view their mental health and psychotherapy-related health information Mental health and psychotherapy/psychiatric records do not have to be released to patients even if they request those records. Otherwise, any type of medical records can be released if requested by the health insurance or health plan for billing purposes and reimbursement. HIPAA applies to all health care providers, health plans, health insurance companies, medical clearinghouses, and others who bill electronically and transmit health information over the Internet.

511. C) Inner ear Sensorineural hearing loss (i.e., presbycusis) involves damage to the hair cells in the cochlea (sensory portion) and may involve cranial nerve VIII (neural).

512. B) Tdap, MCV4, and the HPV vaccines Vaccine questions usually are not this complicated, but there are several lessons that can be learned with this question. The 2017 Centers for Disease Control and Prevention (CDC) recommendations for individuals 13 to 18 years of age are the Tdap catch-up (if not received at age 11–12 years), human papillomavirus (HPV) catch-up (if not received at age 11–12 years), and the MCV4 or meningococcal conjugate vaccine (Menactra). Thereafter, the Td form of the vaccine is indicated every 10 years. The DTaP (diphtheria–tetanus–acellular pertussis) and DT (diphtheria–tetanus) forms of the tetanus vaccine are not given after the age of 7 years.

513. A) Report the patient's grandson for elder abuse to the state protective health services Speaking with the grandson and warning him about elder abuse and being reported to authorities may result in harm to the patient and/or refusal to return to the clinic in the future for follow-up of the patient. Advising the patient to call his son as soon as possible is vague (for what?) and may benefit the patient but it is not the best option in this case.

514. B) Dyspnea Dyspnea is a symptom. The stem of the question is asking for pulmonary function test results, which includes TLC, RV, FEV1, and others. In chronic obstructive pulmonary disease (COPD), there is a reduction of the FEV1 (forced expiratory volume in 1 second) with increase in the TLC (total lung capacity) and RV (residual volume). The lungs of patients with emphysema have lost their elastic recoil (reduced FEV1). The lungs are always full of air that is hard to "squeeze out" of the lungs (this increases residual volume and total lung capacity). To summarize, COPD = reduction in FEV1 with increases RV and TLC.

515. **B) Start the patient on levothyroxine (Synthroid) 0.25 mcg PO daily** The patient is symptomatic (weight gain, lack of energy, and irregular periods) with low free T4. Even though the thyroid-stimulating hormone (TSH) level decreased slightly, the free T4 remains low. An elevated TSH and low free T4 are indicative of hypothyroidism. The next step is to start the patient on levothyroxine (Synthroid) 0.25 mcg daily and recheck the TSH in 6 weeks. The goal is to normalize the TSH (between 1.0 and 3.5) and to ameliorate the patient's symptoms (increased energy, feels better, etc.). Armour thyroid (desiccated thyroid) is a natural supplement composed of dried (desiccated) pork thyroid glands. It is used in alternative medicine as an alternative to synthetic levothyroxine/T4 (Synthroid).

516. **A) Prostate feels rubbery and uniformly enlarged** The prostate should feel rubbery and uniformly enlarged in BPH. A boggy and warm prostate with tenderness is suggestive of acute prostatitis. Hard nodules and indurated areas are highly suggestive of prostate cancer.

517. **C) Blood glucose** Checking the blood glucose is indicated for patients with syncopal and near-syncopal episodes. The nurse practitioner should also perform a thorough history of the incident. Possible causes of syncope are cardiac arrhythmia, vasovagal, hypoglycemia, orthostatic hypotension, seizure, accidental fall, and others.

518. **D) Affected testicle is swollen and feels cold to the touch** The affected testicle will be swollen, but it will feel very warm to the touch. A cold testicle is abnormal and is indicative of gangrene (after 24 hours).

519. **B) N** The correct symbol to indicate total number of subjects in a study (total population) is N. For example, a research study has a total number of subjects or total population of 100 (N = 100). The small letter n is used to indicate a subpopulation. For example, a study uses a total population of N = 100 that is divided into two groups of 50 subjects (n = 50).

520. **B) 27%** This patient's burns have a total body surface areas (TBSA) of 27% and he should be referred to the emergency department as soon as possible. Check the "ABCs" and monitor the patient for shock. Do not puncture bullae.

521. **A) Instability of the knee caused by damage to the anterior cruciate ligament of the knee** A positive Lachman sign is highly suggestive of damage to (i.e., rupture of) the anterior cruciate ligament (ACL) of the knee. The anterior drawer sign may also be positive. The examiner notes laxity of the abnormal knee joint compared with the normal knee. The Lachman test or maneuver is considered more sensitive for ACL damage than the anterior drawer test.

522. **A) Hypocalcemia** Chvostek's sign refers to contraction of the facial muscles when the facial nerve is tapped briskly in front of the ear (anterior to the auditory canal). Low

calcium levels cause tetany and neuromuscular disturbances. Acute hypocalcemia with symptoms (tetany, weakness, arrhythmias) should be referred to the emergency department. Conditions, such as acute or chronic renal failure, vitamin D or magnesium deficiency, or acute pancreatitis, increase the risk of hypocalcemia.

523. B) When the nurse practitioner is unable to speak with the patient directly, she should leave a message with her name and telephone number and instruct the patient to call back Unless it is a secure voicemail system, leaving voicemails that contain personal health information (PHI) is a violation of HIPAA. These regulations have been updated recently so that if a patient lists a phone number as a contact number, he or she has given permission to the health care team to call that number and leave a message. It is best if the patient is asked about whom to contact to relay laboratory or procedure results, only if the patient has signed over authority to leave messages as stated in HIPAA policy of institution.

524. D) Atomoxetine (Strattera) Strattera is classified as a norepinephrine reuptake inhibitor. It is not a stimulant or an amphetamine. Strattera is contraindicated during/within 14 days of taking a monoamine oxidase inhibitor (MAOI) in patients with narrow-angle glaucoma or a heart disorder that will worsen with increases in blood pressure or heart rate, or in those with pheochromocytoma. Children and teenagers should be monitored for suicidal thoughts/plans.

525. A) Fasting blood glucose, fasting lipid profile, and weight Patients on atypical antipsychotics commonly gain weight and are at risk for obesity, hyperglycemia, and type 2 diabetes. Zyprexa will increase lipids (cholesterol, low-density lipoprotein [LDL], and triglycerides). Atypical antipsychotics also increase the risk of death among frail elders and older adults living in nursing homes.

526. B) A punishment by the "spirits" for wrongful actions against others or for failure to follow spiritual rules Native Americans believe that illness is punishment by the spirits for wrong actions or from failure to follow spiritual rules. Shamans "cure" the illness by performing rituals and using herbal medicines. Medicine pouches that are tied to the patient by a string are believed to help cure the illness. Do not remove such pouches without the patient's (or parent's) permission.

527. D) Ulcerative colitis The most important clue for ulcerative colitis is bloody stools that are covered with mucus and pus along with the systemic symptoms (fatigue, low-grade fever).

528. C) Health care providers are mandated by law to report certain types of diseases to the local health department even if the patient does not give permission Physicians and laboratories are legally mandated to report certain types of diseases. Sexually transmitted diseases, HIV infection/AIDS, gonorrhea, and syphilis must be reported to the local health department even if the patient does not give permission. Partner tracing and notification are done by the local health department. The Centers for Disease Control and Prevention (CDC) website contains a list of nationally reportable diseases. Other diseases that are on the CDC 2017 list of reportable diseases (i.e., diseases that must be reported) are tuberculosis; diphtheria; hepatitis A, B, and C; measles; mumps; pertussis; Lyme disease; Rocky Mountain spotted fever; and many others.

529. **D) Calls patients by using their first name only** Patients who are in waiting rooms or rooms with other people should be called by their first names only, to protect their privacy.

530. **B) The NP should advise the patient that a peer who is working with the NP can help answer the patient's questions more thoroughly** In general, discussing personal beliefs is considered unprofessional behavior. Respecting the patient's right to choose is an example of supporting patient autonomy.

531. **A) The spleen is not palpable in the majority of healthy adults** The spleen is located in the left upper quadrant of the abdomen under the diaphragm and is protected by the lower ribcage. In the majority of adults, it is not palpable. The spleen's longest axis is 11 to 20 cm. Any spleen larger than 20 cm is enlarged. The best test for evaluating splenic (or hepatic) size is the abdominal ultrasound. Disorders that can cause splenomegaly include mononucleosis, sickle cell disease, congestive heart failure, bone marrow cancers (myeloma, leukemia), and several other diseases.

532. **C) Thiazide diuretics** Thiazide diuretics have been used to treat hypertension for many decades and numerous placebo-controlled studies have documented their effectiveness as antihypertensive drugs.

533. **D) 10 days** The minimum number of days to quarantine an animal suspected of rabies is 10 days. If the animal is healthy and has no symptoms of rabies at 10 days, it is not infected with the rabies virus and can be returned to the owner.

534. **A) Thiazide diuretics decrease calcium excretion by the kidneys and stimulate osteoclast production** This positive side effect of thiazides results in a decrease in calcium bone loss and an increase in bone mineral density.

535. **D) It is a condition, characteristic, or factor that is being measured** A variable is a condition, characteristic, or factor that is being measured. An independent variable is the one being manipulated that is not affected by the others. A dependent variable changes depending on the manipulation of the independent variable.

536. **A) Take one pill every 1 to 2 hours until relief is obtained or adverse gastrointestinal effects occur, such as abdominal pain, nausea, or diarrhea** Colchicine acts as an anti-inflammatory and helps to suppress gouty attacks. It is usually taken as one tablet (0.6 mg) every 1 to 2 hours until relief is obtained (or adverse gastrointestinal [GI] effects occur, such as abdominal pain, nausea, or diarrhea). The patient should be prescribed only 10 tablets at a time (do not refill) during a flare-up. The maximum dose is 6 mg/day. Many patients will develop adverse GI effects even before the pain is relieved. Colchicine can also be taken daily in small amounts for prophylaxis.

537. **D) Comprehensive eye exam** A comprehensive eye exam by an ophthalmologist is recommended because hydroxychloroquine can adversely affect the retina (scotomas or visual field defects, loss of central vision, loss of color vision). Higher doses and long-term use increase the risk of retinal toxicity.

538. **B) T-score between –1. 0 and –2.5** Osteopenia is defined as a T-score between –1. 0 and –2.5. Osteoporosis is defined as a T-score of –2.5 or below. The T-score is sometimes called the Z-score.

539. **A) *Clostridium difficile*-associated diarrhea** An important risk factor for *Clostridium difficile*-associated diarrhea (CDAD) and *C. difficile* colitis is antibiotic therapy and hospitalization. Almost any antibiotic can cause the condition, but the most common are clindamycin, cephalosporins, and fluoroquinolones. Diarrhea can occur during therapy as well as after therapy (5–10 days; up to 10 weeks). Pseudomembranous colitis is a complication of *C. difficile* colitis.

540. **B) 25-year-old Chinese patient** Alpha thalassemia minor/trait or disease is more prevalent among Asians such as Chinese and Filipinos. Beta thalassemia minor/trait or disease is more common in the countries in the Mediterranean area, such as Greece and Italy.

541. **B) Ovulation disorders** Ovulation disorders are the top cause of female infertility (25%). Affected women may have no ovulation (anovulation) or infrequent ovulation that results in oligomenorrhea (i.e., polycystic ovarian syndrome [PCOS]). The second cause is endometriosis (15%). About 10% of women in the United States (ages 15–44 years) have difficulty getting pregnant (Centers for Disease Control and Prevention, 2009). PCOS is one of the most common causes of female infertility. Infertility in men is often caused by a varicocele (heats up the testes) and abnormal and/or low sperm count.

542. **B) Ménière's disease** The classic triad of symptoms of Ménière's disease is episodic vertigo, tinnitus, and sensorineural hearing loss (low frequency). Tinnitus is usually low pitch (like listening to a conch shell). One may have a strong sensation of ear fullness. The condition can resolve spontaneously or may be chronic. Pathologic lesion in the middle ear is called *endolymphatic hydrops*. Vasovagal syncope does not cause hearing loss or tinnitus, nor is it episodic. Hypoglycemia is not associated with episodic vertigo, tinnitus, and hearing loss.

543. **C) Increased lung compliance** Lung compliance decreases as we get older; therefore, the FEV1 also decreases. There is minimal change in the total lung volume. Airways tend to collapse earlier (than in young patients) with shallow breathing, which increases the risk of pneumonia.

544. **A) Addison's disease** Addison's disease is also known as *primary adrenal insufficiency*. The most common cause of damage to the adrenal cortex (the outer layer of the gland) is autoimmune destruction. The adrenal cortex produces glucocorticoids (cortisol) and mineralocorticoids (aldosterone). Aldosterone regulates sodium retention and potassium excretion through the kidneys (affects blood pressure). Electrolyte abnormalities are high potassium and low sodium. In primary disease (Addison's), the serum cortisol level is low, adrenocorticotropic hormone (ACTH) is high, and serum aldosterone is low. If the patient is not treated, severe stress (illness, accident) may cause an adrenal crisis ("Addisonian" crisis), which can be fatal.

545. **C) The patient has a TBSA of 27% with partial-thickness burns on the left arm and left hand, and superficial burns on the anterior chest and abdominal area** Using the

rule of nines, the anterior thorax is 18% and the left arm/hand is 9%, totaling 27%. A standard Lund–Browder (rule of nines) chart is readily available in most emergency departments. A partial-thickness burn is the same as a second-degree burn. A superficial burn is a first-degree burn.

546. C) The health insurance companies, health plans, Medicare, and Medicaid Third-party payers are health insurance companies, health plans (health maintenance or preferred provider organizations [HMOs or PPOs]), Medicare, and Medicaid. The "first party" is the patient. The "second party" is the health care provider.

547. D) Celiac disease Celiac disease is also known as *celiac sprue*. Patients should avoid foods containing gluten, which causes malabsorption (diarrhea, gas, bloating, and abdominal pain). Foods to avoid are wheat, rye, and barley. Oats do not damage the mucosa in celiac disease. Antigliadin IgA and IgG are elevated in almost all patients (90%).

548. B) Zolpidem (Ambien) Zolpidem (Ambien) has a quick onset of action (15 minutes) and a short half-life of 2 hours. Avoid diphenhydramine (Benadryl) in the elderly, as there is a higher incidence of adverse effects (confusion, prolonged sedation) in this population. Avoid long-acting benzodiazepines such as diazepam (Valium; half-life 12 hours) and temazepam (Restoril; half-life of 10 hours). Hypnotics can be used as needed up to 2 weeks; otherwise, benzodiazepines can cause addiction and withdrawal symptoms.

549. C) Multiply the treatment PSA value by 2 Before starting a prescription of finasteride (Proscar), obtain the baseline prostate-specific antigen (PSA) value. Recheck the PSA again within 2 to 3 months during treatment to assess the patient's response (treatment PSA). For this example, the corrected treatment PSA is 20 (multiply $10 \times 2 = 20$). When comparing the corrected treatment PSA (20) with the baseline PSA (30), the value is lower (means the prostate has shrunk in size). The patient's symptoms will also show improvement, including less nocturia, less dribbling, and stronger urinary stream.

550. D) The nurse practitioner has an ethical duty to provide quality health care to patients Currently, health caregivers are not legally required to report illegal aliens to the state or local authorities. This patient does not have the signs and symptoms of active tuberculosis (TB) disease (cough, weight loss, night sweats) and has a negative chest x-ray. Therefore, he has latent TB infection and is not contagious. Only patients with active TB disease (has signs/symptoms) must be reported to the state public health department.

551. D) Scopolamine patch (Transderm Scop) Scopolamine patch (Transderm Scop) is a prescription medicine that is used for motion/sea sickness. It is a small, circular patch that is placed behind the ear and is effective for 3 days. Advise the patient to apply it 4 hours before the trip to be effective. Because the question is asking about a "prescribed" medication, an over-the-counter (OTC) medicine, such as Dramamine, is an incorrect response. Zofran is indicated for cancer-related nausea and vomiting (chemotherapy, radiation, surgery).

552. **A) *Mal ojo* or *mal de ojo*** *Mal ojo* or *mal de ojo* is a spiritual illness that can cause symptoms such as loss of appetite, crying, diarrhea, colic, fear, weakness, or death. A *curandero* or *curandera* is usually consulted and does spiritual cleansing of the patient. It may take several cleansings (*limpia*) to cure the patient. *Trabajo* means "work" and *malo* means "bad" in Spanish; these are included as distractors.

553. **B) Assess the patient for respiratory distress** Assess the patient for respiratory distress as soon as possible. Follow the "ABCs" and assess the patient for any life-threatening symptoms. Smoke inhalation lung injury is the main cause of death in thermal burn victims.

554. **C) Triazolam (Halcion)** Triazolam (Halcion) has an average half-life of about 2 hours. Alprazolam (Xanax) has a half-life of 12 hours. Lorazepam (Ativan) has a half-life of 15 hours. Clonazepam (Klonopin) has a half-life of 34 hours.

555. **C) Plasma cells** Myeloma is a cancer of the plasma cells (or mature B-cells/ lymphocytes) that affects the bone marrow. Plasma cells produce antibodies and reside mainly in the bone marrow. Signs and symptoms are bone pain, fractures, hypercalcemia, depressed immunity, and anemia. The bone marrow produces white blood cells (neutrophils, lymphocytes, eosinophils, basophils), red blood cells, and platelets. The typical patient is an adult who is age 60 years or older.

556. **C) Continue ipratropium bromide (Atrovent) and add two inhalations of an albuterol (Ventolin) inhaler QID** Treatment of chronic obstructive pulmonary disease (COPD) starts with an anticholinergic (ipratropium bromide [Atrovent]). The next step is to add a short-acting beta-2 agonist (albuterol [Ventolin]).

557. **C) Inform the co-worker that you cannot release any information about this patient because the co-worker is not directly involved in the patient's care** Releasing any information about this patient to a co-worker who is not directly involved in the patient's care would violate the HIPAA privacy rules.

558. **A) IgE-mediated reaction** Anaphylaxis is an immunoglobulin E (IgE)-mediated reaction (also known as *IgE-mediated type 2*). IgE immediate reactions, such as anaphylaxis, trigger mast cell degranulation and release of potent mediators, such as histamines, leukotrienes, and prostaglandins, that immediately induce constriction of smooth muscle, swelling, vasodilation, and other pathological changes in the body that may be fatal.

559. **C) Polymyalgia rheumatica (PMR)** PMR is a rheumatic condition that involves joints and arteries. It is associated with a high risk of giant cell arteritis (GCA) or temporal arteritis (15%–30%). The new onset of vision loss and the location of the pain (neck, both shoulders/hips) are the most important clues. Temporal arteritis can cause permanent blindness. Patients with PMR have a very high (40–100 mm/hr) sedimentation rate. Almost all will have elevated C-reactive protein levels (up to 99%). These patients are managed by rheumatologists by means of long-term steroids.

560. **B) Protecting the rights of the human subjects who participate in research done at the institution** Every research institution has an institutional review board (IRB) whose

job is to review all the research that is conducted in that institution. The IRB's most important role is to protect the rights of the human subjects who participate in research done at the institution of which the IRB is a part (e.g., research hospitals, universities).

561. C) Peripheral arterial disease The ankle–brachial index (ABI) is a test that is used to stratify the severity of arterial blockage in the lower extremities for patients with peripheral arterial disease (PAD). An ABI score of 1.0 to 1.4 is normal. Any value less than 1.0 is abnormal. A score of 0.5 or less is indicative of severe PAD.

562. D) Oral prednisone (Medrol Dose Pack) Symptomatic treatments for a viral upper respiratory infection are saline nasal sprays (e.g., Ocean spray), decongestants (e.g., pseudoephedrine), nonsteroidal anti-inflammatory drugs (NSAIDs; e.g., ibuprofen), increased fluid intake, and alternative herbal remedies (Echinacea, astragalus, elderberry syrup, high doses of vitamin C).

563. A) Rice cereal Patients can eat any food except those that contain the protein gluten. Foods containing wheat, barley, and rye should be avoided.

564. A) Minor surgery in a walk-in surgical center Medicare Part A will pay for medically necessary inpatient care and supplies. Therefore, any type of surgery that is done in outpatient settings, such as a walk-in surgical center, will not be reimbursed. If plastic surgery is medically necessary (e.g., plastic surgery to repair facial damage from a burn), then it will be reimbursed. Costs for organ transplantation, such as kidney transplants, are reimbursed.

565. D) Clean the wound with soap and water and prescribe amoxicillin–clavulanate (Augmentin) 500 mg PO BID × 10 days Cat bites are more likely to become infected than dog bites, and this bite is located on an extremity. These facts justify the prescription of Augmentin 500 mg PO BID × 10 days for the patient. Because the last tetanus booster was given at age 13 years, it has only been 4 years since the patient's last tetanus booster. This incident falls within the 5-year time period in which the previous booster would offer protection; hence there is no need for a tetanus booster at this visit.

566. A) Small, smooth testicles with no pubic or facial hair Small, smooth testicles with no pubic or facial hair (Tanner stage I) is a worrisome finding at the age of 14 years because it signifies that the boy is not in the pubertal stage yet. The average age of onset of puberty among boys is 12 years (range, 10–14 years). The maximum growth spurt in boys occurs about 2 years after the onset of puberty. Boys start about 1 year later than girls and continue to grow until their early 20s (college).

567. C) Hemoglobin electrophoresis The gold standard for diagnosis of thalassemia (or sickle cell anemia) is the hemoglobin electrophoresis.

568. B) Meclizine (Antivert) The case is describing vertigo. Meclizine (Antivert) 12.5 mg to 50 mg TID to QID is used to treat vertigo. Do not forget to also treat nausea, which can be severe. Antinausea medicines, such as dimenhydrinate (Dramamine) or prochlorperazine (Compazine), are effective. Advise the patient that these drugs can cause drowsiness.

569. **C) It is a progesterone-only method of birth control and does not contain estrogen** Seasonale is an extended-cycle form of birth control. It contains both levonorgestrel and ethinyl estradiol. There are 84 pink tablets (active) and seven white pills (inert). In general, more spotting (breakthrough bleeding) is experienced with extended-cycle pills during the first few months of use (compared with the monthly birth control pills).

570. **C) Polymyalgia rheumatica (PMR)** Giant cell arteritis (also known as *temporal arteritis*) is more common among patients with PMR. It can cause permanent blindness if it is not treated. PMR patients are taught how to recognize it. The quick onset of vision loss in one eye, accompanied by a tender indurated artery and scalp tenderness on the same side, are classic symptoms. Patients are screened using the erythrocyte sedimentation rate (ESR) and C-reactive protein (CRP) test. Both will be markedly elevated.

571. **C) Body areas where skin rubs together, such as under breasts or in groin area** Candidal intertrigo infections are more common in obese individuals and in women with pendulous breasts. It is found in areas where skin rubs against skin (under breasts, in the groin area, and on stomach folds in the obese). It is more common in warm and humid weather (summer).

572. **D) Perform 10 exercises each time three times a day** Weak pelvic floor muscles increase the risk of urinary and fecal incontinence. Educate a female patient that the pelvic floor muscles are the ones that she uses when she consciously holds/stops the flow of urine when she urinates. Warn her that the anal sphincter will also tighten with the vaginal muscles. Advise the patient to relax the abdomen and the thighs when doing the exercises. Kegel exercises are also recommended as conservative treatment for patients (male and female) with fecal incontinence.

573. **C) The ovaries are sensitive to deep palpation but they should not be painful** The ovaries are usually slightly sensitive to deep palpation, but they should not be painful. Unilateral adnexal pain accompanied by cervical motion tenderness and purulent endocervical discharge is suggestive of pelvic inflammatory disease (PID).

574. **D) Surgical procedures are regarded as important treatment for many illnesses** Some Asian cultures regard surgery as a last resort and consider loss of blood as depleting the vital forces of the body and causing illness. Western medicine is considered to be "hot," and patients may discontinue or reduce the doses of their medicine without asking. An imbalance of the hot and cold (yin/yang) is believed to cause illness. Treating a "yin" disease (common cold) means avoiding eating yin foods (melons, cucumbers) because they will worsen it. Instead, yin diseases are treated with yang foods (meat, spicy foods) so that the body becomes more balanced.

575. **D) Tdap** The Centers for Disease Control and Prevention (CDC) recommends that one of the tetanus boosters be replaced with the Tdap (once in a lifetime). Thereafter, the Td form of the vaccine is indicated every 10 years. The DTaP (diphtheria–tetanus–acellular pertussis) and DT (diphtheria–tetanus) forms of the tetanus vaccine are not given after the age of 7 years. Puncture wounds are at higher risk for tetanus because *Clostridium*

tetani bacteria are anaerobes (deep puncture wounds are not exposed to air compared with superficial wounds).

576. D) Tinea versicolor Acanthosis nigricans is a benign skin condition that is a sign of insulin resistance. It appears as hyperpigmented velvety areas that are usually located on the neck and the axillae. It is rarely associated with some types of adenocarcinoma of the gastrointestinal tract. Tinea versicolor is a superficial infection of the skin (stratum corneum layer) that is caused by dermatophytes (fungi) of the tinea family. Another name for it is *sunspots*.

577. C) Antinuclear antibody (ANA) The ANA test is usually positive in lupus patients. Other types of autoantibody testing recommended for these patients, in addition to ANA tests, are antiphospholipid antibodies, antibodies to double-stranded DNA, and anti-Smith (Sm) antibodies. Patients with suspected lupus should be referred to a rheumatologist. The erythrocyte sedimentation rate (ESR) and the C-reactive protein (CRP) are nonspecific findings of inflammation and are elevated in patients with autoimmune diseases, infections, and others.

578. A) Educate the patient about hypertension, how the medicine works on his body, and the importance of taking his pill daily When Hmong (an ethnic group prevalent in Thailand, Myanmar, Laos, and Vietnam) see a medical doctor for a symptom, they expect to be treated and "cured" of their illness after one visit. When the symptoms disappear, many will stop taking the medicine. When medication is to be taken on a long-term basis, it is important to educate the patient (and the patient's family) about the disease (in this case, hypertension), how the medicine works on the body, and the reason why the patient has to take the medicine as prescribed (in this case, daily). Many Southeast Asians are very polite and consider speaking in a loud voice, staring, or confrontation to be rude behavior.

579. B) Oral prednisone Patients with polymyalgia rheumatica (PMR) are treated with oral corticosteroids such as prednisone. . One of the hallmarks of the disorder is the dramatic improvement of symptoms after starting treatment with oral prednisone. Usually, the symptoms can be controlled with long-term (2–3 years) low-dose oral prednisone, which can be tapered when symptoms are under control. For most patients, PMR is a self-limiting illness (from a few months to 3 years).

580. D) After a drug is taken by the oral route, it is absorbed in the small intestines and enters the liver through the portal circulation, where it is metabolized before being released into the general circulation First-pass metabolism (first-pass effect) determines how much of the active drug is available to the body (bioavailability). Depending on the drug and other factors, a drug may be poorly metabolized or extensively metabolized by the liver.

581. C) A bluish discoloration or bruising that is located on the umbilical area Cullen's sign is the acute onset of bluish discoloration that is located on the umbilical/periumbilical area, caused by bruising underneath the skin. A bluish discoloration located on the flank area is called the *Grey–Turner's sign*. It is a sign of a severe case of pancreatitis.

582. **B) Osteoarthritis** Glucosamine sulfate has been found to have a beneficial effect on cartilage growth and repair. It may also have an anti-inflammatory effect. Many patients with OA who take it claim that it helps to relieve joint pain. Effects may not be felt for 1 to 3 months after starting the medicine. Glucosamine is a compound made up of glucose and an amino acid.

583. **A) Primary prevention** A community youth center with good staffing can be an effective method of drawing the children out of the streets into a safer environment. It can reduce the risk of children becoming victims of gang violence. In addition, staff members can serve as role models or mentors for the older children.

584. **B) Tuberculosis** The bacillus Calmette-Guérin (BCG) vaccine is given routinely in some countries where tuberculosis (TB) is endemic (or epidemic). One of the few exceptions for the BCG vaccine in the United States is for health care workers, who see a high percentage of patients infected with *Mycobacterium tuberculosis* strains resistant to both isoniazid and rifampin. BCG is considered a biohazardous material (U.S. black box warning) and proper handling and disposal must be followed.

585. **D) Report the child abuse to the department of child protective services** There are several "helping" professions (nurses, teachers, mental health) that are required to report suspected or actual child/elderly abuse to authorities. The nurse practitioner is legally required to report the case to child protective services (CPS). If the child is in danger, CPS may ask for a court order to take the child away for protection until the investigation is completed. Talking about the boyfriend's behavior will not be effective and may put the child and/or mother in danger if the boyfriend suspects that he is being watched.

586. **B) Instruct the patient to lift her head off the table while tensing her abdominal muscles to visualize any masses and then palpate the abdominal wall** An abdominal wall mass will become more prominent when the abdominal wall muscles are tense. If it is an intra-abdominal mass, it will be pressed down by the muscles and will become less obvious or disappear. Some of the most common abdominal wall masses are hernias (epigastric, umbilical, incisional). This patient has a periumbilical hernia (soft lump on her abdomen that is located on the periumbilical area that is painless).

587. **C) Cones** Rods and cones are photoreceptor cells of the retina. The cones of the eyes are responsible for color vision. Cones are very sensitive to colors (red, blue, or green) and work better in brighter light. Rods are good for night vision and for vision in low-light conditions because they are sensitive to light and dark. To remember them, note that both cone and color start with the letters "co."

588. **B) B_{12}-deficiency anemia** Intrinsic factor is made by the parietal cells, which are located on the fundus of the stomach. Intrinsic factor is needed to effectively absorb vitamin B_{12} (found in dairy and meat). Because the gastric fundus is damaged in patients who have undergone gastrectomy, they are at higher risk of B_{12}-deficiency anemia (mean corpuscular volume [MCV] >100).

589. **D) Actinic keratosis** The precursor lesion of squamous cell skin cancer is actinic keratosis. It is caused by chronic sun exposure and is usually found on areas of the body exposed to the sun such as the face, ears, and the dorsum of the arms. Regarding

mortality, the skin cancer that causes the most deaths (from skin cancer) is melanoma (65% of skin cancer deaths).

590. **B) It is the middle number in a group of numbers** The median is the middle value in a given set of numbers (arranged from lowest to highest). For example, for a group of numbers that consists of 2, 3, 6, 7, 7, 8, and 10, the number "7" is the median value.

591. **B) Using limited societal financial resources on programs that will positively affect the largest number of people and have the lowest possible negative outcomes** Generally, the utilitarian principle refers to societal programs that will affect or benefit the largest number of people in a positive manner. It is not used to refer to an individual or to one person.

592. **D) Oral temperature >101°F (>38°C)** Pelvic inflammatory disease (PID) is a clinical diagnosis. The presence of at least one of the major criteria (cervical motion tenderness, adnexal tenderness, uterine tenderness) when combined with the history is highly suggestive of PID. Minor criteria are not necessary, but they help to support the diagnosis of PID (oral temperature >101°F [>38°C]), mucopurulent cervical or vaginal discharge, elevated sedimentation rate, elevated C-reactive protein, large amount of WBCs on saline microscopy of the vaginal fluid, or laboratory documentation of cervical infection with *Neisseria gonorrhoeae* or *Chlamydia trachomatis*).

593. **D) Fovea of the macula** The fovea is located in the center of the macula and is responsible for the sharpest vision ("20/20 vision") in the eyes. In the fovea, the only receptors are the cones, which allow us to see in color and in detail. The macula is responsible for central vision.

594. **B) Consultative relationship** A consultative relationship involves an informal process between two or more providers who exchange information about a patient occasionally.

595. **B) Secondary prevention** The nurse practitioner is evaluating the teenager for major depression. Secondary prevention includes detecting disease at an early stage to halt or slow its progress. All screening tests and lab tests (e.g., mammography, Pap smears) are secondary prevention activities.

596. **C) Hypertension** Drugs with strong anticholinergic properties include diphenhydramine, scopolamine, tricyclic antidepressants (TCAs), and antipsychotics, among others. The mnemonic for anticholinergic overdose signs/symptoms is "dry as a bone, red as a beet, mad as a hatter, blind as a bat." Look for flushing, fever, urinary retention, delirium/hallucinations, and mydriasis (pupillary dilation).

597. **B) Diastolic murmur** Diastolic murmurs are more likely to be pathological. The heart is displaced in a more transverse position that is lateral to the midclavicular line. The systolic ejection murmur is due to increased stroke volume caused by increased cardiac output and higher basal heart rate.

598. **A) Abdominal aortic aneurysm** Elderly males who are ex-smokers are at higher risk for abdominal aortic aneurysm. The aneurysm is usually asymptomatic and is discovered incidentally during a routine chest x-ray or abdominal ultrasound. Although small aneurysms are usually not detectable during abdominal exams, the larger aneurysms

may be palpable during an abdominal exam, but abdominal obesity will obscure the findings. The symptoms in this case point toward a rapidly dissecting aneurysm. The best action is to call 911 *stat*.

599. **D) A filled-in circle** A filled-in circle indicates a diseased or affected female and an empty circle indicates a healthy female. A tip to remember is that females make eggs (or follicles), which resemble a circle. By default, the square symbol is the male.

600. **B) Magnetic resonance imaging (MRI) scan** MRIs provide good visualization of soft tissues of the body (most cancers, brain, cartilage, muscles, inflammation, etc.). They are best used to evaluate tissues with high water content. Patients with metal implants, such as cochlear implants and cardiac pacemakers, should be carefully screened. The MRI does not use radiation, but uses strong magnetic and radio waves to visualize body structures.

601. **C) Information that a research subject can voluntarily withdraw from the study at any time without any penalties or adverse consequences** It should be written on the consent forms that the research subject can voluntarily withdraw from the study at any time without any penalties or adverse consequences. In addition, the human subject should be verbally informed of this right.

602. **C) Obesity** Obesity is not a risk factor for bone loss. But being female, older age, in menopause, having a small thin frame, being of Caucasian or Asian race, family history of osteoporosis, excessive alcohol use, and long-term cigarette smoking are risk factors.

603. **D) Provision of custodial care** Custodial care is provided by nursing homes. SNFs are reimbursed by Medicare and can provide skilled nursing and medical care. If a patient is discharged from a hospital, but needs therapy and skilled care, he or she is usually transferred to an SNF. SNFs have transfer agreements with local hospitals. Nursing home patients are usually medically stable and need skilled or medical care. These patients are unable to perform from two to six activities of daily living (ADL). Patients with Alzheimer's and other types of dementia are usually cared for in nursing homes.

604. **D) Grocery shopping** Grocery shopping, housework, and managing one's finances are considered instrumental activities of daily living (IADL).

605. **B) Acute appendicitis** Both the psoas and obturator signs are associated with acute appendicitis. When the appendix becomes inflamed or ruptured, the blood and pus irritate the psoas and/or obturator muscles, which are both located in the retroperitoneal area. Both muscles are hip flexors and assist with hip movement.

606. **C) The elderly are no longer interested in sexuality** Some studies have shown that older adults in their 80s can remain sexually active. By the age of 70 years, about 80% of males have erectile dysfunction.

607. **A) Selective serotonin reuptake inhibitors (SSRIs)** A common side effect of SSRIs (e.g., fluoxetine [Prozac], paroxetine [Paxil], sertraline [Zoloft], others) is sexual

dysfunction in males. For depressed males, atypical antidepressants, such as bupropion (Wellbutrin), cause less sexual dysfunction.

608. C) Finasteride (Proscar) Finasteride (Proscar) belongs to the drug class called *5-alpha reductase inhibitors*. It helps to lower serum testosterone, which helps to decrease the size of the prostate. It is also used for male-pattern baldness. A smaller prostate results in less obstructive voiding symptoms such as weak stream, frequency, and nocturia. Both terazosin (Hytrin) and tamsulosin (Flomax) are alpha-blockers and may start to control symptoms in as little as 3 days. They work by relaxing the smooth muscle tissue of the prostate gland, which enlarges the diameter of the urethra.

609. C) 5-year-olds By 5 years of age, a child can draw a stick person with six body parts, can copy a triangle, can print some letters and numbers, and can count to 10 or more.

610. C) 12 months By the age of 12 months, an infant is expected to have tripled its birth weight. At 6 months, the infant has doubled his or her birth weight. Birth weight is regained by the second week of life (14 days).

611. A) Acute pancreatitis Grey–Turner's sign is the acute onset of bluish discoloration located on the flank area that is caused by bruising. It is usually associated with severe acute pancreatitis, but it can also be found in some cases of ruptured ectopic pregnancy.

612. B) Collaborative relationship A collaborative relationship is a formal process of sharing responsibility for treating a patient together (sharing progress reports); for example, referring a patient to a specialist or for rehabilitation.

613. A) *Pseudomonas aeruginosa* The most common bacterium is *Pseudomonas*. The second most common bacterium is *Staphylococcus aureus*. Polymyxin and neomycin combination ear drops (Cortisporin) are the first-line treatment for otitis externa. Other ear drops that are also effective are the quinolone ear drops (ofloxacin, ciprofloxacin topical drops).

614. B) The health plan ensures that all Americans have health insurance coverage The national health insurance plan officially known as the Patient Protection and Affordable Care Act, and unofficially nicknamed *Obamacare*, was enacted in March 2010 with the goal of expanding health insurance for the millions of Americans who were uninsured. It prohibits an insurance company from rejecting people with preexisting health conditions. There is also a penalty for employers (and individuals) who choose not to participate in the national health plan. Although increased numbers of Americans gained insurance as a result of the law's passage, many millions more still lack coverage.

615. C) Grooming and hygiene Grooming and hygiene are classified as basic activities of daily living (ADL). Grocery shopping, paying bills, using telephones, and driving a car are all instrumental activities of daily living (IADL).

616. C) CN VIII The Rinne and Weber tests are used to assess cranial nerve VIII (acoustic nerve). The patient's hearing is tested by air conduction (Rinne and Weber) and bone conduction (Rinne only).

617. D) Stress incontinence The signs and symptoms of stress incontinence occur when the increased abdominal pressure caused by sneezing, laughing, and/or straining results in the leaking of a small amount of urine through a weakened sphincter. It is more common in younger women (45–49 years old). The urethra and bladder neck fail to close completely due to loss of connective tissue support.

618. **B) Prescription drugs** Medicare Part D is a voluntary program that charges a premium. Like all Medicare services, patients need to enroll during the "open enrollment" periods during the year (there is a penalty for late enrollment). There is a drug formulary and not all drugs are available or reimbursed. Use of generic drugs is preferred, as there is a spending limit. Medicare Part B will reimburse for alcohol misuse/abuse treatment.

619. **A) Check the thyroid profile** The upper limit of the serum thyroid-stimulating hormone (TSH) level is about 4.0 mU/L. With an elevated TSH of 10, it is important to rule out hypothyroidism. The next step in this patient's evaluation is to order a thyroid profile or thyroid panel test. Serum assays measure bound and unbound (free) forms of thyroxine (T4) and triiodothyronine (T3). Classic findings of hypothyroidism are a low free T4, low T3-resin uptake (THBI), and low free T4 index.

620. **C) Abdominal ultrasound** The ultrasound or sonogram is used as an initial imaging test for abdominal tumors and other types of masses. A CT scan is not considered an initial imaging test in the primary care area. But in many emergency departments, it is used as the initial imaging test in certain cases of abdominal trauma, suspected appendicitis, and other conditions.

621. **A) Fragile X disorder** Fragile X syndrome is the most common form of inherited intellectual disability. The disorder is associated with a higher incidence of autism (especially boys). Males are affected more severely than females. The facial features can vary. The classic facie is long and narrow with a prominent forehead and chin and large ears. Other features include hyperlaxity of the joints, flat feet, high arched palate, and others. Definitive diagnosis is by genetic testing.

622. **B) Tuberculosis** This is a radiograph of a lung infected by *Mycobacterium tuberculosis*, the causative agent in tuberculosis (TB). The upper lobe is the most common location of a TB infection of the lungs. The typical findings are cavitation (round black holes due to local loss of lung tissue), fibrosis, lymphadenopathy, and calcifications.

623. **D) Upper lobes** The upper lobes are the most common location of a tuberculosis infection of the lungs. The typical findings are cavitation (round black holes due to local loss of lung tissue), fibrosis, lymphadenopathy, and calcifications.

624. **D) Pap smear** The U.S. Preventive Services Task Force (USPSTF; 2012) does not recommend Pap smears (cytology) in women younger than 21 years of age because cervical cancer is rare before this age. A history of sexual intercourse or multiple sex partners is not considered to be an indication for a Pap smear in this age group. There is evidence that screening earlier than age 21 years, regardless of sexual history, would lead to more harm than benefit (USPSTF, 2012). Instead, testing for sexually transmitted disease/infection is the best choice for this age group. The USPSTF recommends screening for cervical cancer in women aged 21 to 65 years with cytology (Pap smear) every 3 years.

Another option for women aged 30 to 65 years who want to lengthen the screening interval is a combination of cytology with HPV testing (cotesting) every 5 years.

625. **C) Serum interferon-gamma release assay (IGRA)** The preferred method of testing for tuberculosis (TB) infection in persons who have received the bacillus Calmette-Guérin (BCG) vaccine in the past was a TB blood test—the interferon-gamma release assay—such as the QuantiFERON-TB Gold (Centers for Disease Control and Prevention, 2016). Unlike the TB skin tests (purified protein derivative [PPD], Mantoux), the blood tests are not affected by prior BCG vaccination.

626. **B) Heart failure patients** Thiazolidinediones (TZD) cause fluid retention and can cause or exacerbate heart failure in some patients. They are contraindicated in patients with New York Heart Association Class III or VI heart failure. After initiating a TZD, watch patients for signs and symptoms of heart failure (rapid weight gain, dyspnea, and/or edema).

627. **C) Low-dose computed tomography (LDCT)** The U.S. Preventive Services Task Force recommends annual screening for lung cancer with low-dose computed tomography in adults aged 55 to 80 years who have a 30-pack-year smoking history and currently smoke (or quit within the past 15 years). Discontinue screening once a person has not smoked for 15 years or develops a health problem that substantially limits life expectancy or willingness to have curative lung surgery.

628. **B) A1C of 5.9%** Do not confuse the criteria for diabetes with those for prediabetes. For prediabetes, look for an A1C between 5.7% to 6.4%, fasting plasma glucose (FPG) of 100 to 125 mg/dL, and/or 75-g oral glucose tolerance test (OGTT) 2-hour postprandial glucose of 140 to 199 mg/dL. To diagnose diabetes, look for random blood glucose ≥200 mg/dL with polyuria, polydipsia, and polyphagia, or A1C ≥6.5%, FPG of ≥126 mg/dL, or 2-hour OGTT ≥200 mg/dL (American Diabetes Association, 2016).

629. **A) Selective serotonin reuptake inhibitors (SSRIs)** First-line drug treatment for posttraumatic stress disorder (PTSD) is SSRIs. The Food and Drug Administration has approved sertraline (Zoloft) and paroxetine (Paxil) for PTSD.

630. **A) It is caused by an arteriole crossing a venule, which compresses the venule and causes it to bulge on each side** AV nicking is one of the most common eye findings found in hypertensive retinopathy.

631. **A) Vitamin D drops** According to the American Academy of Pediatrics (APA), all infants should be given vitamin D supplementation within the first few days of life. Mothers who plan to breastfeed their infants should be taught how to use vitamin D drops. Infant formula is supplemented with vitamin D (and many other vitamins, minerals, and omega-3 oil), so there is no need to give it separately.

632. **B) Tanner stage** The stem of the question is asking for the important areas to evaluate in this patient "during this visit." This is a priority-type question. The priorities to evaluate in this patient are depression, sexually transmitted disease (STD) testing, and sexual history. The Tanner staging does not have to be done "during this visit."

633. **B) Roseola infantum (exanthema subitum)** Roseola infantum is a common viral rash that is caused by the human herpesvirus. The most common ages of onset are between 6 months and 2 years. The rashes are maculopapular (small round pink-colored) rashes that first appear on the trunk and then spread to the extremities.

634. **C) The testicles become larger and the skin of the scrotum starts to become darker with straight, fine, countable hairs on the genitals and the axilla** Tanner stage II is when the testicles start to grow. The scrotal skin becomes thicker and starts to get darker (hyperpigmentation). The pubic hair is of a fine texture and straight and there are few countable hairs on the genitals and the axilla.

635. **B) Hand, foot, and mouth disease (HFMD)** HFMD is caused by the coxsackievirus. The virus is found in the saliva, sputum, nasal mucus, feces, and blister fluid. It is transmitted through direct contact of the secretion or in fomites (e.g., preschool toys). Treatment is symptomatic.

636. **C) Identity versus role confusion** Adolescents (aged 12–18 years) are in the stage known as *identity versus role confusion*. At this time, the teen is transitioning into adulthood and reexamining his or her identity and beliefs. The teen wonders about himself or herself (e.g., "who am I?"). Peers are highly valued.

637. **D) 5 to 6 years of age** At about the age of 5 to 6 years, most children can ride a bicycle with training wheels. Helmets should always be worn (primary prevention).

638. **A) Ultrasound of the sacrum** An infant with tufts of fine dark hair on the sacrum should be evaluated for occult spina bifida. The first imaging test to order is an ultrasound of the lower spine.

639. **B) The CDC does not recommend the HPV vaccine for males** The HPV vaccine is now recommended for both males and females. If it is given before age 14 years, only two doses are required, But if the child is older than 14 years, three doses are required to be given over 6 months. The vaccine can be given until the age of 26 years, especially if the individual is at high risk. Do not use the vaccine in children younger than 9 years. There are two types of HPV vaccine (Gardasil and Cervarix). Gardasil can be used for both genders, but Cervarix can only be used for females.

640. **D) Depressed affect** Depression is not included in the criteria for diagnosing autistic spectrum disorders. Signs and symptoms include avoidance of eye contact and social interaction, marked delay or absence of verbal communication, repetitive movements, fixed rituals, and so on. Autism can range from mild to severe. Early diagnosis is important. For evaluation, refer the patient for psychological testing by a psychologist who specializes in autistic spectrum disorders.

641. **A) Write a prescription for the same PPI and give a 1-week supply without refills** This patient is having severe rebound symptoms caused by abrupt cessation of the proton-pump inhibitor (PPI). In addition, he has Barrett's esophagus, which increases the risk of esophageal cancer. Neither an antacid nor an H2 blocker is likely to be effective in controlling his symptoms. This question is a good example of the ethical concept of beneficence.

642. **D) Aortic stenosis** The murmur of aortic stenosis occurs during systole (S1). The aortic area is in the second intercostal space to the right side of the sternum. The murmur can radiate to the right side of the neck if it is severe.

643. **A) Acute lymphoblastic leukemia** Acute lymphoblastic leukemia, a malignancy of the bone marrow, accounts for 34% of all cancers in children. It is more common in boys, and in children between the ages of 2 and 4 years. Aplastic anemia is bone marrow suppression (not cancer) usually caused by medications or a viral infection. Multiple myeloma and non-Hodgkin's lymphoma are more common in older adults.

644. **D) Round olive-like mass located in the right upper quadrant of the abdomen** The stem is asking about the "possible cause of the infant's vomiting" (it is not asking about symptoms). Projectile or forceful vomiting after feeding (postprandial vomiting) is a classic symptom of infantile hypertrophic pyloric stenosis. A hypertrophied pylorus is a pathognomonic finding of the disease. An ultrasound of the pylorus is the imaging study of choice. The other signs and symptoms are dehydration (sunken anterior fontanel, dry lips, weight loss), irritability, and crying (usually due to hunger). A positive rooting reflex is a normal finding in a 4-week-old infant.

645. **B) HIV infection** HIV is the most powerful known risk factor for the development of active tuberculosis (TB). All HIV-infected persons should receive TB testing. People living with HIV are 20 to 30 times more likely to develop TB than those without HIV. Treatment of HIV-infected persons with latent TB infection (LTBI) is a high priority.

646. **C) Color blindness** The Ishihara chart (or Ishihara Color Test) is used to evaluate color blindness and can be used in patients ranging from school-aged children to adults. It displays colored numbers with different colored dots in the background. A pediatric color vision test for preschool children (3–6 years of age) uses shapes instead of numbers.

647. **A) At the height of the symphysis pubis** The uterus at 12 weeks is approximately the size of a grapefruit. Between 12 and 16 weeks, the uterus will rise above the symphysis pubis, and at 24 weeks is at the level of the umbilicus. Between 16 and 36 weeks, the fundal height in centimeters roughly equals the number of weeks of gestation.

648. **C) Paroxetine (Paxil)** Paroxetine (Paxil) is a selective serotonin reuptake inhibitor (SSRI) that causes sexual adverse effects (impotence, inability to reach orgasm) in up to 50% of men who take it. Of all the SSRIs, it seems to be the one with the highest risk of erectile dysfunction. It can also affect a woman's ability to achieve orgasm. The other medications have a lower incidence of adverse sexual effects. Lamotrigine (Lamictal) is an anticonvulsant, clonazepam (Klonopin) is a benzodiazepine, and doxepin (Sinequan) is a tricyclic antidepressant.

649. **B) Bone pain** Rhabdomyolysis is the rapid breakdown of skeletal muscle; it releases large amounts of myoglobin, which is toxic to the kidneys. It can result in acute kidney injury or acute renal failure. There are many causes such as severe exercise, traumatic crush injuries, medicines (statins, fibrates especially if combined), illicit drugs, and others. The signs and symptoms of rhabdomyolysis are muscle pain (shoulders, thighs, calves, lower back), muscle weakness, dark-red or brown urine, fever, tachycardia, and/or decreased urination. Almost half of patients report no muscular symptoms.

650. **C) Anterior epistaxis** Trauma to the small blood vessels in Kiesselbach's triangle (or plexus), located inside the nose anteriorly, causes anterior nosebleeds (anterior epistaxis). This is the most common type of nosebleed and is usually self-limited. Up to 10% of nosebleeds are posterior nosebleeds (hemoptysis, melena, nausea, anemia), which can result in hemorrhage. Posterior nosebleeds can cause significant hemorrhage. If suspected, call 911. Trauma to Kiesselbach's triangle does not cause stroke or subdural hematoma.

651. **C) Basal cell carcinoma** Basal cell carcinoma is caused by chronic ultraviolet (UV) skin damage (i.e., by sunlight), not human papillomavirus (HPV) infection. It is the most common type of skin cancer. HPV infection increases the risk of precancer and cancer of the oropharynx/larynx, anus, penis, and cervix.

652. **B) Bisphosphonates** A T-score of –2.8 means that the patient has osteoporosis. Bisphosphonates are considered the first-line treatment for osteoporosis. They include alendronate (Fosamax), risedronate (Actonel), ibandronate (Boniva), and others with chemical names that end in "–dronate." Dual-energy x-ray absorptiometry (DEXA) scores are reported as either T-scores or Z-scores, but T-scores are more commonly used. A T-score of –1 or higher is normal. A T-score between –1 and –2.5 indicates osteopenia. A T-score of –2.5 or lower indicates osteoporosis.

653. **A) Fifth disease** Fifth disease (erythema infectiosum) is caused by infection with the human parvovirus. It is spread by aerosolized droplets (cough, sneeze). The most commonly affected age group is children and adolescents between the ages of 5 and 15 years. Symptoms may take 1 to 3 weeks to resolve. There are three stages: The first stage is characterized by a bright-red rash on the cheeks/face with slight fever and coldlike symptoms (coryza); the second stage by a generalized rash that appears lacelike; and in the third stage the rash disappears but reoccurs when the child is exposed to sunlight, heat, or exercise. Treatment is symptomatic.

654. **D) Rhinovirus** Infection with rhinovirus causes the common cold and is not associated with serious sequelae in pregnant women or their fetuses. Infection during pregnancy with human parvovirus B19 can cause severe fetal anemia (hemolysis), fetal hydrops (hydrops fetalis), fetal death, and spontaneous abortions. Most women with B19 infection in pregnancy do not suffer serious sequelae. Congenital rubella infection in early pregnancy causes severe birth defects, fetal demise, miscarriages, and stillbirths. Congenital varicella infection is extremely rare but affects the skin, extremities, and brain, and also causes low birth weight.

655. **C) Albendazole (Albenza)** Albendazole can be given in one dose initially, and then another single dose in 2 weeks (to kill eggs not killed in first treatment). If more than one member of the household is infected, it is recommended that all members be treated at the same time. Emphasis on strict handwashing is important, but it is not a treatment method. Washing clothes and bedsheets is recommended for scabies infections.

656. **B) HPV subtypes 16 and 18** Human papillomavirus (HPV) types 16 and 18 are high-risk oncogenic strains. If an HPV-typing test shows one or both strains, the next step is to refer the patient for colposcopy and biopsy. About 70% of cervical cancers worldwide

are due to types 16 and 18 (Centers for Disease Control and Prevention, 2014). HPV types that are low risk cause warts in the cervix, vagina, vulva, penis, anus, and rectum.

657. **C) Prescribe ophthalmic topical antibiotic eye drops, two to three drops to be applied in each eye QID for 7 days** Treatment for viral keratoconjunctivitis (pink eye) is symptomatic. Cold compresses and slightly chilled artificial tears may help with the itching. Educate the parent and/or child to avoid touching the eyes with hands, avoid sharing towels, to perform frequent handwashing, and use tissues if touching the eyes. Viral keratoconjunctivitis is usually caused by an adenovirus (but other viruses can also cause it). It is contagious for 10 to 12 days after onset of symptoms and is a self-limiting condition. It can be transmitted through swimming pools, fomites, and by hands. Children should not attend school until symptoms resolve.

658. **A) Chadwick's sign** The bluish discoloration of the cervix and vagina, known as Chadwick's sign, is caused by increased blood flow. It is seen between 6 and 8 weeks after conception along with Hegar's sign, which is softening of the uterine isthmus (lower uterine segment). Chadwick's sign is considered one of the probable signs of pregnancy. The S3 heart sound, mild edema of ankles and hands, and increase in urinary frequency are seen in the third trimester, along with low-back pain, striae, and shortness of breath.

659. **D) HMG-CoA reductase inhibitors** The HMG-CoA (hydroxy-methylglutaryl coenzyme A) reductase inhibitors, commonly referred to as *statins*, include simvastatin, atorvastatin, and others. High-dose statins or combining statins with fibrates and/or niacin will increase the risk of rhabdomyolysis and drug-induced hepatitis. Rhabdomyolysis can cause acute renal failure. If this complication is suspected, refer the patient to a physician or the emergency department. Biguanides (metformin), thiazolidinediones (pioglitazone), and tetracyclines (doxycycline) do not cause rhabdomyolysis.

660. **D) Mitral regurgitation** The murmur of mitral regurgitation occurs during systole (holosystolic) and is located in the mitral area of the chest. The location of the mitral area (fifth intercostal space on the left side of the midclavicular line) is near the left axilla, so that a loud murmur can radiate to the left axilla. The causes can be congenital or it may a be sequela of rheumatic fever, mitral valve prolapse, or papillary muscle dysfunction secondary to acute or prior myocardial infarction.

661. **A) Straight leg raising test** The straight leg raising test is used to evaluate for sciatica. Classic findings are mid-buttock burning or sharp pain, which may radiate down the thigh, lower leg, and foot. A severe case of sciatica can result in "foot drop," which is why the patient is complaining of weakness of the foot that interferes with walking. This type of sciatica patient needs to be referred to a neurologist to rule out nerve root compression. Sciatica is a type of lumbar radiculopathy. The imaging test of choice is an MRI of the lower spine. The McMurray test is used to assess meniscus damage of the knees. The Lachman test assesses damage to the anterior cruciate ligament. The Markle test (or heel jar test) is used to assess for pelvic inflammatory disease or peritonitis.

662. **C) Auspitz sign** Auspitz sign is observed when a psoriatic lesion is scraped or scratched multiple times, resulting in pinpoint areas of bleeding on the psoriatic plaque.

Lichenification is thickened skin caused by chronic irritation (itching). It is considered a secondary lesion. Another type of secondary skin lesion is an erosion, which occurs with loss of epidermis (but not the dermis). It can resemble a shallow ulcer. The Koebner phenomenon refers to lesions (often linear) that appear on the skin of patients with psoriasis as a result of trauma to the skin (e.g., scratching).

663. **D) Fibromyalgia** The American College of Rheumatology (2010) uses several criteria to diagnose fibromyalgia: widespread pain index, symptoms present at a similar level for at least 3 months, and presence of pain or tenderness at certain body sites. The locations in the body (widespread pain index) are neck, jaw, shoulder girdle, upper and lower arm, chest, abdomen, upper and lower back, upper and lower leg, and hip (trochanters). Other criteria include fatigue, sleep problems, and cognitive symptoms. The exact cause of fibromyalgia is unknown. Treatment is symptomatic.

664. **B) Sciatica** Sciatica is a radiculopathy of the sciatic nerve, which is part of the sacral nerves of the cauda equina. A radiculopathy is spinal nerve root irritation or inflammation that is caused by compression of one (or more) of the five spinal nerve roots. Some of the most common causes of sciatica are protruding or ruptured disk, osteoarthritis of the spine, and metastases. Radiculopathy symptoms include burning pain or sensation, numbness, tingling, and/or weakness.

665. **C) Trephination by using a large paperclip or 18-gauge needle** A subungual hematoma is bleeding that collects under the nail due to trauma of the big toe. One method of draining the blood is called *nail bed trephination*. To perform this procedure, straighten one end of a large paperclip (or use an 18-gauge needle) and heat up the tip with a flame. Then drill downward on the nail surface until a pinpoint hole appears so that the blood underneath the nail can drain. Press gently on the nail. If not treated, the pressure from the blood underneath the nail can cause permanent damage to the root of the nail, with the result that a toenail cannot grow back again.

666. **A) Histamine-2 receptor antagonist** A histamine-2 receptor antagonist (H2 receptor antagonist) is the initial drug considered in treating a patient with GERD whose symptoms are not responding to lifestyle changes. If a patient's symptoms do not respond to the H2 receptor antagonist, the next step is a trial of a proton-pump inhibitor.

667. **D) Odynophagia and early satiety** Worrisome symptoms in patients with gastroesophageal reflux disease (GERD) include odynophagia, early satiety, weight loss, iron-deficiency anemia, gastrointestinal bleeding, and recurrent vomiting. Symptoms of odynophagia and early satiety in a patient with GERD should prompt a workup to rule out esophageal cancer.

668. **B) Ofloxacin ear drops** Ofloxacin ear drops are not considered to be ototoxic. However, aminoglycoside otic drops (gentamycin, tobramycin) are ototoxic and should not be used to treat otitis media or perforation of the tympanic membrane (TM). In addition, ear drops with alcohol, benzocaine, or olive oil should be avoided in patients with TM perforation. Swimming or water inside the ear should be avoided until the TM is healed. Topical therapy with topical quinolone drops may be equivalent to oral therapy, but some experts prefer oral antibiotic therapy, such as amoxicillin or amoxicillin-clavulanate (Augmentin) for 10 days, to treat TM perforations.

669. D) Rubeola Rubeola, also known as *measles*, is caused the rubeola virus. It is very contagious and is transmitted via droplets like the common cold. Koplik's spots (tiny white spots in buccal mucosa) are present during the prodromal period. The blotchy pink rash is also known as a *morbilliform rash*. Treatment is symptomatic and most people recover in 2 to 3 weeks. Measles outbreaks caused by poor MMR (measles, mumps, rubella) vaccination rates have been reported in some areas of the United States. Do not confuse rubeola with rubella (German measles).

670. B) Grand mal seizure *Grand mal seizure* is the older term for generalized tonic–clonic seizure. It starts with abrupt loss of consciousness and stiffening of the muscles (tonic phase). After about a minute, the muscles start to jerk for 1 to 2 minutes (clonic phase). Cessation of muscle twitching signals the start of the postictal period. During this period, the person may be asleep (and gradually wake up) or may become agitated or confused. Do not insert anything in the mouth such as tongue blades. Help the person lay on the floor on his or her side.

671. A) Medial tibial stress fracture Medial tibial stress fracture and medial tibial stress syndrome (MDSS, or "shin splints") are more common in individuals who participate in sports that involve running and/or jumping (track and field, soccer, basketball). Medial tibial stress fracture is more common in female athletes. It is caused or exacerbated by excessive training, sudden increase in training intensity, or overuse. The symptoms of medial tibial stress fracture can resemble MDSS, but the pain is more persistent and worsens until it also occurs at rest. The physical exam findings reveal a focal area of tenderness on the anterior medial aspect of the tibia. The imaging test of choice is MRI. A radiograph (x-ray) will not show a stress fracture. If a medial tibial stress fracture is suspected, the patient should be advised to stop the sport/activity, use RICE (rest, ice, compression, elevation) to relieve symptoms, and should be referred to an orthopedic specialist.

672. B) Thumb spica cast The scaphoid bone is located on the radial aspect of the wrist (same side as the thumb). Another term for scaphoid fracture is *navicular space fracture of the wrist*. In patients with this injury, palpating in the anatomic snuffbox area reveals local tenderness. A thumb spica cast is used to stabilize fractures of the wrist. It is applied below the elbow (forearm in neutral position) and extends to the hand (wrist and thumb are immobilized). Sometimes, this type of fracture is stabilized with a screw (surgery) because it has a higher rate of nonunion.

673. C) Right middle lobe pneumonia This is a chest radiograph (x-ray) of a patient diagnosed with right middle lobe pneumonia. It shows lobar consolidation. The white opaque area is seen on the right middle lobe. A large part of the right middle lobe is located on the anterior aspect of the chest at breast level, extending to the right axillary area.

674. C) Check serum carcinoembryonic antigen (CEA) and cancer antigen (CA) 125 levels The patient is a woman who is of Ashkenazi Jewish background with a positive family history of breast cancer (mother, sister). She is at very high risk for *BRCA1* or *BRCA2* mutations (hereditary breast cancer). The U.S. Preventive Services Task Force (2013) recommends that primary care providers screen women for a family history of breast, ovarian, tubal, or peritoneal cancer. Women with positive screening results should receive genetic screening, and, if indicated after counseling, *BRCA* testing. These high-risk women are screened with a mammogram and breast MRI and are best managed by breast cancer specialists.

675. **A) Mitral valve prolapse** A systolic murmur that is accompanied by a mid systolic click located at the apical area is a classic finding of mitral valve prolapse (MVP). Most cases of MVP are asymptomatic. To detect MVP, order an echocardiogram with Doppler imaging.

676. **B) Bone conduction (BC) > air conduction (AC)** The sound is heard louder by bone conduction versus air conduction (BC>AC) in serous otitis media and other types of conductive hearing loss. This is because when the affected ear is filled with fluid, the tympanic membrane cannot move in response to the sound waves due to the fluid trapped inside the middle ear. Because the sound waves are blocked, the sound is heard better by bone conduction.

677. **D) Budesonide (Rhinocort) one to two sprays in each nostril twice a day** The first-line treatment for allergic rhinitis is topical glucocorticoid nasal sprays such as budesonide (Rhinocort). It will decrease swelling and open the Eustachian tubes so that the middle ear can drain. The other medications (cetirizine, azelastine, nasal saline) are not considered first-line agents for allergic rhinitis, but they can be added if the symptoms are not well controlled. Azelastine (Astelin) is a topical antihistamine. Cetirizine (Zyrtec) is a second-generation systemic antihistamine. Do not combine it with azelastine (Astelin) because both are antihistamines and taken concurrently will cause excessive drowsiness. Topical nasal steroid sprays, cetirizine, and nasal saline sprays are sold over the counter. But azelastine (Astelin) is available only by prescription.

678. **D) Alprazolam (Xanax)** Alprazolam (Xanax) and other benzodiazepines cause sedation and promote sleep. But selective serotonin reuptake inhibitors (SSRIs), such as sertraline (Zoloft), can cause insomnia in some patients. Other drug classes with stimulating effects are decongestants, such as pseudoephedrine (Sudafed), and methylxanthines such as theophylline (Theo-Dur) and caffeine.

679. **C) Wet smear with microscopy** The best method of diagnosing vaginal trichomonas infection in primary care is by wet smear with microscopy. Trichomonas is a protozoan; it is a unicellular organism with flagella. Place a small amount of vaginal discharge on a glass slide, add a few drops of normal saline, and place the cover slip on top. Do not use potassium hydroxide (KOH) as it will rupture the organisms. Trichomonas can be visualized by microscopy.

680. **D) Acute otitis media** Acute otitis media is more common in children. Macular degeneration, osteoporosis, and Parkinson's disease are more common in the geriatric population.

681. **D) Penicillins** Levothyroxine does not interact with penicillins. But it does have numerous drugs it interacts with such as anticoagulants, tricyclic antidepressants, antacids and calcium, iron, multivitamins, proton-pump inhibitors, estrogens, statins, metformin, and others. Certain foods interfere with absorption (calcium-fortified foods, dietary fiber, walnuts, soy). Patients should avoid taking them together, and should space

these foods and drugs several hours apart. Levothyroxine (Synthroid) is a synthetic form of T4.

682. **A) A "clunk" sound heard while performing the Ortolani maneuver** The "clunk" sound during the Ortolani maneuver is a positive finding and signifies a possible hip abnormality (hip dysplasia) in infants. Refer the infant to a pediatric orthopedist. Infants start to babble at 6 months. At 12 months, babies learn to "cruise" or to hold onto furniture while walking. Some boys and girls may have "growing pains" on both legs (or both thighs, calves, or behind the knees), which are usually felt in the late afternoon, evening, and/or at night. These symptoms should not interfere with the child's ability to play and affect children from age 3 to 12 years. Stretching exercises of the thighs and hamstrings, massaging the area, and warm packs are helpful. If pain affects only one leg or hip, it is abnormal (rule out bone cancer, sarcoma, leukemia, hip abnormalities). In such cases, refer the patient to a pediatric orthopedist.

683. **D) Xanthelasma** Xanthelasma is a benign subcutaneous lesion composed of cholesterol that usually develops around the eyelids (Ghosh & Ghosh, 2017). Approximately 50% of patients with xanthelasma have hyperlipidemia. Order a fasting lipid profile. If the patient desires treatment, the lesions can be removed by laser, application of trichloroacetic acid (TCA), or surgery. *Xerosis cutis* is a medical term for extremely dry skin. Psoriasis lesions can occur on the eyelid area. Use of Elidel cream won't cause glaucoma and is effective on eyelids but may sting the first few days of use. Warts are usually not located on the inner canthus or eyelids bilaterally and are not yellow in color.

684. **A) Osteoarthritis and rheumatoid arthritis** Bouchard's nodes are seen in both osteoarthritis (or degenerative joint disease) and rheumatoid arthritis. They are located on the proximal interphalangeal (PIP) joints on the hands.

685. **D) Claims against the nurse practitioner are covered if both the incident and claim happen when the policy is still active** Therefore, both the incident and the claim have to be filed when the policy is active (during the coverage time period). When the nurse practitioner stops paying the premiums for this type of policy, it is no longer active.

686. **D) Love and belonging** Family and friendships are highly valued. The act of giving gifts to her grandchildren is an expression of love by the grandmother. According to Abraham Maslow, only a very small percentage of people reach the highest level, self-actualization.

687. **D) Transient ischemic attack (TIA)** A TIA is a transient episode of neurologic dysfunction due to focal brain, spinal cord, or retinal ischemia, without acute infarction. Originally, TIA was defined as sudden onset of focal neurologic signs and/or symptoms lasting fewer than 24 hours. Patients with suspected TIA require urgent evaluation due to the high risk of stroke. An MRI of the brain is preferred to a CT of the brain. A search for the cause of the TIA includes conditions such as hypertension, blood clot from the heart, carotid blockage, and so forth. For secondary prevention, aspirin therapy and statin therapy are recommended. Some patients may need antithrombotics. Symptoms of a TIA are the same as a stroke but last only a short time. The mnemonic is "FAST" with F (one side of face is drooping), A (ask patient to raise both arms, does one arm drift downward?), S (slurred speech), and T (time; if present, call 911). These signs are seen in stroke along with change in level of consciousness, confusion or memory loss, difficulty

swallowing, difficulty writing, inability to recognize objects/people, incontinence, and trouble speaking or understanding others.

688. D) Clarithromycin (Biaxin) BID, amoxicillin BID, and omeprazole (Prilosec) daily This combination is known as "triple therapy" for the treatment of peptic ulcer disease caused by the bacterium *Helicobacter pylori*. The original quadruple therapy consists of bismuth subcitrate (Pepto Bismol), metronidazole, and tetracycline with a proton-pump inhibitor (PPI) or H2 blocker. The antibiotics are taken for 14 days with a PPI or an H2 blocker, and then the PPI or H2 blocker is continued for 2 to 4 weeks after. Currently, there are several regimens for treating *H. pylori* infection. To confirm eradication, order a urea breath test or fecal antigen test.

689. A) Calcium channel blockers and thiazide diuretics Calcium channel blockers (CCBs) and thiazide diuretics are preferred for treatment of isolated systolic hypertension of the elderly. There is no preference of one over the other, and therapy may be started with either a thiazide diuretic or a CCB. Isolated systolic hypertension of the elderly is caused by hardening of the arteries, resulting in increased peripheral vascular resistance. The goal for patients aged 60 years or older is blood pressure less than 150/90 mmHg unless diabetic or they have chronic kidney disease (goal BP <140/90 mmHg). Watch for orthostatic hypotension (or decrease in systolic blood pressure of >20 mmHg), which is a risk factor for falls.

690. C) Basal cell carcinoma This is a photograph of basal cell carcinoma, the most common type of skin cancer. Although the lesion does not have central ulceration, it contains telangiectasia with a waxy or pearly (shiny) appearance. The gold-standard diagnosis for any type of skin cancer is a biopsy of the lesion that is sent to the lab for pathological evaluation.

691. A) 1, C) 2, B) 3 HPV strains 16 and 18 are highly oncogenic. This patient has cervical cancer and requires immediate biopsy, excisional treatment, and staging for cervical cancer. The correct order of these actions is: (1) Refer the patient for a colposcopy, (2) obtain cervical biopsy specimens for pathological evaluation, and (3) perform loop electrosurgical excision procedure (LEEP) for removal of cancerous cervical tissue.

692. D) Melanoma This is a photograph of melanoma. Think of the "ABCD" rule for pigmented lesions that are highly suspicious: A (asymmetry), B (irregular borders), C (three or more colors such as black, blue, tan, red, white), and D (diameter >6 mm or >¼ inch).

693. B) Raynaud's phenomenon Raynaud's phenomenon involves an interruption in the blood flow to fingers and toes (sometimes nose and ears), due to spasms in the blood vessels. During a Raynaud's attack, the affected area typically turns white, and, as oxygen fails to reach the extremities, they can turn blue, tingle, or throb painfully, and the affected area may swell. Symptoms may resolve quickly or last for hours. Raynaud's disease is more common in women, is not curable, and it is associated with increased risk of other autoimmune diseases such as rheumatoid arthritis or lupus, but treatment can decrease symptoms. The preferred drug is a calcium channel blocker such as nifedipine (Norvasc) or amlodipine (Procardia).

694. B) Hemoglobin electrophoresis Alpha thalassemia and sickle cell anemia are both conditions that affect the hemoglobin molecule. The gold-standard test for these types of diseases (hemoglobinopathies) is the hemoglobin electrophoresis.

695. B) Musculoskeletal system The musculoskeletal system is not damaged by nonsteroidal anti-inflammatory drugs (NSAIDs). In fact, NSAIDs are used to treat muscle and/or joint pain and inflammation. The systems adversely affected by NSAIDs are the cardiovascular, gastrointestinal, renal, hematological (because aspirin affects platelets), and dermatological (e.g., Stevens–Johnson syndrome).

696. D) Neovascularization Patients with diabetes often develop ophthalmic complications, such as neovascularization, which is the formation of new fragile blood vessels in the retina. Other signs of diabetic retinopathy are dot and blot hemorrhages, microaneurysms, and "cotton wool" spots (soft exudates). In the initial stages of diabetic retinopathy, patients are generally asymptomatic, but in more advanced stages of the disease patients may experience floaters, as well as distortions, blind spots (scotomas) and/or blurred vision. Diabetic retinopathy is the most common cause of blindness in adults. Screening for diabetic retinopathy is recommended for type 2 diabetics at the time of diagnosis. Arteriovenous nicking (AV nicking), copper wire arterioles, and flame hemorrhages are associated with hypertensive retinopathy.

697. D) Macrocytic and normocytic red blood cells Vitamin B_{12}-deficiency adversely affects myelin, leading to neuropathy. The most common cause of B_{12}-deficiency anemia is pernicious anemia. Anemia resulting from vitamin B_{12} or folate deficiency is referred to as *macrocytic* or *megaloblastic* anemia because the red blood cells (RBCs) are larger than normal. Deficiency in folate and B_{12} does not affect the color of RBCs (normochromic). The RBCs have large cytoplasm because folate and B_{12} are necessary for normal DNA synthesis and cytoplasmic maturation. The mean corpuscular volume (MCV) measures the size of the RBCs. An MCV greater than 100 is seen in macrocytic anemias (folate or B_{12}-deficiency anemia). The mean corpuscular hemoglobin concentration (MCHC) is a measure of color, but number values are not used on the exam. Instead, color is described as normochromic or hypochromic.

698. A) Diarrhea with blood mixed in the stool Irritable bowel syndrome (IBS) is considered a functional disorder because the colon tissue is normal. There is no inflammation or bleeding in IBS. Patients report chronic abdominal pain, flatulence, bloating, and changes in bowel movements. IBS is more common in women than men. Rectal bleeding, blood in stool, anemia, fatigue, and weight loss are associated with inflammatory bowel disease (IBD), such as Crohn's disease or ulcerative colitis.

699. B) Intussusception The "classic triad" of intussusception—currant jelly stools, sausage-like mass, and pain (an infant with inconsolable crying, who draws up knees to abdomen)—is seen in less than 15% of patients. A sausage-shaped abdominal mass may be palpated on the right side of the abdomen. One third of patients do not pass blood or mucus or develop an abdominal mass. Older children may present with pain alone (Kitagawa & Miqdady, 2016).

700. D) Ankylosing spondylitis Ankylosing spondylitis (AS) is a lifelong autoimmune disease and form of arthritis that causes inflammation, pain, and stiffness, mainly in the spinal joints. The typical patient is a young adult. In the early stages of AS, the pain and stiffness often start in the lower back, but over time may move up the spine and into the neck. Most people with AS experience episodes of acute pain—known as *flares*—followed by periods when symptoms temporarily subside. There are no specific lab tests to identify ankylosing spondylitis. The erythrocyte sedimentation rate (ESR) is increased by the inflammation. There is a high risk of uveitis (red eyes, blurred to decreased vision, photophobia, floaters).

701. B) Schedule the patient for uterine ultrasound and endometrial biopsy Postmenopausal bleeding should always be investigated because it could be a sign of endometrial carcinoma. Although endometrial carcinoma is the most serious cause of postmenopausal bleeding, an atrophic endometrium with dyssynchronous shedding is the most common cause. A less common cause is cervical or endometrial polyps. A uterine ultrasound is ordered to evaluate the lining of the endometrium and rule out polyps. A uterine biopsy is ordered to sample for pathology.

702. A) Combination HIV-1 and HIV-2 antibody immunoassay with p24 antigen The Centers for Disease Control and Prevention (CDC) recommend screening with the combination antigen/antibody immunoassay with p24 antigen test. Previously, the ELISA (enzyme-linked immunosorbent assay) was used as the screening test, and the Western blot was the confirmatory test. The ELISA and Western blot tested only for the HIV antibody. The CDC recommends testing everyone between the ages of 13 and 64 years for HIV at least once as part of routine health care. If risk factors are present, the patient should be tested for HIV annually. For sexually active gay and bisexual men, the CDC recommends more frequent testing, perhaps every 3 to 6 months (CDC, 2016).

703. A) Acoustic nerve damage Labyrinthitis is also known as *vestibular neuritis*. It is caused by viral or postviral inflammation that affects the vestibular portion of cranial nerve VIII (acoustic nerve). It is usually a self-limiting disorder. The other symptoms listed are common with labyrinthitis and are made worse with moving the head, sitting up, rolling over, or looking upward. Treatment is corticosteroids (methylprednisone), antivirals (valacyclovir), and antihistamines such as meclizine (Antivert) or dimenhydrinate (Dramamine).

704. A) Transfusion of blood is prohibited even in cases of emergency The Watch Tower Society (the governing body of the Jehovah's Witnesses) recommends that its members should not accept whole blood or its primary components in any form. Jehovah's Witnesses believe that the Bible commands them "not to eat blood" and they regard accepting transfusions as equivalent to eating blood. In 2000, a ruling stated that they can accept "minor" components of blood, but they cannot accept a "major" blood component. In the 1980s, organ transplants became acceptable. Patients who identify as Jehovah's Witness should be asked about their preferences regarding blood transfusion before surgical procedures.

705. A) Sinusitis and hydrocele Transillumination is used for evaluation of the frontal and maxillary sinus as well as for a hydrocele. Because light is able to pass through the delicate skin covering the hollow sinus cavities, a light source held against the upper cheek will produce a red dot on the palate if the sinuses are normal (filled with air rather than obstructed). The transillumination test is used to differentiate a hydrocele from hernia—an illuminated scrotum will show the testicle in the center surrounded by water in the hydrocele.

706. C) Cauda equina syndrome Acute cauda equina syndrome is a surgical emergency. It requires decompression surgery of the spine to prevent permanent nerve damage of the affected nerve roots. The cauda equina contains 18 nerve roots. MRI is the best imaging test. The most common cause of compression is a herniated nucleus pulposus. Most herniations occur either at L4–L5 or L5–S1. The spinal nerves can also become infected (e.g., in tuberculosis, herpes, cytomegalovirus infections). Symptoms include low-back pain, sciatica (unilateral or bilateral), saddle pattern paresthesias, bladder and/or bowel incontinence, and lower extremity motor and sensory abnormalities. Sciatic pain is typically described as sharp or searing, rather than dull; some patients experience a "pins-and-needles" sensation, numbness or weakness, or a prickling sensation down the leg.

707. A) *Clostridium difficile*-associated diarrhea (CDAD) Important risk factors for CDAD and *C. difficile* colitis are antibiotic therapy and hospitalization. Almost any antibiotic can cause the condition, but the most common are clindamycin, cephalosporins, and fluoroquinolones. Diarrhea can occur during as well as after therapy (5–10 days; up to 10 weeks). Pseudomembranous colitis is a complication of *C. difficile* colitis.

708. B) Azithromycin 1 g PO in a single dose There are two regimens for treatment of non-gonococcal urethritis: either azithromycin 1 g PO in a single dose or doxycycline 100 mg PO BID for 7 days. Before treatment, test the patient for chlamydia and gonorrhea. Use the first urine of the day to test the patient with a nucleic acid amplification test (NAAT). The bacteria that may cause this condition are *Chlamydia trachomatis*, *Ureaplasma urealyticum*, *Mycoplasma genitalium*, and *Trichomonas vaginalis*. There is no test for the last three pathogens mentioned.

709. B) Croup The "barky" cough of croup is harsh, loud, and worse at night. Other symptoms are fever, hoarse or raspy voice, and stridor. A warm steamy room (let hot water run in shower with door closed) or a mist humidifier help. Croup is caused by several types of viruses, but parainfluenza types 1, 2, and 3 are the most common viruses.

710. C) Use the spirometer to assess severity of symptoms The patient is having an acute asthmatic exacerbation. The patient's vital signs reveal a respiratory rate of 14 breaths/min and pulse of 88 beats/min, which are within normal limits (not in respiratory distress). Before administering nebulized albuterol, use the spirometer to quantify the degree of impairment and listen to the breath sounds. Then after the treatment, recheck spirometry to evaluate the patient's response. The nebulizer treatment can be repeated in 20 minutes as needed. Change the patient's prescription to a combination steroid and long-acting beta-agonist inhaler plus a Medrol dose pack.

711. B) Angiotensin-converting enzyme (ACE) inhibitors or angiotensin receptor blockers (ARBs) The preferred drugs for treatment of patients with stable heart failure are ACE inhibitors or ARBs, usually in combination with beta-blockers, a diuretic, and/or spironolactone.

712. B) 7.5% or higher The estimated 10-year ASCVD risk score is 7.5% or higher. The 2013 ACC/AHA guidelines recommend treatment with high-intensity statins for patients aged 40 to 75 years with very high low-density lipoprotein (LDL) values who have a score of 7.5% or higher.

713. C) High-intensity statin This patient fulfills the criteria for high-intensity statin dosing criteria from the 2013 American College of Cardiology/American Heart Association

(ACC/AHA) blood cholesterol guideline. He already has heart disease (angina), type 2 diabetes, low-density lipoprotein (LDL) of 195 mg/dL, and low high-density lipoprotein (HDL) of 25 mg/dL. This patient is at very high risk for heart disease and warrants a high-intensity dose of statin. There are only two choices at this level: atorvastatin (Lipitor) 40 to 80 mg or rosuvastatin (Crestor) 20 to 40 mg.

714. **D) Encourage sexual abstinence and condom use** *Healthy People 2020* has four overarching goals: (1) attain high-quality longer lives free of preventable disease, disability, injury, and premature death; (2) achieve health equity and eliminate disparities, and improve health for all groups; (3) create social and physical environments that promote good health for all; and (4) promote quality of life, healthy development, and healthy behaviors across life stages. Sexual abstinence is only one specific area of sexual health promotion.

715. **D) Initiate cardiopulmonary resuscitation (CPR) immediately** Although the patient is in obvious respiratory distress, CPR is not yet warranted. This patient is at very high risk for acute respiratory failure.

716. **C) HIV antibodies** The ELISA (enzyme-linked immunosorbent assay) and Western blot tests detect only HIV antibodies. That is why there is a "window period" with HIV infection. If the test is performed too early in the infection, it will be falsely negative because there may not yet be enough antibodies against HIV to trigger a positive result.

717. **A) Discontinue atorvastatin (Lipitor) and order a liver function profile** The patient has symptoms of liver damage, including fatigue, anorexia, jaundice, and darker colored urine. The statin should be discontinued, and a liver function profile is indicated. This patient is taking high-dose atorvastatin (60 mg) plus a high-dose B-complex vitamin (which contains niacin or vitamin B_3). The combination of a statin with niacin raises the risk of drug-induced hepatitis and rhabdomyolysis.

718. **D) Vascular dementia** Vascular dementia (multi-infarct dementia) is the second most common type of dementia. It is caused by stroke, large artery infarctions, small artery infarctions (lacunes), and chronic subcortical ischemia of the brain. Symptoms vary depending on the location of the damaged tissue in the brain. Common symptoms are memory loss, impaired judgment, apathy (loss of motivation), and impaired decision-making function. The most common type of dementia in the United States is Alzheimer's disease.

719. **A) Trigeminal neuralgia** Trigeminal neuralgia is a rare nerve disorder that causes a stabbing or electric shock-like pain in parts of the face. It is more common in older adults. Symptoms are very painful, sharp electric-like spasms that usually last a few seconds or minutes, but can become constant. Pain is usually only on one side of the face, often around the eye, cheek, and lower part of the face. Pain may be triggered by touch or sounds. Painful attacks of trigeminal neuralgia can be triggered by common, everyday activities.

720. **A) Giardiasis** *Giardia lamblia* is a protozoan with flagella that infects the small intestine. Giardiasis is common in the developing world and rural areas and can cause acute and chronic infection. Campers, hunters, backpackers, and travelers to endemic areas are at highest risk. The incubation period is 7 to 14 days, and symptoms can last for 2

to 4 weeks. Chronic infection can result in malabsorption and significant weight loss. First-line antibiotics are tinidazole (Tindamax) or nitazoxanide (Nizonide). Alternative antibiotics are metronidazole (Flagyl) and others.

721. D) Expert opinion Expert opinions and professional society opinions are considered to offer the lowest level of evidence because they are subjective and not based on research. Cohort studies are used to investigate risk factors and causes of disease. An example of a cohort study is the Framingham Study. An experiment that uses randomization, control group, and intervention group(s), offers a lower level of evidence than randomized controlled trial. The ranking of options for this question is as follows: (1) randomized controlled trial, (2) experiments, (3) cohort studies, and (4) expert opinions. The best method of correctly answering this type of question is to memorize the categories for the best level of evidence (meta-analysis and/or systematic review and/or RCTs) and the lowest form of evidence (opinions, editorials).

722. A) Meta-analysis Meta-analyses and systematic reviews offer the highest level of evidence. The ranking of options for this question is as follows: (1) meta-analysis, (2) randomized controlled trial, (3) cohort study, and (4) expert opinion. The best method of correctly answering this type of question is to memorize the categories for the best level of evidence (meta-analysis and/or systematic review and/or randomized controlled trials) and the lowest form of evidence (opinions, editorials). Cohort studies are used to investigate risk factors and causes of disease. An example of a cohort study is the Framingham Study.

723. D) Refer the infant to a pediatric neurosurgeon Premature closure of the fontanels is called *craniosynostosis*. Premature closure of the anterior fontanel ("soft spot") is serious because the brain cannot grow properly. The anterior fontanel usually closes within 9 to 18 months of life. The sutures will have to be surgically separated in the operating room. There are numerous causes for craniosynostosis such as thyroid disease, genetic diseases, metabolic diseases, and so on.

724. C) Anterior cruciate ligament damage A positive anterior drawer sign occurs when there is damage to the anterior cruciate ligament. The patient is tested in supine position with knees flexed at 90 degrees and feet flat on the exam table. Hold the proximal lower leg (upper tibia) and push the leg anteriorly. The test is positive if the affected knee slides or has laxity when compared with the uninjured knee. Refer patient to an orthopedic specialist if the knee is unstable. The best imaging test for joints is the MRI.

725. A) Metronidazole (Flagyl) 500 mg orally TID × 10 to 14 days The first-line antibiotic for patients with mild to moderate *Clostridium difficile* colitis is metronidazole. Vancomycin is reserved for patients with severe cases.

Abbreviations and Acronyms

AAA	abdominal aortic aneurysm
AACN	American Association of Colleges of Nursing
AAHSA	American Association of Homes and Services for the Aging
AAI	atlantoaxial instability
AANP	American Association of Nurse Practitioners
AANPCB	American Academy of Nurse Practitioners Certification Board
AAP	American Academy of Pediatrics
ABCs	airway–breathing–circulation
ABI	ankle–brachial index
ABR	auditory brainstem response
ABRS	acute bacterial rhinosinusitis
AC	air conduction
ACA	Affordable Care Act of 2010
ACCP	American College of Chest Physicians
ACD	anemia of chronic disease
ACE	angiotensin-converting enzyme
ACEI	angiotensin-converting enzyme inhibitor
ACIP	Advisory Committee on Immunization Practices
ACL	anterior cruciate ligament
ACNP	acute care nurse practitioner
ACS	acute coronary syndrome
ACTH	adrenocorticotropic hormone
ADD	attention deficit disorder
ADHD	attention deficit hyperactivity disorder
ADL	activities of daily living
AF	atrial fibrillation
AFB	acid-fast bacillus
AFP	alpha-fetoprotein
AGNP	adult-gerontology nurse practitioner
AGPCNP	adult-gerontology primary care nurse practitioner
AGS	American Geriatrics Society
ALF	assisted-living facility
ALL	acute lymphocytic leukemia
ALT	alanine aminotransferase
AMA	American Medical Association
AMD	age-related macular degeneration/atrophic macular degeneration
AML	acute myelogenous leukemia
ANA	American Nurses Association; antinuclear antibody; antinuclear antigen
ANC	absolute neutrophil count
ANCC	American Nurses Credentialing Center
ANENP	American Association of Emergency Nurse Practitioners
ANP	adult nurse practitioner
Anti-HBc	antibody to hepatitis B core antigen

Anti-HBs antibody to hepatitis B surface antigen
Anti-HCV antibody to hepatitis C virus
Anti-TNF anti–tumor necrosis factor
AOA Administration on Aging
AOM acute otitis media
A1C hemoglobin A1C test for diabetes
AP acute pancreatitis
A–P anterior–posterior
APMHNP adult psychiatric mental health nurse practitioner
APRN advanced practice registered nurse
APS adult protective services
aPTT activated partial thromboplastin time
ARB angiotensin receptor blocker
ARNP advanced registered nurse practitioner
ARR absolute risk reduction
ART antiretroviral therapy
AS ankylosing spondylitis
ASA acetylsalicylic acid
ASCVD atherosclerotic cardiovascular disease
ASCUS atypical squamous cells of undetermined significance
ASMP arthritis self-management program
AST aspartate aminotransferase
ATS American Thoracic Society
AUC area under the curve
AUDIT alcohol use disorders identification
AV atrioventricular
AZT azidothymidine
BC bone conduction
BCC basal cell carcinoma
BCG bacillus Calmette-Guérin
BDTC black dot tinea capitis
BG blood glucose
BID *bis in die* (twice a day)
BLS Basic Life Support
BM bowel movement
BMD bone mineral density
BMI body mass index
BMR basal metabolic rate
BP blood pressure
BPH benign prostatic hyperplasia
BPV benign positional vertigo
BSE breast self-examination
BTB breakthrough bleeding
BUN blood urea nitrogen
BV bacterial vaginosis
CA cancer
CABG coronary artery bypass graft
CAD coronary artery disease
CAM complementary and alternative medicine
CAP community-acquired pneumonia
CBC complete blood count
CBT computer-based test
CCB calcium channel blocker
CCNE Commission on Collegiate Nursing Education
CCRC continuing-care retirement community
CDAD *Clostridium difficile*-associated diarrhea
CDC Centers for Disease Control and Prevention

CD4	helper T lymphocyte express cluster determinant 4
CDI	*Clostridium difficile* infection
CE	continuing education
CF	cystic fibrosis
CFU	colony-forming unit
CHADS2	congestive heart failure, hypertension, age, diabetes, stroke score
CHD	coronary heart disease
CHESS	changes in health, end-stage disease, symptoms and signs
CHF	congestive heart failure
CHIP	Children's Health Insurance Program
CHIPRA	Children's Health Insurance Program Reauthorization Act
CINAHL	Cumulative Index to Nursing and Allied Health Literature
CK	creatinine kinase
CKD	chronic kidney disease
CMA	certified medical assistant
CMS	Centers for Medicare & Medicaid Services
CMV	cytomegalovirus
CNA	certified nurse's aide
CNS	central nervous system; clinical nurse specialist
CO	cardiac output
COBRA	Consolidated Omnibus Budget Reconciliation Act
COC	combined oral contraceptive
CON	certificate of need
COPD	chronic obstructive pulmonary disease
CPK	creatinine phosphokinase
CPPS	chronic pelvic pain syndrome
CPR	cardiopulmonary resuscitation
CPT	Current Procedural Terminology
CR	caloric restriction [theory]
CRH	corticotropin-releasing hormone
CRP	C-reactive protein
C&S	culture and sensitivity
C-section	cesarean section
CSF	cerebrospinal fluid
CT	computed tomography
cTnT	cardiac troponin
CTS	carpal tunnel syndrome
CVA	cerebrovascular accident; costovertebral angle
CVS	chorionic villus sampling
CXR	chest x-ray
CYP450 system	cytochrome P450 system
DASH	dietary approaches to stop hypertension
D&C	dilation and curettage
DDH	developmental dysplasia of the hip
DDS	doctor of dental surgery
DEA	Drug Enforcement Administration
DEET	N, N-diethyl-meta-toluamide
DES	diethylstilbestrol
DFA-TP	direct fluorescent antibody testing
DGI	disseminated gonorrheal infection
DHEA	dehydroepiandrosterone
DHHS	Department of Health and Human Services
DHT	dihydrotestosterone
DIC	disseminated intravascular coagulation
DIP	distal interphalangeal (joint)
DJD	degenerative joint disease
DKA	diabetic ketoacidosis

DM	diabetes mellitus
DMARD	disease-modifying antirheumatic drug
DMD	doctor of medicine in dentistry
DME	durable medical equipment
DMPA	depot medroxyprogesterone acetate
DMV	department of motor vehicles
DNA	deoxyribonucleic acid
DNP	doctor of nursing practice
DO	doctor of osteopathy
DON	director of nursing
DOT	directly observed treatment
DPP-4	dipeptidyl peptidase-4
DRE	digital rectal examination
DS	Down syndrome
DSM-5	*Diagnostic and Statistical Manual of Mental Disorders* (5th edition)
DTaP	diphtheria–tetanus–acellular pertussis
DTR	deep tendon reflex
DVT	deep vein thrombosis
DXA	dual x-ray absorptiometry
EBM	evidence-based medicine
EBV	Epstein–Barr virus
ED	emergency department
EDD	estimated date of delivery
EEG	electroencephalogram
EES	erythromycin estolate
EF	ejection fraction
EFT	electronic fund transfer
eGFR	estimated glomerular filtration rate
EIA	enzyme immunoassay
EKG	electrocardiogram
ELISA	enzyme-linked immunosorbent assay
EOM	extraocular (eye) movement
EPA	Environmental Protection Agency
EPO	erythropoietin
EPT	Expedited Partner Therapy
ERT	estrogen replacement therapy
ESR	erythrocyte sedimentation rate
ETOH	ethanol
FAS	fetal alcohol syndrome
FBG	fasting blood glucose
FDA	Food and Drug Administration
FEV1	forced expiratory volume in 1 second
FHT	fetal heart tone
5-FU	5-fluorouracil
fL	femtoliter
FNP	family nurse practitioner
FOBT	fecal occult blood test
FPMHNP	family psychiatric mental health nurse practitioner
FPR	fasting plasma glucose
FSH	follicle-stimulating hormone
FTA–ABS	fluorescent antibody–absorption antibody
FTT	failure to thrive
FVC	forced vital capacity
GAD	generalized anxiety disorder
GBS	group B *Streptococcus*
GCA	giant cell arteritis
GERD	gastroesophageal reflux disease

GFR	glomerular filtration rate
GGT	gamma glutamyl transpeptidase *or* gamma glutamyl transferase
GH	growth hormone
GHRH	growth-hormone releasing hormone
GI	gastrointestinal
GITT	Geriatric Interdisciplinary Team Training
GLP-1	glucagonlike contransporter-2
GNP	gerontologic nurse practitioner
GnRH	gonadotropin-releasing hormone
GSE	genital self-examination
G6PD	glucose-6-phosphate dehydrogenase
gtts	*guttae* (drops/minute)
GU	genitourinary
HA	headache
HAART	highly active antiretroviral therapy
HbeAg	hepatitis B e- antigen
HbF	fetal hemoglobin
HBIG	hepatitis B immune globulin
HBM	Health Belief Model
HbS	sickle hemoglobin
HBsAG	hepatitis B surface antigen
hCG	human chorionic gonadotropin
HCP	health care personnel
HCT	hematocrit
HCTZ	hydrochlorothiazide
HCV	hepatitis C virus
HDL	high-density lipoprotein
HDTZ	hydrochlorothiazide
HEENT	head, ear, eye, nose, throat
HELLP	hemolysis, elevated liver enzymes, low platelets
HEPA	high-efficiency particulate air
HF	heart failure
HGH	human growth hormone
H&H	hemoglobin and hematocrit
Hib	*Haemophilus influenzae* type b
HIPAA	Health Insurance Portability and Accountability Act
HIV	human immunodeficiency virus
HMG-CoA	5-hydroxy-3-methylglutaryl-coenzyme A
HMO	health maintenance organization
HPA	hypothalamic–pituitary–adrenal (axis)
HPL	human pancreatic lipase
HPV	human papillomavirus
HRT	hormone replacement therapy
HS	half strength
HSV	herpes simplex virus
HTN	hypertension
HUD	Department of Housing and Urban Development
HZ	herpes zoster
Hz	hertz
HZO	herpes zoster ophthalmicus
IADL	instrumental activities of daily living
IBS	irritable bowel syndrome
IC	infective endocarditis
ICD-10	*International Classification of Diseases* (10th edition)
ICP	intracranial pressure
ICS	inhaled corticosteroid; intercostal space
ICU	intensive care unit

I&D	incision and drainage
IDA	iron-deficiency anemia
IDSA	Infectious Disease Society of America
IDU	intravenous drug user
IE	infective endocarditis
IF	intrinsic factor
IFA	indirect immunofluorescence assay
IFG	impaired fasting glucose
IgE	immunoglobulin E
IgG	immunoglobulin G
IgG Anti-HAV	hepatitis A antibody IgG type
IgM	immunoglobulin M
IGRA	interferon–gamma release assay
IGT	impaired glucose tolerance
IM	intramuscular
INH	isoniazid; isonicotinoylhydrazine
INR	international normalized ratio
I&O	intake and output
IOP	intraocular pressure
IPV	intimate partner violence; inactivated polio vaccine
IRB	institutional review board
ITP	idiopathic thrombocytopenic purpura
IU	international unit
IUD	intrauterine device
IUGR	intrauterine growth restriction
IV	intravenous
IVP	intravenous pyelogram
JCAHO	The Joint Commission on the Accreditation of Health care Organizations
JNC	Joint National Committee
JVD	jugular venous distention
K/DOQI	Kidney Disease Outcomes Quality Initiative
KOH	potassium hydroxide
KUB	kidney, ureter, and bladder x-ray study
LABA	long-acting beta agonist
LAIV	live attenuated influenza vaccine
LCL	lateral collateral ligament
LDCT	low-dose computed tomography
LDH	lactate dehydrogenase
LDL	low-density lipoprotein
LEEP	loop electrosurgical excision procedure
LFT	liver function test
LGBT	lesbian–gay–bisexual—transgender
LH	luteinizing hormone
LLW	left lower quadrant
LMP	last menstrual period
LOC	level of consciousness
LPN	licensed practical nurse
LSIL	low-grade squamous intraepithelial lesion
LTBI	latent TB infection
LTCF	long-term care facility
LTRA	leukotriene receptor antagonist
LUV	left upper quadrant
LV	left ventricular
LVEF	left ventricular ejection fraction
LVH	left ventricular hypertrophy
MAOI	monoamine oxidase inhibitor
MCH	mean corpuscular hemoglobin

MCHC	mean corpuscular hemoglobin concentration
MCL	medial collateral ligament
MCV	mean corpuscular volume
MCV4	meningococcal conjugate vaccine quadrivalent
MDI	metered-dose inhaler
MDMA	3, 4-methylenedioxy-N-methamphetamine
MDRD	modification of diet in renal disease
MDS	Minimum Data Set
MDS–CHESS	Minimum Data Set—Changes in Health, End-stage disease, Symptoms and Signs (scale)
MEE	middle ear effusion
MHA-TP	microhemagglutination test for antibodies to *T. pallidum*
MHC	mean hemoglobin concentration
MI	myocardial infarction
MIC	minimum inhibitory concentration
MMA	methylmalonic acid
MMPI-2	Minnesota Multiphasic Personality Inventory, 2nd ed.
MMR	measles, mumps, rubella
MMSE	Mini-Mental State Examination
MODY	maturity-onset diabetes of the young
MR	mitral regurgitation
MRI	magnetic resonance imaging
MRSA	methicillin-resistant *Staphylococcus aureus*
MS	multiple sclerosis
MSG	monosodium glutamate
MSH	melanocyte-stimulating hormone
MSM	men who have sex with men
MSW	master of social work
MTP	metatarsophalangeal (joint)
MVI	multivitamin
MVP	mitral valve prolapse
MVTR	moisture vapor transmission rate
NAAT	nucleic acid amplification test
NAFLD	nonalcoholic fatty liver disease
NAMS	North American Menopause Society
NASH	nonalcoholic steatohepatitis
NCEA	National Center on Elder Abuse
NCOA	National Council on Aging
NG	nasogastric
NGU	nongonococcal urethritis
NICU	neonatal intensive care unit
NL	normal limits
NLM	National Library of Medicine
NLNAC	National League for Nurses Accrediting Commission
NNT	number needed to treat
NONPF	National Organization of Nurse Practitioner Faculty
NP	nurse practitioner
NPDR	nonproliferative diabetic retinopathy
NPH	neutral protamine Hagedorn
NPI	national provider identifier
NPPES	National Plan and Provider Enumeration System
NPV	negative predictive value
NRTI	nucleoside reverse transcriptase inhibitor
NSAID	nonsteroidal anti-inflammatory drug
NTD	neural tube defect
N/V	nausea/vomiting
NYHA	New York Heart Association

OA	osteoarthritis
OAE	otoacoustic emission
OBRA	Omnibus Budget Reconciliation Act
OC	oral contraceptive
OCD	obsessive-compulsive disorder
OFC	occipitofrontal circumference
OD	*oculus dexter* (right eye)
OGTT	oral glucose tolerance test
OHL	oral hairy leukoplakia
OS	*oculus sinister* (left eye)
OSHA	Occupational Safety and Health Administration
OT	occupational therapy
OTC	over the counter
OU	*oculus uterque* (both eyes)
PA	pernicious anemia; physician assistant
PAD	peripheral artery disease
PAT	paroxysmal atrial tachycardia
PCL	posterior cruciate ligament
PCMH	patient-centered medical home
PCOS	polycystic ovarian syndrome
PCP	phencyclidine; *Pneumocystis carinii* pneumonia; primary care provider
PCR	polymerase chain reaction
PCV	pneumococcal vaccine
PDL	pulse-dye laser
PE	pulmonary embolism
PEF	peak expiratory flow
PEFR	peak expiratory flow rate
PEP	postexposure prophylaxis
PET	positron emission tomography
PFT	pulmonary function test
PHN	postherpetic neuralgia
PID	pelvic inflammatory disease
PIP	proximate interphalangeal (joint)
PKU	phenylketonuria
PMB	postmenopausal bleeding
PMDD	premenstrual dysphoric disorder
PMI	point of maximal impulse
PMR	polymyalgia rheumatica
PO	*per os* (by mouth)
PPD	purified protein derivative
PPI	proton-pump inhibitor
PPO	preferred provider organization
PPSV	pneumococcal polysaccharide vaccine
PPV	positive predictive value
PrEP	preexposure prophylaxis
PRN	*pro re nata* (as needed)
PSA	prostate-specific antigen
PSVT	paroxysmal supraventricular tachycardia
PT	physical therapy; prothrombin time
PTH	parathyroid hormone
PTSD	posttraumatic stress disorder
PTT	partial thromboplastin time
PUD	peptic ulcer disease
PUSH	Pressure Ulcer Scale for Healing
PVD	peripheral vascular disease
PVR	peripheral vascular resistance
QID	*quarter in die* (four times a day)

RA	rheumatoid arthritis
RADT	rapid antigen detection testing
RAI	resident assessment instrument
RAIV	radioactive iodine uptake
RBC	red blood cell
RCA	root cause analysis
RCT	randomized controlled trial
RDW	red blood cell distribution width
RF	rheumatoid factor
RIV	recombinant inactivated virus
RLV	right lower quadrant
RMSF	Rocky Mountain spotted fever
RNA	ribonucleic acid
ROM	range of motion
RPR	rapid plasma reagin (test)
RRR	relative risk reduction
RSV	respiratory syncytial virus
RUQ	right upper quadrant
RV	residual volume
SABA	short-acting beta-agonist
SAH	subarachnoid hemorrhage
SBON	state board of nursing
SC (or SQ)	subcutaneous
SCA	sickle cell anemia
SD	standard deviation
SDH	subdural hematoma
SE	sentinel event
SERM	selective estrogen receptor modulator
SGLT2	sodium-glucose cotransporter-2
SGOT	serum glutamic oxaloacetic transaminase
SGPT	serum glutamic pyruvic transaminase
SIDS	sudden infant death syndrome
SJS	Stevens–Johnson syndrome
SOB	short of breath
SoFAS	solid fats and added sugars
SLE	systemic lupus erythematosus
SMAST	Short Michigan Alcoholism Screening Test
SNF	skilled nursing facility
SNRI	selective norepinephrine reuptake inhibitor
SOAPE	subjective, objective, assessment planning, and evaluation
SPF	sun protection factor
SQ (or SC)	subcutaneous
SSHL	sudden sensorineural hearing loss
SSNI	selective norepinephrine reuptake inhibitor
SSRI	selective serotonin reuptake inhibitor
STD	sexually transmitted disease
STEMI	ST-elevation myocardial infarction
STI	sexually transmitted infection
SVTC	supraventricular tachycardia with aberrant conduction
TA	temporal arteritis
TB	tuberculosis
TBG	thyroid-binding globulin
TBSA	total body surface area
TCA	tricyclic antidepressant
TCH	trichloroacetic acid
TCM	traditional Chinese medicine
TCO	Test Content Outline

Td	tetanus–diphtheria
Tdap	tetanus–diphtheria–pertussis
TED	thromboembolitic deterrent
TEN	toxic epidermal necrolysis
TIA	transient ischemic attack
TIBC	total iron binding capacity
TID	*ter in die* (three times a day)
TIG	tetanus immunoglobulin
TIV	trivalent inactivated vaccine
TLC	total lung capacity
TM	tympanic membrane
TMP/SMX	trimethoprim–sulfamethoxazole
TNF	tumor necrosis factor
TNM	tumor–nodes–metastasis
TnT	troponin
TPA	third-party administrator
TPO	thyroid peroxidase antibody
TPPA	*T. pallidum* agglutination assay
TRAb	thyrotropin receptor antibody
TRH	thyroid-releasing homrone
TSH	thyroid-stimulating hormone
TSI	thyroid-stimulating immunoglobulin
TST	tuberculin skin test
TTM	Transtheoretical Model
TZDs	thiazolidinediones
UA	urinalysis
URI	upper respiratory infection
USDA	U.S. Department of Agriculture
USPSTF	U.S. Preventive Services Task Force
UTI	urinary tract infection
UV	ultraviolet
VAERS	Vaccine Adverse Event Reporting System
VDRL	Venereal Disease Research Laboratory (test)
VT	ventricular tachycardia
VTE	venous thromboembolism
VZV	varicella zoster virus
WBC	white blood bell
WHO	World Health Organization
WHR	waist-to-hip ratio
WIC	Special Supplemental Food Program for Women, Infants, and Children
WNL	within normal limits
WPW	Wolff–Parkinson–White (syndrome)
ZDV	zidovudine

Resources

Administration on Aging, Administration for Community Living, U.S. Department of Health and Human Services. (2016). A profile of older Americans: 2016. Retrieved from https://www.acl.gov/sites/default/files/Aging%20and%20Disability%20in%20America/2016-Profile.pdf

Agency for Healthcare Research and Quality. (n.d.). Patient centered medical home resource center: Defining the PCMH. Retrieved from https://pcmh.ahrq.gov/page/defining-pcmh

Agency for Healthcare Research and Quality, National Guideline Clearinghouse, & American Geriatrics Society. (2015). 2015 updated Beers criteria for potentially inappropriate medication use in older adults. Retrieved from https://guideline.gov/summaries/summary/49933/American-Geriatrics-Society-2015-updated-Beers-Criteria-for-potentially-inappropriate-medication-use-in-older-adults

AIDS Education and Training Center. (n.d.). Issues of ethnopharmacology in AIDS management. Retrieved from https://www.aetcnmc.org/curricula/ethnopharmacology/mod4_2.html

AIDSinfo. (2016). The stages of HIV infection. Retrieved from https://aidsinfo.nih.gov/understanding-hiv-aids/fact-sheets/19/46/the-stages-of-hiv-infection

AIDSinfo. (2017). The basics of HIV prevention. Retrieved from https://aidsinfo.nih.gov/understanding-hiv-aids/fact-sheets/20/48/the-basics-of-hiv-prevention

American Academy of Dermatology. (n.d.). Role of diet in acne: Recommendations. Retrieved from https://www.aad.org/practicecenter/quality/clinical-guidelines/acne/role-of-diet-in-acne

American Academy of Nurse Practitioners. (n.d.). AANPCP 2015 statistics. Retrieved from https://www.aanpcert.org/resource/documents/AANPCP%202015%20Pass%20Rate%20Report.pdf

American Academy of Nurse Practitioners National Certification Board. (2017, August). Family Nurse Practitioner. Adult-Gerontology Nurse Practitioner. FNP & AGNP Certification. Candidate Handbook. Retrieved from https://www.aanpcert.org/resource/documents/AGNP%20FNP%20Candidate%20Handbook.pdf

American Academy of Pediatrics. (2008). Red reflex examination in neonates, infants, and children. *Pediatrics, 122*(6). Retrieved from http://pediatrics.aappublications.org/content/122/6/1401

American Academy of Pediatrics. (2010, March 3). Vitamin D supplementation for infants. Retrieved from https://www.aap.org/en-us/about-the-aap/aap-press-room/pages/Vitamin-D-Supplementation-for-Infants.aspx

American Cancer Society. (n.d.). Can ovarian cancer be found? Retrieved from https://www.cancer.org/cancer/ovarian-cancer/detection-diagnosis-staging/detection.html

American Cancer Society. (n.d.). Key statistics for lung cancer. Retrieved from https://www.cancer.org/cancer/non-small-cell-lung-cancer/about/key-statistics.html

American Cancer Society. (n.d.). Skin cancer facts. Retrieved from https://www.cancer.org/cancer/skin-cancer.html

American Cancer Society. (2015). Cancer facts & figures 2015. Retrieved from http://www.cancer.org/acs/groups/content/@editorial/documents/document/acspc-044552.pdf

American Cancer Society. (2016). Lung cancer fact sheet. Key statistics for lung cancer.Retrieved from https://www.cancer.org/cancer/non-small-cell-lung-cancer/about/key-statistics.html

American College of Cardiology, & American Heart Association. (2014). ACC/AHA release updated guideline on the treatment of blood cholesterol to reduce ASCVD risk. *American Family Physician, 90*(4), 260–265.

American College of Obstetricians and Gynecologists. (2015). Committee opinion, no. 651. Menstruation in girls and adolescents: Using the menstrual cycle as a vital sign. Reaffirmed 2017. Retrieved from https://www.acog.org/Resources-And-Publications/Committee-Opinions/Committee-on-Adolescent-Health-Care/Menstruation-in-Girls-and-Adolescents-Using-the-Menstrual-Cycle-as-a-Vital-Sign

American College of Obstetricians and Gynecologists. (2016). Abnormal cervical cancer screening test results. Retrieved from https://www.acog.org/Patients/FAQs/Abnormal-Cervical-Cancer-Screening-Test-Results

American College of Rheumatology. (2012). Recommendations for management of hand, hip, and knee OA. Retrieved from https://www.rheumatology.org

American Diabetes Association. (2016). National Diabetes Education Initiative. Diabetes management guidelines. Standards of medical care in diabetes—2016. *Diabetes Care, 39*(Suppl. 1), S1–S106.

American Diabetes Association. (2017). Standards of medical care in diabetes: Summary of revisions. *Diabetes Care, 40*(Suppl.), S4–S5.

American Diabetes Association Clinical Practice Recommendations. (2016). FNP exam. *Diabetes Care, 37* (Suppl. 1).

American Heart Association. (n.d.). Heart attack or a stroke? Call 911 first. And fast. Retrieved from http://www.heart.org/HEARTORG/General/Heart-Attack-or-Stroke-Call-911-First-And-Fast_UCM_435652_Article.jsp#.Wd6lF2hSz7w

American Heart Association. (2017). A patient's guide to taking warfarin. Retrieved from http://www.heart.org/HEARTORG/Conditions/Arrhythmia/PreventionTreatmentofArrhythmia/A-Patients- Guide-to-Taking-Warfarin_UCM_444996_Article.jsp#.WXDP1ra1vcs

American Lung Association. (n.d.). Lung capacity and aging. Retrieved from http://www.lung.org/lung-health-and-diseases/how-lungs-work/lung-capacity-and-aging.html

American Lung Association. (2016). Lung cancer fact sheet. Retrieved from http://www.lung.org/lung-health-and-diseases/lung-disease-lookup/lung-cancer/resource-library/lung-cancer-fact-sheet.html?referrer=https://www.google.com

American Nurses Credentialing Center. (2012). Certification: ANCC alternative item demo. Retrieved from http://ancc.nursecredentialing.org/certification/ExamResources/SampleQuestions/FamilyNP

American Nurses Credentialing Center. (2015, December). Adult-Gerontology Primary Care Nurse Practitioner Board Certification Examination. *Test content outline*. Retrieved from http://nursecredentialing.org/Exam61-AdultGeroPrimaryCareNP-TCO

American Nurses Credentialing Center. (2015). Test content outline: Adult-gerontology primary care nurse practitioner board certification examination. Retrieved from http://www.nursecredentialing.org/Documents/Certification/TestContentOutlines/AGPCNP-Dec2015-TCO.pdf

American Nurses Credentialing Center. (2016). 2016 ANCC certification data (pass rates). Retrieved from http://www.nursecredentialing.org/Certification/FacultyEducators/FacultyCategory/Statistics/2015-CertificationStatistics.pdf

American Nurses Credentialing Center. (2016). Family nurse practitioner (22) reference list. Retrieved from http://nursecredentialing.org/Exam22-FamilyNP-TRL

American Nurses Credentialing Center. (2016). Test content outline: Family nurse practitioner board certification examination. Retrieved from htttp://www.nursecredentialing.org/Documents/Certification/TestContentOutlines/FamilyNP-TCO-2015.pdf

American Nurses Credentialing Center. (2016, February). Family Nurse Practitioner Board Certification Examination. *Test content outline*. Retrieved from http://nursecredentialing.org/FamilyNP-TCO2016

American Nurses Credentialing Center. (2017). Certification: Adult-gerontology primary care nurse practitioner. Retrieved from http://nursecredentialing.org/AdultGeroPrimaryCareNP

American Nurses Credentialing Center. (2017). Certification: Family nurse practitioner. Retrieved from http://nursecredentialing.org/FamilyNP

American Nurses Credentialing Center. (2017). Certification: General testing and renewal handbook. Retrieved from http://nursecredentialing.org/GeneralTestingandRenewalHandbook

American Psychiatric Association. (2013). *Diagnostic and statistical manual of mental disorders* (5th ed.). Arlington, VA: American Psychiatric Publishing.

American Urological Association. (2016, July). Medical student curriculum: Urinary incontinence. Retrieved from http://www.auanet.org/education/auauniversity/medical-student-education/medical-student-curriculum/urinary-incontinence

Apicella, M. (2017). Treatment and prevention of meningococcal infection. In E. L. Baron (Ed.), *UpToDate*. Retrieved from http://www.uptodate.com/contents/treatment-and-prevention-of-meningococcal-infection?to

Archer, S. M. (2016, March 17). Nonsurgical treatment of nasal polyps clinical presentation. In A. D. Meyers (Ed.), *Medscape*. Retrieved from http://emedicine.medscape.com/article/861353-clinical#b4

Armstrong, C. (2014, October 1). JNC 8 guidelines for the management of hypertension in adults. *American Family Physician, 90*(7), 503–504. Retrieved from http://www.aafp.org/afp/2014/1001/p503.html

Association of Reproductive Health Professionals. (2014). Quick reference guide for clinicians. Choosing a birth control method. Retrieved from http://www.arhp.org/publications-and-resources/quick-reference-guide-for-clinicians/choosing

Ball, J. W., Dains, J. E., Flynn, J. A., Solomon, B. S., & Stewart, R. W. (2015). *Seidel's guide to physical examination* (8th ed.). St. Louis, MO: Mosby/Elsevier.

Bastian, L. A., & Brown, H. L. (2017). Clinical manifestations and diagnosis of early pregnancy. In V. A. Barrs (Ed), *UpToDate*. Retrieved from https://www.uptodate.com/contents/clinical-manifestations-and-diagnosis-of-early-pregnancy

Berul, C., Seslar, S. P., & Zimetbaum, P. J. (2017). Acquired long QT syndrome. *UpToDate*. Retrieved from https://www.uptodate.com/contents/acquired-long-qt-syndrome?source=search_result&search=long%20QT&selectedTitle=1~150

Berul, C. (2018). Acquired long QT syndrome: Definitions, causes, and pathophysiology. In S. Asirvatham & P. J. Zimetbaum (Eds.), *UpToDate*. Retrieved from https://www.uptodate.com/contents/acquired-long-qt-syndrome-definitions-causes-and-pathophysiology

Bickley, L.S. (2017). *Bates' guide to physical examination and history-taking* (12th ed.). Philadelphia, PA: Wolters Kluwer.

Bickford, C. J., Marion, L., & Gazaway, S. (2015). *Nursing: Scope and standards of practice* (3rd ed.). Silver Spring, MD: American Nurses Association. Retrieved from http://www.augusta.edu/nursing/cnr/documents/seminar-files/pp8.28.pdf

Bienfang, D. C. (2017). Overview and differential diagnosis of papilledema. *UpToDate*. Retrieved from https://www.uptodate.com/contents/overview-and-differential-diagnosis-of-papilledema?source=search_result&search=overview%20and%20differential%20diagnosis%20of%20papilledema&selectedTitle=1~150

Biggs, H. M., Behravesh, C. B., Bradley, K. K., Dahlgren, F. S., Drexler, N. A., Dumler, S., … Traeger, M. S. (2016). Diagnosis and management of tickborne rickettsial diseases: Rocky mountain spotted fever and other spotted fever group rickettsioses, ehrlichioses, and anaplasmosis—United States: A practical guide for health care and public health professionals. *MMWR Recommendations and Reports*, *65*(2), 1–44. Retrieved from http://www.cdc.gov/mmwr/volumes/65/rr/rr6502a1.htm

Blanda, M. (2017). Cluster Headache. Retrieved from http://emedicine.medscape.com/article/1142459-overview#a4

Bondy, C. A. (2007). Care of girls and women with Turner syndrome: A guideline of the Turner Syndrome Study Group. *Journal of Clinical Endocrinology & Metabolism*, *92*(1), 10–25. doi:10.1210/jc.2006-1374

Bor, D. H. (2016). Etiologies of fever of unknown origin in adults. In A. R. Thorner (Ed.), *UpToDate*. Retrieved from http://www.uptodate.com/contents/etiologies-of-fever-of-unknown-origin-in-adults?source=preview&search=define+fever&language=en-US&anchor=H1&selectedTitle=2~150#H1

Borson, S., Scanlan, J., Brush, M., Vitaliano, P., & Dokmak, A. (2000). The Mini-Cog: A cognitive "vital signs" measure for dementia screening in multi-lingual elderly. *International Journal of Geriatric Psychiatry*, *15*(11), 1021–1027.

Branson, B. M., Owen, S. M., Wesolowski, L. G., Bennett, B., Werner, B. G., Wroblewski, K. E., & Pentella, M. A. (2014). Laboratory testing for the diagnosis of HIV infection: Updated recommendations. Atlanta, GA: Centers for Disease Control and Prevention. doi:10.15620/cdc.23447

Brusch, J. L. (2015, August 17). Pathophysiology of complicated urinary tract infections. In M. S. Bronze (Ed.), *Medscape*. Retrieved from http://emedicine.medscape.com/article/2039975-overview

Buppert, C. (2012). Is it a HIPAA violation to leave biopsy results on voicemail? *Medscape Family Medicine*. Retrieved from https://www.medscape.com/viewarticle/770258

Cefalu, W. T. (Ed.). (2016). American Diabetes Association standards of medical care in diabetes—2016. *Diabetes Care*, *39*(Suppl. 1). Retrieved from http://care.diabetesjournals.org/content/suppl/2015/12/21/39.Supplement_1.DC2/2016-Standards-of-Care.pdf

Center for Generational Kinetics. (n.d.) Generational breakdown: Info about all of the generations. Retrieved from http://genhq.com/faq-info-about-generations

Centers for Disease Control and Prevention. (n.d.). Cervical cancer screening guidelines for average-risk women. Retrieved from https://www.cdc.gov/cancer/cervical/pdf/guidelines.pdf

Centers for Disease Control and Prevention (n.d.). Summary chart of U.S. medical eligibility criteria for contraceptive use. Retrieved from https://www.cdc.gov/reproductivehealth/contraception/pdf/summary-chart-us-medical-eligibility-criteria_508tagged.pdf

Centers for Disease Control and Prevention. (2012) *Principles of epidemiology in public health practice: An introduction to applied epidemiology and biostatistics* (3rd ed.). Atlanta, GA: U.S. Department of Health and Human Services.

Centers for Disease Control and Prevention. (2014). Contraindications and precautions for varicella vaccination. Retrieved from https://www.cdc.gov/vaccines/vpd-vac/varicella/hcp-contraindications.htm

Centers for Disease Control and Prevention. (2014). Latent tuberculosis infection: A guide for primary health care providers. Retrieved from https://www.cdc.gov/tb/publications/ltbi/diagnosis.htm

Centers for Disease Control and Prevention. (2015). 2015 sexually transmitted diseases treatment guidelines: Bacterial vaginosis. Retrieved from https://www.cdc.gov/std/tg2015/bv.htm

Centers for Disease Control and Prevention. (2015). Chlamydial infections. Retrieved from https://www.cdc.gov/std/tg2015/chlamydia.htm

Centers for Disease Control and Prevention. (2015). STD treatment guidelines: Human papillomavirus (HPV) infection. Retrieved from https://www.cdc.gov/std/tg2015/hpv.htm

Centers for Disease Control and Prevention. (2015). Vitamin D. Retrieved from https://www.cdc.gov/breastfeeding/recommendations/vitamin_d.htm

Centers for Disease Control and Prevention. (2016). Adult obesity facts. Retrieved from https://www.cdc.gov/obesity/data/adult.html

Centers for Disease Control and Prevention. (2016). Flu vaccine and people with egg allergies. Retrieved from http://www.cdc.gov/flu/protect/vaccine/egg-allergies.htm

Centers for Disease Control and Prevention. (2016). HIV/AIDS: HIV basics Retrieved from https://www.cdc.gov/hiv/basics/index.html

Centers for Disease Control and Prevention. (2016). Important milestones: Your baby by four months. Retrieved from https://www.cdc.gov/ncbddd/actearly/milestones/milestones-4mo.html

Centers for Disease Control and Prevention. (2016). Important milestones: Your baby by nine months. Retrieved from https://www.cdc.gov/ncbddd/actearly/milestones/milestones-9mo.html

Centers for Disease Control and Prevention. (2016). Important milestones: Your baby by six months. Retrieved from https://www.cdc.gov/ncbddd/actearly/milestones/milestones-6mo.html

Centers for Disease Control and Prevention. (2016). Important milestones: Your baby by two months. Retrieved from https://www.cdc.gov/ncbddd/actearly/milestones/milestones-2mo.html

Centers for Disease Control and Prevention. (2016). Important milestones: Your child by five years. Retrieved from https://www.cdc.gov/ncbddd/actearly/milestones/milestones-5yr.html

Centers for Disease Control and Prevention. (2016). Important milestones: Your child by four years. Retrieved from https://www.cdc.gov/ncbddd/actearly/milestones/milestones-4yr.html

Centers for Disease Control and Prevention. (2016). Important milestones: Your child by one year. Retrieved from https://www.cdc.gov/ncbddd/actearly/milestones/milestones-1yr.html

Centers for Disease Control and Prevention. (2016). Important milestones: Your child by three years. Retrieved from https://www.cdc.gov/ncbddd/actearly/milestones/milestones-3yr.html

Centers for Disease Control and Prevention. (2016). Important milestones: Your child by two years. Retrieved from https://www.cdc.gov/ncbddd/actearly/milestones/milestones-2yr.html

Centers for Disease Control and Prevention. (2016). Tuberculosis (TB): Testing in BCG-vaccinated persons. Retrieved from http://www.cdc.gov/tb/topic/testing/testingbcgvaccinated.htm

Centers for Disease Control and Prevention. (2016). Tuberculosis (TB): Treatment. Retrieved from https://www.cdc.gov/tb/topic/treatment/default.htm

Centers for Disease Control and Prevention. (2016). Vaccines and preventable diseases. Pneumococcal vaccine recommendations. Retrieved from https://www.cdc.gov/vaccines/vpd/pneumo/index.html

Centers for Disease Control and Prevention. (2017). 2015 sexually transmitted diseases treatment guidelines: Summary. Retrieved from https://www.cdc.gov/std/tg2015/default.htm

Centers for Disease Control and Prevention. (2017). 2017 national notifiable conditions (historical). Retrieved from https://wwwn.cdc.gov/nndss/conditions/notifiable/2017

Centers for Disease Control and Prevention. (2017). About HIV/AIDS. Retrieved from https://www.cdc.gov/hiv/basics/whatishiv.html

Centers for Disease Control and Prevention. (2017). Cancer among men. Retrieved from http://www.cdc.gov/cancer/dcpc/data/men.htm

Centers for Disease Control and Prevention. (2017). Cancer among women. Retrieved from http://www.cdc.gov/cancer/dcpc/data/women.htm

Centers for Disease Control and Prevention. (2017). Frequently asked flu questions 2017-2018 influenza season. Retrieved from https://www.cdc.gov/flu/about/season/flu-season-2017-2018.htm

Centers for Disease Control and Prevention. (2017). Gateway to health communication & social marketing practice: Violence and homicide among youth. Retrieved from https://www.cdc.gov/healthcommunication/toolstemplates/entertainmented/tips/ViolenceYouth.html

Centers for Disease Control and Prevention. (2017). Health of American Indian or Alaska Native population. Retrieved from https://www.cdc.gov/nchs/fastats/american-indian-health.htm

Centers for Disease Control and Prevention. (2017). HIV among people aged 50 and over. Retrieved from https://www.cdc.gov/hiv/group/age/olderAmerican's/index.html

Centers for Disease Control and Prevention. (2017). HIV basics. Retrieved from https:// www.cdc.gov/hiv/basics/index.html.

Centers for Disease Control and Prevention. (2017). Immunization schedules: Catch-up immunization schedule for persons aged 4 months through 18 years who start late or who are more than 1 month behind. Retrieved from https://www.cdc.gov/vaccines/schedules/hcp/imz/catchup.html

Centers for Disease Control and Prevention. (2017). Influenza antiviral medications: Summary for clinicians. Retrieved from https://www.cdc.gov/flu/professionals/antivirals/summary-clinicians.htm

Centers for Disease Control and Prevention. (2017). Legal status of expedited partner therapy (EPT). Retrieved from https://www.cdc.gov/std/ept/legal/default.htm

Centers for Disease Control and Prevention. (2017). Lung cancer statistics. Retrieved from https://www.cdc.gov/cancer/lung/statistics/index.htm

Centers for Disease Control and Prevention. (2017). Lyme disease home. Retrieved from http://www.cdc.gov/lyme/healthcare

Centers for Disease Control and Prevention. (2017). Recommendations for HIV screening of gay, bisexual, and other men who have sex with men—United States, 2017. *Morbidity and Mortality Weekly Report*, *66*(31), 830–832.

Centers for Disease Control and Prevention. (2017). Recommended immunization schedule for adults aged 19 years or older, United States, 2018. Retrieved from https://www.cdc.gov/vaccines/schedules/downloads/adult/adult-combined-schedule.pdf

Centers for Disease Control and Prevention. (2017). Teen drivers: Get the facts. Retrieved from http://www.cdc.gov/motorvehiclesafety/teen_drivers/teendrivers_factsheet.html

Centers for Disease Control and Prevention. (2017). Tuberculosis (TB): Fact sheet: Treatment options for latent tuberculosis infection. Retrieved from https://www.cdc.gov/tb/publications/factsheets/treatment/ltbitreatmentoptions.htm

Centers for Disease Control and Prevention. (2017). Tuberculosis (TB): Testing & diagnosis. Retrieved from https://www.cdc.gov/tb/topic/testing/default.htm

Centers for Disease Control and Prevention. (2017). Tuberculosis (TB): Testing for TB infection. Retrieved from https://www.cdc.gov/tb/topic/testing/tbtesttypes.htm

Centers for Disease Control and Prevention. (2017). Tuberculosis (TB): Treatment regimens for latent TB infection (LTBI). Retrieved from https://www.cdc.gov/tb/topic/treatment/ltbi.htm

Centers for Disease Control and Prevention. (2018). Influenza (flu): Influenza vaccines—United States, 2017–18 influenza season. Retrieved from https://www.cdc.gov/flu/protect/vaccine/vaccines.htm

Centers for Disease Control and Prevention. (2018). Rocky Mountain spotted fever: deadly, but preventable. Retrieved from http://www.cdc.gov/features/rmsf

Centers for Disease Control and Prevention & Association of Public Health Laboratories. (2014, June). Quick reference guide—Laboratory testing for the diagnosis of HIV infection: Updated recommendations. Retrieved from https://stacks.cdc.gov/view/cdc/23446

Centers for Medicare & Medicaid Services. (2016). Welcome to Medicare coverage database. Retrieved from https://www.cms.gov/medicare-coverage-database

Centers for Medicare & Medicaid Services. (2017). Medicaid & CHIP: Strengthening coverage, improving health. Retrieved from https://www.medicaid.gov/medicaid/program-information/downloads/accomplishments-report.pdf

Chow, A. W., & Doron, S. (2016). Evaluation of acute pharyngitis in adults. In S. Bond (Ed.), *UptoDate*. Retrieved from http://www.uptodate.com/contents/evaluation-of-acute-pharyngitis-in-adults

Colucci, W. S. (2017). Treatment of acute decompensated heart failure: Components of therapy. In S. B. Yeon (Ed.), *UpToDate*. Retrieved from https://www.uptodate.com/contents/treatment-of-acute-decompensated-heart-failure-components-of-therapy?source=search_result&search=treatment%20of%20acute%20decompensated%20heart%20failure&selectedTitle=1~150

Colucci, W. S. (2018). Use of angiotensin converting enzyme inhibitors in heart failure with reduced ejection fraction. In S. B. Yeon (Ed.), *UpToDate*. Retrieved from https://www.uptodate.com/contents/ace-inhibitors-in-heart-failure-with-reduced-ejection-fraction-therapeutic-use?source=machineLearning&search=ace+inhibitors+heart+failure&selectedTitle=1~150§ionRank=1&anchor=H21135813#H21135813

Colucci, W. S. (2018). Overview of the therapy for heart failure with reduced ejection fraction. In S. B. Yeon (Ed.), *UpToDate*. Retrieved from https://www.uptodate.com/contents/overview-of-the-therapy-of-heart-failure-with-reduced-ejection-fraction

Colyar, M. R. (2015). *Advanced practice nursing procedures*. Philadelphia, PA: F. A. Davis.

Committee on Infectious Diseases, American Academy of Pediatrics. (2017, September 4). Recommendations for prevention and control of influenza in children, 2017-2018. *Pediatrics, 140*(4). Retrieved from http://pediatrics.aappublications.org/content/pediatrics/early/2017/09/06/peds.2017-2550.full.pdf

Derrow, P. (2016). Seniors, sex, and STDs. Retrieved from http://www.berkeleywellness.com/self-care/sexual-health/article/seniors-sex-and-stds

Domino, F. J., Baldor, R. A., Golding, J., & Stephens, M. B. (Eds.). (2016). *The 5-minute clinical consult standard 2016* (24th ed.). Philadelphia, PA: Lippincott Williams & Wilkins.

Domino, F. J., Baldor, R. A., Golding, J., & Stephens, M. B. (Eds.). (2017). *The 5-minute clinical consult standard 2017* (25th ed.). Philadelphia, PA: Lippincott Williams & Wilkins.

Donovan, D., & McDowell, I. (2017). *AFMC primer on population health: A virtual textbook on public health concepts for clinicians*. Ottawa, ON, Canada: The Association of Faculties of Medicine of Canada. Retrieved from http://phprimer.afmc.ca/Part1-TheoryThinkingAboutHealth/Chapter4BasicConceptsInPreventionSurveillanceAndHealthPromotion/Thestagesofprevention

Drugs.com. (n.d.). FDA pregnancy categories: FDA pregnancy risk information: An update. Retrieved from https://www.drugs.com/pregnancy-categories.html

Duderstadt, K. G. (2014). *Pediatric physical examination* (2nd ed.). St. Louis, MO: Mosby/Elsevier.

EBSCO Nursing Resources. (n.d.). CINAHL Databases. Retrieved from https://www.ebscohost.com/nursing/products/cinahl-databases

Engorn, B., & Flerlage, J. (Eds.). (2015). *The Harriet Lane handbook* (20th ed.). Philadelphia, PA: Saunders/Elsevier.

Epstein, B., & Turner, M. (2015). The nursing code of ethics: Its value, its history. *Online Journal of Issues in Nursing, 20*(2). doi:10.3912/OJIN.Vol20No02Man04

Ergene, E. (2016). Adult optic neuritis. In E. Ing (Ed.), *Medscape*. Retrieved from http://emedicine.medscape.com/article/1217083-overview

European Pressure Ulcer Advisory Panel and National Pressure Ulcer Advisory Panel. (2009). *Prevention and treatment of pressure ulcers: Quick reference guide*. Washington DC: National Pressure Ulcer Advisory Panel.

Ferguson, G. T., & Make, B. (2017). Management of stable chronic obstructive pulmonary disease. In H. Hollingsworth (Ed.), *UpToDate*. Retrieved from https://www.uptodate.com/contents/management-of-stable-chronic-obstructive-pulmonary-disease?source=search_result&search=management%20of%20stable%20copd&selectedTitle=2~150

Ferri, F. F. (Ed.). (2016). *Ferri's clinical advisor 2016: 5 books in 1*. Philadelphia, PA: Elsevier.

Ferri, F. F. (Ed.). (2017). *Ferri's clinical advisor 2017: 5 books in 1*. Philadelphia, PA: Elsevier.

Fishbach, F., & Dunning, M. B. (2015). *A manual of laboratory and diagnostics tests* (9th ed.). Philadelphia, PA: Lippincott Williams & Wilkins.

Folstein, M. F., Folstein, S. E., McHugh, P. R. (1975). "Mini-mental state": A practical method for grading the cognitive state of patients for the clinician. *Journal of Psychiatric Research, 12*(3), 189–198.

Fowler, M. D. M. (2015). *Guide to the code of ethics for nurses with interpretive statements: Development, interpretation, and application* (2nd ed.). Silver Spring, MD: American Nurses Association.

Frandsen, B. (2014). 6 leadership types: The pros and cons for nurse leaders. Retrieved from https://www.aadns-ltc.org/Resources/Nurse-Leader-Blog/details/post/6-leadership-types-the-pros-and-cons-for-nurse-leaders/2014-03-11

Frandsen, B. (2014). Nursing leadership: Management & leadership styles. Retrieved from https://www.aanac.org/docs/white-papers/2013-nursing-leadership---management-leadership-styles.pdf?sfvrsn=4

Frechtling, J., & Sharp, L. (1997). *User-friendly handbook for mixed method evaluations*. Collingdale, PA: Diane Publishing. Retrieved from https://www.nsf.gov/pubs/1997/nsf97153

Gabbe, S. G., Niebyl, J. R., Simpson, J. L., Landon, M. B., Galan, H. L., Jauniaux, E. R. M., … Grobman, W. A. (Eds.). (2017). *Obstetrics: Normal and problem pregnancies* (7th ed.). Philadelphia, PA: Elsevier.

Ghosh, C., & Ghosh, T. (2017). Eyelid lesions. In J. Trobe (Ed.), *UptoDate*. Retrieved from https://www.uptodate.com/contents/eyelid-lesions

Gilbert, D. N., Chambers, H. F., Eliopoulos, G. M., Saag, M. S., & Pavia, A. T. (Eds.). (2016). *The Sanford guide to antimicrobial therapy* (46th ed.). Sperryville, VA: Antimicrobial Therapy.

Gilbert, D. N., Chambers, H. F., Eliopoulos, G. M., Saag, M. S., & Pavia, A. T. (Eds.). (2017). *The Sanford guide to antimicrobial therapy* (47th ed.). Sperryville, VA: Antimicrobial Therapy.

Gilpin, L. (2016, June). Why Native American women still have the highest rates of rape and assault. High Country News. Retrieved from http://www.hcn.org/articles/why-native-american-women-still-have-the-highest-rates-of-rape-and-assault

Global Initiative for Chronic Obstructive Lung Disease. (2015). Pocket guide to COPD diagnosis, management, and prevention. A guide for health care professionals. Retrieved from http://goldcopd.org

Global Initiative for Chronic Obstructive Lung Disease. (2017). *GOLD 2017 Global strategy for the diagnosis, management and prevention of COPD*. Retrieved from http://goldcopd.org

Goldstein, A. O., & Goldstein, B. G. (2017). Dermatophyte (tinea) infections. In A. O. Ofori (Ed.), *UpToDate*. Retrieved from https://www.uptodate.com/contents/dermatophyte-tinea-infections?source=search_result&search=dermatophyte%20infection&selectedTitle=1~134

Gorman, C. R. (2017). Roseola infantum clinical presentation. In W. D. James (Ed.), *Medscape*. Retrieved from http://emedicine.medscape.com/article/1133023-clinical#b2

Graber, E. (2017, March 24). Treatment of acne vulgaris. In A. O. Ofori (Ed.), *UpToDate*. Retrieved from http://www.uptodate.com/contents/treatment-of-acne-vulgaris?topicKey?=DERM%2F2&e

Grove, S. K., Gray, J. R., & Burns, N. (2015). *Understanding nursing research: Building an evidence-based practice* (6th ed.). St. Louis, MO: Saunders/Elsevier.

Gupta, K., Hooton, T. M., Naber, K. G., Wullt, B., Colgan, R., Miller, L. G., … Soper, D. E. (2011). International clinical practice guidelines for the treatment of acute uncomplicated cystitis and pyelonephritis in women: A 2010 update by the Infectious Disease Society of America and the

European Society for Microbiology and Infectious Diseases. *Clinical Infectious Diseases, 52*(5), e103–e120. Retrieved from http://cid.oxfordjournals.org/content/52/5/e103.full.pdf+html

Guttmacher Institute. (2017). State laws and policies: Minors' access to contraceptive services. Retrieved from http://www.guttmacher.org

Guyatt, G. H., Akl, E. A., Crowther, M., Gutterman, D. D., & Schuünemann. (2012). Executive summary: Antithrombotic therapy and prevention of thrombosis, 9th ed: American College of Chest Physicians evidence-based clinical practice guidelines. *Chest, 141*(2 Suppl.), 7S–47S. doi:10.1378/chest.1412S3

Harris, M., Taylor, G., & Jackson, D. (2014). *Clinical evidence made easy*. Bandburry, UK: Scion Publishing.

Haugen, B. R., Alexander, E. K., Bible, K. C., Doherty, G. M., Mandel, S. J., Nikiforov, Y. E., ... Wartofsky, L. (2016). 2015 American Thyroid Association management guidelines for adult patients with thyroid nodules and differentiated thyroid cancer. *Thyroid, 26*(1), 1–133. doi:10.1089/thy.2015.0020

Heron, M. (2016). Deaths: Leading causes for 2013. *National Vital Statistics Reports, 65*(2), 1–95. Retrieved from http://www.cdc.gov/nchs/data/nvsr/nvsr65/nvsr65_02.pdf

HIPAA Journal. (2015). FCC confirms rules regarding HIPAA and patient telephone calls. *HIPAA Journal*. Retrieved from http://www.hipaajournal.com/fcc-confirms-rules-regarding-hipaa-and-patient-telephone-calls-8048

Hooton, T. M. (2016). Acute uncomplicated cystitis and pyelonephritis in men. In A. Bloom (Ed.), *UpToDate*. Retrieved from http://www.uptodate.com/contents/acute-uncomplicated-cystitis-and-pyelonephritis-in-men?source=see_link#H12809622

Hooton, T. M., & Gupta, K. (2016). Acute uncomplicated cystitis and pyelonephritis in women. In A. Bloom (Ed.), *UpToDate*. Retrieved from https://www.uptodate.com/contents/acute-uncomplicated-cystitis-and-pyelonephritis-in-women?source=preview&search=%2Fcontents%2Fsearch&anchor=H899949262#H899949198

Hull, R. D., & Garcia, D. A. (2017). Management of warfarin-associated bleeding or supratherapeutic INR. In J. S. Tirnauer (Ed.), *UpToDate*. Retrieved from https://www.uptodate.com/contents/management-of-warfarin-associated-bleeding-or-supratherapeutic-inr?source=search_result&search=management%20of%20warfarin%20assoc%20bleeding&selectedTitle=1~150

Immunization Action Coalition. (2017). Ask the experts: Diseases & vaccines: Influenza. Retrieved from http://www.immunize.org/askexperts/experts_inf.asp

Indian Health Service. (2017). Disparities. Retrieved from https://www.ihs.gov/newsroom/factsheets/disparities

Inker, L. A., & Perrone, R. D. (2017). Assessment of kidney function. In J. P. Forman (Ed.), *UpToDate*. Retrieved from https://www.uptodate.com/contents/assessment-of-kidney-function?source=machineLearning&search=blood+urea+nitrogen+adult&selectedTitle=1~150§ionRank=2&anchor=H25#H25

Innes, J. A. (Ed.), & Maxwell. S. (2016). *Davidson's essentials of medicine* (2nd ed.). London, UK: Elsevier.

Isaacs, C., & Peshkin, B. N. (2016, October 11). Management of patients at high risk for breast and ovarian cancer. In A. B. Chagpar & B. Goff (Eds.), *UptoDate*. Retrieved from https://www.uptodate.com/contents/management-of-patients-at-high-risk-for-breast-and-ovarian-cancer

James, P. A., Oparil, S., Carter, B. L., Cushman, W. C., Dennison-Himmelfarb, C., Handler, J., ... Ortiz, E. (2014). 2014 evidence-based guideline for the management of high blood pressure in adults: Report from the panel members appointed to the Eighth Joint National Committee (JNC 8). *Journal of the American Medical Association, 311*(5), 507–520. doi:10.1001/jama.2013.284427

Kansky, C. (2016). Normal and abnormal puerperium. In C. Isaacs (Ed.), *Medscape*. Retrieved from http://emedicine.medscape.com/article/260187-overview

Kaufman, C. A. (2016). Treatment of oropharyngeal and esophageal candidiasis. In J. Mitty (Ed.), *UptoDate*. Retrieved from https://www.uptodate.com/contents/treatment-of-oropharyngeal-and-esophageal-candidiasis

Kaunitz, A. M. (2017). Progestin-only pills (POPs) for contraception. In C. A. Schreiber (Ed.), *UptoDate*. Retrieved from http://www.uptodate.com/contents/progestin-only-pills-pops-for-contraception

Kersey-Matusiak, G. (2013). *Delivering culturally competent nursing care*. New York, NY: Springer Publishing.

Kitagawa, S., & Miqdady, M. (2016). Intussusception in children. In J. I. Singer & B. UK Li (Eds.), *UpToDate*. Retrieved from https://www.uptodate.com/contents/intussusception-in-children?source=search_result&search=intussusception&selectedTitle=1~112

Kleinman, A. (1988). *The illness narratives: Suffering, healing, and the human condition*. New York, NY: Basic Books. Retrieved from https://www.amazon.com/Illness-Narratives-Suffering-Healing-Condition/dp/0465032044

Kleinman, A., Eisenberg, L., & Good, B. (1978). Culture, illness, and care. *Annuls of Internal Medicine, 88*, 251–258.

Kobayashi, M., Bennett, N. M., Gierke, R., Almendares, O., Moore, M. R., Whitney, C. G., & Pilishvili, T. (2015). Intervals between PCV13 and PPSV23 vaccines: Recommendations of the Advisory Committee on Immunization Practices (ACIP). *Morbidity and Mortality Weekly Report*, *64*(34), 944–947.

Kübler-Ross, E. (1969). *On death and dying*. New York, NY: Macmillan.

LeBlond, R.F., Brown, D.D., Suneja, M., & Szot, J. F. (Eds.). (2015). *DeGowin's diagnostic examination* (10th ed.). New York, NY: McGraw-Hill.

Leininger, M. (2014). Sunrise enabler. Retrieved from http://www.madeleine-leininger.com/resources.shtml

Lerma, E. V. (2014). Blood urea nitrogen (BUN). In E. B. Staros (Ed.), *Medscape*. Retrieved from http://emedicine.medscape.com/article/2073979-overview

Levin, J., Chatters, L. M., & Taylor, J. (2007). Religion, health and medicine in African Americans: Implications for physicians. *Journal of the National Medical Association, 97*(2), 237-247. Retrieved from http:// www.baylorisr.org/wp-content/uploads/levin_african.pdf

Lim, W. S., van der Eerden, M. M., Laing, R., Boersma, W. G., Karalus, N., Town, G. I., . . . Macfarlane J. T. (2003). Defining community acquired pneumonia severity on presentation to hospital: an international derivation and validation study. *Thorax, 58*(5), 377–382. doi:10.1136/thorax.58.5.377

Llamas, M. (2016). FDA says risks may outweigh benefits for antibiotics Levaquin, Cipro. Retrieved from https://www.drugwatch.com/2016/05/16/fda-black-box-warning-for-levaquin-cipro-antibiotic-risk

Lowy, F. D. (2017). Methicillin-resistant *Staphylococcus aureus* (MRSA) in adults: Treatment of skin and soft tissue infections. In E. L. Baron (Ed.), *UpToDate*. Retrieved from http://www.uptodate.com/contents/methicillin-resistant-staphylococcus-aureus-mrsa-in-adults-treatment-of-skin-and-soft-tissue-infections?source=search_result&search=methicillin+resistant+staphylococcus+aureus+mrsa+in+ad&selectedTitle=5~150

Mandell, L. A, Wunderink, R. G., Anzueto, A., Bartlett, J. G., Campbell, G. D., Dean, N.C., … Whitney, C. G. (2007). Infectious Diseases Society of America/American Thoracic Society consensus guidelines on the management of community-acquired pneumonia in adults. *Clinical Infectious Disease, 44* (Suppl. 2), S27–S72. doi:10.1086/511159

Mann, J. F. E. (2017). Choice of drug therapy in primary (essential) hypertension. In J. P. Forman (Ed.), *UpToDate*. Retrieved from https://www.uptodate.com/contents/choice-of-drug-therapy-in-primary-essential-hypertension?source=search_result&search=hypertension%20treatment&selectedTitle=1~150

Marah, J.-P. (2013). Cervicitis ectropion and true erosion: Causes, symptoms, diagnosis, treatment and ongoing care. Retrieved from http://tipsdiscover.com/health/cervicitis-ectropion-and-true-erosion-causes-symptoms-diagnosis-treatment-and-ongoing-care

Mayo Clinic. (2017). Posterior prolapse (rectocele). Retrieved from https://www.mayoclinic.org/diseases-conditions/rectocele/basics/definition/con-20027826?.p=1

Mayo Clinic. (2017). Small bowel prolapse (enterocele). Retrieved from https://www.mayoclinic.og/diseases-conditions/enterocele/basics/symptoms/con-20025707?=1

Mayo Clinic. (2017). Urinary incontinence. Retrieved from https://www.mayoclinic.org/diseases-conditions/urinary-incontinence/basics/definition/con-20037883?p=1

Mayo Clinic Mayo Medical Laboratories. (2017). Gamma-glutamyltransferase (GGT), serum. Retrieved from https://www.mayomedicallaboratories.com/test-catalog/Clinical+and+Interpretive/8677

McCulloch, D. K., & Bakris, G. L. (2016). Moderately increased albuminuria (microalbuminuria) in type 2 diabetes mellitus. In R. J. Glossock & D. M. Nathan (Eds.), *UptoDate*. Retrieved from http://www.uptodate.com/contents/moderately-increased-albuminuria-microalbuminuria-in-type-2-diabetes-mellitus

Medicare Learning Network. (2017). Evaluation and Management Services. Retrieved from https://www.cms.gov/Outreach-and-Education/Medicare-Learning-Network-MLN/MLNProducts/Downloads/eval-mgmt-serv-guide-ICN006764.pdf

MedicineNet. (2017). Urinary retention facts. Retrieved from http://www.medicinenet.com/script.main/art.asp?articlekey=113304

MedlinePlus. (n.d.). Aging changes in body shape. Retrieved from https://medlineplus.gov/ency/article/003998.htm

Morris, J. G., Jr. (2017). *Vibrio vulnificus* infections. In A. Bloom (Ed.), *UptoDate*. Retrieved from http://www.uptodate.com/contents/vibrio-vulnificus-infections

Mount, D. B. (2016). Clinical manifestations and treatment of hypokalemia in adults. In J. P. Forman (Ed.), *UpToDate*. Retrieved from https://www.uptodate.com/contents/clinical-manifestations-and-treatment-of-hypokalemia-in-adults?source=machineLearning&search=give+potassium+supplement+with+diuretics&selectedTitle=1%7E150§ionRank=3&anchor=H419957#H419957

Munoz, F. M. (2017). Treatment and prevention of giardiasis. In P. F. Weller & S. L. Kaplan (Eds.), *UpToDate*. Retrieved from http://www.uptodate.com/contents/treatment-and-prevention-of-giardiasis

National Asthma Education and Prevention Program Coordinating Committee. (2007). *Expert panel report 3: Guidelines for the diagnosis and management of asthma*. Bethesda, MD: National Institutes of Health. Retrieved from https://www.nhlbi.nih.gov/files/docs/guidelines/asthgdln.pdf

National Center for Biotechnology Information Resources. (n.d.). PubMed help. FAQs. PubMed quick start. Retrieved from https://www.ncbi.nlm.nih.gov/books/NBK3827/#pubmedhelp.FAQs

National Center for Health Statistics. (2017). Leading causes of death. Retrieved from http://www.cdc.gov/nchs/fastats/leading-causes-of-death.htm

National Center for Health Statistics. (2017). Older persons' health. Retrieved from https://www.cdc.gov/nchs/fastats/older-american-health.htm

National Congress of American Indians. (n.d.). An introduction to Indian Nations in the United States. Retrieved from http://www.ncai.org/about-tribes/indians_101.pdf

National Council of State Boards of Nursing. (n.d.) Nurse Practice Act, rules & regulations: Nurse Practice Acts guide and govern nursing practice. Retrieved from https://www.ncsbn.org/nurse-practice-act.htm

National Eye Institute. (n.d.). Facts about retinal detachment. Retrieved from https://nei.nih.gov/health/retinaldetach/retinaldetach

National Guideline Clearinghouse. (2012). Guideline summary: Evidence-based management of anticoagulant therapy: Antithrombotic therapy and prevention of thrombosis, 9th ed: American College of Chest Physicians evidence-based clinical practice guidelines. Retrieved from https://www.guideline.gov/summaries/summary/35262/evidencebased-management-of-anticoagulant-therapy-antithrombotic-therapy-and-prevention-of-thrombosis-9th-ed-american-college-of-chest-physicians-evidencebased-clinical-practice-guidelines

National Heart, Lung, and Blood Institute. (2012). Asthma care quick reference: Diagnosing and managing asthma (NIH Publication No. 12-5075). Retrieved from https://www.nhlbi.nih.gov/files/docs/guidelines/asthma_qrg.pdf

National Institute of Aging. (2002). Driving and dementia: Health professionals can play important role. Retrieved from https://www.nia.nih.gov/alzheimers/features/driving-and-dementia-health-professionals-can-play-important-role

National Institute of Arthritis and Musculoskeletal and Skin Diseases. (2016). Questions and answers about vitiligo. Retrieved from http://www.niams.nih.gov/health_info/vitiligo/#7

National Institute of Diabetes and Digestive and Kidney Diseases. (2017). Bladder control medicines. Retrieved from https://www.niddk.nih.gov/health-information/urologic-diseases/bladder-control-medications

National Institute of Diabetes and Digestive and Kidney Diseases. (2017). Cystocele (prolapsed bladder). Retrieved from https://www.niddk.nih.gov/health-information/cystocele-prolapsed-bladder

National Institute on Drug Abuse. (2017). Methamphetamine. Retrieved from https://www.drugabuse.gov/publications/drugfacts/methamphetamine

National Institutes of Health, U.S. National Library of Medicine. (n.d.). Fact sheet: MEDLINE. Retrieved from https://www.nlm.nih.gov/pubs/factsheets/medline.html

National Institutes of Health, U.S. National Library of Medicine. (n.d.). FAQ: Finding medical information in Medline. Retrieved from https://www.nlm.nih.gov/services/usemedline.html

National Organization for Rare Disorders. (n.d.). Essential tremor. Retrieved from https://rarediseases.org/rare-diseases/essential-tremor

NephCure Kidney International. (n.d.) Renal diet. Retrieved from https://nephcure.org/livingwithkidneydisease/diet-and-nutrition/renal-diet/

New York State Nursing Board Office. (2013). Practice information: Collborative practice with physicians. Retrieved from http://www.op.nysed.gov/prof/nurse/npcollab.htm

Nishimura, R. A., Otto, C. M., Bonow, R. O., Carabello, B. A., Erwin, J. P., 3rd, Guyton, R. A., ... Thomas, J. D. (2014). 2014 AHA/ACC guideline for the management of patients with valvular heart disease: A report of the American College of Cardiology/American Heart Association Task Force on Practice Guidelines. *Journal of the American College of Cardiology, 63*(22), e57–e185.

O'Brien, J. M. (2003). How nurse practitioners obtained provider status: Lessons for pharmacists. *American Journal of Health-System Pharmacy, 60*(22), 2301–2307. Retrieved from http://www.ajhp.org/content/60/22/2301

Office of Disease Prevention and Health Promotion (n.d.). Healthy people 2020. Retrieved from https://www.healthypeople.gov

OpenAnesthesia. (n.d.). Herbal medicines: Anticoagulation effects. Retrieved from https://www.openanesthesia.org/herbal_medicines_anticoagulation_effects

Pagana, K. D., Pagana, T. J., & Pagana, T. N. (2015). *Mosby's diagnostic and laboratory test reference* (12th ed.). St. Louis, MO: Mosby/Elsevier.

Papadakis, M. A., McPhee, S. J., & Rabow, M. W. (Eds.). (2016). *Current medical diagnosis & treatment 2016* (55th ed.). New York, NY: McGraw-Hill.

Papp, J. R., Schachter, J., Gaydos, C. A., & Van Der Pol, B. (2014). Recommendations for the laboratory-based detection of *chlamydia trachomatis* and *Neisseria gonorrhoeae*. *Morbidity and Mortality Weekly Report, 63*(RR02), 1–19. Retrieved from https://www.cdc.gov/mmwr/preview/mmwrhtml/rr6302a1.htm

Patel, A., & Stewart, F. (2015). On hypertension in the elderly: An epidemiologic shift. Retrieved from http://www.acc.org/latest-in-cardiology/articles/2015/02/19/14/55/on-hypertension-in-the-elderly

Pemberton, J. H. (2017) Acute colonic diverticulitis: Medical management. In W. Chen (Ed.), *UpToDate*. Retrieved from https://www.uptodate.com/contents/acute-colonic-diverticulitis-medical-management?source=machineLearning&search=diverticulitis+treatment&selectedTitle=1%7E39§ionRank=3&anchor=H26#H26b

Pharmacist's Letter/Prescriber's Letter. (2014). Magic mouthwash recipes. Retrieved from http://pharmacistsletter.therapeuticresearch.com/pl/ArticleDD.aspx?nidchk=1&cs=&s=PL&dd=230703&cat=4313&pt=2

Population Reference Bureau. (n.d.) Fact sheet: Aging in the United States. Retrieved from http://www.prb.org/Publications/Media-Guides/2016/aging-unitedstates-fact-sheet.aspx

Press, D., & Alexander, M. (2017, March 14). Treatment of dementia. In S. T. DeKosky & K. E. Schmader (Eds.), *UptoDate*. Retrieved from http://www.uptodate.com/contents/treatment-of-dementia

Prometric. (n.d.). For test takers: Schedule. Retrieved from https://www.prometric.com/en-us/for-test-takers/pages/schedule.aspx?Type=schedule

Realin, A. P. (2012). *A desk reference to personalizing patient care*. Maitland, FL: Florida Hospital.

Rice, S. G., & Council on Sports Medicine and Fitness. (2008). Medical conditions affecting sports participation. *Pediatrics, 121*(4), 841–848. Retrieved from http://pediatrics.aappublications.org/content/pediatrics/121/4/841.full.pdf

Rogers, R. G., & Fashokun, T. B. (2017). Pelvicorgan prolapse in women: Epidemiology, risk factors, clinical manifestations, and management. In K. Eckler (Ed.), *UptoDate*. Retrieved from https://www.uptodate.com/contents/pelvic-organ-prolapse-in-women-an-overview-of-the-epidemiology-risk-factors-clinical-manifestations-and-management?source=search_result&search=uterine%20prolapse&selectedTitle=1~54

Rosenstock, I. M., Strecher, V. J., & Becker, M. H. (1988). Social learning theory and the Health Belief Model. *Health Education Quarterly, 15*(2), 175–183.

Ross, J., & Chacko, M. R. (2016). Pelvic inflammatory disease: Clinical manifestations and diagnosis. In A. Bloom (Ed.), *UptoDate*. Retrieved from https://www.uptodate.com/contents/pelvic-inflammatory-disease-clinical-manifestations-and-diagnosis?source=see_link§ionName=Perihepatitis&anchor=H1112643159#H8

Rovin, B. H. (2017). Assessment of urinary protein excretion and evaluation of isolated non-nephrotic proteinuria in adults. In A. Q. Lam (Ed.), *UpToDate*. Retrieved from https://www.uptodate.com/contents/assessment-of-urinary-protein-excretion-and-evaluation-of-isolated-non-nephrotic-proteinuria-in-adults?source=search_result&search=functional+proteinuria&selectedTitle=1~150

RxList. (n.d.). Aldactone. Retrieved from http://www.rxlist.com/aldactone-drug/warnings-precautions.htm#P

Sackett, D. L., Rosenberg, W. M. C., et al. (1996). Evidence-based medicine: What it is and what it isn't. *British Medical Journal, 312*(71). doi:10.1136/bmj.312.7023.71

Scibella, B. (2015). Analyzing qualitative data, part 2: Chi-square and multivariate analysis [Blog post]. Retrieved from http://blog.minitab.com/blog/applying-statistics-in-quality-projects/analyzing-qualitative-data-part-2-chi-square-and-multivariate-analysis

Sexton, D. J. (2017) Treatment of Rocky Mountain spotted fever. In J. Mitty (Ed.), *UpToDate*. Retrieved from http://www.uptodate.com/contents/treatment-of-rocky-mountain-spotted-fever?topicKey=I...

Sexton, D. J., & Chu, V. H. (2017). Antimicrobial prophylaxis for bacterial endocarditis. In C. Otto (Ed.), *UptoDate*. Retrieved from https://www.uptodate.com/contents/antimicrobial-prophylaxis-for-bacterial-endocarditis?source=search_result&search=endocarditis%20guidelines&selectedTitle=3~150

Sexuality Information and Education Council of the United States. (n.d.). Large scale survey investigates the sexual behavior of Americans. Retrieved from http://www.siecus.org/index.cfm?fuseaction=Feature.showFeature&featureID=1947

Skin Cancer Foundation. (2017). Skin cancer facts & statistics. Retrieved from http://www.skincancer.org/skin-cancer-information/skin-cancer-facts

Sofronescu, A. G. (2015, July 16). Thyroid-stimulating hormone. In T. M Wheeler (Ed.), *Medscape*. Retrieved from http://emedicine.medscape.com/article/2074091-overview

Stewart, A., & Graham, S. (2013). Sexual risk behavior among older adults. *Clinical Advisor*. Retrieved from http://www.clinicaladvisor.com/features/sexual-risk-behavior-among-older-adults/article/283811

Stone, N. J., Robinson, J. G., Lichtenstein, A. H., Bairey Merz, C. N., Blum, C. B., Eckel, R. H., … Wilson, P. W. F. (2014). ACC/AHA guideline on the treatment of blood cholesterol to reduce atherosclerotic cardiovascular risk in adults: A report of the American College of Cardiology/American Heart Association Task Force on Practice Guidelines. *Journal of the American College of Cardiology, 63*(25 Part B): 2889–2934.

Taffet, G. E. (2017). Normal aging. In D. J. Sullivan (Ed.), *UptoDate*. Retrieved from https://www.uptodate.com/contents/normal-aging?source=search_result&search=changes%20in%20lungs%20aging&selectedTitle=1~150#H23810938

Taylor, E. J. (Ed.). (2012). *Religion: A clinical guide for nurses*. New York, NY: Springer Publishing.

The Joint Commission. (n.d.). Patient safety systems chapter, sentinel event policy and RCA2. Retrieved from https://www.jointcommission.org/sentinel_event.aspx

The Joint Commission. (2017). Sentinel event policy and procedures. Retrieved from https://www.jointcommission.org/sentinel_event_policy_and_procedures

Thompson, E. G., & Vachharajani, T. J. (n.d.). Prerenal acute kidney injury: Topic overview. Retrieved from http://www.webmd.com/a-to-z-guides/prerenal-acute-kidney-injury-topic-overview

Touhy, T. A., & Jett, K. F. (Eds.). (2010). *Ebersole and Hess' gerontological nursing & healthy aging* (3rd ed.). St. Louis, MO: Mosby Elsevier.

Treat, J. R. (2017). Tinea capitus. In A. O. Ofori (Ed.), *UpToDate*. Retrieved from http://www.com/contents/tinea-capitis?topicKey=DERM%2F99983&elapsedTime

University of Ottawa. (n.d.). Sensitivity, specificity, predictive values and likelihood ratios. Retrieved from http://www.med.uottawa.ca/sim/data/Sensitivity_e.htm

University of Southern California. Clinician Consultation Center. (2017). PEP quick guide for occupational exposures. Retrieved from http://nccc.ucsf.edu/clinical-resources/pep-resources/pep-quick-guide

University of Twente. (n.d.) Health belief model. Retrieved from https://www.utwente.nl/en/bms/communication-theories/sorted-by-cluster/Health%20Communication/Health_Belief_Model

Urology Health. (2017). What is urinary incontinence? Retrieved from http://www.urologyhealth.org/urologic-conditions/urinary-incontinence

U.S. Cancer Statistics Working Group. (2017). *United States cancer statistics: 1999–2014 incidence and mortality web-based report*. Atlanta, GA: U.S. Department of Health and Human Services, Centers for Disease Control and Prevention and National Cancer Institute.

U.S. Census Bureau. (n.d.). QuickFacts. Retrieved from https://www.census.gov/quickfacts/fact/table/US/PST045217

U.S. Census Bureau. (n.d.). Statistical brief. Sixty-five plus in the United States. Retrieved from https://www.census.gov/population/socdemo/statbriefs/agebrief.html

U.S. Department of Health and Human Services. (n.d.). About Healthy People. *HealthyPeople.gov*. Retrieved from https://www.healthypeople.gov/2020/About-Healthy-People

U.S. Department of Health and Human Services. (2017). Guidelines for the prevention and treatment of opportunistic infections in HIV-infected adults and adolescents. (pp. B-1–B-18). *AIDSinfo.gov*. Retrieved from https://aidsinfo.nih.gov/contentfiles/lvguidelines/adult_oi.pdf

U.S. Department of Health and Human Services & U.S. Food and Drug Administration. (n.d.). Hepatitis B and C treatments. Retrieved from https://www.fda.gov/forpatients/illness/hepatitisbc/ucm408658.htm

U.S. Department of Veterans Affairs. (n.d.). HIV/AIDS: Epstein-Barr virus (EBV)/oral hairy leukoplakia (OHL). Retrieved from https://www.hiv.va.gov/provider/image-library/epstein-barr.asp?post=1&slide=264

U.S. Food & Drug Administration. (2016). Institutional review boards frequently asked questions: Information sheet. Retrieved from http://www.fda.gov/RegulatoryInformation/Guidances/ucm126420.htm

U.S. Food & Drug Administration. (2016). Notice to industry: Final guidance for over-the-counter products that contain acetaminophen. Retrieved from http://www.fda.gov/Drugs/DrugSafety/ucm310469.htm

U.S. Food & Drug Administration. (2016). Pregnancy and lactation labeling (drugs) final rule. Retrieved from https://www.fda.gov/drugs/developmentapprovalprocess/developmentresources/labeling/ucm093307.htm

U.S. Food & Drug Administration. (2017). CFR-Code of Federal Regulations Title 21. Part 1308 - Schedule of Controlled Substances. Schedule II. Retrieved from https://www.accessdata.fda.gov/scripts/cdrh/cfdocs/cfcfr/cfrsearch.cfm?fr=1308.12

U.S. Preventive Services Task Force. (2012, March). Cervical cancer: Screening. Retrieved from https://www.uspreventiveservicestaskforce.org/Page/Document/UpdateSummaryFinal/cervical-cancer-screening

U.S. Preventive Services Task Force. (2012). Clinical summary: Ovarian cancer: Screening. Retrieved from https://www.uspreventiveservicestaskforce.org/Page/Document/ClinicalSummaryFinal/ovarian-cancer-screening

U.S. Preventive Services Task Force. (2016, January). Breast cancer: Screening. Retrieved from http://www.uspreventiveservicestaskforce.org/Page/Document/UpdateSummaryFinal/breast-cancer-screening1

U.S. Preventive Services Task Force. (2016, April). Final recommendation statement: Aspirin use to prevent cardiovascular disease and colorectal cancer: Preventive medication. Retrieved from https://www.uspreventiveservicestaskforce.org/Page/Document/RecommendationStatementFinal/aspirin-to-prevent-cardiovascular-disease-and-cancer

U.S. Preventive Services Task Force. (2017). Recommendations for primary care practice. Retrieved from https://www.uspreventiveservicestaskforce.org/Page/Name/recommendations

U.S. Preventive Services Task Force. (2017). USPSTF A and B recommendations. Retrieved from https://www.uspreventiveservicestaskforce.org

U.S. Preventive Services Task Force. (2016, November). Statin use for the primary prevention of cardiovascular disease in adults: Preventive medication. Retrieved from https://www.uspreventiveservicestaskforce.org/Page/Document/UpdateSummaryFinal/statin-use-in-adults-preventive-medication1

Vargas, J. M. (2008). Pterygium Slitlamp.jpg: Severe Pterygium reaching the pupil. [Image]. Retrieved from https://commons.wikimedia.org/wiki/File:Pterygium_Slitlamp.jpg

Vasavada, S. P. (2017, December 12). Urinary incontinence medication. In E. D. Kim (Ed.), Medscape. Retrieved from https://emedicine.medscape.com/article/452289-medication

Vinchinsky, E. P., & Mahoney, D. H. (2016). Diagnosis of sickle cell disorders. In J. S. Tirnauer (Ed.), *UpToDate*. Retrieved from https://www.uptodate.com/contents/diagnosis-of-sickle-cell-disorders?source=search_result&search=diagnosis%20of%20sickle%20cell&selectedTitle=1~150

Welt, C. K. (2017). Evaluation of the menstrual cycle and timing of ovulation. R. F. Barbieri & W. F. Crowley (Eds.), *UptoDate*. Retrieved from https://www.uptodate.com/contents/evaluation-of-the-menstrual-cycle-and-timing-of-ovulation

Williams, B. A., Chang, A., Ahalt, C., Chen, H., Conant, R., Landefeld, C. S., ... Yukawa, M. (Eds.). (2014). *Current diagnosis and treatment: Geriatrics* (2nd ed.). New York, NY: McGraw-Hill.

Williamson, M. A., & Snyder, L. M. (Eds.). (2011). *Wallach's interpretation of diagnostic tests* (9th ed.). Philadelphia, PA: Lippincott Williams & Wilkins.

Wilson, W., Taubert, K. A., Gewitz, M., Lockhart, P. B., Baddour, L. M., Levison, M., ... Durack, D. T. (2007, April 19). Prevention of infective endocarditis: Guidelines from the American Heart Association: A guideline from the American Heart Association Rheumatic Fever, Endocarditis, and Kawasaki Disease Committee, Council on Cardiovascular Disease in the Young, and the Council on Clinical Cardiology, Council on Cardiovascular Surgery and Anesthesia, and the Quality of Care and Outcomes Research Interdisciplinary Working Group. *Circulation, 116*(15), 1736–1754.

Winland-Brown, J., Lachman, V. D., & O'Connor Swanson, E. (2015). The new "Code of Ethics For Nurses with Interpretive Statements" (2015): Practical clinical application, Part I. *MEDSURG Nursing, 24*(4), 268–271. Retrieved from http://www.nursingworld.org/MainMenuCategories/EthicsStandards/CodeofEthicsforNurses/Code-of-Ethics-2015-Part-1.pdf

Wolfe, M. M. (2017). Proton pump inhibitors: Overview of use and adverse effects in the treatment of acid related disorders. In S. Grover (Ed.), *UpToDate*. Retrieved from https://www.uptodate.com/contents/overview-and-comparison-of-the-proton-pump-inhibitors-for-the-treatment-of-acid-related-disorders?source=search_result&search=proton%20pump%20inhibitors%20adult&selectedTitle=1~150

Workowski, K. A., & Bolan, G. A. (2015). Sexually transmitted diseases treatment guidelines, 2015. *MMWR Recommendations and Reports, 64*(3), 1–137. Retrieved from https://www.cdc.gov/std/tg2015/tg-2015-print.pdf

World Health Organization. (2016). *ICD-10: International statistical classification of diseases and related health problems* (10th ed.). Geneva, Switzerland: Author. Retrieved from http://apps.who.int/classifications/icd10/browse/2016/en

Zane, R. D., & Kosowsky, J. M. (2015). *Pocket emergency medicine* (3rd ed.). Philadelphia, PA: Wolters Kluwer.

Index

Note: Page numbers followed by "f" and "t" denote figures and tables respectively.
Numbers that appear in bold italics denote Practice Test question numbers, the rationales for which appear in chapter 32.

Note: Page numbers followed by "f" and "t" denote figures and tables respectively.
Numbers that appear in bold italics denote Practice Test question numbers, the rationales for which appear in chapter 32.

Note: Page numbers followed by "f" and "t" denote figures and tables respectively.
Numbers that appear in bold italics denote Practice Test question numbers, the rationales for which appear in chapter 32.

Note: Page numbers followed by "f" and "t" denote figures and tables respectively.
Numbers that appear in bold italics denote Practice Test question numbers, the rationales for which appear in chapter 32.

Note: Page numbers followed by "f" and "t" denote figures and tables respectively.
Numbers that appear in bold italics denote Practice Test question numbers, the rationales for which appear in chapter 32.

Note: Page numbers followed by "f" and "t" denote figures and tables respectively.
Numbers that appear in bold italics denote Practice Test question numbers, the rationales for which appear in chapter 32.

Note: Page numbers followed by "f" and "t" denote figures and tables respectively.
Numbers that appear in bold italics denote Practice Test question numbers, the rationales for which appear in chapter 32.

Note: Page numbers followed by "f" and "t" denote figures and tables respectively.
Numbers that appear in bold italics denote Practice Test question numbers, the rationales for which appear in chapter 32.

Note: Page numbers followed by "f" and "t" denote figures and tables respectively.
Numbers that appear in bold italics denote Practice Test question numbers, the rationales for which appear in chapter 32.

Note: Page numbers followed by "f" and "t" denote figures and tables respectively.
Numbers that appear in bold italics denote Practice Test question numbers, the rationales for which appear in chapter 32.

Note: Page numbers followed by "f" and "t" denote figures and tables respectively.
Numbers that appear in bold italics denote Practice Test question numbers, the rationales for which appear in chapter 32.

Note: Page numbers followed by "f" and "t" denote figures and tables respectively.
Numbers that appear in bold italics denote Practice Test question numbers, the rationales for which appear in chapter 32.

Note: Page numbers followed by "f" and "t" denote figures and tables respectively.
Numbers that appear in bold italics denote Practice Test question numbers, the rationales for which appear in chapter 32.

Note: Page numbers followed by "f" and "t" denote figures and tables respectively.
Numbers that appear in bold italics denote Practice Test question numbers, the rationales for which appear in chapter 32.

Note: Page numbers followed by "f" and "t" denote figures and tables respectively.
Numbers that appear in bold italics denote Practice Test question numbers, the rationales for which appear in chapter 32.

Note: Page numbers followed by "f" and "t" denote figures and tables respectively.
Numbers that appear in bold italics denote Practice Test question numbers, the rationales for which appear in chapter 32.

Note: Page numbers followed by "f" and "t" denote figures and tables respectively.
Numbers that appear in bold italics denote Practice Test question numbers, the rationales for which appear in chapter 32.

Note: Page numbers followed by "f" and "t" denote figures and tables respectively.
Numbers that appear in bold italics denote Practice Test question numbers, the rationales for which appear in chapter 32.

Note: Page numbers followed by "f" and "t" denote figures and tables respectively.
Numbers that appear in bold italics denote Practice Test question numbers, the rationales for which appear in chapter 32.